Image-Guided Aesthetic Treatments

Robert L. Bard
Editor

Image-Guided Aesthetic Treatments

Springer

Editor
Robert L. Bard
The Angio Foundation and Bard Diagnostics
New York, NY, USA

ISBN 978-3-031-36264-4 ISBN 978-3-031-36266-8 (eBook)
https://doi.org/10.1007/978-3-031-36266-8

This Springer imprint is published by the registered company Springer Nature Switzerland AG
The registered company address is: Gewerbestrasse 11, 6330 Cham, Switzerland

To my wife, Loreto, whose vision allowed the creation of this international collaboration and whose steadfast guidance coalesced advanced noninvasive imaging with newer aesthetic treatments supporting breakthrough therapeutic outcomes.

Foreword

Dr. Robert Bard is one of the world's experts in ultrasound technology. More specifically he has pioneered ultrasound imaging of the skin for malignant and benign lesions and has taken this technology from concept to an integral part of a medical practice.

In the aesthetic arena there has been a major emphasis in recent years on procedural safety in fillers, fat grafting, and laser treatments. Dr. Bard has brought the masters in imaging and aesthetic treatment together to teach the rest of us how to perform safer more effective aesthetic treatments with adjunctive imaging.

Image guidance allows the physician to measure the skin thickness and the depth of fat tissue as well as evaluate the elasticity of the skin and subcutaneous tissues. Medical imaging maps the arteries, veins, and nerves providing preoperative landmarks reducing postoperative bleeding and avoiding nerve damage.

Intraarterial filler injection has led to irreversible blindness and skin loss. Imaging permits safer therapeutics with increased effectiveness and decreased treatment times. Image-guided treatment greatly reduces patient anxiety even by simply helping to avoid bruising and the possibility of postoperative disfigurement.

Benign disease and cosmetic treatment options are further improved by 3-D volumetric mapping of regional anatomic structures. This data set allows for serial accurate comparison in follow-up exams for comparison and research studies.

The ability to follow the course of nerves allows for ultrasound-guided nerve block anesthesia and decreases the possibility of nerve injury during treatment. New cryoprobes/thermi-needles target nerves of the face producing muscle relaxation similar to Botox injections without the cost and bruising sequelae.

Imaging may noninvasively identify subdermal fillers or implants as to content and location. Translocation of fillers/implants may be observed and corrected by real-time interventions.

The book combines the use of optical media including dermoscopy, confocal microscopy, OCT (optical coherence tomography), high-resolution 3D ultrasound, real-time 4D Doppler histogram analysis, dermal MDCT, and DCE-MRI scanning. This is the first time these modalities have been discussed in one format for aesthetic purposes. Some of this technology is currently expensive and beyond the scope of most practitioners. However, historically these procedures become less expansive and more mainstream over time and in the future we will be referencing this publication for advances that will be used by aesthetic practitioners on a daily basis.

Boca Raton, FL, USA Jason Pozner

Acknowledgments

Mark Lebwohl
Cristian Navarrete-Dechent
Jill Waibel
Julia Welzel
Gaston Roustan
Fernanda Cavallieri
Orlando Catalano
Giovanni Pellacani
Ximena Wortsman
Fernando Alfageme
Luigi Solbiati
Mona Darwish
Manu Jain
Babar Rao
Ellen Marmur
Gary Goldenberg
David Goldberg
Andrew Rossi
Bruce Katz
John Melnick
Orit Markowitz
Andrew Alexis

Staff
Maryann St Rita
Aimee Arceo
Soraya Behzadi—assistant editor

The original version of the book was inadvertently published without the "Acknowledgment" section. This has now been amended across all versions of the book.

Contents

Industry Review of the Aesthetic Industry

1

January E. Howard and Lennard M. Gettz

Abstract

The history of cosmetics is reviewed with technologies unfolding less invasive options and more functional solutions involving neutraceutical supplementation with natural resources. Minimally invasive options are documented as is the adaptation of therapy to the Covid-19 pandemic. This chapter dives into the positive and negative implications of aesthetic procedures and how minimally invasive tactics could help advance all procedures focusing on the sake of performance, safety, and longevity.

Keywords

History · Aesthetic · Nutraceuticals · PRP · Antioxidants · Rose petals · Minimally invasive · Anti-aging · Microneedling

J. E. Howard (✉)
Cellular Medicine Association,
Ft. Lauderdale, FL, USA

L. M. Gettz
Deer Park, NY, USA
e-mail: lg@321image.com

1.1 Introduction

Conducting an industry review on the current state of the aesthetic industry would be incomplete without shedding a spotlight on social outlook and how it drives consumer activity trends. All aesthetic procedures are promoted to enhance one's overall look and public appeal and are often theorized to elevate one's self-appreciation. The public desire to achieve this is what supports this multi-million dollar industry to self-generate constant energy to acquire new market support each year (Fig 1.1).

Historically, the study of human nature has shown consistent evidence of aesthetic personalization throughout every social class as part of natural human desire and need for visually expressing personal pride and individualism. To date, there is an ever-growing list of solutions to enhance and improve a person's image, from PRP injections, microneedling, chemical peels, Botox, and fillers. These procedures have widely grown in popularity throughout the global community because of their affordable cost to the client/patient, their easy access, and their immediate performance and effectiveness.

The future of minimally invasive modalities has projected a major market growth without any signs of slow down. Introducing aesthetic procedures to just about ANY practitioner, let it be a dentist, an OB/GYN, a plastic surgeon, or a urologist offers a natural add-on, exponentially wid-

R. L. Bard (ed.), *Image-Guided Aesthetic Treatments*, https://doi.org/10.1007/978-3-031-36266-8_1

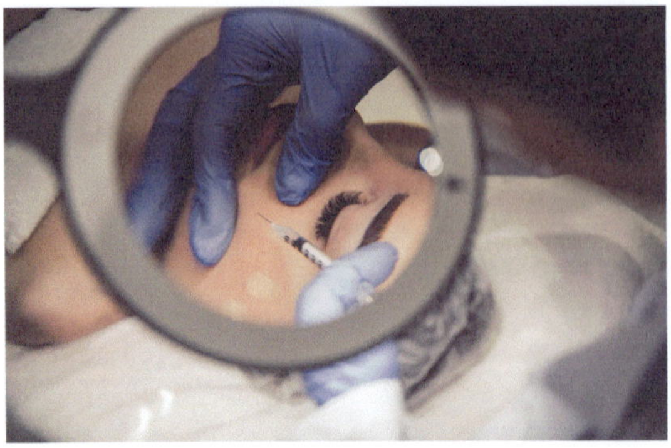

Fig. 1.1 Facial injections may avoid nerve and vascular structures under ultrasound image guidance. (© T-Photo | Shutterstock.com)

ening the access of these treatments to the community at large. Where dentists and plastic surgeons clearly have their specialized work intact, aesthetic procedures offer a supplemental income and a lucrative addition to their existing service set. For the practitioner, these procedures are a sensible upgrade by adding fairly recognizable protocols and equipment from prior training.

Practitioners find the integration and learning curve of adapting aesthetic modalities into their existing practice to be quite comfortable and cost-effective. For example, one can be trained to produce their own dermal filler or bio filler by extracting PRP (which is the client's own biologic) by "cooking" the platelet poor plasma. This is instead of purchasing bio filler from any of the existing manufacturers, offering a savings of anywhere from $300 to $800 per box.

As the industry concepts of beautification evolved and expanded toward clinical procedures, a sensible upgrade is the implementation of IMAGE GUIDANCE—a valuable tool forged by medical diagnostics. For over 30 years, ultrasound imaging has offered great value in clinical applications and is now adding great directive support to injection situations whereby knowing where the veins and bones truly are could be very helpful as a matter of safety. Whether someone is new to conducting injectable treatments or is a seasoned professional, having the reassurance of visual confirmation lowers the likelihood of hitting a vein or creating an occlusion. Reducing or eliminating risk to the client from pain or the stress of a "land mine" event is a major selling point for imaging devices in pre and post procedures.

1.2 The Modern Age of Clinical Aesthetics

Throughout the twentieth century, economic and medical industry reports have traced major activity in cosmetic procedures as part of a global consumer trend of personal enhancement investments. Where elective surgical procedures like breast augmentation, liposuction, and rhinoplasty once dominated the aesthetic media, the early 1980s brought forth a new wave of *Minimally Invasive* procedures which forged an entire industry of cosmetic self-rejuvenation. In 1981, bovine collagen was the first agent approved by the FDA for cosmetic injection. It was developed to induce a youthful appearance (as well as address facial deformities) to target smile lines and improve the presence of facial acne scars. The first regulatory approval gave way for dozens of injectable cosmetic filling agents as well as technologies in pursuit of "anti-aging" or facial enhancement. This minimally invasive treatment trend includes chemical peel, dermal fillers, laser skin resurfacing, hair removal techniques, microdermabrasion, and others [1, 2] (Fig. 1.2).

We can track the history of cosmetic enhancement and aesthetic rejuvenation through the

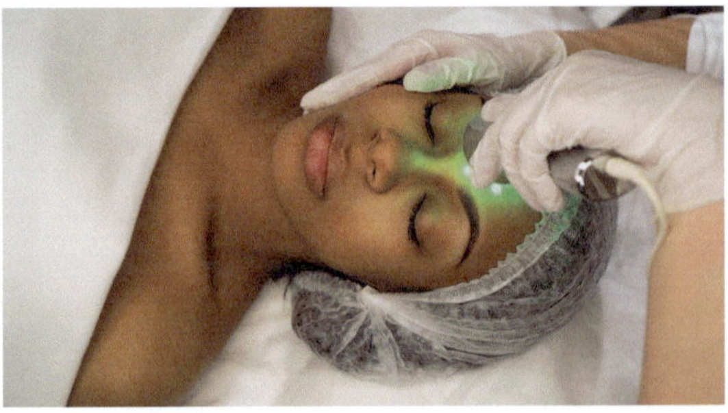

Fig. 1.2 Optical and thermal energy devices build collagen and firm tissue characteristics. (© Vagengeym | Dreamstime.com)

timeline of cosmetic body art as the earliest tribal rituals, to the old testament (840 BC) from the book of Esther to ancient Egypt (1320 BC) [3]. Since ancient times, the concept of cosmetics and facial enhancement has been part of personal essence—especially for the elite. Often, they were used in religious ceremonies—as seen in ancient Egypt—or as cultural identification [4]. Cosmetic products such as creams, lotions, and talcum powders became more globally accessible to the human zeitgeist, supporting pursuits of cultural acceptance, personal enhancement, and beauty. Tracking the aesthetic market in the west, skin care products including skin lotions, powders, creams, bleaches, ointments, and cleansers have historically accounted for a large percentage of the American cosmetics and hygiene industry. The claims and perceived notion of smoother, whiter skin is aligned with better health, and beauty has become the impression of beauty since the 1800s. Concealing and removing imperfections like freckles, rashes, and pimples are also part of the aesthetic objectives [5].

1.3 The Demand for Aesthetic Surgeries

The history of plastic surgery goes back as far as between 1000 and 800 BC with Sushruta—considered the "Father of Plastic Surgery" from ancient India. He was responsible for the advancement of medicine, and his early teachings of anatomy, pathophysiology, and therapeutic strategies were achievements linked to nasal reconstruction. Sushruta's surgical studies led to his development of the cheek flap for nasal reconstruction. His surgical concepts and his creative approaches still apply today [6].

The term PLASTIC surgery is traditionally a clinical term often used for reconstructive treatment of parts of the body affected by disease, injury, infection, birth defects, or trauma. COSMETIC or aesthetic surgery is an elective procedure that enhances or reshapes parts of the body to support the patient's pursuit for self-esteem. Analysts identified the many influences of opting for cosmetic surgery—covering perceived advantages of the likelihood of a more fulfilled life. Where one's self-confidence is linked by societal behavior with an attractive appearance through surgical enhancement, studies emphasized exposure to the media may have significant influence in pursuing cosmetic surgery [7].

One of the oldest cosmetic procedures has been Rhinoplasty (nose job) dating back to the sixth century. Within the recent decade, surgeons have perfected this process such that in 2014, Rhinoplasty has been recognized as the second most popular procedure in the USA with over 215,000 cases within a total estimate of 15M cosmetic procedures. This procedure is second in popularity only to breast enhancement. Other aesthetic procedures that fill this public demand is for gluteal implants, liposuction, and eyelid uplift [8].

The demand for enhancement procedures directly aligns with the worldwide human ambition to fight the many foibles of natural affliction of the aging process. To pursue the ability to improve one's personal health and appearance is heavily driven by the desire to look and feel young again—such that "the battle to reverse time" has expanded this multi-million dollar market. This trend includes the increase in demand for facial aesthetics products such as anti-aging, anti-wrinkle, oxygenation, and rejuvenation neurotoxin free botulinum as well as the growing industry of minimally invasive procedures.

Additionally, dental implants have been added to the list of cosmetic procedures, addressing the treatment of dental imperfections and congenital defects. More recent dermal solutions cover technology-driven laser treatments of lesions, skin toning, and the removal of tattoos, hair, and scars [8].

1.4 Risks and Complications

By now, we all understand the set of risks that exist within any surgical procedure. Not only are all patients prone to different healing rates and capacities, but there may be a wide array of possible complications associated with cosmetic/plastic surgeries—including infection, post-op internal bleeding, reactions to foreign materials or anesthesia, and complex issues during the healing process such as nerve damage, fluid buildup, and blood clotting [9].

2020 news headlines published a major health alert with women who invested in textured breast implants to potentially cause breast implant-associated anaplastic large cell lymphoma (BIA-ALCL)—an uncommon and treatable type of large cell lymphoma that can develop around breast implants. BIA-ALCL is not a cancer of the breast tissue itself. In a 2020 FDA study, there have now been 733 unique confirmed cases worldwide which included 36 known deaths [10, 11].

1.5 Minimally Invasive/ Injectable Treatments

According to international studies, the market of non-invasive aesthetic treatment has been a steady boom at an estimated USD 53B since the early 2020s with a projected growth of 15%+ for the next 10 years. This continued consumer demand for improving physical appearance in adults gained an uptick in the induction of the more affordable and more accessible non-invasive and minimally invasive aesthetic procedures within this period.

INJECTABLE procedures also gained significant popularity especially in the 50+ year old age group. A high population of women are recorded to request aesthetic fillers including Botox. In 2018, an est. $2.8 billion minimally invasive cosmetic procedures were conducted domestically (according to the Grand View Research), showing a consistent rise each year of 9%—identifying its major growth in demand and popularity. These procedures rose sharply by an est 228% within 2000–2018 in the USA, and they now account for 95% of all cosmetic treatments undertaken for NSFA treatments with a 5% decrease in surgical procedures. Minimal invasiveness results in faster recovery, lesser scarring, limited stress, and better patient satisfaction [5, 8, 12, 13] (Fig. 1.3).

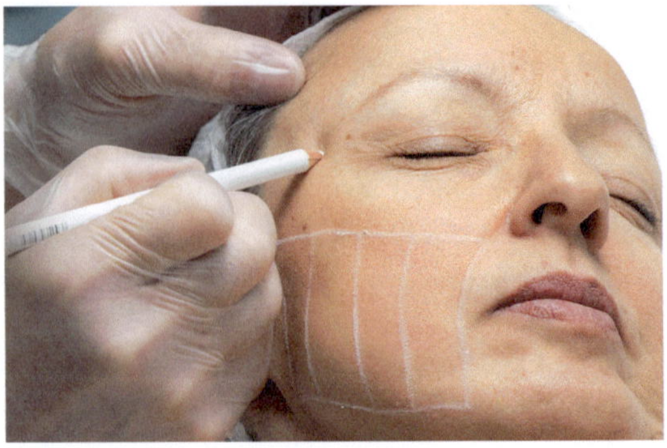

Fig. 1.3 Variations on injections including microneedling procedures are useful in scar and keloid treatments. (© Karel Noppe I Dreamstime.com)

Within the last two decades, the widening term "Medical Aesthetics" has become a trend representing physical corrections and restoration beyond cosmetic applications. Injectable techniques have expanded to clinically support the aesthetic dermatologist to repair facial texture structurally through contouring, lifting, volumizing, improving muscle and tissue tone, or implement focal fat reduction. The professional may apply a host of materials into the skin including inert fillers, platelet-rich plasma (PRP), stem cells, and lipolytic agents. As the expansion of agents and injecting materials continue to grow with its demand, the inducing clinician must undergo comprehensive safety and procedural training alongside a solid understanding of the elements used in these injectable treatments in order to achieve proper outcomes [14].

1.6 The Covid-19 Pandemic and Self-Enhancement

Global analytics of the aesthetics community during the coronavirus outbreak (COVID-19) in 2019 resulted in the freeze of all non-emergency/elective hospital procedures. It is this suspension alongside the societal distress caused by the lockdown that created a backlog of procedures and an increased demand for self-enhancement. Also, other influential factors driving the rise in

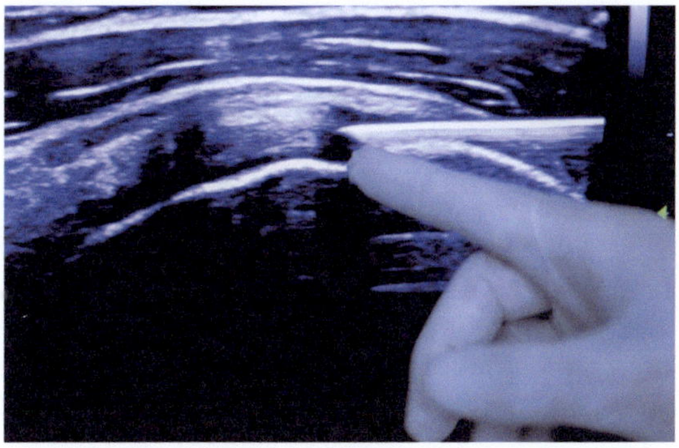

Fig. 1.4 Real-time imaging may better demonstrate blood flow and thin facial nerves and provides a preop map of danger sites. (© Edward Olive | Dreamstime.com)

cosmetic surgery during the pandemic were attributed to the vast exposure to video conferencing, where more individuals are forced to view themselves (and grow critical of their appearance) during video meetings (Fig 1.4).

Global studies have been implemented on adults observing behaviors and concerns while undergoing multiple video conferencing usage, including the use of video-enhancement tools to improve picture quality and focus of visual attention while on video calls. A significant percentage of participants identified appearance concerns while on video-associated with self-focused attention and increasing appearance concerns due to their time on video calls. The report concluded a large number of interest in acquiring future beauty treatments and nonsurgical aesthetic procedures such as anti-wrinkle injections. A recent colloquialism for this is the "Zoom Face Phenomenon" driven by the covid-driven boom of video conferencing (tying this issue with the Zoom video brand) [15–18].

1.7 Phasing Out the "Anti-aging" Terminology

More than a definition, applying the term REJUVENATION is truly the goal vs. ANTI-AGING. For decades, the term "anti-aging" has been a phrase that represented the entire marketing lexicon describing products, services, and procedures to promote aesthetic enhancement. Further review of this Ageism is seen as more about stereotyping and/or discrimination against individuals or groups on the basis of their age.

The science is not about recapturing the fountain of youth—alluding to a criticism of one's natural aging process—but about firming, tightening, polishing, or skin conditioning. A commentary on social appeal dictates that beauty and attraction is defined not necessarily on looking younger but having a radiant appearance. The recent trending term identifies today's aesthetic procedures as REGENERATIVE or AESTHETIC ENHANCEMENT, implying a more objective-based category. Where wrinkles, shadows, and loose skin render a fatigued and worn impression, it is the million dollar industry of ENHANCEMENT that has taken on what tolls of time has done to the physical self—both the face and body [7, 19].

1.8 Overview on Minimally Invasive Procedures

The value of aesthetics in our community exists throughout all social groups. The market recognizes one popular focus group in particular to include the parent community—whose exhaustive commitments to countless physical demands may oftentimes appear in their features. Investing in facial enhancements offers a sense of personal satisfaction about their renewed public appearance. In addition, such procedures have been studied to bring personal empowerment from experiencing that natural facial glow from having improved skin texture. Psychologists and counselors identify the means of having a rested appearance as looking and feeling optimized could actually support an emotional uplift by motivating the self to manifest a healthier lifestyle.

1.9 Face Lifts

A facelift, technically known as a rhytidectomy (rooted from the word rhytis or "wrinkle," and ektome "excision"—or the surgical removal of wrinkles), is a cosmetic process dedicated to providing a more youthful facial appearance. To achieve this, there are various surgical and minimally invasive techniques available. Surgery could mean the extraction of loose, sagging skin (often from age) and the skin tightening on the patient's face, neck, cheeks, or eyelids. Non-surgical enhancement strategies that address these and issues like frown lines and other facial wrinkles can also be achieved with other modern techniques such as the injection of bio fillers and the performance of laser skin resurfacing or photodynamic therapy for the removal of wrinkles, spots, and textures.

1.10 Microneedling

Microneedling is a procedure using small needles to prick the skin in order to generate new collagen and healthier tissue for more toned skin. The concept of microneedling was widely used on a commercial level since the 1900s in Europe to address acne and skin scars. The technology continues in popularity throughout the aesthetics community and has evolved from manual applications to electric microneedling that may help with a wide set of issues such as fine lines and wrinkles, oversized pores, acne, dark spots, hair loss, and stretch marks [20].

As a working arsenal to dermatologists, aestheticians, and other trained clinical subscribers, microneedling is recognized to be far less costly than other skin therapeutic technologies including laser treatments, which by comparison can cost about 3–4 times. The entire process is usually around 15–20 min and may commonly require 4–6 treatments depending on need.

1.11 The PRP Process

In recent years, the success of platelet-rich plasma (PRP) treatment protocols is growing in popularity, capturing an expanding share of the aesthetics market. To date, the history of the PRP therapeutic process has been recorded from Equine (Horses) Medicine since the early 1990s. Veterinary medicine applied the use of PRP to treat ligament damage such as tears or inflammation in the tendons. This process has also been applied in horses with osteoarthritis both showing significant success for continued research both in animals and early human studies. The evolution and success of the PRP relied on the preparation of the plasma, including volume and percentages applied and the quality and consistency of the extracted matter [21–23].

Clinical professionals find its benefits to be easily integrated within their practices to expand their services. From dentists, dermatologists, and cosmetic surgeons to most non-medical cosmetic practices, training and adopting PRP systems into a practice or aesthetic-related business has been found to require a low level of commitment and investment.

The vast appeal of offering a minimally invasive (non-surgical) regenerative enhancement solution provides a great alternative to the consumer while adding a much lower cost alternative to acquiring PRP is now being used to treat chronic osteoarthritis and other orthopedic injuries and is also more widely marketed in the aesthetics channels. PRP is widely applied in various areas of the medical field for its proven properties of regenerative therapy as well as in many areas of clinical aesthetics. In dermatology, there has been significant success in PRP's expanded use from wound healing, scar reduction, skin and tissue regeneration, and skin enhancement.

The science of PRP originated in hematology IN THE 1970S as part of plasma transfusion for thrombocytopenia patients or those with low platelet count in their blood. The biological concept of plasma extraction by centrifugation of autologous blood (sourced from oneself) offers 1-to-1 cellular compatibility by accessing one's own healing properties [24].

In aesthetics, the PRP extraction and application process forge the healing properties of the plasma—extracting the usable "platelet-rich plasma" from the "platelet poor plasma" to be used TOPICALLY in applications similar to microneedling. It is also widely applied as

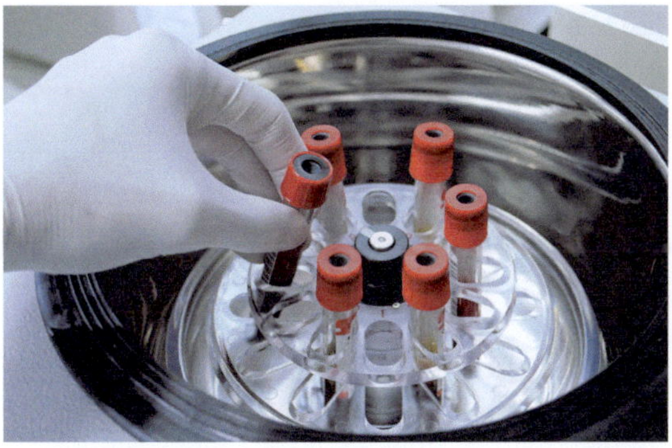

Fig. 1.5 PRP and other injectable biologics are improving blood perfusion to treated areas. (© T-Photo I Shutterstock.com)

SUBCUTANEOUS injections such as breast lifts or to increase collagen on the facial skin's surface. PRP also offers restorative and tissue healing value for follicles in hair restoration procedures (Fig. 1.5).

Under clinical supervision, PRP treatment of facial enhancement and wrinkle removal involves drawing approximately 20–60 mL of blood. The practitioner would centrifuge this to separate plasma from blood cells, capturing the injectable YELLOW matter known to be "rich in platelets." However, in larger aesthetic services, like a vampire breast lift, or a P-shot (Priapus Shot), you actually need to draw an estimated minimum of 60 mL of blood to a rough minimum of 6–10 tubes. Upon the centrifuging process, once the PRP is harvested, in most cases, platelet poor plasma is discarded [25–27].

1.12 Historical Context of Natural Aesthetics

Four thousand years ago, the Egyptians used plants especially rose petal extracts for aesthetic enhancement. The treatment of the flower of R*osa Gallica,* organically grown in France, pesticide free, and chemically balanced with antioxidants, is currently used in clinical practice as an extract of whole fresh or cut and dried rose petals and rose petal tinctures: organically distilled.

Traditional usage has been as follows:

- Anti-inflammatory.
- Anti-mutagenic.
- Anti-oxidant.
- Cellular regeneration.
- Collagen accelerator.
- Internal detoxification.
- Dermal rehydration.

1.13 Medicinal Overview

Chinese medicine recommends rose petal extract for regulating vital energy or "qi," for strengthening blood circulation, purifying the liver, and alleviating joint pains. The high concentration of anthocyanins in the petals is known for their ability to strengthen the vascular system, prevent blood platelet stickiness (blood clots), and also have powerful antioxidant, antibacterial, and anti-inflammatory activity.

Rose petal essential oils were used as a dermal rehydrator to beautify the skin by the ancient Egyptians. In Roman times, people treated breast diseases, skin conditions, and even wound infections with orally ingested preparations. Research has shown that an extract from Rosa Gallica strikingly increases the effectiveness of several antibiotics against methicillin-resistant *Staphylococcus aureus*. Two active compounds from the extract have been identified as tellimagrandin I and rugosin B. Other studies have demonstrated strong activity of Rosa Gallica extract against strains of *Candida albicans* isolated from overtreatment with antibiotics. Additionally, the effect of an anthocyanin preparation isolated from the flower petals of Rosa Gallica demonstrated strong effects of Rosa extracts against abnormal cells. A 3-year research study by the BioFoundation for Angiogenesis Research preceded the development of the chemical constituents of the ProRose+ formulation. Scientific evaluation has shown the antioxidant effect to be 10× (ten times) more powerful than green tea preparations and resveratrol formulations. Collagen regeneration has been observed clinically and documented with high resolution sonograms. Improved blood flow to hair follicles has been demonstrated with vascular imaging technologies. The 2011 World Anti-Aging Conference showed poor dermal penetration of creams and good tissue regeneration with internal antioxidants. A 20-year study by the AngioFoundation revealed that the curative effects appeared in other glandular sites, such as the breast, prostate, and thyroid which was presented at the international 2021 Inflammatory Skin Disease Symposium as it showed improvement in cutaneous inflammatory processes such as psoriasis, rosacea, lupus, hidradenitis, and related collagen type diseases.

1.14 Active Ingredients

Rose petals contain anthocyanins and proanthocyanidins, tellimagrandin I and rugosin B; carotenoids, and plant acids including gallic acid and essential oils. The liquid portion of oil of rose contains as its chief constituent the alcohol geraniol. Geraniol, with a rose-like odor, is a primary alcohol and yields, upon oxidation, the aldehyde citral, also present in rose petals. Rose oil furthermore contains about 20% of L-citronellol. A proprietary blend of balancing antioxidants has been added to the extract. Rose petals as concentrated extract/elixir with the recommended dosage of 10–20 drops twice per day. Drug Interactions: None known Contraindications: None known except alcohol dependence.

Side Effects: Allergic reactions are possible in susceptible persons.

Synergism: When combined with Coenzyme Q10 and resveratrol, the treatment benefit is enhanced.

1.15 Epilogue

The modern age of aesthetic procedures has much to thank the medical scientific community when it comes to their approach and strategies behind clinical treatments. Recent visionary concepts such as injectable bio-fillers are clearly rooted from the same delivery of therapeutic material, showing similar logic, tools, and applications. Also, medical innovations such as laser, ultrasound, radiotherapies, and other non-invasive electronic devices have also added a major foothold to the aesthetics movement.

The evolution in clinical aesthetics continues to advance all procedures especially for the sake of performance, safety, and longevity. Over time, this level of evolution also reflects on the economics and access of these procedures—where the major BOOM in aesthetic modalities has clearly engaged the global market. And as the global market maintains a major uptick in demand for aesthetic procedures, so continues the introduction of new protocols, strategies, and improvements in treatment options and opportunities.

References

1. Breaking down the most popular noninvasive cosmetic treatments, American Society of Plastic Surgeons, Rod Rohrich I Dallas, TX Friday, June 16, 2017. https://www.plasticsurgery.org/news/blog/breaking-down-the-most-popularnoninvasive-cosmetic-treatments.
2. Kontis TC, Rivkin A. The history of injectable facial fillers. Facial Plast Surg. 2009;25(2):67–72. https://pubmed.ncbi.nlm.nih.gov/19415573/.
3. History of cosmetics. https://en.wikipedia.org/wiki/History_of_cosmetics.
4. Library of Congress. History of the beauty business. https://guides.loc.gov/business-of-beauty/history.
5. Cosmetics and personal care products in the medicine and science collections. https://americanhistory.si.edu/collections/object-groups/health-hygiene-and-beauty/skin-care.
6. Sushruta: father of plastic surgery. https://pubmed.ncbi.nlm.nih.gov/23788147/.
7. Colbert S. University of Missouri. https://www.muhealth.org/our-stories/cosmetic-vs-plastic-surgery-whats-difference.
8. Worldwide Medical Aesthetics Industry—market is expected to grow at a CAGR of 9.9% between 2021 to 2029. https://www.globenewswire.com/news-release/2021/03/05/2187849/28124/en/Worldwide-Medical-Aesthetics-IndustryMarket-is-Expected-to-Grow-at-a-CAGR-of-9-9-Between-2021-to-2029.html.
9. Complications of reconstructive plastic surgery. Stanford Healthcare. https://stanfordhealthcare.org/medicaltreatments/r/reconstructive-plastic-surgery/complications.html.
10. BIA-ALCL Physician Resources. American Society of Plastic Surgeons. https://www.plasticsurgery.org/for-medical-professionals/health-policy/bia-alcl-

physicianresources#:~:text=The%20August%20 20%2C%202020%2C%20FDA,which%20 included%2036%20known%20deaths.
11. Bia-ALCL: American Society of Plastic Surgeons. https://www.plasticsurgery.org/for-medical-professionals/health-policy/biaalcl-physician-resources/summary-and-quick-facts.
12. GVR report: non-invasive aesthetic treatment market size, share & trends report, non-invasive aesthetic treatment market size, share & trends analysis report by procedure. https://www.grandviewresearch.com/industry-analysis/non-invasive-aesthetic-treatmentmarket#:~:text=According%20to%20the%20American%20Society,the%20market%20in%20the%20country.
13. Characteristics of patients seeking and proceeding with non-surgical facial aesthetic procedures. NIH. https://www.ncbi.nlm.nih.gov/pmc/articles/PMC7935348/.
14. Trends for facial injectable therapies in medical aesthetics. https://www.ncbi.nlm.nih.gov/pmc/articles/PMC6128160/.
15. Medical aesthetics market to reach USD 16,034.87 million, globally, by 2028 at 12.5% CAGR- - COVID-19 impact and global analysis by the insight partners. https://www.prnewswire.com/news-releases/medical-aesthetics-market-to-reach-usd-16-034-87-million-globally-by-2028-at-12-5-cagr%2D%2D%2D%2Dcovid-19-impact-and-global-analysis-by-the-insight-partners-301387695.html.
16. The zoom effect: exploring the impact of video calling on appearance dissatisfaction and interest in aesthetic treatment during the COVID-19 pandemic. NIH. https://pubmed.ncbi.nlm.nih.gov/34146086/.
17. 'Zoom face' phenomenon has people eyeing plastic surgery—by Sandy Cohen February 3, 2022, UCLA. https://connect.uclahealth.org/2022/02/03/zoom-face-phenomenon-has-people-eyeing-plastic-surgery/.
18. Commentary on: The Zoom Boom: how video calling impacts attitudes towards aesthetic surgery in the COVID-19 era. https://pubmed.ncbi.nlm.nih.gov/34232299/.
19. Toxic terminology: why we're over "anti-aging". https://www.intoxicatingbeauty.com/intoxicating-lifestylemagazine/why-we-are-over-anti-aging/.
20. WebMD. https://www.webmd.com/beauty/what_is_microneedling.
21. A critical overview of the use of platelet-rich plasma in equine medicine over the last decade. https://www.frontiersin.org/articles/10.3389/fvets.2021.641818/full.
22. What is the potential use of platelet-rich-plasma (PRP) in cancer treatment? A mini review. NIH/PUBMED. https://www.ncbi.nlm.nih.gov/pmc/articles/PMC7113436/.
23. CEH horse report/Prp—improving treatment of tendon & ligament injuries. https://ceh.vetmed.ucdavis.edu/sites/g/files/dgvnsk4536/files/local_resources/pdfs/pubs-HR29-1-bkm.sec.pdf.
24. Platelet-rich plasma: where are we now and where are we going? https://www.ncbi.nlm.nih.gov/pmc/articles/PMC3445108/.
25. Availability of platelet-rich plasma for treatment of erectile dysfunction and associated costs and efficacy: a review of current publications and Canadian data. https://www.ncbi.nlm.nih.gov/pmc/articles/PMC8195577/.
26. Principles and methods of preparation of platelet-rich plasma: a review and author's perspective. https://www.ncbi.nlm.nih.gov/pmc/articles/PMC4338460/.
27. Healthline: "what to expect from a vampire breast lift (VBL)". https://www.healthline.com/health/vampire-breast-lift.

Facial Danger Zones: Ultrasound Anatomy

2

Cameron P. Christiansen and Elie M. Ferneini

Abstract

Soft tissue fillers are a common cosmetic procedure to correct unwanted facial feature discrepancies. The use of these fillers has grown significantly over the last few years. When proper technique is used, facial fillers typically have a successful outcome with minor complications. However, due to the high vascularity of the head and neck, major complications can occur. With any procedure, it is crucial to know how to manage complications when they arise, but more importantly, how to reduce the risk of major complications occurring. New technology and techniques have been discovered to help aid in reducing the risk, including ultrasound for visualization of important anatomical structures and soft tissue filler after placement. This chapter explores proper technique for soft tissue filler placement in the head and neck while reviewing the various filler materials and introducing ultrasound as an aid in placement.

Keywords

Soft tissue fillers · Head · Neck · Ultrasound · Facial danger zones

2.1 Introduction

The use of soft tissue fillers as a nonsurgical cosmetic procedure has only continued to gain popularity. In 2020, the American Society of Plastic Surgeons reported that 3.4 million soft tissue filler procedures were performed, making it the second most common cosmetic surgery procedure in the United States. With the rise of social media, online meetings, and the desire for achieving the ideal facial contour, it can be assumed that these procedures will only continue to be in high demand. Injecting soft tissue fillers in facial regions is a safe and predictable procedure, but the clinician must be trained and take caution when performing these procedures. This chapter will explore soft tissue fillers, the proper technique for placement, complications, and new technologies using ultrasound in assisting the placement of soft tissue fillers.

C. P. Christiansen
Oral and Maxillofacial Surgery, Nassau University Medical Center, East Meadow, NY, USA

E. M. Ferneini (✉)
Beau Visage Med Spa, Cheshire, CT, USA

R. L. Bard (ed.), *Image-Guided Aesthetic Treatments*, https://doi.org/10.1007/978-3-031-36266-8_2

2.2 Soft Tissue Fillers

Soft tissue fillers can be classified as temporary (absorbable) or permanent (nonabsorbable) [1]. Temporary fillers include those composed of hyaluronic acid (HA), collagen, HA with dextranomer beads, poly-L-lactic acid, and calcium hydroxylapatite. Permanent fillers include silicone preparations, polymethylmethacrylate (PMMA) microspheres, polyacrylamide hydrogels (PAHGs), and polyalkylimide gels [2]. The most common type of soft tissue filler placed is hyaluronic acid [3, 4]. While these soft tissue fillers have varying clinical applications and properties, the technique and principles are generally the same.

2.3 Hyaluronic Acid (HA)

HA is a complex sugar molecule that naturally occurs in the body [2]. It attracts water molecules and gives volume to the skin. As we age, the collagen, elastin fibers, fat, and HA found in the dermis break down resulting in wrinkles. HA fillers are used to correct these wrinkles by providing the skin with the HA needed to attract water to the area and replace the depleted volume. The HA gels in the fillers are produced by *Streptococcus* and cross-linked with 1,4-butanediol diglycidyl ether. The gels are then mixed with a phosphate buffer saline solution at varying concentrations [2]. The cross-linking of the HA fillers is increased in comparison to human HA which allows the fillers to be more resistant to degradation. However, these HA molecules do breakdown over time, but clinical results can be expected for up to 18 months after initial placement of the HA filler [2, 5]. Common HA fillers include Restylane, Juvederm, and Belotero. The difference between the various HA fillers are the particle size, the degree of cross-linking, and the concentration of the HA gel to saline. Fillers with increased cross-linking and higher concentration of HA gel result in increased longevity. The filler particle size contributes to the amount of volume replaced. Fillers with larger particle sizes are used when significant volume replacement is needed. Fillers with smaller particle sizes are used when minimal volume replacement is needed and yield smoother, more natural results. If large particle fillers are used to replace minimal volume, patients could complain of the treated areas appearing bumpy and unaesthetic.

2.4 Injection Technique

When placing soft tissue fillers, it is crucial to understand which type of material and which technique is ideal to achieve the desired patient outcome. Decisions need to be made concerning the amount of volume to be replaced and the corresponding anatomy in the area of replacement. Proper selection of syringe, needles, and cannulas should also be taken into consideration with which technique is to be used for placement.

The placement of fillers occurs at varying depths depending on which type of filler you are using. Fillers with large particles are placed in the subdermis area. If these fillers are placed too superficially, a lack of aesthetic outcome can be achieved. This can occur as a result of the area appearing bulky and bumpy, or the area can appear as a blue discoloration due to the Tyndall effect. If these fillers are placed too deep, the fillers are unable to adequately replace the volume needed. Fillers with smaller sized particles are placed more superficially just below the dermis. These fillers are less likely to contribute to the Tyndall effect due to their smaller particle size and allowing the light to scatter properly.

Soft tissue injections can be made with a variety of needles and cannulas. The gauge of the needle is dependent on the size of the filler particle. If needles are to be used for placement, aspiration is crucial as the facial regions are highly vascularized. One way to minimize the risk of injection into vasculature is by using blunt-tipped cannulas [2]. The initial access port is made through the skin using a 25 G needle followed by the insertion of the cannula. These cannulas are typically longer than traditional needles as well allowing for deeper placement and access to differing sites through the same access point, decreasing the number of initial injections.

Serial injections are multiple injections made close to each other in a continuous line. It is important to ensure that there are no gaps between the injected materials, so close placement of the material is crucial to maximize esthetics [2, 6]. If minor voids are noticed after placement, the filler material can be gently massaged along the line of placement to ensure the material is unified [2, 4]. This type of injection technique is helpful in replacing minimal volume in highly esthetic areas such as the glabella, philtral column, and fine wrinkles.

Linear threading is a technique in which a needle is inserted fully at the midpoint of the wrinkle in a parallel fashion. This full insertion creates a channel for the material to be deposited in. The needle is then slowly withdrawn as the clinician deposits the material in a continuous manner. This technique is useful in nasolabial folds and vermilion-cutaneous borders [2].

Cross-hatching is similar to linear threading, but the material is deposited over a larger area. Cross-hatch lines are first determined and defined. The grid should follow the appropriate contour of the injection site. The material is then deposited in a series of injections along the defined grid in the same fashion as the linear threading technique [6, 7]. This technique is used for correction of large areas, especially perioral [2].

Fanning is another technique that can be used. This technique is achieved by first inserting the needle and injecting the material. The needle is then moved to a different location in a clockwise or counter-clockwise manner without being fully withdrawn, leaving the needle tip in the skin and placing more filler [2]. Moving in this direction allows for proper contour and even distribution. Fanning also reduces the number of times a patient needs to have their skin penetrated, decreasing discomfort. This technique is used in deep nasolabial folds, marionette lines [7], and deep malar injections [2].

2.5 Complications

With any surgical and non-surgical procedure, there is always the risk of complications. Soft tissue fillers are no different, and patients should be fully informed of the possibility of complications, both minor and major. Minor and more common complications include swelling, bruising, tenderness, erythema, and itching [2].

Major complications include infection [1], hypersensitivity [2], necrosis [2, 4, 8], and blindness [4, 8]. Infection rates are estimated to be around 0.004–0.02% [1] and are most commonly associated with insufficient disinfection of the site prior to injection. It is important to use an alcohol wipe to clean the area to reduce the chance of infection. Hypersensitivity reactions are not as common due to the improved purity of the filler product. Trace proteins were more commonly found in older fillers and contributed to this complication [2]. Skin necrosis in the site of the injection is typically seen when filler is injected in large quantities around or in vasculature [2]. It has been found that the incidence in all soft tissue filler procedures resulting in tissue necrosis is 0.001% [8]. High risk areas of tissue necrosis include the glabella, nasal ala, lip, and nasolabial fold. Blindness is the most severe complication reported with soft tissue fillers. A literature review was performed in 2015, and 98 cases of vision changes were reported [9]. High risk areas included the glabella (38.8%), nasal region (25.5%), nasolabial fold (13.3%), and the forehead (12.2%). While the risk of blindness is low, clinicians must ensure they take every precaution to avoid this life altering complication. Aspiration prior to injection is crucial to ensure that the tip of the needle is not located in an artery, allowing the retrograde travel of filler through the bloodstream to the eye [10].

2.6 Facial Danger Zones

With all facial fillers, understanding the anatomy of the areas where you are injecting is crucial. Understanding this anatomy and the various danger zones of the face is vital in decreasing the risk of complications.

2.7 Upper Face

The supraorbital artery is a branch of the ophthalmic artery and exits the supraorbital notch which is located about 11 mm lateral to the medial canthus of the eye. It enters the corrugator muscle at the level of the supraorbital rim and travels in a medial-to-lateral direction. The supraorbital artery also has multiple branches: a deep and a superficial branch. The superficial branch anastomoses with supratrochlear artery and frontal branch of the superficial temporal artery. The supratrochlear artery also arises from the ophthalmic artery and exits the supratrochlear notch about 3 mm lateral to the medial canthus. The supratrochlear artery is a relatively superficial artery and is typically located 1–2 mm deep in the frontalis muscle. A pertinent and important anastomosis for injection of facial fillers is where the supraorbital and supratrochlear vessels anastomose with the angular artery in the nasal glabellar area. Injections in the glabellar area should be performed superficially and aspiration is essential.

The central retinal artery supplies blood to the optic nerve and is a branch of the ophthalmic artery. This artery performs an anastomosis with the supraorbital, supratrochlear, and angular artery, and blockage of this artery can result in the feared complication of blindness. If the surgeon suspects any compromise to these vessels, ophthalmic evaluation should be considered. Patients might complain of vision changes, ocular pain, headache, nausea, vomiting, and lack of extraocular movements. Clinically, the signs of central retinal artery occlusion are a pale swollen retina and a chief complaint of inability to see out of the affected eye. A recent review identified 190 documented cases of blindness following injection of facial fillers [11], so while the risk is minimal, the complication still occurs and surgeons need to be aware (Figs. 2.1 and 2.2).

The superficial temporal artery is the terminal branch of the external carotid artery. It originates

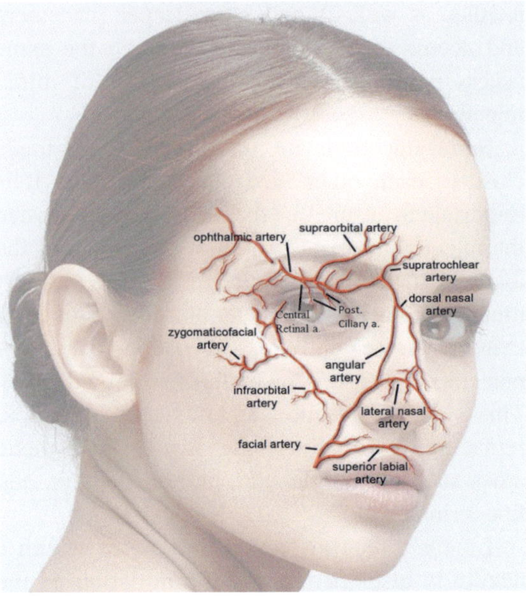

Fig. 2.1 Critical vessels of the upper and lower face

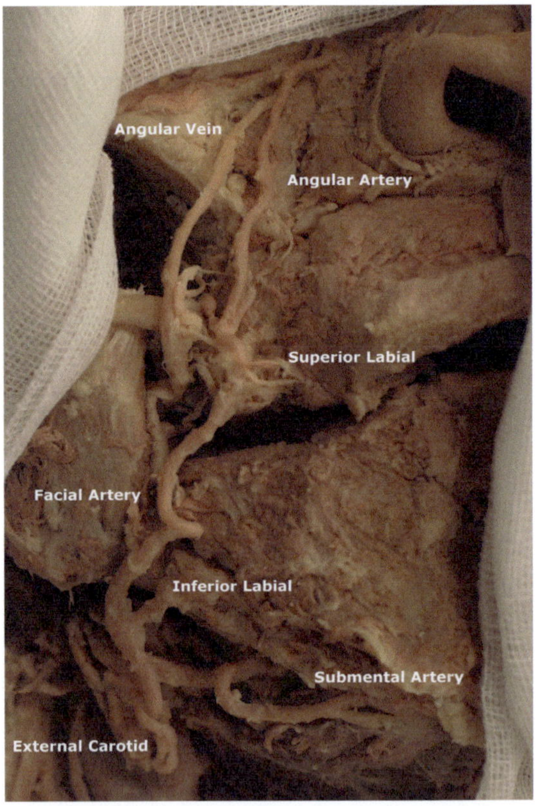

Fig. 2.2 Anatomic specimen of arteries

at the level of the mandibular ramus and extends superiorly traversing the parotid gland and running superficially to the zygomatic process and temporal bone. The artery has two branches: the parietal and frontal, which are located superficial to the frontalis muscle. With regards to facial fillers, the frontal branch of the superficial temporal artery is an important vessel to be cognizant of and it has been found to have an average diameter of 2 mm. When injecting fillers, the surgeon should place them deep in the periosteal plane or take extra care and precaution when placing the fillers more superficial.

2.8 Midface

The midface is highly vascularized with all major arteries forming anastomoses with each other. For injections in this area, fillers should be placed deep to avoid vascular compromise. The dorsal nasal arteries, or external nasal arteries, arise from the ophthalmic artery, supplying the upper eyelid and lateral nose and eventually anastomosing with the angular arteries on each side of the nose. The angular artery is the terminal end of the facial artery and can be detected around 5 mm medial to the medial canthal vertical line. The lateral nasal artery is a branch of the facial artery and travels parallel to the ala of the nose toward the tip of the nose. The artery forms anastomoses with the septal branches of the superior labial artery, angular artery, ophthalmic artery, internal maxillary artery, and smaller nasal surface arteries. It also forms an anastomosis with the contralateral lateral nasal artery. These arteries perfuse the skin and cartilage of the nose, along with other deeper structures in the nose.

The infraorbital artery is a branch of the maxillary artery and exits the infraorbital foramen. The infraorbital foramen is located approximately 1/3 the distance between the medial and lateral canthi. The distance inferiorly between the infraorbital rim and the infraorbital foramen is about 11 mm. The infraorbital artery is responsible for supplying the skin of the lower eyelid and middle face. As it travels in the inferior direction after emerging from the infraorbital foramen, it is located deep to the levator labii superioris muscle and superficial to the levator anguli oris muscle. Prior to placement of facial fillers in this area, surgeons should palpate the infraorbital foramen and avoid injections medial to it toward the medial canthus. If the surgeon determines that filler should be placed medial to the infraorbital foramen, filler can be placed laterally and pushed medially to the desired location.

2.9 Lower Face

The lower face is the location of the main artery of the face, the facial artery. The facial artery is a branch of the external carotid artery, traversing through the submandibular gland at the lower border of the mandible and continuing in a superior medial oblique fashion across the face. While traveling, the facial artery gives off branches including the submental, inferior labial artery, and superior labial artery. The terminal end of the facial artery becomes the angular artery, as discussed previously. The main trunk of the facial artery travels deep to the platysma, which can act as a safety barrier when injecting.

The inferior labial artery is commonly located posterior to the mucosal-muscular interface and below the superior border of the lip. Injections in this area should be made superficially and no greater than 2 mm deep. The needle should be inserted at the vermillion border or within the dry vermillion. Injections of the upper lip should also be made superficially in the submucosa later in a fanning technique. The superior labial artery is largest in diameter at the labial commissure and smallest in diameter at the midline. The artery is also deepest at the branch point of the facial artery and most superficial at the peak of Cupid's bow. Intravascular injection of filler material around the lips can lead to tissue and lip necrosis (Fig. 2.3).

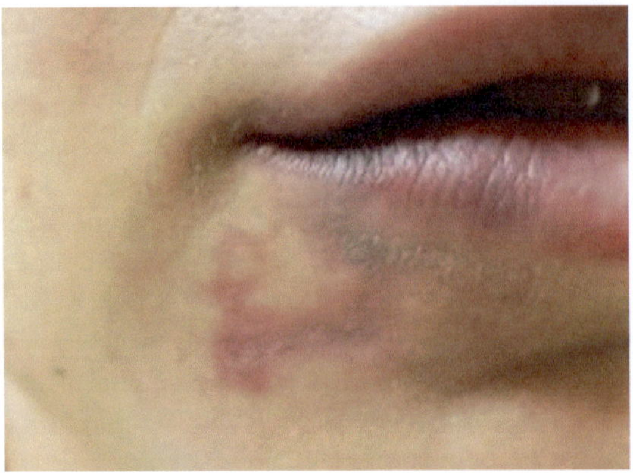

Fig. 2.3 Lower lip discoloration due to arterial insufficiency from aberrant filler placement

2.10 Ultrasound in Soft Tissue Filler Placement

When placing soft tissue fillers, knowing where you are injecting is crucial. Ultrasound has been used for many years to view soft tissue and subcutaneous structures. It is an easy-to use, noninvasive modality that works as sound waves from the ultrasound transducer travel through the body. As these sound waves encounter a structure, tissue, or material, they are reflected back to the transducer at varying strengths. Materials or structures higher in density reflect stronger and produce a bright or white (hyperechogenic) signal. Low density structures reflect a gray (hypoechogenic) signal or black signal (anechoic) [12]. Ultrasound can be used to identify important anatomic structures and also examine the placement of fillers postoperatively.

Prior to injecting filler material, sonography can be used to visualize the epidermis, underlying dermis, subcutaneous tissues, muscles, vessels, and other structures. The first layer visible is the epidermis, and it appears as a hyperechoic line. However, this line is not actually the epidermis and is called the epidermal echo. The epidermal echo is created by reflections of the ultrasound gel on the skin. The dermis is the next visible layer and is recognized as an area of heterogeneity with varying strengths of hyperechoic reflections of the collagen and hypoechoic reflections of the extracellular matrix between the collagen fibers. Small vessels, hair follicles, and glands potentially can also be observed based on the type of transducer being used and the area observing. The third layer seen is the subcutaneous layer and is typically visualized as a hypoechoic area with linear hyperechoic areas. Muscles are also able to be visualized by ultrasound and appear anechoic or hypoechoic. Blood vessels appear anechoic under ultrasound and are important to recognize when using ultrasound prior to filler injection. If desiring to better identify vessels, Doppler ultrasound can be used. This type of ultrasound is used to monitor the flow of liquid in a vessel. Depending on the direction of the flow, the Doppler signal is either red or blue [13].

Hyaluronic acid fillers are able to be visualized with sonography and appear as scattered anechoic round structures localized to the area where they were deposited immediately after placement. As time passes, the fillers are resorbed and appear smaller; however, they remain localized to the same location and maintain their anechoic status. After a period of 12–18 months, the filler can become very difficult to visualize with sonography due to resorption [14, 15]. Doppler ultrasound can also be used for patients who have been injected with HA filler mixed with lidocaine to better visualize these fillers. Oftentimes you will see blood flow as indicated by the red and blue colors surrounding the filler deposits [13]. Correction of incorrect placement or reactions to fillers can also be aided with the use of ultrasound.

2.11 Conclusion

Overall, the use of soft tissue fillers in the head and neck is a safe and effective procedure, when trained properly and safety is taken. These fillers will only continue to become more common and surgeons need to become proficient and skilled in their delivery. Minor side effects are common and are not typically a medical emergency, but it is crucial to know how to manage and recognize the signs of critical complications. Because the face is highly vascularized, it is crucial that clinicians aspirate prior to injection and also deposit the material slowly and in control. Using tools such as ultrasound can only aid in the placement and safety of these procedures. Identifying important anatomical structures prior to placement can help decrease the risk of major unwanted complications. If patients are managed appropriately, patients can expect desired esthetic results with minor complications.

References

1. Ferneini EM, Beauvais D, Aronin SI. An overview of infections associated with soft tissue facial fillers: identification, prevention, and treatment. J Oral Maxillofac Surg. 2017;75(1):160–6. https://doi.org/10.1016/j.joms.2016.09.004.
2. Ferneini E, Boynton T, Almunajed H, Dimitrov K, Banki M. Review of facial fillers and injectable neurotoxins. Am J Cosmet Surg. 2013;30(2):53–60. https://doi.org/10.5992/AJCS-D-12-00028.1.
3. Ramanadham SR, Rohrich RJ. Newer understanding of specific anatomic targets in the aging face as applied to injectables: superficial and deep facial fat compartments—an evolving target for site-specific facial augmentation. Plast Reconstr Surg. 2015;136(5 Suppl):49S–55S. https://doi.org/10.1097/PRS.0000000000001730.
4. Rohrich RJ, Bartlett EL, Dayan E. Practical approach and safety of hyaluronic acid fillers. Plast Reconstr Surg Glob Open. 2019;7(6):e2172. https://doi.org/10.1097/GOX.0000000000002172.
5. Newman J. Review of soft tissue augmentation in the face. Clin Cosmet Investig Dermatol. 2009;2:141–50. https://doi.org/10.2147/ccid.s3631.
6. Vedamurthy M, Vedamurthy A. Dermal fillers: tips to achieve successful outcomes. J Cutan Aesthet Surg. 2008;1(2):64–7. https://doi.org/10.4103/0974-2077.44161.
7. Bass LS. Injectable filler techniques for facial rejuvenation, volumization, and augmentation. Facial Plast Surg Clin North Am. 2015;23(4):479–88. https://doi.org/10.1016/j.fsc.2015.07.004.
8. Ferneini EM, Ferneini AM. An overview of vascular adverse events associated with facial soft tissue fillers: recognition, prevention, and treatment. J Oral Maxillofac Surg. 2016;74(8):1630–6. https://doi.org/10.1016/j.joms.2016.03.009.
9. Beleznay K, Carruthers JDA, Humphrey S, Jones D. Avoiding and treating blindness from fillers: a review of the world literature. Dermatol Surg. 2015;41(10):1097–117. https://doi.org/10.1097/DSS.0000000000000486.
10. Ferneini EM, Hapelas S, Watras J, Ferneini AM, Weyman D, Fewins J. Surgeon's guide to facial soft tissue filler injections: relevant anatomy and safety considerations. J Oral Maxillofac Surg. 2017;75(12):2667.e1–5. https://doi.org/10.1016/j.joms.2017.08.026.
11. Chatrath V, Banerjee PS, Goodman GJ, Rahman E. Soft-tissue filler–associated blindness: a systematic review of case reports and case series. Plast Reconstr Surg Glob Open. 2019;7(4):e2173. https://doi.org/10.1097/GOX.0000000000002173.
12. Schelke LW, Van Den Elzen HJ, Erkamp PPM, Neumann HAM. Use of ultrasound to provide overall information on facial fillers and surrounding tissue. Dermatol Surg. 2010;36(Suppl 3):1843–51. https://doi.org/10.1111/j.1524-4725.2010.01740.x.
13. Schelke LW, Decates TS, Velthuis PJ. Ultrasound to improve the safety of hyaluronic acid filler treatments. J Cosmet Dermatol. 2018;17(6):1019–24. https://doi.org/10.1111/jocd.12726.
14. Romana Grippaudo F, Mattei M. The utility of high-frequency ultrasound in dermal filler evaluation. Ann Plast Surg. 2011;67(5):469–73. https://doi.org/10.1097/SAP.0b013e318203ebf6.
15. Micheels P, Besse S, Flynn TC, Sarazin D, Elbaz Y. Superficial dermal injection of hyaluronic acid soft tissue fillers: comparative ultrasound study: fillers. Dermatol Surg. 2012;38(7):1162–9.

Intense Pulse Light Technologies for Aesthetic Procedures and Beyond

3

Michelle P. Zappas

Abstract

LASER stands for light amplification by stimulated emission of radiation. Lasers interact with the skin in different ways: via reflection, absorption, scattering, or transmission of energy. Dispersion of photons occurs when the light from the laser is absorbed by the tissue. Intense Pulse Light (IPL) technology works by transmitting the energy to the chromophores; the absorption of energy generates heat and destroys the target by thermocoagulation (Raulin et al., Lasers Surg Med. 32:78–87, 2003). The main chromophores are hemoglobin, melanin, and water. These biomolecules are responsible for many of the pigment and vascular changes that are treated with IPL. This chapter explores the usefulness of IPL treatment regarding its non-invasive healing of many aesthetic dermatologic conditions.

Keywords

Intense pulse light · Rosacea · Acne · Malignant lesions · Skin rejuvenation · Aesthetic

M. P. Zappas (✉)
University of Southern California, Los Angeles, CA, USA
e-mail: zappas@usc.edu

3.1 Introduction to IPL Technology

There are a variety of lasers usually named by the lasing medium [1]. Different lasers are used to treat different skin conditions as determined by the wavelength and energy output. For example, the carbon dioxide (CO_2) and erbium:yttrium-aluminum garnet (Er:YAG) are often used in skin resurfacing; however, down time is often an issue [1]. IPL is often used to treat vascular and pigment changes. Table 3.1 details different examples of laser types, wavelengths, and clinical uses (adapted with permission from Haney [1]) (Fig. 3.1).

The majority of IPL have settings that can be adjusted to treat specific conditions [2]. The pulse duration, energy fluence, and wavelengths are adjusted by the clinician depending on the patient's skin type and condition to be treated. Wavelengths between 400 and 1000 nm are absorbed by chromophores [3]. The IPL device incorporates various cutoff filters; the filter cuts off the lower wavelengths, and the emitted light with the longer wavelengths is used to pass to the treated area [3]. As an example, the 560 nm filter will emit wavelengths longer than 560 nm and works to target more shallow lesions (see Fig. 3.2).

Patient selection is fundamental to the IPL consultation. It ensures the efficacy and safety of treatment. The Fitzpatrick Skin Type Classification

R. L. Bard (ed.), *Image-Guided Aesthetic Treatments*, https://doi.org/10.1007/978-3-031-36266-8_3

system was originally developed by physician Thomas Fitzpatrick in the 1970s. At first, Dr. Fitzpatrick differentiated four types to determine the tendency of an individual to burn or tan when exposed to the sun. The lower the Fitzpatrick score, the more likely the patient is to experience a burn. The classification system is as follows: skin phototype I is an individual who burns easily and does not tan at all; skin phototype II burns easily and tans with difficulty (often red haired, freckled individuals), and phototype III burns

Table 3.1 Differences between laser types used in aesthetics

Laser type	Wavelength	Clinical use
Pulsed dye	577–695	Vascular, pigment
Ruby	694 nm	Pigment, hair reduction
Alexandrite	755 nm	Hair reduction, pigment, tattoo removal
Diode	800 nm	Hair reduction
Neodymium (Nd): YAG	1064 nm, 1320 m	Hair reduction, non-ablative skin resurfacing
Erbium (Er): glass	1540–1550 nm	Non-ablative skin resurfacing
Er: YAG	2940 nm	Skin resurfacing
CO_2	10,600 nm	Skin resurfacing, tissue cutting, coagulation, vaporization

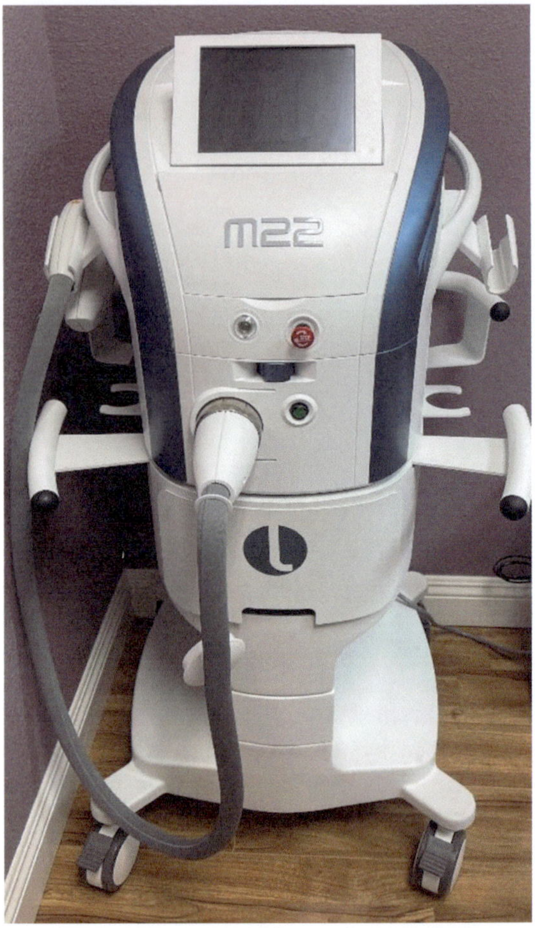

Fig. 3.1 Example of an intense pulsed light (IPL) device

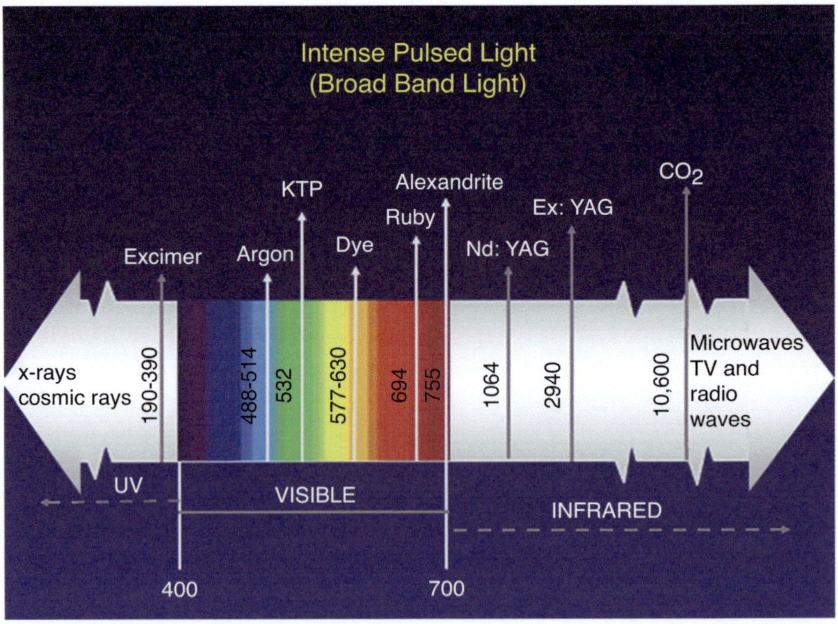

Fig. 3.2 IPL spectrum. (Reprinted with per mission from DiBernardo and Pozner [4])

moderately, shows immediate pigment darkening reactions, and tans moderately after 60 min of sun [5]. In 1988, the classification system is expanded to types V and VI [5]. In the United States, the most common Fitzpatrick types are 1–III; 48% of the population can be classified as type III, and types I and II make up 35% of the population [6]. Initially, category VI was made for patients with black skin. Patients with mixed races fit into the category range from IV to VI.

This classification system is subjective in nature but can be useful in the diagnosis and management of skin conditions. IPL generally works best on patients with Fitzpatrick scores between I and III. Individuals with higher Fitzpatrick scores tend to need longer pulse durations, higher wavelength filters, and decreased energy fluence to ensure safe conditions.

3.2 Treatment Procedure

Before IPL, patients should sign a treatment and photograph consent as well as a post care instruction form. As part of the informed consent, patients should be made aware of the alternatives to treatment, including topical agents, laser resurfacing, and chemical peels. The ability for the patient to comply with sun avoidance before, after, and in between treatments and to complete the series should be discussed.

Imaging can be a powerful tool in the treatment of the patient with IPL. Patients should first be cleansed of all facial cosmetics and placed in a supine position. At least three photographs should be taken, one head on and each profile. It is important to get all sides/angles of the face when treating with IPL because for many patients the dyschromia is on the cheeks or side of face. Oftentimes, the most significant photodamage is on the left cheek because of exposure to ultraviolet (UV) radiation while driving. These photographs can be used in the consultation with the patient to ensure that the clinician and patient are in agreement with regard to treatment expectations.

A topical anesthetic may be used to ensure patient comfort. Once that is washed off, eye protection should be placed on the patient, the clinician, and everyone else in the room. A clear, cooling gel is placed on the treatment area. A test spot with one or two pulses in the treatment area should be performed, and the skin reaction should be observed. Parameters can be adjusted when necessary. Usually, three to five treatments spaced 4 weeks apart are recommended to achieve the best clinical results.

3.3 Vascular Lesions

Vascular malformations can be treated with IPL. Because of its ability to target vascular structures, IPL has been used regularly in the treatment of hemangiomas, vascular malformations, and telangiectasias. The pulse light is absorbed by hemoglobin within the blood vessels. A positive clinical endpoint that is seen immediately after the treatment is a dark blue to gray discoloration of the vascularity.

3.3.1 Port Wine Stains

Port wine stains (PWS) are cutaneous vascular malformations which appear as pink, red, violaceous dermal patches [7]. Three in 1000 children are born with PWS; all racial groups and genders are equally affected [7]. Most malformations occur on the face, particularly along the trigeminal nerve and neck. PWS is associated with Sturge-Weber syndrome (SWS), Klippel-Trenaunay syndrome, Cobb syndrome, and Proteus [7]. Although PWS are often benign, complications such as nodules, bleeding, granulomas, and tissue hypertrophy can occur. Treatment modalities such as cryotherapy, electrocautery, and excision can lead to unnecessary scarring and should be avoided. IPL has shown to be effective in the treatment of PWS improving the physical and psychological manifestations. A split face comparison study showed significant improvement of PWS with IPL [8]. Improvement was additionally noted in PWS resistant to treatment [9]. A larger retrospective analysis found 70% of patients achieved 70–100% reduction in PWS after 1 and 4 treatments [10]. Ho et al. found 90% of patients achieved 25% clearance, 50% achieved 25–50%, 40% greater than 50%, and 9% greater than 75% clearance [11].

3.3.2 Telangiectasias and Poikiloderma

Telangiectasias are widened venules, approximately 0.1 to −1 mm in diameter, that form thin red or blue lines and fine web-like clusters on the skin. They may occur independently but are often associated with connective tissue disease, liver disease, rosacea, aging, varicose veins, sun exposure, and the overuse of steroid creams. Progressive disseminated telangiectasias is a rare skin condition characterized by a gradual dispersal of superficial telangiectasias progressing to widespread erythema [12]. Telangiectasias do not need to be treated but can be cosmetically distressing.

Poikiloderma or erythrosis interfollicularis colli is a common skin in middle-aged patients caused by UV exposure [12] and cosmetics. Erythema, telangiectasias, and dyschromia usually occur on the neck and chest and are sometimes accompanied by increased sensitivity. Pulsed dye lasers are most effective, but telangiectasias are also responsive to YAG and IPL. In a large study of 1000 patients with telangiectasias, 89.7% experience 75–100% improvement [13].

In a study looking at IPL in the treatment for these vascular lesions, patients with poikiloderma received 2.8 treatments [12]. These patients showed excellent results with a 76–90% improvement in symptoms [12]. Two open-labeled uncontrolled studies and retrospective study IPL treatment in 334 patients with poikiloderma of Civatte resulted in good to excellent reduction in vascular pigmentation in atrophic skin changes in 81–82% of patients after 3–5 sessions [14, 15] (see Fig. 3.3).

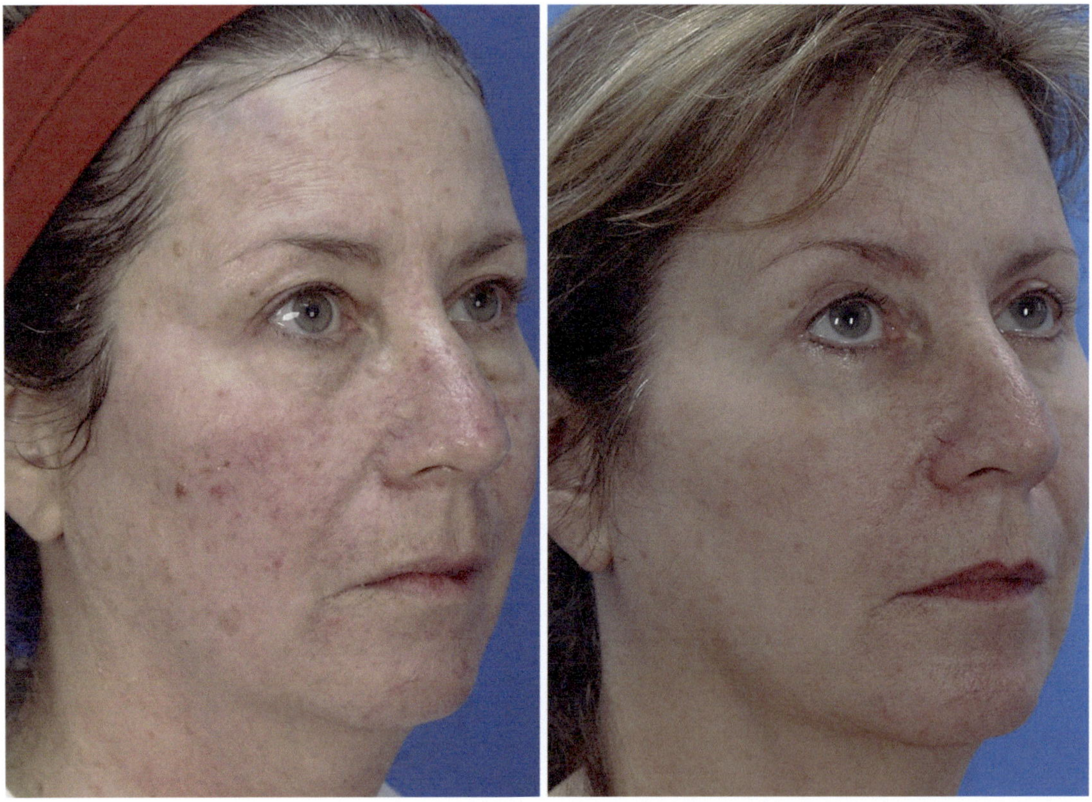

Fig. 3.3 Before and after facial vasculature treatment with IPL. (Reprinted with permission from DiBernardo and Pozner [4])

3.3.3 Rosacea

Rosacea is a chronic, inflammatory disorder with cutaneous and ocular manifestations characterized by erythema, telangiectasias, papules, and pustules. Overtime, phymas and rhinophyma can develop. The pathogenesis of rosacea is not well understood and thought to be multifactorial secondary to UV radiation, reactive oxygen species, vascular hyperreactivity, neuropeptides, and exacerbation of immune response [16]. Microbes, such as *H. pylori* and demodex mites, also play a role [16]. Women and young adults seem to be affected by this disease; triggers include sun exposure and alcohol. Avoidance of environmental triggers is the first step in relieving symptoms. Patients with type I rosacea have erythematous macules due to dilated capillaries and inflammation on the nose and cheeks [17]. Transient flushing and erythema can progress to chronic, persistent erythema in type II. In type III, hyperplasia of the sebaceous glands on the nose results in rhinophyma [17]. Ocular rosacea occurs in more than 50% of cases, resulting in meibomian gland dysfunction (MGD) and related dryness, irritation, and conjunctivitis [17]. This can also be treated with IPL as discussed later.

Topical brimonidine, topical oxymetazoline, azelaic acid, and metronidazole are modalities often used to treat mild to moderate rosacea. Systemic agents such as oral tetracyclines and oral isotretinoin can be used for moderate to severe disease. IPL also plays a role in the management of rosacea. A study conducted on 227 patients with rosacea, treated with 540 nm wavelength, resulted in significant improvement in the erythema and telangiectasias compared to control groups [18]. These patients were followed over 2 years and showed a reduction in recurrence of symptoms. Similar studies with varying patient sizes showed the same beneficial response [19–22]. Combination of IPL with radiofrequency may improve results.

3.3.4 Hemangiomas

Hemangiomas are benign tumors of the endothelium mainly occurring on the face, neck, or upper chest [23]. They may be superficial, deep, or mixed. Hemangiomas are often not present at birth but rapidly grow within the first year of life. Many begin to resolve spontaneously after the first year, but others require intervention for cosmetic reasons. Oral propranolol is first-line therapy for large lesions at risk of scarring or disfigurement [24]. IPL is better in small, superficial, or ulcerated lesions [24]. IPL has shown a clinical improvement with 75% to 100% clearance of hemangiomas in 61.29% of the patients [23]. Approximately 21% of patients had between 50% and 74% clearance [23]. Eighteen percent had only a slight improvement 25% to 49% in symptoms [23]. With all these treatments, there were minimal side effects and no scarring [23].

3.4 Acne

Acne is the result of hyperactive sebaceous glands, follicle obstruction, follicular hyperkeratinization, and *Propionibacterium acnes* (*P. acnes*) colonization. It can manifest as with open and closed comedones as well as papules and pustules. Noninflammatory acne includes comedones and responds well to over-the-counter treatments, such as salicylic acid and benzoyl peroxide. Erythematous papules, pustules, nodules, and cysts characterize inflammatory acne [25] and *P. acnes* colonization plays a prominent role. Although clearly not life threatening, acne can cause severe psychological distress and even suicidal ideation [26]. Mild to moderate acne is often treated with topical agents, such as retinoids, benzoyl peroxide, and antibiotics. Moderate to severe lesions often require systemic therapies such as oral isotretinoin, antibiotics, hormonal contraceptives, and spironolactone.

Multiple studies have shown improvement of acne with IPL [27–30]. There is conflicting evidence as to whether inflammatory vs non inflammatory lesions respond best. Chang [27] conducted a split face, open label, prospective trial of 30 women with mild to moderate acne. IPL resulted in improvement of dyschromia and skin tone but did not improve inflammatory lesions [27]. Sami reported 90% clearance of inflammatory acne lesions with four to eight sessions of IPL [30]. IPL efficacy ranged from 34 to 88.3% improvement depending on the type of acne lesions (inflammatory vs. non-inflammatory); more commonly, it fell between 40 and 60% [2].

The results in treatment of acne are more efficacious when IPL is combined with photodynamic therapy (PDT). IPL is used as an activator of aminolevulinic acid HCl (ALA) and results in significant improvement of moderate to severe facial acne. At 12 weeks, there was a 75% to 85% improvement in the ALA-PDT group versus 50%–60% improvement in the IPL alone group [31]. More commonly efficacy ranged between 60% and 80% [2]. IPL can be considered a safe and effective option for acne vulgaris, especially in patients intolerant of or resistant to oral retinoids and antibiotics.

3.5 Premalignant and Malignant Lesions

Actinic keratosis (AK) are cutaneous lesions resulting from the proliferation of atypical epidermal keratinocytes. They are manifested by erythematous scaling, macules, papules, and plaques found in sun-exposed areas [32]. AKs are precancerous, early lesions on the continuum of squamous cell carcinoma (SCC) to basal cell carcinoma (BCC), and therefore, most providers treat them [32]. First-line treatment is topical fluorouracil, imiquimod, and the photosensitizing agents in PDT. PDT plays a prominent role in the treatment of precancerous and cancerous lesions. Laser-assisted PDT increases its efficacy. IPL seems to be an effective treatment of AKs, but results are enhanced when combined with ALA- or methyl aminolevulinate (MAL)-PDT. Four studies [33–36] resulted in a 50%–91% resolution of AKs. Avram and Goldman [33] showed that 68% of the AKs resolved after one treatment with ALA-PDT [33]. Another study from 2005 showed that 42% of AKs resolved with one treatment [37]. Follow-up and longitudinal studies are needed to confirm complete remission.

There are limited, small studies looking at the use of PDT for other malignant lesions. There is evidence that PDT may also be safe and effective for BCC, SCC, and AKs, as well as Bowen's. One study examined use of MAL-PDT in patients with AKs, BCC, and Bowen's disease [34]. After two treatments, the (ten) patients with BCC and (nine) with Bowen's had complete resolution of their lesions [34]. In the treatment of melanoma, however, the conclusions are not as straightforward. There is potential for lasers to increase cell proliferation, and treatment of melanoma with IPL could worsen the lesion [38]. In general, any raised lesion suspected of melanoma should not be treated with IPL.

3.6 Photoaging and Skin Rejuvenation

IPL is the fifth most common aesthetics procedure, behind Botox, soft tissue fillers, laser skin resurfacing, and chemical peels [39]. Dyschromia and skin rejuvenation are common reasons for treatment with IPL resulting in an improvement in texture, fine lines, vascularity, and pigmentation [40–43].

3.6.1 Lentiginous Disorders

Many patients, particularly older patients, with fair skin or those who have spent a lot of time in the sun will develop solar lentigos. Nine studies with an aggregate of 199 patients were reviewed documenting the use of IPL for the treatment of solar lentigines. All studies reported improved efficacy in treatment of solar lentigines and ephelides on the face and bodies after an average of 3 to 5 treatments [44–51]. Micro-crusting is often seen after treatment of pigmented lesions, histological analysis of these crusts reveals they are composed of melanin [46]. The crusting and sloughing leads to less melanin in basal layer of the dermis and subsequent resolution of lentigines [46]. A high quality randomized observer blinded split face comparison study of 32 women (17 with ephelides and 15 with solar lentigines) compared IPL with

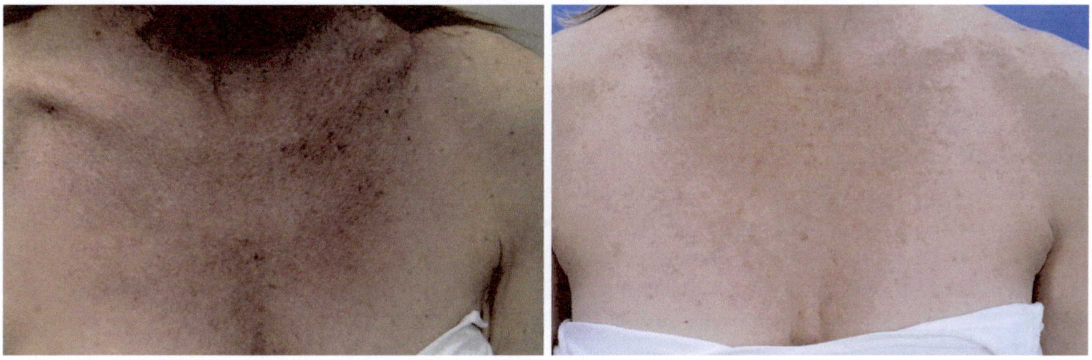

Fig. 3.4 Before and after three IPL treatments of decollete. (Reprinted with permission from DiBernardo and Pozner [4]

another established treatment option of lentigines: quality switched alexandrite laser (QSAL) [52]. This study showed significant improvement in lentigines (see Fig. 3.4). Post-inflammatory hyperpigmentation (PIH) occurred in eight patients with ephelides and one with lentigines on QSAL site, but not the IPL. IPL is effective and safe in patients when compared to QSAL—particularly in Asian patients due to the tendency toward PIH in this patient population [52].

3.6.2 Melasma

Melasma can be a frustrating, chronic, recurring condition affecting women. It is often called the "mask of pregnancy" and leads to brown gray macules coalescing into patches on the face. An increase in melanin biosynthesis underlies all hyperpigmentation. When triggered by UV exposure, this often spontaneously resolves. The pathogenesis of melasma is more complicated. There seems to be a genetic predisposition, in addition to hormones, heat, and sun exposure. There is downregulation of the H19 gene in patients with melasma inducing tyrosinase expression resulting in increased melanin synthesis [53]. Estrogen results in an additional tyrosinase overexpression [53]. Hyper-functional melanocytes deposit excess melanin in the epidermis and dermis [54].

Melasma is challenging to treat. First-line treatment is topical bleaching agents, such as hydroquinone 4%, and sun protection. Other skin bleaching agents such as azelaic acid, kojic acid, and niacinamide can be used as alternative or in combination. In moderate to severe melasma, triple therapy (fluocinolone acetonide 0.01%, hydroquinone 4%, tretinoin 0.05%) can be used. IPL also has good efficacy. Seven studies showed moderate efficacy of IPL in the treatment of refractory or recurrent melasma. Wang and colleagues conducted a randomized controlled trial (RCT) IPL showing significant improvement when compared to standard of care which is topical hydroquinone and sunscreen [55]. The group treated with IPL had a 39.8% improvement compared to 11.6% in the control group, but these results were only partially maintained at 24 weeks. Another RCT showed an improvement in IPL compared to triple combination treatment and sunscreen [56]. The IPL groups had a reduction in symptoms from 17.6% to 9.7% which was significantly superior to control group [56]. In patients who have not shown improvement in other modalities, IPL at low energy/joules may be an option.

3.7 Meibomian Gland Dysfunction

More recently, IPL therapy has expanded from dermatologic conditions. As previously mentioned, patients with rosacea often have meibomian gland dysfunction (MGD). Sixteen million Americans have been diagnosed with dry eye disease [57]; however, many more are likely afflicted with symptoms. The meibomian glands are located in the upper and lower eyelids and secrete an oily substance, meibum, which helps lubricate the eye. MGD occurs when these glands become obstructed, resulting in tear film abnormalities [58]. Symptoms associated with this condition are dryness, grittiness, irritation, burning, watering, soreness, and eye fatigue [58].

The effect of IPL on MGD was discovered accidentally. Patients with rosacea were treated with IPL and noticed a reduction in the MGD, dry eye symptoms [58]. IPL is thought to work by causing thrombosis of the telangiectatic blood vessels in the eyelids, reducing demodex eyelid infestation and increasing the temperature of meibum [58]. This results in an augmentation of the structure of the meibomian glands and the fluid from a semi-solid to liquid state [58]. A randomized, double-masked placebo-controlled trial notes significant improvement in MGD after three sessions [59]. IPL combined with meibomian gland expression also significantly improved dry eye symptomatology and safely and effectively treated MGD [60]. There is minimal data on this topic, but IPL may be useful in the treatment of MGD.

3.8 Safety, Risks, and Contraindications

Complications of IPL are relatively rare and include hypo-, hyperpigmentation, burning, and checkerboard mottling. Hyperpigmentation is often resolved with avoidance of sun and topical regimens. Checkerboard patterns can be treated with additional treatment topical skin care and sun protection/avoidance. Burns usually occur when wrong filters, energies, or pulse durations are used. Patient selection can also play a role, high Fitzpatrick scores, and tanning, including self-tanner. Post treatment cooling with towels, burn gels, and topical antibiotics can help prevent and treat the burns. Hypopigmentation may occur after treatment, particularly after a burn. Hypopigmentation is more difficult to treat, and complete resolution may not occur.

3.9 Monitoring Treatment Progression with Images

Consistent before and after photos are a critical part of any aesthetics treatment, especially IPL. Pre-consultation, post treatment, and long-term patient management are invaluable assets to help ensure an accurate detailed record of the patients' treatment history. Pre-existing issues that may affect treatment need to be documented and discussed with the patient. Providers struggle with reproducibility when it comes to before and after photos. Using a consistent background, lighting and position can help. Side by side before and after photos allow you and the patient to view their transformation. Images can help reassure the patient and allow them to view improvements in a clear manner.

3.10 Conclusions

IPL is a useful treatment modality to treat a wide range of dermatologic conditions. It is non-invasive and effective in treating many aesthetic conditions. With the proper settings, pre-, and post-treatment instructions, IPL offers a high rate of patient satisfaction with few side effects or adverse events.

References

1. Haney B. Aesthetic procedures: nurse practitioner's guide to cosmetic dermatology. Berlin: Springer; 2020. https://doi.org/10.1007/978-3-030-19948-7.
2. Wat H, Wu DC, Rao J, Goldman MP. Application of intense pulsed light in the treatment of dermatologic disease: a systematic review. Dermatol Surg. 2014;40(4):359–77. https://doi.org/10.1111/dsu.12424.
3. Raulin C, Greve B, Grema H. IPL technology: a review. Lasers Surg Med. 2003;32:78–87.
4. DiBernardo BE, Pozner JN. Intense pulsed light therapy for skin rejuvenation. Clin Plast Surg. 2016;43(3):535–40. https://doi.org/10.1016/j.cps.2016.03.008.
5. Fitzpatrick TB. The validity and practicality of sun-reactive skin types I through VI. Arch Dermatol. 1988;124(6):869–71.

6. Keiser E, Linos E, Kanzler M, Lee W, Sainani KL, Tang JY. Reliability and prevalence of digital image skin types in the United States: results from National Health and Nutrition Examination Survey 2003-2004. J Am Acad Dermatol. 2012;66(1):163–5.
7. Ortiz AE, Nelson JS. Port-wine stain laser treatments and novel approaches. Facial Plast Surg. 2012;28:611–20.
8. Babilas P, Schreml S, Eames T, Hohenleutner U, Szeimies RM, Landthaler M. Split-face comparison of intense pulsed light with short- and long-pulsed dye lasers for the treatment of port-wine stains. Lasers Surg Med. 2010;42:720–7.
9. Bjerring P, Christiansen K, Troilius A. Intense pulsed light source for the treatment of dye laser resistant port-wine stains. J Cosmet Laser Ther. 2003;5:7–13.
10. Raulin C, Schroeter CA, Weiss RA, Keiner M, et al. Treatment of port-wine stains with a noncoherent pulsed light source. A retrospective study. Arch Dermatol. 1999;135:679–83.
11. Ho WS, Ying SY, Chan PC, Chan HHL, et al. Treatment of port wine stains with intense pulsed light: a prospective study. Dermatol Surg. 2004;30:887–91.
12. Wenzel SM, Hohenleuter U, Landthaler M. Progressive disseminated essential telangiectasia and erythrosis interfollicularis colli as examples for successful treatment with a high intensity flashlamp. Dermatology. 2008;217:286–90. https://doi-org.libproxy1.usc.edu/10.1159/000151273.
13. Clementoni MT, Gilardino P, Muti GF, Signorini M, et al. Intense pulsed light treatment of 1,000 consecutive patients with facial vascular marks. Aesthet Plast Surg. 2006;30:226–32.
14. Rusciani A, Motta A, Fino P, Menichini G. Treatment of poikiloderma of civatte using intense pulsed light source: 7 years of experience. Dermatol Surg. 2008;34:314–9.
15. Weiss RA, Goldman MP, Weiss MA. Treatment of poikiloderma of civatte with an intense pulsed light source. Dermatol Surg. 2000;26:823–8.
16. McAleer MA, Fitzpatrick P, Powell FC. Papulopustular rosacea: prevalence and relationship to photodamage. J Am Acad Dermatol. 2010;63:33.
17. Anzengruber F, Czernielewski J, Conrad C, et al. Swiss S1 guideline for the treatment of rosacea. J Eur Acad Dermatol Venereol. 2017;31(11):1775–91. https://doi.org/10.1111/jdv.14349.
18. Luan X, Zhang J, Wu L, Zhou N. Improved telangiectasia and reduced recurrence rate of rosacea after treatment with 540 nm-wavelength intense pulsed light: a prospective randomized controlled trial with a 2-year follow-up. Exp Ther Med. 2020;19(6):3543. http://libproxy.usc.edu/login?url=https://www-proquest-com.libproxy1.usc.edu/scholarly-journals/improved-telangiectasia-reduced-recurrence-rate/docview/2399083439/se-2?accountid=14749.
19. Schroeter CA, Haaf-von Below S, Neumann HA. Effective treatment of rosacea using intense pulse light system. Dermatol Surg. 2005;31:1285–9.
20. Papageorgiou P, Clayton W, Norwood S, Chopra S, Rustin M. Treatment of rosacea with intense pulsed light: significant improvement and long-lasting results. Br J Dermatol. 2008;159:628–32.
21. Mark KA, Sparacio RM, Voigt A, Marenus K, Sarnoff DS. Objective and quantitative improvement of rosacea-associated erythema after intense pulsed light treatment. Dermatol Surg. 2003;29:600–4.
22. Liu J, Liu J, Ren Y, Li B, Lu S. Comparative efficacy of intense pulsed light for different erythema associated with rosacea. J Cosmet Laser Ther. 2014;16:324–7.
23. Li DN, Gold MH, Sun ZS, Tang AR, Wang HB, Sheng-Kang L. Treatment of infantile hemangioma with optimal pulse technology. J Cosmet Laser Ther. 2010;12(3):145–50. https://doi.org/10.3109/14764172.2010.487908.
24. Krowchuk DP, Frieden IJ, Mancini AJ, et al. Clinical practice guideline for the management of infantile hemangiomas. Pediatrics. 2019;143:e20183475.
25. Lu L, Shi M, Chen Z. Efficacy of IPL therapy for the treatment of acne vulgaris: a meta-analysis. J Cosmet Dermatol. 2020;19:2596–605.
26. Halvorsen JA, Stern RS, Dalgard F, Thoresen M, Bjertness E, Lien L. Suicidal ideation, mental health problems, and social impairment are increased in adolescents with acne: a population-based study. J Investig Dermatol. 2011;131(2):363–70.
27. Chang SE, Ahn SJ, Rhee DY, Choi JH, et al. Treatment of facial acne papules and pustules in Korean patients using an intense pulsed light device equipped with a 530- to 750-nm filter. Dermatol Surg. 2007;33:676–9.
28. Kawana S, Tachihara R, Kato T, Omi T. Effect of smooth pulsed light at 400 to 700 and 870 to 1,200 nm for acne vulgaris in Asian skin. Dermatol Surg. 2010;36:52–7.
29. Choi YS, Suh HS, Yoon MY, Min SU, et al. Intense pulsed light vs. pulsed-dye laser in the treatment of facial acne: a randomized split-face trial. J Eur Acad Dermatol Venereol. 2010;24:773–80.
30. Sami NA, Attia AT, Badawi AM. Phototherapy in the treatment of acne vulgaris. J Drugs Dermatol. 2008;7:627–32.
31. Mei X, Shi W, Piao Y. Effectiveness of photodynamic therapy with topical 5-aminolevulinic acid and intense pulsed light in Chinese acne vulgaris patients. Photodermatol Photoimmunol Photomed. 2013;29:90–6.
32. Criscione VD, Weinstock MA, Naylor MF, Luque C, Eide MJ, Bingham SF, Department of Veteran Affairs Topical Tretinoin Chemoprevention Trial Group. Actinic keratoses: natural history and risk of malignant transformation in the veterans affairs topical treinoin chemoprevention trial. Cancer. 2009;115(11):2523.
33. Avram DK, Goldman MP. Effectiveness and safety of ALA-IPL in treating actinic keratoses and photodamage. J Drugs Dermatol. 2004;3(1 Suppl):S36–9.
34. Downs AMR, Bower CB, Oliver DA, Stone CA. Methyl aminolaevulinate-photodynamic therapy for actinic keratoses, squamous cell carcinoma in

situ and superficial basal cell carcinoma employing a square wave intense pulsed light device for photoactivation. Br J Dermatol. 2009;161:189–90.
35. Haddad A, Santos ID, Gragnani A, Ferreira LM. The effect of increasing fluence on the treatment of actinic keratosis and photodamage by photodynamic therapy with 5-aminolevulinic acid and intense pulsed light. Photomed Laser Surg. 2011;29:427–32.
36. Kim HS, Yoo JY, Cho KH, Kwon OS, et al. Topical photodynamic therapy using intense pulsed light for treatment of actinic keratosis: clinical and histopathologic evaluation. Dermatol Surg. 2005;31:33–6; discussion 36–37.
37. Willey A, Anderson RR, Azpiazu JL, Bakus AD, Barlow RJ, Dover JS, Garden JM, Kilmer SL, Landa N, Manstein D, Ross EV Jr, Sadick N, Tanghetti EA, Yaghmai D, Zelickson BD. Complications of laser dermatologic surgery. Lasers Surg Med. 2006;38:1–15.
38. Ash C, Town G, Whittall R, Tooze L, Phillips J. Lasers and intense pulsed light (IPL) association with cancerous lesions. Lasers Med Sci. 2017;32(8):1927–33. https://doi.org/10.1007/s10103-017-2310-y.
39. American Society of Plastic Surgeons. Plastic surgery statistics report. https://www.plasticsurgery.org/documents/News/Statistics/2020/plastic-surgery-statistics-full-report-2020.pdf. Accessed 2 Aug 2021.
40. Bitter PH. Noninvasive rejuvenation of photodamaged skin using serial, full-face intense pulsed light treatments. Dermatol Surg. 2000;26:835–42.
41. Kligman DE, Zhen Y. Intense pulsed light treatment of photoaged facial skin. Dermatol Surg. 2004;30(8):1085–90.
42. Sadick NS, Weiss R, Kilmer S, et al. Photorejuvenation with intense pulsed light: results of a multicenter study. J Drugs Dermatol. 2004;3:41–9.
43. Weiss RA, Weiss MA, Beasley KL. Rejuvenation of photoaged skin: 5 years results with intense pulsed light of the face, neck, and chest. Dermatol Surg. 2002;28:1115–9.
44. Bjerring P, Christiansen K. Intense pulsed light source for treatment of small melanocytic nevi and solar lentigines. J Cutan Laser Ther. 2000;2:177–81.
45. Kawada A, Asai M, Kameyama H, Sangen Y, et al. Videomicroscopic and histopathological investigation of intense pulsed light therapy for solar lentigines. J Dermatol Sci. 2002;29:91–6.
46. Kawada A, Shiraishi H, Asai M, Kameyama H, et al. Clinical improvement of solar lentigines and ephelides with an intense pulsed light source. Dermatol Surg. 2002;28:504–8.
47. Kent Remington B, Remington TK. Treatment of facial lentigines in Peutz-Jeghers syndrome with an intense pulsed light source. Dermatol Surg. 2002;28:1079–81.
48. Kontoes PP, Vlachos SP, Marayiannis KV. Intense pulsed light for the treatment of lentigines in LEOPARD syndrome. Br J Plast Surg. 2003;56:607–10.
49. Kawana S, Ochiai H, Tachihara R. Objective evaluation of the effect of intense pulsed light on rosacea and solar lentigines by spectrophotometric analysis of skin color. Dermatol Surg. 2007;33:449–54.
50. Konishi N, Kawada A, Kawara S, Oiso N, et al. Clinical effectiveness of a novel intense pulsed light source on facial pigmentary lesions. Arch Dermatol Res. 2008;300(Suppl 1):S65–7.
51. Sasaya H, Kawada A, Wada T, Hirao A, et al. Clinical effectiveness of intense pulsed light therapy for solar lentigines of the hands. Dermatol Ther. 2011;24:584–6.
52. Wang CC, Sue YM, Yang CH, Chen CK. A comparison of Q-switched alexandrite laser and intense pulsed light for the treatment of freckles and lentigines in Asian persons: a randomized, physician-blinded, split-face comparative trial. J Am Acad Dermatol. 2006;54:804–10.
53. Kim NH, Lee CH, Lee AY. H19 RNA downregulation stimulated melanogenesis in melasma. Pigment Cell Melanoma Res. 2010;23(1):84.
54. Grimes PE, Yamada N, Bhawan J. Light microscopic, immunohistochemical, and ultrastructural alterations in patients with melasma. Am J Dermatopathol. 2005;27(2):96.
55. Wang CC, Hui CY, Sue YM, Wong WR, et al. Intense pulsed light for the treatment of refractory melasma in Asian persons. Dermatol Surg. 2004;30:1196–200.
56. Figueiredo Souza L, Trancoso Souza S. Single-session intense pulsed light combined with stable fixed-dose triple combination topical therapy for the treatment of refractory melasma. Dermatol Ther. 2012;25:477–80.
57. Farrand KF, Fridman M, Stillman IO, Schaumberg DA. Prevalence of diagnosed dry eye disease in the United States among adults aged 18 years and older. Am J Ophthalmol. 2017;182:90–8.
58. Cote S, Zhang A, Ahmadzai V, Maleken A, Li C, Oppedisano J, Nair K, Busija L, Downie LE. Intense pulsed light (IPL) therapy for the treatment of meibomian gland dysfunction. Cochrane Database Syst Rev. 2020;(3):CD013559. https://doi.org/10.1002/14651858.CD013559.
59. Craig JP, Chen YH, Trunbull PR. Cumulative effect of intense pulsed light (IPL) therapy for meibomian gland dysfunction (MGD) confirmed in prospective, double-masked, placebo controlled trial. Investig Ophthalmol Vis Sci. 2015;56(7):6194.
60. Rong B, Tang Y, Tu P, Liu R, Qiao J, Song W, et al. Intense pulsed light applied directly on eyelids combined with meibomian gland expression to treat meibomian gland dysfunction. Photomed Laser Surg. 2018;36(6):326–32. https://doi.org/10.1089/pho.2017.4402.

4 Facial Danger Zones in Aesthetics

Beth Haney and Michelle P. Zappas

Abstract

Dermal fillers are an integral part of aesthetic practice, but there are serious complications that can arise during the procedure, especially if the practitioner has little experience or familiarity with innate structures of the face such as glands, nerves, arteries, and veins. Imaging devices using infrared and ultrasound can identify these structures and guide placement of the filler or assist in surgical procedures. These devices are an invaluable tool that can be used in aesthetic procedures, but on occasion, immediate correction or emergency intervention might be warranted. A benefit of using hyaluronic acid (HA) dermal fillers is they can be easily dissolved when necessary, with hyaluronidase.

Keywords

Injectable facial fillers · Hyaluronic acid · Hyaluronidase · Silicone · MRI · PET-CT · Granuloma · Facial vessels · Ultrasound · Poly-L-lactic acid · Calcium hydroxyapatite

B. Haney · M. P. Zappas (✉)
Department of Nursing, USC Suzanne Dworak-Peck School of Social Work, Los Angeles, CA, USA
e-mail: bhaney@usc.edu; zappas@usc.edu

4.1 Introduction

Consideration of underlying facial structures, vascularity, and nerves is a crucial part of safely injecting temporary dermal fillers. Different areas are at increased risk for complications due to the underlying anatomical structures. The most severe complications of dermal fillers occur when it is inserted into or pressed against a vessel. This may result in occlusion of the vessel and subsequent ischemia, necrosis, or permanent vision loss. Blindness is a very rare yet debilitating consequence of facial fillers to the upper and lower face. This vision loss presents as ocular pain and reduced vision immediately after injection. It may be accompanied by ptosis, headache, dizziness, nausea, and an extraocular muscle palsy. Intravascular injection can be avoided with understanding of facial anatomy and proper injection technique.

On the face, four main vessels arise from the trunk of the facial artery: the inferior labial artery, superior labial artery, lateral nasal branch (to the nasalis), and the angular artery (Fig. 4.1) [1–3]. These vessels, along with the infraorbital artery, are crucial to avoid during aesthetic procedures because they feed vital structures of the eye, nose, and lips. Occlusion of these vessels can lead to skin necrosis, scarring, blindness, and potentially, in the remote chance, cerebral infarction [4]. Areas at risk of complications include

R. L. Bard (ed.), *Image-Guided Aesthetic Treatments*, https://doi.org/10.1007/978-3-031-36266-8_4

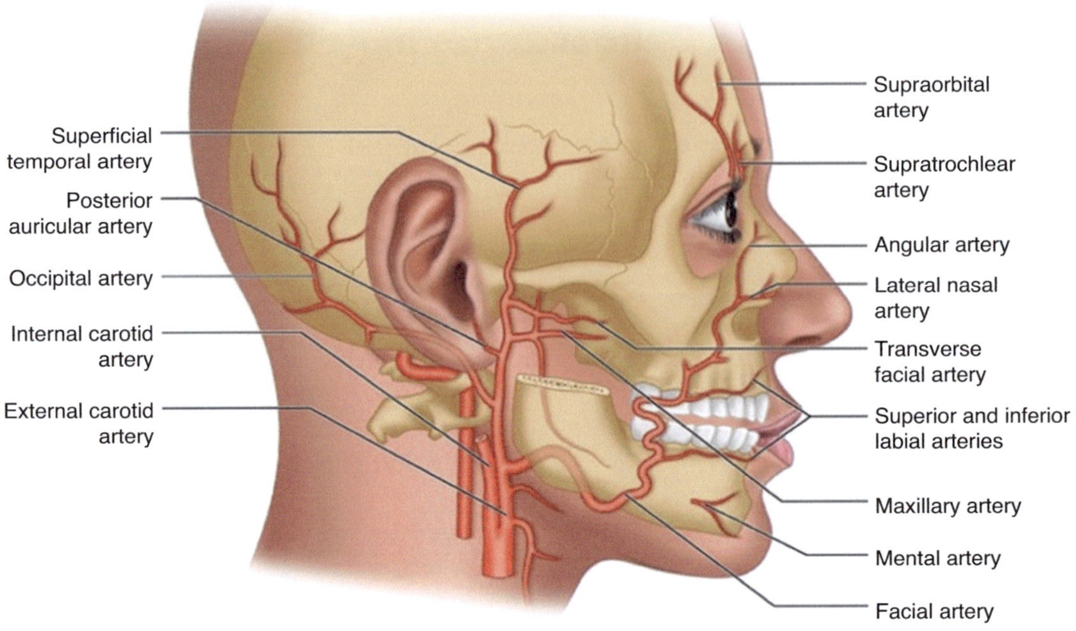

Fig. 4.1 Facial arteries pertinent to facial aesthetic procedures. (Adapted from Ferneini et al. 2021 [3])

virtually any area in the face that is treated with dermal fillers.

During aesthetic procedures, it is essential the facial arteries be avoided to prevent upstream effects related to blood supply. Portable, handheld infrared and/or ultrasound imaging devices can locate facial arteries and other important vessels of the face and are an option for potential prevention of complications.

Due to the wide variability in anatomy between individuals, imaging techniques can help deliver temporary dermal fillers in a safe manner. For example, duplex ultrasound has been used to identify single vessels when injecting in the glabellar, temporal, and nasolabial folds [5, 6]. This non-invasive technique can aid in the visualization and locate the depth of small facial arteries. The complex three-dimensional and variable structure of the vascular network in the face can be imaged with an MRI with a time of light three-dimensional camera. This technique allows for visualization of the facial arteries for safe injections in a contrast and radiation free manner [7]. The available technologies and appropriate imaging techniques are options that can be utilized prior to a procedure to help alleviate potential emergent situations.

4.2 Danger Zones of the Upper Face

4.2.1 Infraorbital Hollows

When injecting the infraorbital region, the major anatomical areas the injector should avoid are the trochlear vessels proximal to the nose and the infraorbital artery. The main branches of the infraorbital artery are the zygomaticofacial and nasal branches. The danger zone for injecting temporary dermal fillers to this area is medial to the pupil and lateral to the nasal wall (Fig. 4.2). Best practices are retromuscular, preorbital fat injections.

The lateral third of the zygomatic bone is also a danger zone. Retrograde embolization of filler into the internal carotid can lead to blindness and cerebral infarction (Fig. 4.2). In order to avoid this vasculature, small amounts of filler injected deep into the suborbicularis plane or at the supra-

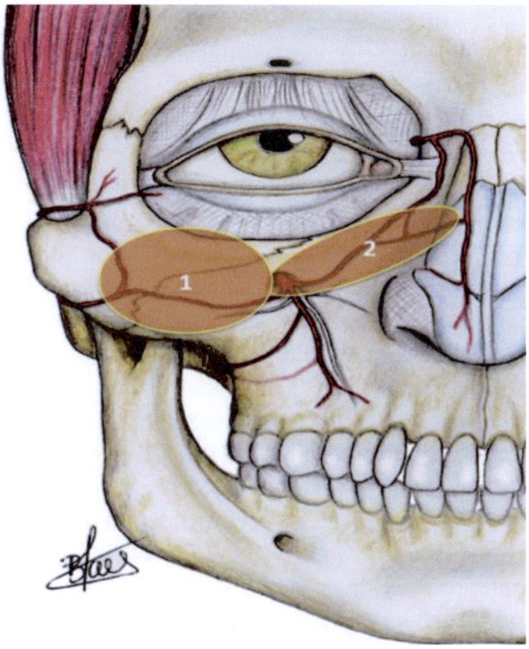

Fig. 4.2 Illustration of danger zones in the infraorbital area: marked area 1 shows involvement of the zygomatic malar branch with risk of skin necrosis through skin perforators, marked area 2 represents risk of arterial embolization into the internal carotid system through retrograde flow into the dorsal nasal or superficial temporal artery, before reaching the ophthalmic, retinal artery, or even cerebral arteries. (Printed with permission from Hufschmidt et al. 2018)

periosteal level with a serial puncture technique is often used [8]. Small boluses of 0.2 cc are injected and then physically pressed down. No more than 1 cc under each eye should be used in one visit in order to avoid occlusion or compression of the vascular supply. The patient can follow-up in 2 to 4 weeks for a touch-up if the desired cosmetic result is not reached with the initial dosing of the product.

The orbital vascular anatomy is multifaceted and highly variable. The ophthalmic artery branches into the lacrimal artery, supraorbital artery, supratrochlear artery, the anterior and posterior ethmoid artery, and nasal artery. The musculature and globe of the eye are supplied by the long ciliary artery, short ciliary artery, anterior artery, central retinal artery, and muscular artery. The blood to the retina is distributed by the central retinal artery and the short posterior ciliary arteries [9]. These arteries originate from the internal carotid artery and branches to the ophthalmic artery which supplies blood, nutrients, and oxygen to the orbit of the eyes, musculature, and eyelids. Tissue necrosis, loss of vision, and even cerebral infarction can occur if these vessels become occluded.

4.2.2 Glabella and Forehead

Caution should be used when injecting temporary facial fillers into the glabella and forehead as there is a risk for vessel puncture while traversing the supraorbital or supratrochlear artery with the needle [8]. These small vessels are at risk because they lack an additional blood supply. Skin necrosis is a possible complication as the result of vascular compromise to the area (Figs. 4.3, 4.4, 4.5, and 4.6). Vision loss can also occur. The risk is greater when deep injection of filler is used to augment the profile of the glabellar region and could result in an injection of filler into the ophthalmic artery or its branches [8]. In a study investigating the glabellar and central forehead, vasculature of cadavers and ultrasound examination of healthy volunteers showed that at the glabellar point, the horizontal distance from the midline to the central artery was 4.7 and 7.8 mm to the paracentral artery and 14.7 and 19.2 mm to the superficial and deep branches of the supra-

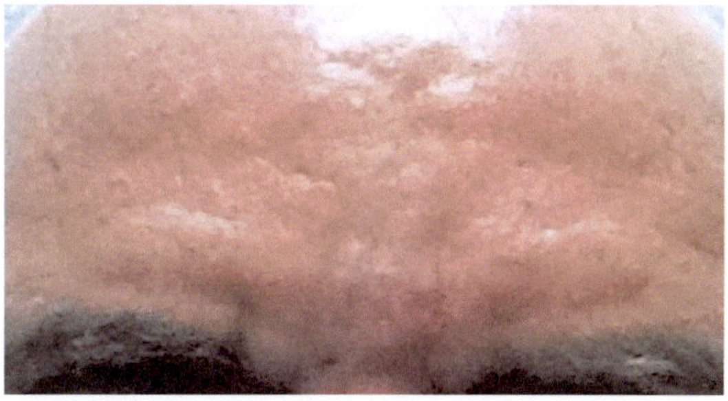

Fig. 4.3 Note the slight discoloration of the right side during the procedure. Pt was treated with 20 units of hyaluronidase and massage to the area. Pt was instructed to use warm packs 5 times a day, take 325 mg aspirin daily (no pre-existing conditions), and return to the clinic every day for follow-up. (Photo courtesy B. Haney, DNP, FNP-C, FAANP, FAAN)

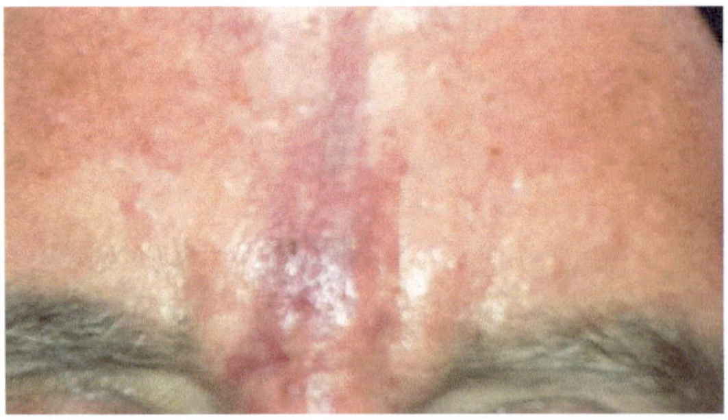

Fig. 4.4 Three days post-treatment of 20 units of hyaluronidase. (Photo courtesy B. Haney, DNP, FNP-C, FAANP, FAAN)

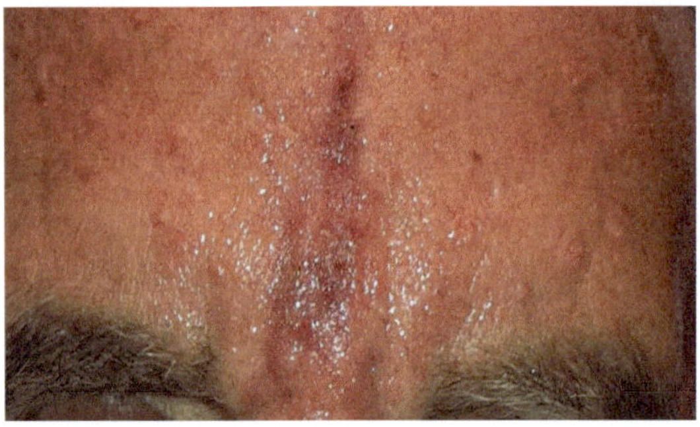

Fig. 4.5 Ten days after hyaluronidase treatment, daily follow-up, and home care by patient. (Photo courtesy B. Haney, DNP, FNP-C, FAANP, FAAN)

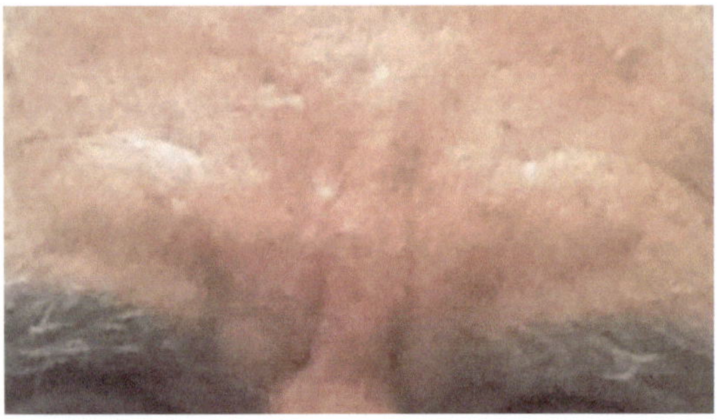

Fig. 4.6 One month after hyaluronidase treatment. After full recovery, the patient returned to the clinic 3 months later for a small amount of HA filler to the same area without any adverse events. (Photo courtesy B. Haney, DNP, FNP-C, FAANP, FAAN)

trochlear artery [10]. From the dermis to the arteries, the depth was between 3.1 and 5.9 mm for the central artery and deep branch of the supratrochlear artery, respectively [10]. Placement of filler subcutaneously or intradermal of the frontalis carries minimal risk of nerve damage since the supraorbital and supratrochlear nerves run in a deeper plane with the vessels running parallel to them [8]. Thus, a superficial, retrograde serial puncture technique is preferred to restore volume to the glabellar rhytids—commonly called the "elevens."

The forehead often has a convex profile appearance with a depression in the suprabrow area that can increase with age. This concavity occurs between the tuber-frontale and the supraciliary arches. The supraorbital nerve exits the supraorbital foramen via the supraorbital notch along the orbital rim and runs parallel to the supraorbital artery. This can be palpated and should be avoided by injecting laterally and 1 cm from the supraorbital foramen since a compression injury to the nerve could result. This injury can be avoided by injecting in a retrograde fashion and laterally at least 1 cm from the supraorbital foramen. Filler should be positioned deep in the supra-periosteal plane for patient safety [8].

4.2.3 Temples

Anatomically, the different layers of the temporal region range from superficial to deep and are the dermis, subcutaneous fat, superficial and deep temporal fascia, and temporal muscle [8]. Vessels run in different planes of these layers. As we age, the temporal region can lose its subcutaneous fat and become convex in appearance. This volume loss results in increased visibility of the temporal crest and lateral orbital rim and the upper zygomatic arch which can be corrected with dermal fillers. There is a higher rate of visual complications with injections here related to the close proximity to the orbit and vascular connections to the carotid artery [11]. The superficial temporal artery and the frontal branch of the cranial nerve (CN) VII nerve are the two major structures to be avoided when injecting the temples. The arrangement of the artery and nerve bundle is located within the superficial temporal fascia, a continuance of the galea aponeurotica scalp [8].

The temporal artery originates from the external carotid artery and branches near the parotid gland into the superficial temporal artery and maxillary artery. The superficial temporal artery's pulse can be felt above the zygomatic arch and in front of the tragus. It can be helpful to put your nondominant finger on this pulse while injecting the temples to ensure you are avoiding this area while depositing filler to this area. The supraorbital and supratrochlear arteries also supply this region, so filler in the ophthalmic artery can lead to a retinal artery occlusion resulting in vision loss [9].

The frontal branch of CN VII innervates the muscle of the forehead and brows. It is located deep in the superficial temporal fascia and is important to prevent brow ptosis [8]. The best way to locate this danger zone is to draw a line from the earlobe to lateral brow and the tragus to the highest forehead rhytid (Fig. 4.7) [8]. That area coincides with the course of the frontal branch.

A safe injection technique for this area positions product in the supra-periosteal plane that is the one up-one over technique. This access is 1 cm up from lateral supra-orbital tubercle and 1 cm over from the temporal crest (Fig. 4.8). The needle should be inserted perpendicularly to the skin surface until contact with the bone is made, aspiration should be performed, and then product slowly injected in a large bolus. The recommended amount is approximately 1.00 cc in each temple but can vary depending on the anatomy of the patient [11].

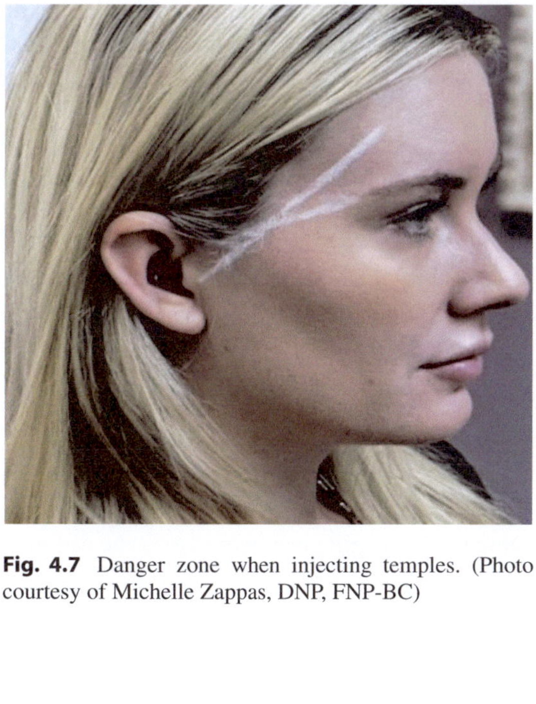

Fig. 4.7 Danger zone when injecting temples. (Photo courtesy of Michelle Zappas, DNP, FNP-BC)

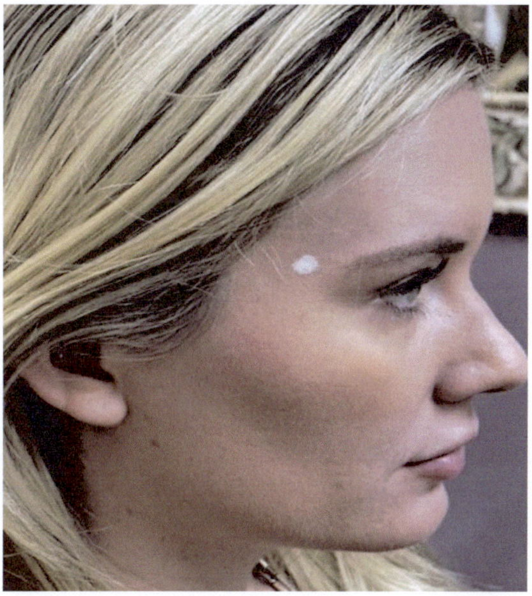

Fig. 4.8 One up one over location for safe injection of temples. (Photo courtesy of Michelle Zappas, DNP, FNP-BC)

4.2.4 Vessels of the Lower Face

When performing aesthetic procedures, the importance of understanding facial anatomy cannot be overemphasized. Structures in facial compartments vary in distribution, and location and the type of dermal filler used can have different ramifications depending on the involvement of those structures. The temporary and absorbable dermal filler class includes HA, calcium hydroxyapatite (CaHA), collagen, autologous fat, and poly-L-lactic acid (PLLA). The permanent filler class includes liquid silicone and polymethylmethacrylate (PMMA). All dermal fillers have the potential for complications including infection, skin necrosis, and vessel occlusion [12–17].

Aesthetic practice often is sought to refresh the patient's appearance through replacing lost facial volume during the aging process. Changes in the tissues of the jawline, lips, cheeks, temples, and infraorbital area cause many people to worry about their appearance and explore options such as laser and dermal filler procedures, neurotoxin, and surgical procedures. Specifically, the infraorbital hollows are a bothersome feature of aging, and many patients complain of looking *tired* when the fat redistribution in this area changes over time. Hence, re-volumization of the under eye and other areas of the face is sought after aesthetic treatments, and most have been performed successfully with dermal filler products. However, treating any facial area with dermal fillers carries risk, and the severity of complications and the locations of pertinent vessels are crucial for the practitioner to understand.

Vessels of the face include those that communicate with the brain, eyes, and muscles of mastication and expression [18, 19]. Caution when augmenting the cheeks, midface, and lateral face with dermal filler must be exercised to avoid the maxillary artery, transverse facial artery, and the facial artery (Fig. 4.1). The facial artery is significant because of its function and multiple branches that feed muscles of the face, including the buccinator, levator anguli oris, levator veli palatini, masseter, mentalis, mylohyoid, nasalis, palatoglossus, palatopharyngeus, platysma, procerus, risorius, styloglossus, and the transverse portion of the nasalis [20]. There are diverging channels between the angular branch of the facial artery and the medial branches of the infraorbital artery on the external carotid side and the dorsal nasal and supratrochlear branches of the ophthalmic artery on the internal carotid side [1]. However, like other vessels throughout the body, the facial artery can have anatomical variations. It may arise as a single vessel from the linguofacial trunk or a thyro-linguofacial trunk [21]. Accordingly, the facial artery may also arise from either the internal carotid artery or common carotid artery if there is no external carotid artery present.

4.2.5 Importance of Imaging in Aesthetics

Facial fillers are common incidental findings on magnetic resonance imaging (MRI) and positron emission tomography–computed tomography (PET-CT) scans, and they have a characteristic appearance and typical anatomic distribution [22]. Although facial filler injections are considered safe, they are associated with several complications such as vascular compromise, blindness, and skin necrosis in severe cases. Because the deposits of filler products might mask malignancy, knowledge of typical imaging features is mandatory and MRI can be a problem-solving tool for unclear cases [22].

According to some experts, the images of different fillers created by MRI have specific features; for example, calcium hydroxylapatite (CaHA) has characteristic calcifications, whereas other injectable fillers have overlapping visual features [22]. The rapidly absorbing fillers, HA and collagen, and the slowly absorbing filler, polyalkylimide and polyacrylamide hydrogels (PAAG), have signal patterns compatible with high water content and have a similar appearance because of the water content. On PET-CT and PET-MRI, most fillers show physiologic high F18-fluorodeoxyglucose (FDG) uptake and are increasingly used to detect inflammation and infection, and it is also used to evaluate fever of unknown origin [22].

These filler characteristics should not be confused with pathology because abscesses, cellulitis, non-inflammatory nodules, and foreign body granulomas are common filler-related complications [16, 17, 23]. FDG should not be used when evaluating filler complications, and astute observation by the practitioner of the patient response is essential to prompt evaluation if necessary. Diagnostic imaging can help clarify the differential diagnosis in emergency cases where a patient notices signs of infection, loss of function, or a change in their facial structure absent or posts a recent procedure. Imaging in cases with suspected deep spread of infection, MRI or contrast-enhanced CT in the emergency setting is essential [22].

4.3 Hyaluronidase Use

Hyaluronidase (HYAL) is an enzyme that catalyzes hyaluronidase fillers and is used to correct occasional lumpiness of treatment, but most importantly, HYAL can prevent skin necrosis and permanent scarring from vascular occlusion due to misplaced HA filler. HYAL dissolves the HA product usually within minutes after injection of the enzyme and does not have to be injected directly into the occluded vessel, and through diffusion it can reinstate vessel circulation quickly [24]. For these reasons, many practitioners choose to use HA dermal filler products.

Certain circumstances in aesthetics, for example, mis-placed filler, vascular compromise, lumpiness, or unexpected outcomes, may require the use of hyaluronidase [17, 25]. Although hyaluronidase is an enzyme that dissolves hyaluronic acid dermal filler, interestingly, it preserves endogenous hyaluronic acid. Even when large doses of hyaluronidase are used, the endogenous hyaluronidase returns to baseline after 48 h [26]. This suggests there is little reason to avoid its use when necessary, even in cases where some time has passed.

Careful and constant observation of the patient's skin response during injections of any type of dermal filler is crucial to enable the practitioner to act quickly in the event of a vascular incident. One important consideration is many of the modern dermal fillers contain an anesthetic agent (lidocaine), and this might mask the symptom of pain when a vessel is accidentally occluded. Accordingly, the signs of impending vascular compromise should be recognized by any novice or expert aesthetic practitioner (Figs. 4.9, 4.10, and 4.11).

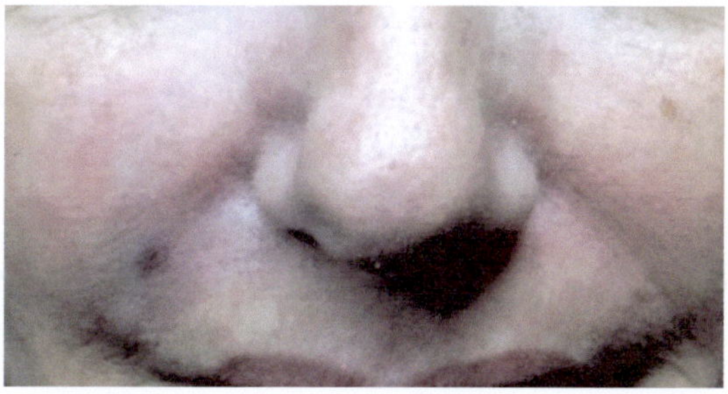

Fig. 4.9 Day of treatment with HA filler into the nasolabial area. Note the bluish discoloration resembling a bruise. (Photo courtesy B. Haney, DNP, FNP-C, FAANP, FAAN)

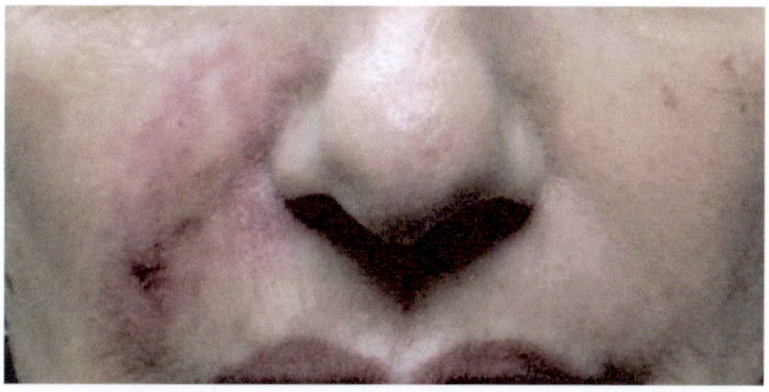

Fig. 4.10 Twenty-four hours after hyaluronidase treatment. Patient was injected with hyaluronidase 100 units diluted with saline 10:1, and the area was massaged until capillary refill of 2 s was observed. Patient home care instructions included daily 325 mg aspirin, warm packs to the area 5 times a day, and daily follow-up. (Photo courtesy B. Haney, DNP, FNP-C, FAANP, FAAN)

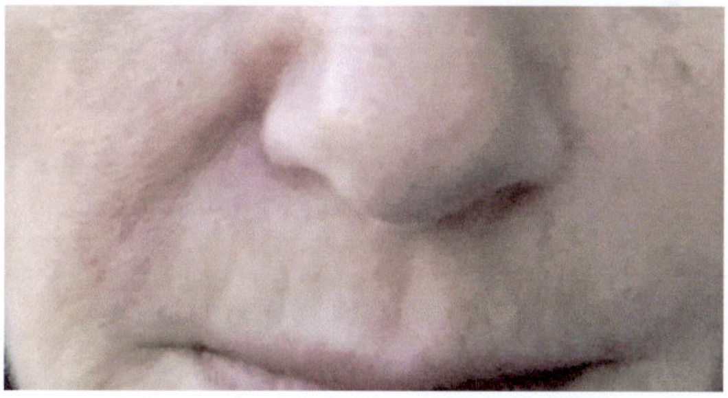

Fig. 4.11 Nine days after hyaluronidase treatment and home care. Complete resolution occurred in 14 days and patient returned 1 month later for subsequent HA filler treatment with excellent results and no adverse reaction. (Photo courtesy B. Haney, DNP, FNP-C, FAANP, FAAN)

The table summarizes the signs, symptoms, and skin changes of vascular occlusion from dermal fillers (Table 4.1)

Table 4.1 Signs and symptoms of a vascular occlusion during dermal filler injections

Timing, signs, and symptoms	Details and clinical aspects
Pain (during the procedure)	Important to note is pain may be absent initially if anesthetics are used; therefore, the absence of pain would be a variable indicator of ischemia. Intensifying pain is felt in areas affected by ischemia, and the patient may then report pain. A common attribute is the pain can be more intense than expected
Pallor or blanching (immediate, lasting tens of seconds)	Blanching or skin color change can occur immediately after arterial compromise as a temporary phase. This can be caused from intra-arterial occlusion or pressure from filler that compresses the vessel. Important to note is if epinephrine was used, there may be temporary skin discoloration in the area
Livedo phase (within minutes, occasionally within hours)	The area of occlusion takes on a blotchy, reddish, or bluish appearance, oftentimes resembling a bruise. It is important to consider the patient response, assess the area closely, and look for a "lacy" aspect to determine the cause of the discoloration. Checking for a slow capillary refill (>2 s) may assist in determining arterial insufficiency
Significant skin discoloration (dark blue or grayish, occurs in minutes to hours)	With occlusion, the skin appears dark blue or gray due to oxygen depletion. Important to consider bruising also takes on this appearance, and careful assessment of the patient is crucial
Sloughing (days to weeks)	This is a late sign. In an area that has progressed to necrosis, redness and ulceration develops and this often leads to a permanent scar

4.4 Conclusion

Practice pearls to avoid complications in the danger zones of dermal fillers include in-depth knowledge of facial anatomy, aspirating before injecting dermal filler product, and injecting slowly in a retrograde fashion. Tenting, or gently lifting and pinching, the skin allows more space between superficial branches of the prominent arteries. Using a small gauge needle and a reversible agent—such as hyaluronic acid (HA) fillers—can help prevent complications since they can be quickly degraded by hyaluronidase (HYAL). Occluding the vessels using pressure or palpating important vessels might help prevent complications. It is imperative that practitioners maintain vigilance when injecting dermal fillers into the facial compartments and be aware of signs of impending vascular compromise. The use of available imaging devices and techniques that identify facial vasculature before and during procedures can increase the level of patient safety and be valuable tools to the aesthetic practitioner.

References

1. Fisher CM. Facial pulses in internal carotid artery occlusion. Neurology. 1970;20(5):476–8.
2. Lee HJ, Won SY, Jehoon O, Hu KS, Mun SY, Yang HM, et al. The facial artery: a comprehensive anatomical review. Clin Anat. 2018;31(1):99–108.
3. Ferneini EM, Goupil MT, McNulty MA, Niekrash CE. Applied head and neck anatomy for the facial cosmetic surgeon. Berlin: Springer International; 2021.
4. Hufschmidt K, Bronsard N, Foissac R, Baque P, Balaguer T, Chignon-Sicard B, et al. The infraorbital artery: clinical relevance in esthetic medicine and identification of danger zones of the midface. J Plast Reconstr Aesthet Surg. 2019;72(1):131–6.
5. Kadouch J, Schelke LW, Swift A. Ultrasound to improve the safety and efficacy of lipofilling of the temples. Aesthet Surg J. 2021;41(5):603–12.
6. Lee W, Moon HJ, Kim JS, Yang EJ. Safe glabellar wrinkle correction with soft tissue filler using Doppler ultrasound. Aesthet Surg J. 2021;41(9):1081–9.
7. Mespreuve M, Waked K, Hendrickx B. Visualization techniques of the facial arteries. J Cosmet Dermatol. 2021;20(2):386–90.
8. Carruthers A, Carruthers J, Dover JS, Alam M. Soft tissue augmentation. 4th ed. Amsterdam: Elsevier; 2018.
9. Li X, Du L, Lu JJ. A novel hypothesis of visual loss secondary to cosmetic facial filler injection. Ann Plast Surg. 2015;75(3):258–60.
10. Phumyoo T, Jiirasutat N, Jitaree B, Rungsawang C, Uruwan S, Tansatit T. Anatomical and ultrasonography-based investigation to localize the arteries on the central forehead region during the glabellar augmentation procedure. Clin Anat. 2020;33(3):370–82.
11. Cotofana S, Gaete A, Hernandez CA, Casabona G, Bay S, Pavicic T, et al. The six different injection techniques for the temple relevant for soft tissue filler

augmentation procedures—clinical anatomy and danger zones. J Cosmet Dermatol. 2020;19(7):1570–9.
12. Allergan. Juvederm XC product insert; 2016.
13. Galderma. Restylane lyft with lidocaine package insert; 2018.
14. Galderma. Sculptra aesthetic prescribing information; 2016.
15. Aesthetics M. Radiesse lidocaine injectable implant. Raleigh: Merz North America Inc.; 2016.
16. Grunebaum LF, Funt D. complications of cosmetic fillers. Aesthet Dermatol. 2018;4:128–40.
17. DeLorenzi C. Complications of injectable fillers, part I. Aesthet Surg J. 2013;33(4):561–75.
18. Vigliante CE. Anatomy and functions of the muscles of facial expression. Oral Maxillofac Surg Clin North Am. 2005;17(1):1–15. v.
19. Seeley RR, Tate P, Stephens TD. Anatomy & physiology. 8th ed. Dubuque, IA: McGraw-Hill; 2008. xxi, 1116 p.
20. Meegalla N, Sood G, Nessel TA, Downs BW. Anatomy, head and neck, facial arteries. Treasure Island, FL: StatPearls; 2021.
21. Mangalgiri A, Namdev LN, Mahore D, Kapre M. The study of higher origin of facial artery and its surgical significance. Indian J Otolaryngol Head Neck Surg. 2015;67(1):72–4.
22. Mundada P, Kohler R, Boudabbous S, Toutous Trellu L, Platon A, Becker M. Injectable facial fillers: imaging features, complications, and diagnostic pitfalls at MRI and PET CT. Insights Imaging. 2017;8(6):557–72.
23. Cohen JL. Understanding, avoiding, and managing dermal filler complications. Dermatol Surg. 2008;34(Suppl 1):S92–9.
24. DeLorenzi C. Complications of injectable fillers, part 2: vascular complications. Aesthet Surg J. 2014;34(4):584–600.
25. Carruthers J, Carruthers A. In: Dover J, editor. Soft tissue augmentation. 3rd ed. Amsterdam: Elsevier; 2017.
26. Casabona G, Marchese PB, Montes JR, Hornfeldt CS. Durability, behavior, and tolerability of 5 hyaluronidase products. Dermatol Surg. 2018;44(Suppl 1):S42–50.

5 Bard: Aesthetics—4D Facial Nerve Biomicroscopy

Robert L. Bard and Paul Dreschnack

Abstract

Avoiding nerve injury is critical with new image-guided treatment procedures. Vascular structures are readily discernible with high-resolution Doppler sonography, but the facial nerves are millimeter or submillimeter in size and better imaged with real-time facial motion techniques and 4D mapping with coordinated skin targeting. This chapter explores the innovative benefits of using 4D mapping with regard to differentiating functionalization of the nerve, fascia, muscle, as well as ligaments and tendons.

Keywords

Skin cancers · Vascular structures · Sonography · Doppler · Autoimmune disease · Treatment

R. L. Bard (✉)
The Angio Foundation and Bard Diagnostics, New York, NY, USA
e-mail: rbard@cancerscan.com

P. Dreschnack
Department of Surgery, St. Joseph's Hospital, Yonkers, NY, USA

5.1 Introduction

2020 arrived with laser technology breakthroughs such as noncontact laser generation of ultrasound images and image-guided reflective confocal/optical coherence laser treatment of nonaggressive skin cancers as well as new treatment protocols. This ushers in the possibility of other therapeutic options such as photon particle intervention targeted by remote laser ultrasound robotics. Treatment options include 1064 laser for minimally invasive tumors or photon irradiation on deeper or highly aggressive cancers. HIFU insonation has been successfully used for 20 years and could supplement other modalities. Near infrared radiation is being intensively investigated.

3D imaging technologies offer one-step image-guided treatment since the size, depth, margins, and tumor aggression parameters are quantifiably displayed. Real-time 3D Doppler treatment verification is critical since aggressive basal cell cancer types (morpheaform) have a 27.7% 5 year recurrence rate suggesting that earlier imaging either missed deep tumor nests or subcutaneous locoregional metastases. Ultrasound biomicroscopy plays a key role since biopsies may miss the most aggressive region thereby underestimating the potential for recurrence. 3D vessel density histogram confirms complete tumor destruction by verification of functional vascular obliteration. 4D is real-

R. L. Bard (ed.), *Image-Guided Aesthetic Treatments*, https://doi.org/10.1007/978-3-031-36266-8_5

time 3D imaging highlighting the differential motility of nerve, fascia, muscle, ligament, and tendons.

5.2 Identifying Skin Cancers

Basal cell cancers (BCC) are the most common malignancy worldwide. BCCs are rarely fatal; however, certain aggressive squamous cell cancer (SCC) types have devastating health consequences via locoregional growth and circulatory dissemination [1]. Metastatic potential of BCC is determined by functional analysis of specific intratumor sonographic findings. Malignant melanoma is the leading cause of death of women in the 25–45 age range and has a 98% diagnostic accuracy using ultrasound 15–24 MHz systems and higher with 30, 48, and 70 MHz frequencies now available. More importantly, there are specific tumor vessel density criteria identifying which melanoma cancer is most aggressive using quantitative Doppler 3D histogram analysis technologies [2].

5.3 Quantifiable Digital Scanning Versus Biopsy

The optical dermatologic modalities of RCM (reflectance confocal microscopy) and OCT (optical coherence tomography) are highly accurate in ruling out malignant disorders and often flag a biopsy on a visually innocent appearing lesion such as amelanotic melanoma or pigmented basal cell cancer. 4D ultrasound imaging is a real-time evaluation of a 3D volume so we know immediately the depth and quickly assess the probability of recurrence. Specific echoes generated by nests of keratin are strong indicators of aggression and analyzed volumetrically. Highly suspect areas are then checked for locoregional spread, and search is performed for draining sentinal node lymphadenopathy so we show our patient that the disease is completely sonographically imaged in real time as the exam proceeds in systematic diagnostic stages. 4D permits image-guided biopsy of the most virulent area of the dermal tumor and allows the pathologist to focus on the most suspicious region of the postoperative lymph node specimen mass excised from the axilla, neck, or groin. In serious cases, the patient is forewarned that the surgical operation may be complex involving skin grafts and advanced tissue reconstruction and can make advanced plans prior to definitive treatment.

5.3.1 Digital Imaging Reduces Complications

Fear of complications deters patients from seeking medical advice and possible disfiguring surgical intervention so many opt for noninvasive options. One out of 33,000 moles is malignant meaning high-resolution imaging reduces unnecessary biopsies. Cancer treatment depends on accurate determination of tumor depth and penetration possibly involving facial nerves, periocular muscles, nasal bone, or ear cartilage. Verified superficial tumors may be treated topically or by low-dose non-scarring radiation therapies. Many cancers provoke a benign local immune response or concomitant inflammatory reaction that simulates a larger tumor burden. There is often cicatrix formation accompanying the body's healing response, and benign disorders may coexist and appear clinically inseparable from the malignant lesion. Precision 4D imaging highlights the true surgical borders of the cancerous tissue resulting in smaller excisional margins, healthy tissue sparing, and reduced scar formation.

5.4 Doppler Applications

Blood vessel mapping using the various Doppler flow modalities is routinely used in both cancer treatment and reconstructive preoperative planning. In cancer surgery, it is important to identify aberrant large veins or significant arteries in the operative site so that hemostasis is maintained and postoperative blood loss is minimized. Before initiating cosmetic procedures or aesthetic treatments, many plastic surgeons routinely perform a screening overview scan of the facial tissues including the eye, nose, jaw, and neck to check for forgotten fillers or post procedure complications such as subdermal scar formation, intradermal calcific deposits from healed previous injuries or retained silicone, and other fillers that may have been injected in the past. Particular attention is focused on the nasal glabellar area because instances of total, permanent blindness have been occurring for over 10 years due to the inadvertent deposition of injectable filler or fat transplant material into the draining veins that supply the back of the eye. Advance warning of this danger zone means injectables may be deposited in a safer location. Fat transplants and silicone pads around the orbit occasionally put pressure on the venous return resulting in tissue discoloration and edema from venous obstruction, while emboli to the ophthalmic arteries cutting off blood supply to facial regions cause death and sloughing of the affected ischemic skin. Vascular occlusion or insufficiency may be documented by Doppler studies and successful therapeutic relief documented in real time. Advanced 3D Doppler systems allow for histogram vessel density measurement of neoplastic angiogenesis (Fig. 5.1). This baseline

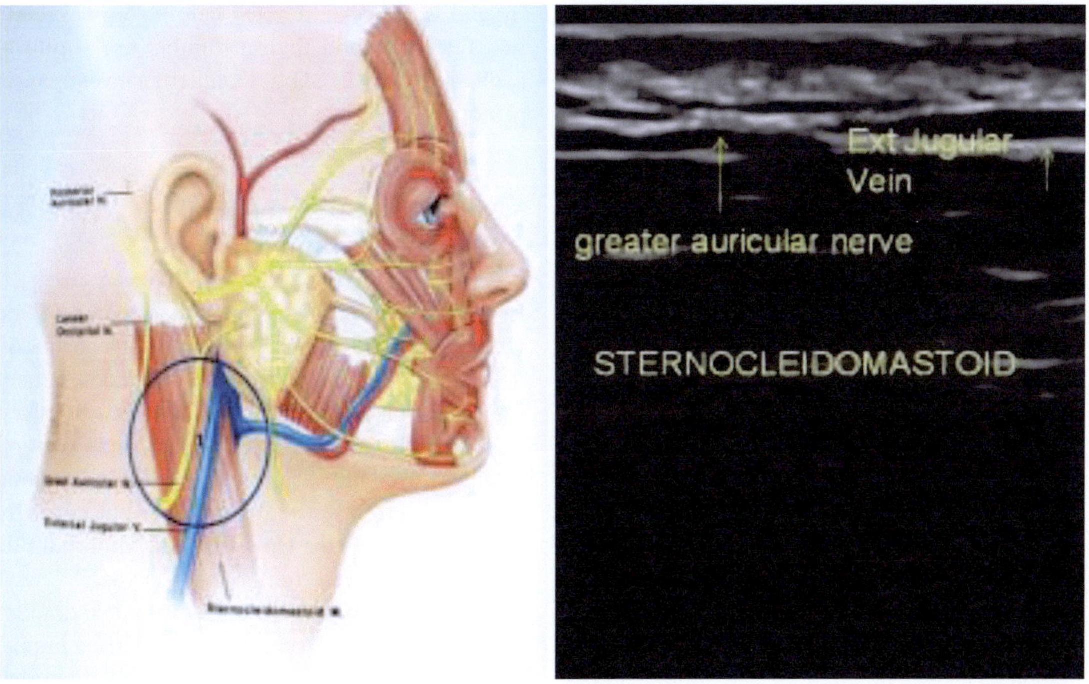

Fig. 5.1 Nerve depicted as echogenic tubular structure

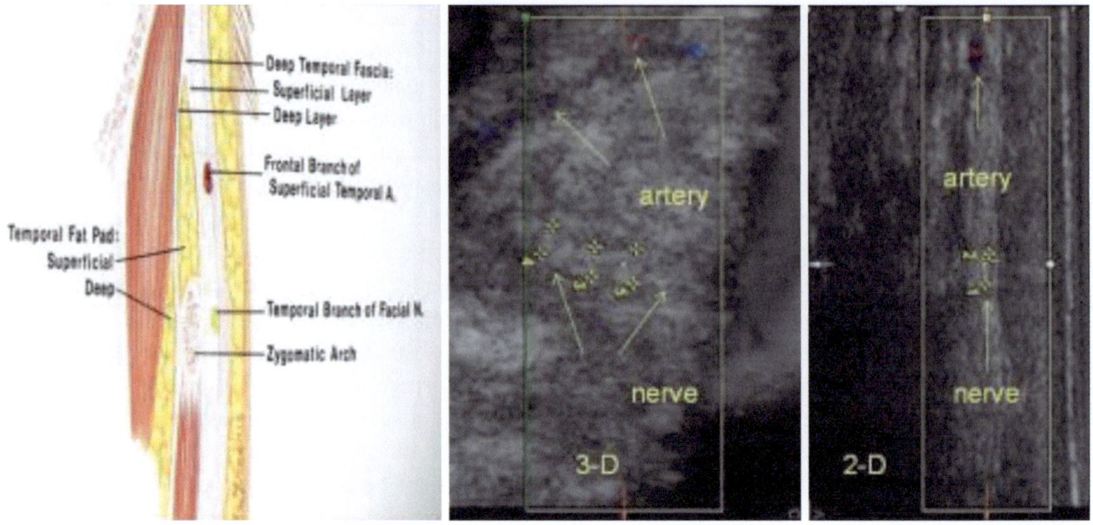

Fig. 5.2 Linear nerve outlined by arrows

neovascularity is used as a treatment surrogate endpoint allowing for image-guided clinical reevaluation and timely correction of therapy (Fig. 5.2) [3].

5.5 Glandular Cancer Imaging Updates

It is well established that non-dermatological malignancies have dermal manifestations either directly or indirectly. Breast cancer invading the lower dermis and nipple discovered with high-resolution probes signifies that the tumor has spread further than clinically anticipated. That finding is essential for detecting the newly discovered entity of breast implant-associated anaplastic large cell lymphoma (BIA-ALCL). This capability is also vital for diagnosing the recent epidemic of male breast cancer occurring in our 9/11 First Responders arising near the mammographically difficult area of the nipple areolar complex.

Prostate cancer clearly identified by 4D delimited by the capsule and of low vessel density is being followed serially in 6-month intervals. Subsequent capsular invasion or increase in vessel density on histogram analysis requires urologic measures. Bladder cancer is evaluated concomitantly with the prostate and neovascularity and wall invasion noted before surgical referral. Testicular and thyroid tumors are similarly evaluated by 3D Doppler investigation protocols.

5.5.1 Contrast Enhanced Ultrasound (CEUS)

In 1990, Dr Rodolfo Campani, director of the University of Pavia Radiology Department, developed ultrasound contrast enhanced cancer imaging for liver tumors followed by Drs. Cosgrove (London), Lassau (Paris), and Catalano (Naples) for breast, prostate, and melanoma. CEUS is currently used worldwide but not fully FDA approved in the United States. Microbubble, safe media show tumor neovascularity with exquisite detail and are used to evaluate therapeutic response in solid organ disease. This is important since the RECIST studies demonstrated that tumor enlargement during treatment may be related to apoptotic cell death with cystic degeneration or immune cell infiltration destroying malignant tissue. Co-existing benign disease may be indistinguishable from and integrated into the tumor mass. Doppler ultrasound or CEUS reliably verifies decreased angiogenesis in these cases instead of using contrast CT or DCE-MRI for confirmation. Thermal treatments such as cryotherapy, HIFU, photodynamic treatment, or laser ablation are designated complete when perfusing cancer arteries are no longer visible.

5.5.2 Margin Delineation

Advances in laser/optical devices allow near microscopic tissue analysis of the cells by rapid, non-invasive testing. Real-time microscopy is performed during surgery to assure that the tumor border is clear in cases of skin cancer, and future use in breast and prostate cancer treatment is under clinical study. Prostate, thyroid, and breast cancers are now treated robotically, and we predict other malignancies to be digitally ablated in the near future [4].

5.6 Autoimmune Disease and Cancer

Abnormal immune responses that initially appear in the skin are associated with increased cancer incidence. Inflammatory vessels in psoriasis and infection are visibly cataloged since successful treatment is quantified by measured decrease in the number and type of abnormal vessels. High vascular immune vessel density is proportional to increased risk of future neoplastic tissue manifestations. Many arthritic conditions have coexistent dermal components alerting us to the probability of more extensive subclinical joint involvement. Botanical and cosmeceutical formulations have ameliorated many inflammatory diseases and possibly prevented malignant conditions, and their effect may be monitored before more aggressive approaches are initiated [5–11].

5.7 Treatment

Standard procedures include surgical excision, photodynamic therapy, curettage with or without electro dissection, and Mohs Micrographic Surgery (MMS). Topical treatments are 5-fluorouracil cream and imiquimod for low risk, superficial lesions. Immunotherapies have proven highly effective in the case of malignant melanoma although accompanied by significant side effects such as confusion and cutaneous disorders.

New options with pulsed electromagnetic field technologies are non-invasive and have been effective in treating inflammatory disorders such as psoriasis, rosacea, and eczema. Minimally invasive injectables using an alternative to stem cells are exosomes to be discussed later in the chapter.

5.8 Radiation History

The discovery of X-rays by Roentgen in 1896 allowed for the application for breast cancer treatment by Dr Emil Grubbe with this therapy in the same year. In 1898, the Curies discovered radium due to its elemental ionizing radiation on film. The first successful treatment of skin cancer occurred in 1899.

The technology evolved from X-ray tubes and radium sources to high energy radioactive elements like cobalt and cesium. Low megavoltage generators and high megavoltage linear accelerators along with particles (electron beam and protons). Brachytherapy (BT) added remote afterloading devices, and miniature X-ray tubes generated electronic brachytherapy (EBT).

5.9 Functional Treatment Biology

Radiation produces free radicals that damage DNA as the electromagnetic energy disrupts mitosis in rapidly dividing cells. While normal cells can repair damage, treated cancer cells cannot divide and are considered inactive or sterilized. This means that cancer cells that grow slowly will die slowly, and the tissues will look like active cancer but are, in fact, "sterile" or biologically inactive or dead, while appearing functional to the pathologist. Therefore, a biopsy may be "positive," while the cancer is biologically inactive and potentially cured. Similarly, the size of a treated tumor poorly correlates with treatment success since edema from dying cells or infiltration with T cells, and other immunologic tissue can transiently enlarge the tumor mass while it is biologically "dead" [12–14].

Superficial radiation therapy (SRT)for non-melanoma skin cancer has been increasing in use with the aging population and portable units suitable for the office-based setting; while in use since the 1900s, it declined in use with the advances in MMS. The precision image-guided radiation technologies are now achieving higher clinical application due to the cosmetic benefit and minimal side effects. While SRT uses low energy photons with limited penetration, the new focused "proton" beams are targeted precisely and limit surrounding tissue damage in spite of very high energy and may be used more frequently in more aggressive subtypes. Of note, 3D Doppler ultrasound not only establishes tumor depth and response to therapy, but assesses the malignant aggression potential using the specific echo pattern and neovascular findings characteristic of dangerous lesions. It has been used as a template for the image guidance coordinates for radiation therapy planning [13, 14]. HIFU and LASER treatments are used sporadically in cases where other options are not feasible and anecdotally have had good results.

5.10 Treatment Verification

The overall recurrence rate analysis by Cognetta of 1715 NMSCs (BCC and SCC) was 1.9% [15]. Another study by Shulte on 1276 NMSCs showed a combined rate of 5.1% [16]. A paper by Zagrodnik using BCC histopathology for superficial, nodular, and sclerosing (morpheaform) cell types revealed a 5 year recurrence rate of 11.8, 2.8, and 27.7%, respectively [17]. More aggressive histopathologic types recurred up to 27%, and this in part may be explained by tumor not treated since it was outside the treatment field as in satellite, in transit, or more distant or deeper subcutaneous metastases not detected by the available imaging technology at the time. The vascular measurement parameters in OCT and RCM add another measure of treatment success by verifying absent blood flow in previously non-treated neovascular tumor tissue. Future tumor neovascularity assessment will use the (off label FDA approved) contrast enhanced ultrasound (CEUS) for advanced quantification.

5.11 Cosmetic Factors

Cancers of the face – ears, eyes, nose, perioral, and other visible areas – are good candidates for SRT where treatment may have significant cosmetic consequences. Common side effects are radiation dermatitis, erythema, and mild discomfort. Late reactions include hyper/hypopigmentation, telangiectasias, and atrophy.

Most patients are elderly and multiple treatments generally are a hardship. Fewer more intense sessions will cause skin damage but must be balanced against longevity, treatment effect, and cosmesis since the curative dosage is difficult to ascertain [18]. Since the cosmetic effect may be better than surgery, there is a trend to SRT use as a first-line treatment, except for deep tumor invasion, aggressive tumor histology, previously irradiated lesions, and some type of NMSC occurring in organ transplant patients. SRT is superior to electron beam radiotherapy (EBRT) and electronic brachytherapy (EBX) for most cases of NMSC. Keloids may be successfully treated with few side effects and good functional return [19]. SRT is contraindicated in micronodular BCC, sclerosing BCC, recurrent BCC, and poorly differentiated SCC or desmoplastic SCC with/without perineural spread [20]. Since most BCC is facial, better results may be obtained with small field MRI [21] and ultrasound fusion-guided MRI targeting [22]. Verification of clinically acceptable treatment response has been studied by Markowitz [23].

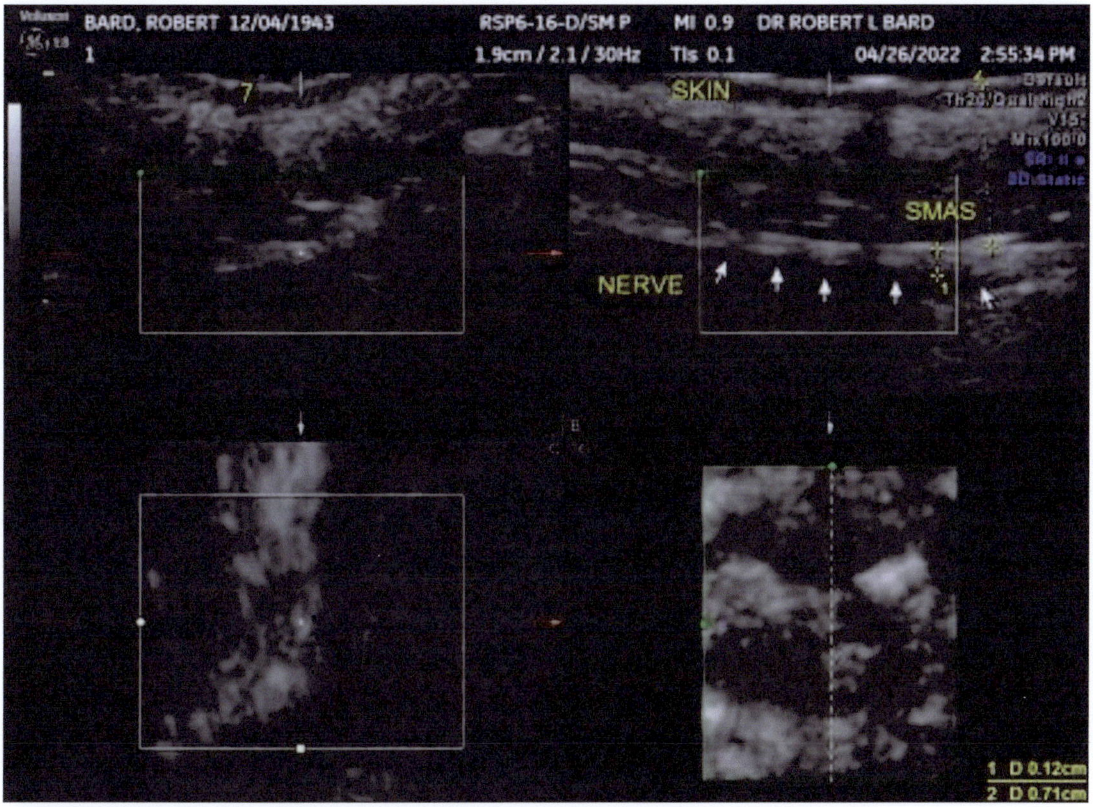

Fig. 5.3 The echogenic facial nerve is demonstrated in 3 orthogonal planes

5.11.1 4D Nerve Mapping

While some nerves course near arterial structures, many diverge at a distance and are hard to differentiate with imaging from the subcutaneous fasci, ligaments, and tendons. Aside from iatrogenic nerve injury, a recent use is the treatment of Bell's Palsy which is the most common form of idiopathic facial paralysis of the 7th cranial nerve thought to be caused by a viral or autoimmune condition. This affects middle-aged patients in the equal distribution between male and female sexes. Although spontaneous resolution within months is usual, some cases may be protracted for years or even a lifetime. Mesenchymal stem cells or exosomes injected around the facial nerve in the preauricular tissue and repeated after interval have been successfully performed diminishing inflammation and promoting recovery [24]. 4D imaging is able to distinguish branches of the extracranial 7th nerve from tendons, fascia, and ligaments with the aid of motion that moves muscle and tendons more vigorously than the relatively fixed submillimeter nerve bundles with very high-resolution imaging.

Exosomes with their regenerative and immunomodulatory properties are used in dermatology for wound healing, stimulating hair growth, psoriasis, and atopic dermatitis [25] and may prove useful in the newly recognized role of nerve cells activation in pruritic conditions (Figs. 5.3, 5.4, 5.5, 5.6, 5.7 and 5.8) [26].

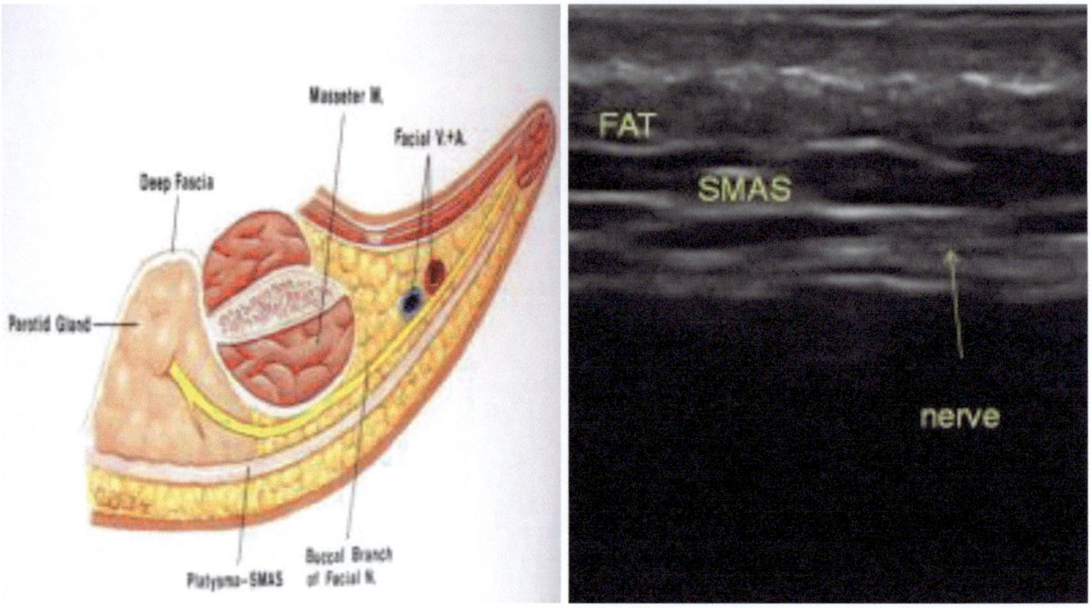

Fig. 5.4 The echogenic nerve is adjacent to the SMAS

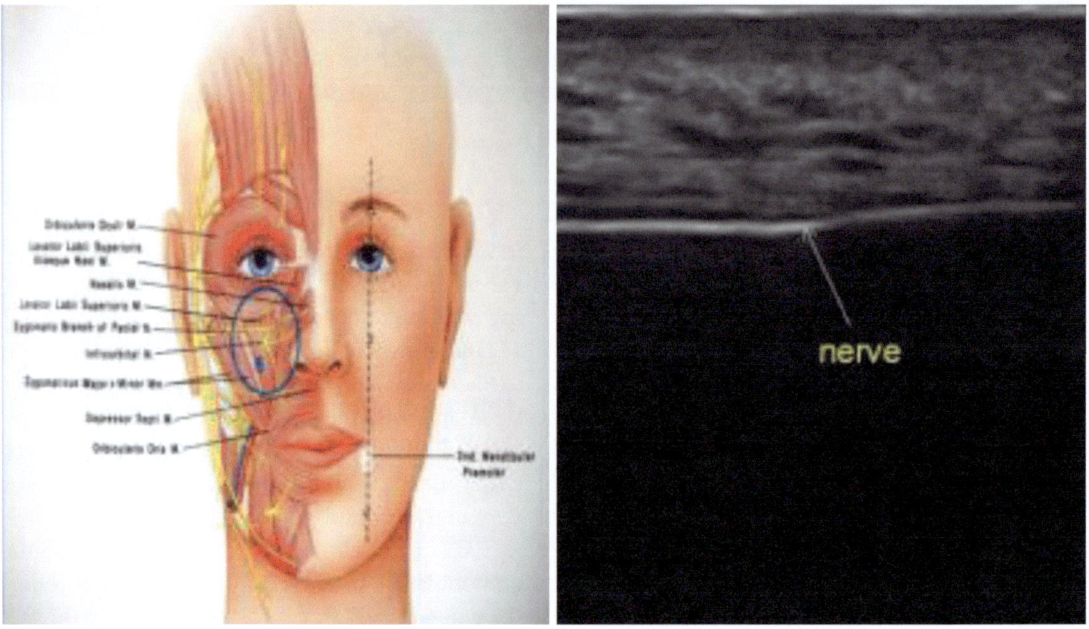

Fig. 5.5 The echogenic linear nerve abuts the boney cortex

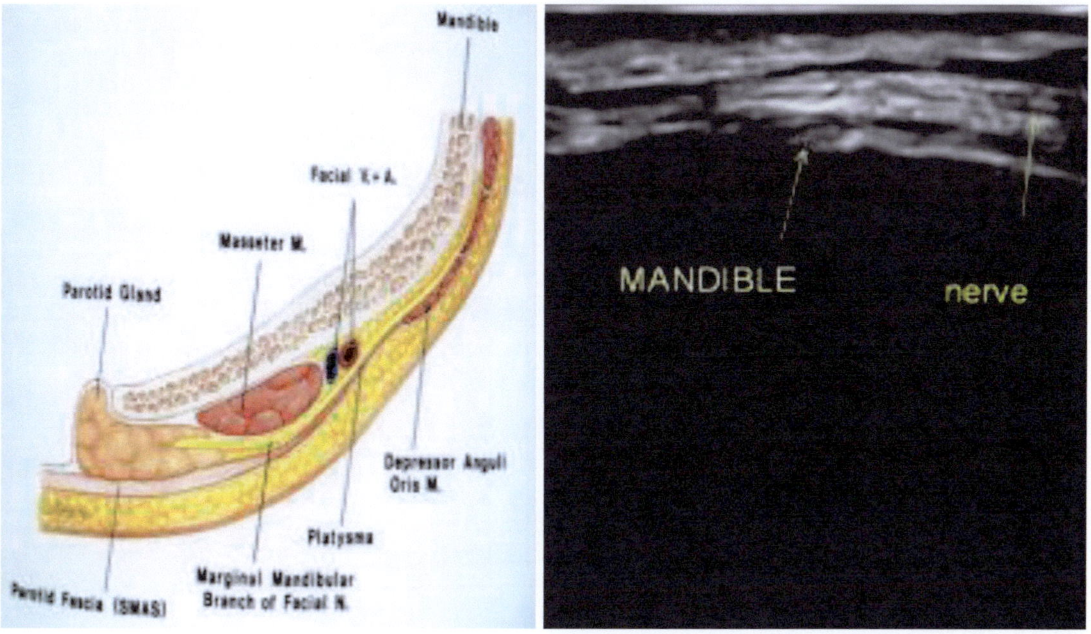

Fig. 5.6 The tubular nerve lies deep to the SMAS

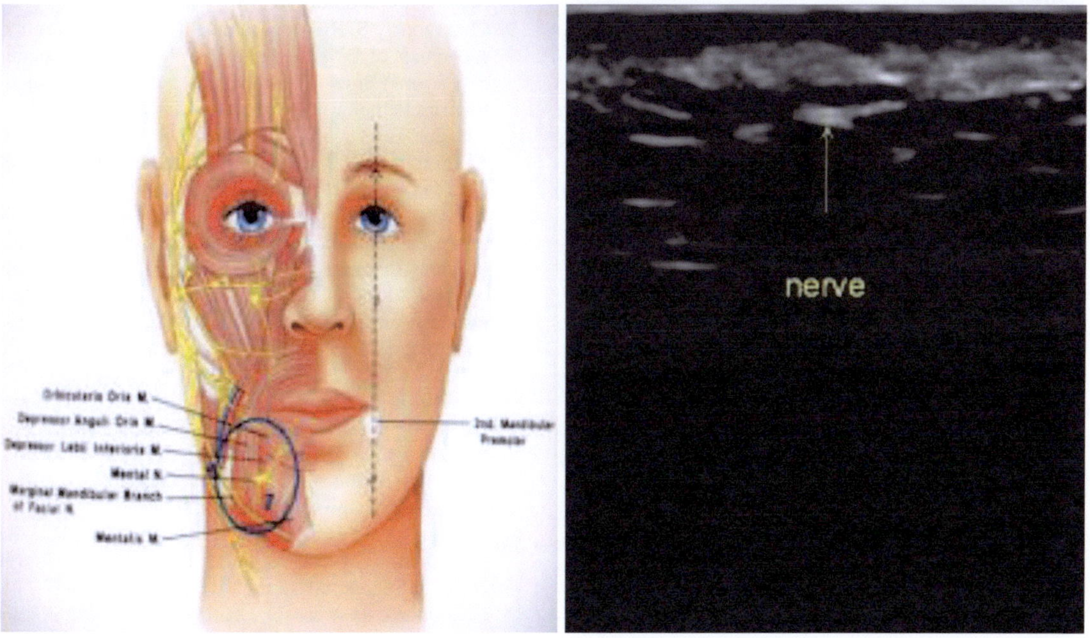

Fig. 5.7 The echogenic nerve lies deep to the muscle

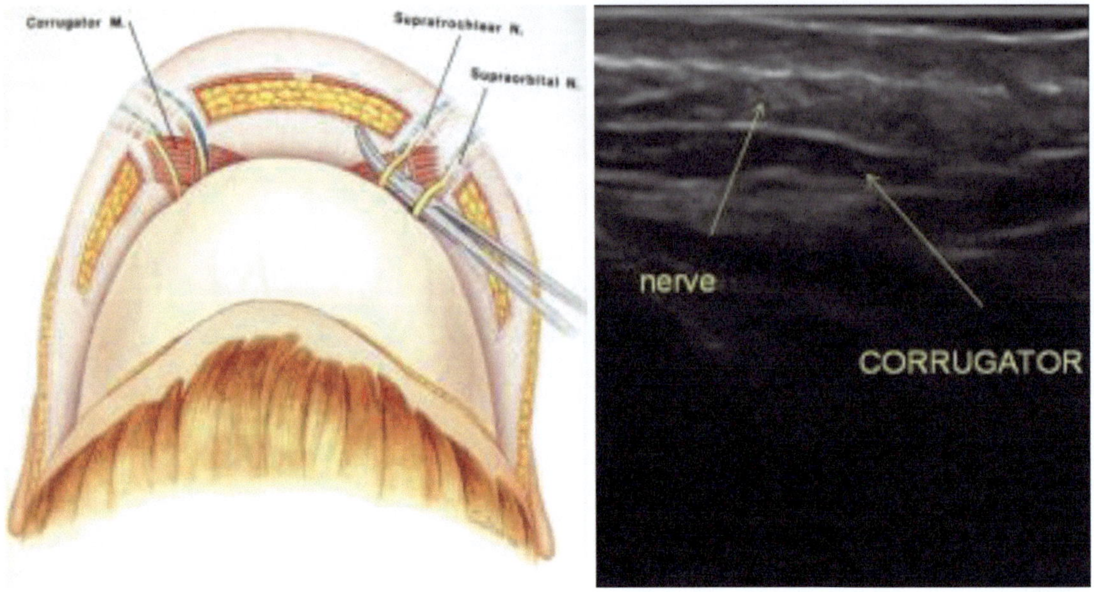

Fig. 5.8 The nerve lies between the muscle layers

References

1. Ewing J. Neoplastic diseases. London: WB Saunders; 1940.
2. Lassau N, Koscielny S, Avril M, Margulis A, Duvillard P, Baere T, Roche A, Leclere J. Prognostic value of angiogenesis evaluated with high frequency and color Doppler sonography for preoperative assessment of melanomas. AJR. 2002;178:1547–51.
3. Cornud F, Hamida K, Flam T, Helenon O, Chretien Y, Thiounn N, Correas J, Casanova J, Moreau J. Endorectal color Doppler sonography and endorectal MR imaging features of non palpable prostate cancer. AJR. 2000;175:1161–8.
4. Bard R. Dynamic contrast enhanced MRI of prostate cancer. New York: Springer; 2009.
5. Awad AB, Fink CS. Phytosterols as anticancer dietary compounds: evidence and mechanism of action. J Nutr. 2000;130(9):2127–30.
6. Toda S, Shirataki Y. Inhibitory effects of Astragali radix, a crude drug in oriental medicines, on lipid peroxidation and protein oxidative modification by copper. J Ethnopharmacol. 1999;68(1–3):331–3.
7. Wang D, Shen W, Tian Y, Sun Z, Jiang C, Yuan S. Protective effect of active components extracted from radix Astragali on human erythrocyte membrane damages caused by reactive oxygen species [article in Chinese]. Zhongguo Zhong Yao Za Zhi. 1996;21(12):746–8, 763.
8. Chan MM, Mattiacci JA, Hwang HS, Shah A, Fong D. Synergy between ethanol and grape polyphenols, quercetin, and resveratrol, in the inhibition of the inducible nitric oxide synthase pathway. Biochem Pharmacol. 2000;60(10):1539–48.
9. Chakraborty S, Roy M, Bhattacharya RK. Prevention and repair of DNA damage by selected phytochemicals as measured by single cell gel electrophoresis. Environ Pathol Toxicol Oncol. 2004;23(3):215–26.
10. Mertens-Talcott SU, Bomser JA, Romero C, Talcott ST, Percival SS. Ellagic acid potentiates the effect of Quercetin on p21waf1/cip1, p53, and MAPKinases without affecting intracellular generation of reactive oxygen species in vitro. J Nutr. 2005;135:609–14.
11. Mertens-Talcott SU, Talcott ST, Percival SS. Low concentrations of quercetin and Ellagic acid synergistically influence proliferation, cytotoxicity and apoptosis in MOLT-4 human leukemia cells. J Nutr. 2003;133:2669–74.
12. McGregor S, Minni J, Herold D, et al. Superficial radiation therapy for treatment of nonmelanoma skin cancers. J Clin Aesthet Dermatol. 2015;8(12):12–4.
13. Bard RJ, editor. Image guided dermatologic treatment. Berlin: Springer; 2019. p. 43–56.
14. Padhani A, Petralia G. Whole body MRI. In: Proceedings of 18th Annual International Cancer Imaging Society, Menton; 2018.
15. Cognetta A, Howard B, Heaton H, et al. Superficial Xray treatment in the treatment of basal and squamous cell carcinoma. JAAD. 2012;67:1237–41.
16. Schulte KE, Lippoid A, Auras C, et al. Soft Xray therapy for cutaneous basal and squamous cell carcinomas. JAAD. 2005;53:993–1001.
17. Zadronik B, Kempt W, Seifert E, et al. Superficial radiotherapy for patients with basal cell carcinoma. Cancer. 2003;98(12):2708–14.

18. Zaorsky N, Lee CT, Zhang E, et al. Hypofractionated radiation therapy for basal and squamous cell skin cancer: a meta-analysis. Radiother Oncol. 2017;125(1):13.
19. Nestor M, Berman B, Goldberg D, et al. Consensus guidelines on the use of superficial radiation therapy for treating nonmelanoma skin cancers and keloids. J Clin Aesthet Dermatol. 2019;12(2):12–8.
20. Hafner J. Superficial radiotherapy to treat skin cancer. In: Proceedings 37th Annual ISDS Meeting 2016, Amsterdam; 2016.
21. Budak M, Weir J, Yaap P, et al. High resolution microscopy-coil MR imaging of skin tumors. Radiographics. 2015;35(4):1077–90.
22. Bard R. MRI imaging of skin cancer. In: Proceedings of the 2020 AIUM Annual Meeting of the American Institute of Ultrasound in Medicine, New York; 2020.
23. Markowitz O. Patient-driven management using same-day noninvasive diagnosis and complete laser treatment of basal cell carcinomas: a pilot study. Lasers Surg Med. 2019;51(10):24–9.
24. Dreschnack P, Scott M, Bochenek C. Bell's Palsy and stem cell therapy. J Regen Med. 2020;9(1):156–8.
25. Quinones M, Sanabria R, Sanchez M, et al. Rôle of exosome derived cells in dermatology. Front Cell Dev Biol. 2021;2(2):12–21.
26. Bard R, Gettz L, Stoff J, et al. 3D Doppler imaging of inflammatory skin disease. In: 4th ISDS Symposium at New York Academy Medicine; 2021.

Facial Rejuvenation/Non-Surgical Procedures

6

Beth Haney

Abstract

Non-surgical aesthetic treatments are popular options for men and women who want to maintain a youthful and healthy appearance without enduring a surgical procedure. The available treatments include neurotoxins, or botulinum neurotoxin type A (BoNT/A) injections, dermal filler injections, laser treatments, radiofrequency procedures, and topical applications. Botulinum neurotoxin type A (BoNT/A) for cosmetic use, commonly known as Botox®, Dysport®, and Xeomin®, is the most commonly performed non-surgical aesthetic procedure in the world. The action of BoNT/A results in smoother skin due to the relaxation of the facial muscle fibers. Alternatively, dermal fillers replace facial volume and are the second most requested, non-surgical aesthetic procedure worldwide. Practical knowledge of BoNT/A and available temporary dermal filler pharmacology are important aspects of aesthetic practice. This chapter will provide information on the use of neurotoxin and temporary dermal filler procedures including mechanisms of action, potential complications, and future uses.

B. Haney (✉)
Department of Nursing, USC Suzanne Dworak-Peck School of Social Work, University of Southern California, Los Angeles, CA, USA
e-mail: bhaney@usc.edu

Keywords

Botox · Dysport · Xeomin · Neurotoxin complications · Botulinum toxin type A (BoNT/A) · Eyelid ptosis · Brow ptosis · Temporary dermal filler · Hyaluronic acid · G-prime · Crosslinked · Poly-L-lactic acid (PLLA) · Calcium hydroxyapatite (CaHA) · Dermal filler pharmacology · NASHA · PLLA · CaHA · Muscle memory · Radiofrequency · Ultrasound · Laser emitting device · LED

6.1 Neurotoxins: Botulinum Toxin Type A (BoNT/A)

6.1.1 Mechanism of Action

The facial muscles are the only muscle group in the human body that insert directly into the skin [1, 2]. The repeated contraction of facial muscles results in lines (rhytids) both at rest and during facial expression. These types of lines are categorized as dynamic lines because they are created by movement. The resting face that is free from lines etched in the skin is a more youthful looking face, and with repeated use, BoNT/A can result in smooth line-free skin. This aesthetically pleasing result is an outcome of the temporary relaxation of facial muscles from BoNT/A treatments.

R. L. Bard (ed.), *Image-Guided Aesthetic Treatments*, https://doi.org/10.1007/978-3-031-36266-8_6

To comprehend how BoNT/A works in the musculature of the face and neck, an understanding of the synaptic communication and neurotransmitter relationship is necessary. The five commercial brands of BoNT/A, Botox®, Dysport®, Xeomin®, Daxxify®, and Jeuveau®, all work in similar ways. Soluble N-ethylmaleimide-sensitive factor adaptor proteins (SNAPs) and SNAP receptors (SNAREs) are the main targets of BoNT/A [3]. Injection of the BoNT/A molecule into the muscle blocks neuromuscular transmission by binding to surface receptors on motor nerve terminals, entering the nerve terminals, and inhibiting the release of acetylcholine [4]. This inhibition occurs as the pH-induced translocation of the toxin light chain to the cell cytosol cleaves SNAP-25, a presynaptic protein that is crucial in the successful docking and release of acetylcholine from vesicles within nerve endings [5]. The result is a decrease in the target muscle activity ultimately resulting in less dynamic line formation (see Figs. 6.1 and 6.2).

In addition, there is some evidence the affected muscle might atrophy, and subsequent re-innervation of the muscle occurs, thus slowly reversing BoNT/A action. Transmission gradually begins as the neuromuscular junction recovers from cleavage of the SNAP-25 and new nerve endings are formed [4–9]. This phenomenon may be associated with the term "muscle memory" when referring to the longer-lasting cosmetic effect of the BoNT/A on select patients [10].

The pharmacological effect of BoNT/A is caused by the cleaving of SNAP25 and subse-

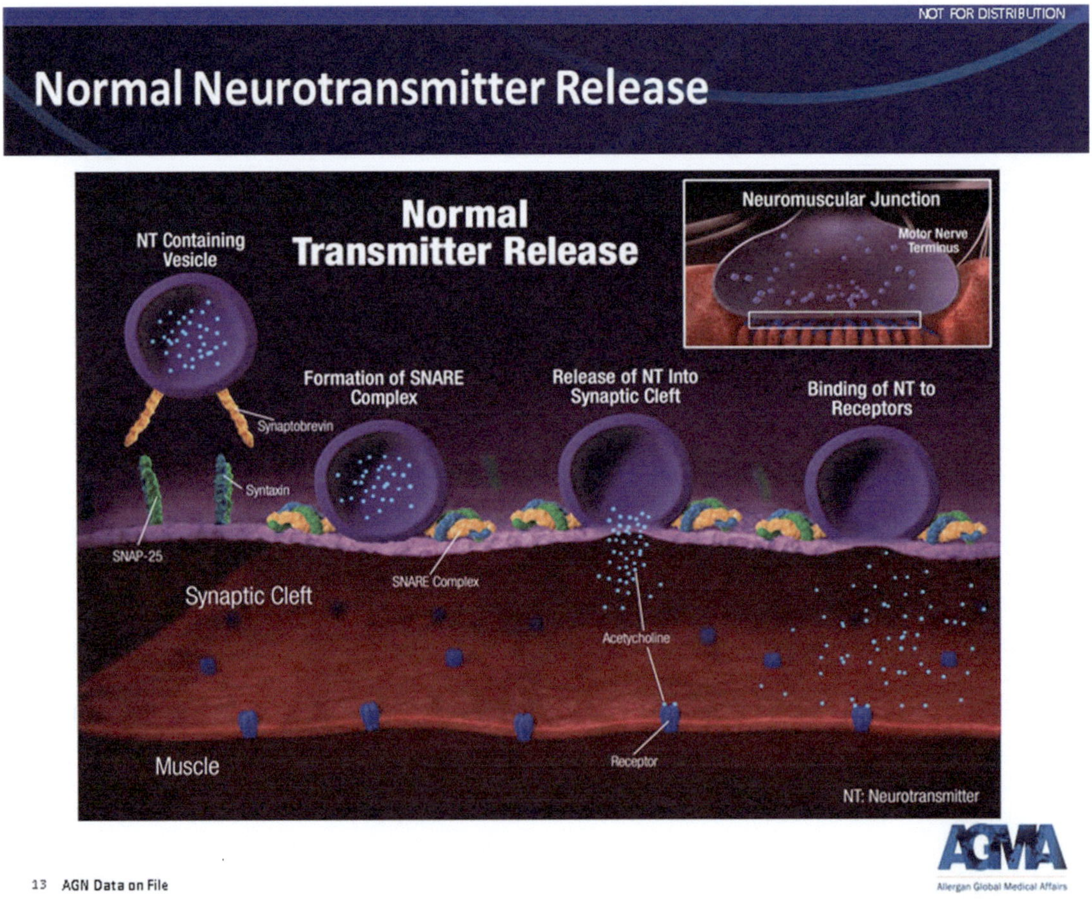

Fig. 6.1 Normal transmitter (acetylcholine) release in muscle. (Used with permission from Professor Bal Ram Singh, PhD, Institute of Advanced Sciences)

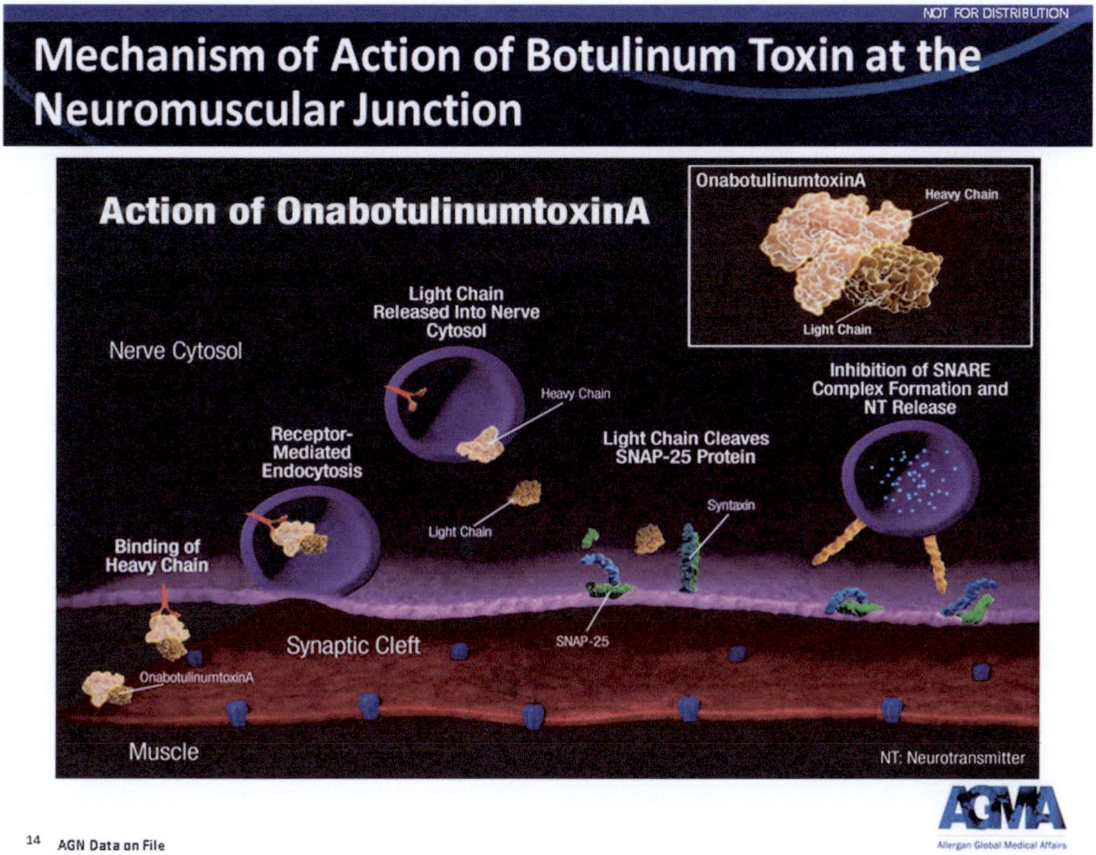

Fig. 6.2 Mechanism of action of onabotulinumtoxinA. Note the cleaving of the SNAP-25 complex. (Used with permission from Professor Bal Ram Singh, PhD, Institute of Advanced Sciences)

quent decrease in the formation of SNARE complexes and blocking acetylcholine release from the peripheral nerve cells into the neuromuscular junction (Figs. 6.1 and 6.2) [3, 5, 11]. Relaxation of the targeted muscle or muscle group temporarily leads to smoother overlying skin because the muscle is no longer able to fully contract and create rhytids. The smoothing results are temporary and last approximately 3 to 4 months, although the medication package insert states up to 6 months [8, 9, 12].

Of the five types of BoNT/A, onabotulinumtoxinA (Botox®) has 28 indications in 100 countries for treatment of a variety of conditions other than cosmetic applications including bladder spasms, hyperhidrosis, cervical dystonia, facial spasms, migraine headaches, blepharospasm, and depression. OnabotulinumtoxinA is also the most widely studied neurotoxin for therapeutic and cosmetic purposes, with over 2800 articles and over 400 peer-reviewed articles worldwide between 1986 and 2013 [8, 13].

6.2 Potential BoNT/A Adverse Reactions and Selected Imaging Technology for Treatment

Treatments with BoNT/A create a more refreshed, smooth, and alert appearance when done correctly. Unwanted side effects such as eyelid or eyebrow ptosis, asymmetry, or hematoma formation can occur if the practitioner is not properly trained or has little experience. However, some less significant side effects can still occur even in experienced hands such as swelling, redness, or bruising. Bruising can be almost entirely avoided with the use of imaging technology such as the laser emitting diode (LED) or near infrared (NIR) devices that use targeted light to illuminate superficial blood vessels under the skin surface. Available devices include AccuVein®, Veinlite®, and Intellivision, among others, and are used in hospitals, medical offices, and private practices to locate vessels for intravenous injection, phlebotomy, or aesthetic work (Fig. 6.3).

These devices work by using near infrared light-emitting diodes (NIR-LED) to visualize superficial veins because the hemoglobin absorbs the emitted light and forms an image on the skin surface. The NIR imaging uses light rays to penetrate into skin and acquire the images of venous structures and allows a deeper look below the skin for better contrast between skin and veins. In the electromagnetic spectrum, there is a low absorption window within NIR region in which light can penetrate deeper into the skin and tissues because of the low absorption range of hemoglobin, oxy-hemoglobin, and water which are main absorbers of radiations in skin [14]. This demonstrates hemoglobin affects visible light absorbance. In another example, a commonly used medical device, the pulse oximeter, measures absorption ratios of different wavelengths of oxygenated and deoxygenated blood and provides useful diagnostic information in the primary and acute care settings [15].

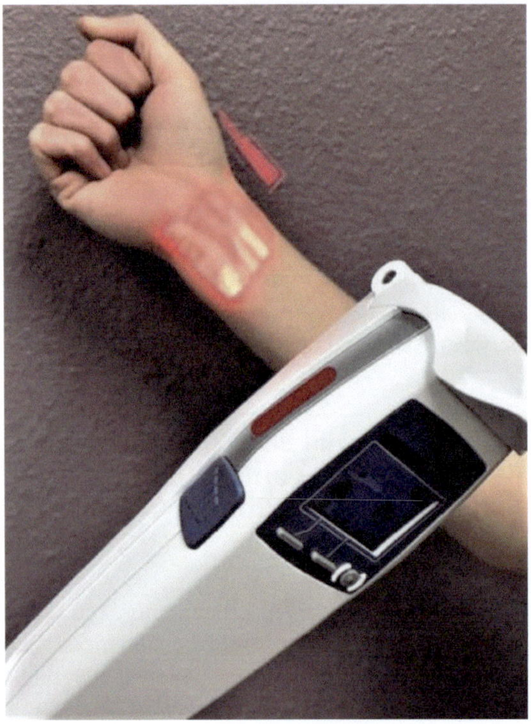

Fig. 6.3 The near infrared (NIR) light illuminates vessels under the skin and can help prevent bruising. (Photo: B. Haney, DNP, FNP-C, FAANP, FAAN)

Light emitting imaging technology devices are very helpful in locating veins through the varying degrees of light absorption and are effective ways to help prevent bruising in aesthetic practice by avoiding vein puncture. The other two common side effects, swelling and redness at injection site(s), are short-lived and do not typically last longer than 24–48 h, whereas bruising can be visible for weeks.

Several more and potentially longer-lasting side effects are eyelid and/or eyebrow ptosis or an asymmetrical outcome. Eyelid ptosis is a potential side effect of BoNT/A treatment that results in a heavy lid sensation and a sleepy appearance and can last for days or weeks. This unfavorable side effect is caused from diffusion of the BoNT/A into the levator palpebrae superioris and can be avoided by using precise injection technique [8–10, 12, 16]. This untoward outcome is easily avoided by accurate placement of the BoNT/A no closer than 1 CM above the bony orbital rim and injecting medial to the mid-pupillary line when treating the glabella area [16, 17]. The application of pressure under the orbital bone during injection of the corrugators may help prevent eyelid ptosis from solution spread during treatment. If necessary, eyelid ptosis can be treated with prescription apraclonidine or oxymetazoline (Upneeq®) drops that help to elevate the upper eyelid through stimulation of an adrenergic muscle located near the levator muscle called Muller's muscle [17–19]. These drops can be used as directed until the ptosis resolves, usually within minutes for oxymetazoline or several weeks for apraclonidine.

Eyebrow ptosis, on the other hand, can last for several months and results from too high a dose in the frontalis or injection sites placed too low. The patient might complain of heavy, flattened, dropped brows, and a completely immobile forehead with possible puffiness to the eyelids. The practitioner can avoid brow ptosis by injecting the procerus and corrugator muscles with the frontalis to ensure the counterbalance of depressor and elevator muscles [10, 16, 20]. In addition, injecting a small amount 1 CM above the orbital rim at the mid-pupillary line will help prevent brow ptosis [17, 21]. Further, injection of a low dose of BoNT/A at the lateral tail of the brow and procerus along with the frontalis can help prevent brow ptosis. Because of the depressor effect of treating the frontalis muscles, it is not recommended to treat the frontalis exclusively [10, 16, 17, 20].

Occasionally, patients might have a naturally asymmetrical appearance, and BoNT/A treatments are an effective option to correcting this issue. However, practitioners must be cautious and mindful that BoNT/A can *create* asymmetry if accurate placement is not used. For example, injections at different heights on the forehead might lead to one brow lower than the other on a patient with naturally symmetrical brows. Or, in addressing lip lines or nasalis lines, if too large a dose is used, lip dysfunction can result from diffusion of too much BoNT/A into the orbicularis oris and/or levator labii superioris muscle fibers. The patient may notice asymmetrical smiling, difficulty pronouncing certain words, inability to whistle or play musical instruments, and/or impaired drinking and eating [17, 22].

6.3 Potential Future Uses for Botulinumtoxin Type A (BoNT/A)

On-label uses of BoNT/A on the face include the glabella and orbital areas. The off-label cosmetic applications of BoNT/A include the infra-orbital muscles to treat fine wrinkles, the platysma to treat banding in the neck, the mentalis to treat dimpling of the chin, the depressor anguli oris to lift the oral commissures, and the nasalis muscle to treat bunny lines [23].

BoNT/A currently has other medical uses and is being studied for approval for a variety of indications by the US Federal Drug Administration (FDA). One novel FDA-approved indication is axillary hyperhidrosis (excessive underarm sweating), and some additional off-label dermatologic uses include acne, rosacea, scar reduction, pain, and psoriasis [24–26].

Researchers are currently considering multiple investigational applications of BoNT/A in medical specialties other than dermatology, including for treatment of psychiatric, gastroenterological, neurologic, gynecologic, and ophthalmic conditions [27]. This section will only focus on potential future uses of BoNT/A in aesthetic practice. However, a chart listing many of the medical conditions currently treated with BoNT/A is included in this section to demonstrate the emerging potential applications of BoNT/A (Table 6.1).

6.3.1 Hyperhidrosis

Excessive underarm sweating (axillary hyperhidrosis) is an approved indication for onabotulinumtoxinA (Botox®) and has been a welcome addition to the group of conditions treated by BoNT/A. Axillary hyperhidrosis (AH) is an embarrassing ailment for affected patients. The condition is the result of an overproduction of sweat beyond necessary body cooling, and approximately 3–5% of people in the United States experience this bothersome disorder [28]. Most people with AH become aware before age 25; however, those who suffer with palmar hyperhidrosis (PH) usually notice excessive palmar sweating prior to puberty [29].

In addition to BoNT/A, there are several approaches used to help control AH including topical application of aluminum chloride products, radiofrequency, or ultrasound treatments; and in intractable cases, surgical intervention. BoNT/A treatment is reserved for patients who fail the more conservative treatments such as antiperspirants [29].

The typical BoNT/A treatment for AH consists of 15–25 subdermal or subcutaneous injec-

Table 6.1 Therapeutic uses for botulinum neurotoxin

Ophthalmology
1. Strabismus[a,b,c]
2. Nystagmus
Neurology
1. Blepharospasm[a,b,c]
2. Cervical dystonia[a,b,c]
3. Writer's cramp[b]
4. Laryngeal dysphonia[c]
5. Hemifacial spasm[a,b,c]
6. Tremor (essential, Parkinsonism)
7. Tics
8. Bruxism
9. Focal spasticity[a,b,c]: Upper and lower limb spasticity
10. Cerebral palsy[a,b]
Hyperhidrosis[a,b,c]
1. Focal: Axillary, palmar, plantar
Hypersalivation
1. Sialorrhea[b] (motor neuron diseases/amyotrophic lateral sclerosis)
2. Drooling[b] (Parkinsonian syndromes)
Aesthetic (muscle)
1. Glabellar rhytids[a,b,c]
2. Lateral canthus (orbital)[a]
Pain
Muscular
1. Temporomandibular disorders
2. Low back pain
Non-muscular
3. Migraine[a]
4. Neuropathic pain
5. Trigeminal pain
6. Pelvic pain
7. Osteoarthritis
Urology
1. Overactive bladder[a,b,c] (idiopathic or neurogenic detrusor over-activity)
2. Urinary retention
3. Bladder pain syndrome
4. Pelvic floor spasms
5. Benign prostate hyperplasia
Gastroenterology
1. Chronic anal fissures
Psychiatry
1. Depression[d]

Adapted from Pirazzini et al. [30]
[a]USA approved indication
[b]EU approved indication
[c]Evidence-based therapeutic indication
[d]To be evaluated

tion sites per axilla of 2 units onabotulinumtoxinA or 5u abobotulinumtoxinA; however, the doses may vary slightly [28–30]. Pain control at injection sites includes ice applied immediately prior to and during treatment or topical anesthetic cream applied 30 min prior to treatment. The duration of the effect of BoNT/A in the axillae tends to be longer than intramuscular injection of the facial muscles, lasting about 6–9 months. The longer duration is likely due to the stimulation by the sympathetic division of the autonomic nervous system on the sweat glands, with acetylcholine acting as neurotransmitter between nerve endings and sweat glands [28, 29].

Palmar hyperhidrosis can also be treated with BoNT/A successfully when topical hyperhidrosis remedies fail; however, studies are limited, and this is an off-label indication. Treatment of PH can be a painful procedure, and topical anesthetic is usually warranted, but BoNT/A treatment is well tolerated and may improve quality of life in people who suffer with hyperhidrosis of the axillae and hands [31].

6.3.2 Acne

Acne is a common and often an embarrassing disease for both genders and can occur at various intervals during the lifespan from puberty through menopause. Treatments include topical and oral medications, acne washes, light-based treatments, and peels. One emerging use for intradermal BoNT/A is as an additional acne treatment, and it is currently being investigated [32].

Acne lesions form in the pilosebaceous unit and are influenced by hormones that lead to increased sebum production, and this increased sebum production leads to acne lesions and flares in susceptible individuals. Pore size has also been associated with sebum production [33]. Sebum production in human skin is increased through acetylcholine signaling; therefore, because BoNT/A blocks acetylcholine, sebum production is decreased. Literature supports that individuals with oily skin are more responsive to acetylcholine than those with normal skin because the concentration of acetylcholine receptors is higher in their sebaceous glands. For these reasons, BoNT/A intradermal injections significantly decrease sebum production in oily skin but not in those with normal skin [32, 34].

Another benefit of BoNT/A treatment in many people was the decrease in pore size [32, 34]. Pore size was found to be influenced by BoNT/A, and this can have a positive impact on the appearance of the skin. Oily skin, large pores, and scars add to the rough, uneven appearance of the skin and are problematic for many people who suffer with acne. Options to alleviate these concerns are increasing with the advancement of new uses and the advent of intradermal BoNT/A injections as an exciting new possibility for the treatment of acne [32, 35, 36].

6.3.3 Facial Scars

Scarring is a concern in those who undergo surgical procedures or closure of traumatic wounds, especially on the face [24, 37]. Scars from facial wounds and incisions can be unsightly, particularly in areas where muscle movement is frequent. The mechanism of BoNT/A results in the relaxation of muscles; therefore, it is postulated that the use of BoNT/A before, during, or after facial surgical procedures would decrease the tension on the closed edges of the incision and result in an improved cosmetic appearance [24, 25, 38].

There is some evidence that injecting surgical sites with the typical pre-procedure anesthetic and vasoconstrictor (lidocaine with epinephrine), mixed with BoNT/A, decreases the number of injections while also resulting in immediate local muscle paralysis [37, 39]. This local paralysis leads to improved cosmesis of facial scars because the surrounding muscle tension is decreased [38]. The reconstitution of BoNT/A with lidocaine and epinephrine did not affect the longevity or effect of the BoNT/A, and muscle function returned after 3 months [39]. Although re-constitution of BoNT/A with an anesthetic and/or vasoconstrictor is not recommended by drug manufacturers, it might be an acceptable option for scar prevention in the future.

6.4 Temporary Dermal Fillers

Globally, temporary dermal fillers are the second most requested, non-surgical facial aesthetic procedure behind BoNT/A treatments [40]. Practical knowledge of temporary dermal filler use, duration, and effect are important aspects of aesthetic practice, and the importance of understanding their intrinsic pharmacological aspects cannot be overemphasized. The practitioner must understand the various type(s) of filler used in the skin and tissues to achieve the most aesthetically pleasing and appropriate outcome.

There are several different categories of fillers, (1) temporary or biodegradable, (2) stimulant, and (3) permanent or non-biodegradable fillers. Each type of filler has specific requisites, and the choice depends on several factors including the desired result, skin condition, and average product longevity to determine which is used on the patient.

Permanent dermal filler discussion is beyond the scope of this chapter; however, temporary dermal fillers will be the focus, and some of the information provided herein will pertain to all types of dermal filler products. The temporary fillers composed of hyaluronic acid (HA), calcium hydroxyapatite (CaHA), and poly-L-lactic acid (PLLA) fillers will be discussed as they are most commonly used by aesthetic practitioners. Although all three of these temporary filler products are popular, only one has the distinguishing property of reversibility, the HA temporary fillers. The ability to reverse HA fillers easily with hyaluronidase makes them an attractive option for many providers and patients.

6.5 Hyaluronic Acid (HA) Fillers

Hyaluronan, or HA, is a naturally occurring linear polysaccharide that is found in the skin, epithelial, connective, and other tissues. Hyaluronan is innate in human skin and lacks a protein component so it does not require allergy skin testing prior to injection, making it a convenient product to use for facial applications. HA is hydrophilic and is able to bind 1000 times its molecular weight in water so it makes a good substance for adding volume to skin and facial tissue [41, 42]. In youth, humans have an abundance of HA in the skin, and it contributes to the fullness in skin appearance. As we age, the amount of naturally occurring HA in skin decreases, and subsequently, we begin to produce less HA. This phenomenon plays an important role in the appearance of aging, wrinkle formation, decreased tissue elasticity, and hydration [41, 43].

In its natural state, HA has an approximate half-life of 24–48 h before it is broken down and metabolized in the liver into water and carbon dioxide [41, 43–46]. In the skin, HA is broken down by hyaluronidase and free radicals [42, 43, 47]. Natural HA injected into the skin would break down quickly through enzymatic action so would not be appropriate for cosmetic purposes due to its short duration and minimal effect in aesthetic patients.

Advanced processes have been developed through available technology that have led to longer-lasting HA products that can endure for months or years. The HA molecules are stabilized using crosslinking technology with hydroxyl groups and provide the long-lasting qualities of modern HA fillers. The crosslinking agent in the Restylane® and Juvederm® HA families of products is 1,4-butanediol diglycidyl ether (BDDE) [42, 43, 48, 49]. These developments have made injectable HA stable and more resistant to break down.

The different HA families of filler are developed using slightly different technologies. The Juvederm® family of products are sterile, biodegradable, non-pyrogenic, viscoelastic, clear, colorless, homogenized gel implant produced by *Streptococcus equi* bacteria, developed through a fermentation process, and crosslinked with BDDE [42, 48]. The Restylane® family of products are made of hyaluronic acid generated by a *Streptococcus* species of bacteria, also chemically crosslinked with BDDE, stabilized and suspended in phosphate buffered saline [49]. Belotero Balance® is a HA product that is sterile, non-pyrogenic, viscoelastic, homogenous, clear gel implant bacterially fermented, manufactured from *Streptococcus* bacteria, and crosslinked with BDDE [50].

The HA fillers also differ in particle size, crosslinking of the HA molecules, the amount of crosslinking in the product, as well as the G-prime or viscosity of the product. These product features guide the practitioner in choosing the appropriate filler for specific effects ranging from smoothing superficial lines to bone augmentation [41, 42, 50].

6.5.1 G-Prime and Particle Size

G-prime is a measurement of the stiffness of the hyaluronic gel product and helps determine the appropriate area and depth for placement in the skin. Generally, thicker products are not suitable for placement in the superficial layers of skin due to the possibility of long-lasting swelling, uneven result, and the Tyndall effect – residual visibility of the product as a bluish tint [41].

G-prime also contributes to the increased longevity of the effect of the HA products, i.e. the higher the G-prime, the longer the filler might last [41, 42, 44, 47]. The modern, crosslinked HA dermal fillers of the Belotero®, Juvederm®, and Restylane® families of products, are frequently used to replace volume or soften fine lines in the face. These fillers include both crosslinked or high weight, *and* non-crosslinked or low weight, HA molecules within their gel vehicle. The higher the concentration of crosslinked HA molecules, the longer the effect will last [41, 42, 47, 51, 52].

After injection into the skin, the non-crosslinked hyaluronic acid is quickly broken down, and only the crosslinked, larger molecular weight polymers are left behind. The reason for the low weight, non-crosslinked molecules in the product allows easier injection through the needle or cannula [42, 43]. If the gel consisted of purely large weight, crosslinked molecules, the product would not be conducive to injection through a small caliber needle [52].

Particle size is another relevant aspect of the HA fillers. Particles are formed into specific sizes through different processes employed by each manufacturer. In one sizing method, particle size is created through a process where crosslinked HA is pushed through a customized screen to create different, specific sizes of the particles. Smaller sizes are made into lower G-prime, or less viscous products, whereas the larger particle sizes are made into the higher G-prime, or more viscous products [42, 44]. To date, there is no scientific data on which process yields the preferred longevity profile or outcome.

The concentration of the different HA products is listed in Table 6.2 [7, 44, 48–50, 53–56].

HA fillers break down slowly over time, but on occasion, a small number of patients may experience a diminished effect within an unreasonably short time period. Comparison of clear, pre-treatment photographs with pre-treatment, post-treatment, and recent photographs generally demonstrates the effect of the filler. Visual documentation is very important to capture objective images, especially in aesthetic practice. The subjective patient perception is one of the myriad of reasons to take pre-treatment photographs.

Table 6.2 Various concentrations and particle sizes of HA fillers

Product	Concentration of HA	Particle size
Restylane	20 mg/mL	250 μm
Restylane Lyft	20 mg/mL	650 μm
Restylane Refyne	20 mg/mL	–
Restylane Defyne	20 mg/mL	–
Juvederm	24 mg/mL	Varies
Juvederm ultra plus	24 mg/mL	Varies
Juvederm Voluma	20 mg/mL	–
Belotero	22.5 mg/mL	N/A

While some have the same concentration, larger particle size create longer-lasting effects

6.6 Calcium Hydroxyapatite (CaHA): Radiesse®

Calcium hydroxyapatite (CaHA) is the generic name for the temporary filler, Radiesse®, and is made of the same compound as human bone [57, 58]. Initially, CaHA was used as a treatment for urinary stress incontinence, as a radiographic marker, and for vocal cord restoration [59–62]. CaHA was first approved in the United States in 2006 for aesthetic treatment of naso-labial folds (NLF) and lipoatrophy of HIV [57].

CaHA is an opaque, sterile, non-pyrogenic, semi-solid, cohesive implant, whose principal component is synthetic calcium hydroxyapatite suspended in a gel carrier of glycerin, sodium carboxymethylcellulose, 0.3% lidocaine hydrochloride, and sterile water [63]. CaHA is made up of 70% carrier gel, and the remaining 30% is CaHA microspheres that are suspended in an injectable gel. These elements of CaHA make it radiopaque and visible on CT scans and x-ray studies [59]. CaHA injectable implant (1.5 cc and 0.8 cc) has a calcium hydroxyapatite particle size range of 25–45 μg and should be injected with a 25 gauge outer diameter to 27 gauge inner diameter needle [41, 63].

During injection of CaHA into the skin, the gel evenly distributes the CaHA microspheres for a uniform placement and dispersal. The product requires no skin testing prior to administration, and this makes it a convenient choice for facial augmentation [58]. The carrier gel dissipates within several weeks, and the CaHA microspheres remain in the tissue at the injection site until they slowly breakdown into calcium and phosphate ions [57]. After injection of the product, the carrier gel is broken down and phagocytized. The remaining CaHA particles act as a support substance or *scaffolding* that allows for new collagen formation [41].

Post-market studies indicate CaHA can last up to 2 years, and it also induces collagenesis when correctly placed in the skin, and in susceptible patients, this collagenesis might contribute to the lasting effect of this filler [41, 57, 63]. However, in older patients with less skin elasticity, collagenesis from CaHA placement may be decreased, and these patients might require larger amounts of product or more frequent treatments.

6.7 Poly-L-Lactic Acid (PLLA): (Sculptra®)

Poly-L-Lactic Acid (PLLA) is the generic name for the temporary filler, Sculptra®, and was first FDA approved in 2004 for treatment of facial lipoatrophy associated with Human Immunodeficiency Virus (HIV) [64, 65]. PLLA is the active and durable ingredient and is a synthetic biodegradable polymer that is used for soft tissue augmentation. It is a freeze-dried powder of PLLA and must be rehydrated with 5 mL sterile water per vial prior to injection. The particle size of PLLA is 40–60 μm [41, 66].

Stimulation of an inflammatory tissue response produced by PLLA leads to collagen deposition in the skin. Sculptra® is composed of PLLA microparticles, sodium carboxymethylcellulose, and nonpyrogenic mannitol [66, 67]. The package insert recommends product rehydration for 2 h; however, 48 h has proven more successful clinically by reducing the incidence of undesired nodule formation. The volume correction outcome with PLLA has been shown to last up to 2 years [67, 68].

After the product is injected, the PLLA component is hydrolyzed into lactic acid monomers that induce a localized foreign body tissue response through the recruitment of monocytes, macrophages, and fibroblasts. Subsequently, a capsule is formed around each microsphere as the lactic acid is metabolized, and the result is collagen deposition by the host fibroblasts. The new tissue volume is the result of dermal fibroplasia and increased dermal thickness [65, 67].

PLLA is biodegradable and biocompatible and has been used in medical devices such as absorbable sutures and mesh [67]. Due to its unique mechanism of action, the volumizing effects of PLLA treatment will not be immediate, although the initial fullness from the sterile water diluent is temporarily noticeable, and patients usually require more than one treatment session [66, 67]. The initial fullness from injection of the sterile water diluent typically resorbs within 24-48 h [68].

The novice injector is wise to avoid the temptation to bring the area to full corrected state when using PLLA because it generally requires more than one treatment session to allow time for adequate collagen formation [65, 67]. Therefore, a series of treatments is recommended to avoid overcorrection. The final outcome is dependent on the number of treatment sessions, and the patient should be informed visible PLLA effects can take up to 2 months.

Patient expectations, possible side effects, and treatment outcomes of dermal fillers should be reviewed with the patient at every visit to ensure the patient understands the characteristics of the appropriate dermal filler for their aesthetic concern. PLLA has a unique mechanism of action and ingredient that requires practitioner knowledge of product handling and injection technique to avoid a poor outcome. Factors that can contribute to poor outcome and nodule/papule formation while using PLLA include the following [41, 68]:

1. Placement of product that is too superficial.
2. Product injected into active muscles.
3. Inadequate product hydration time.
4. Poor suspension of particles.

It is important to note that many aesthetic patients expect to see improvement quickly and they might become anxious or disappointed if the results are not clearly visible within a short amount of time. This concern has led some practitioners to use a HA filler at the same time of PLLA treatment so the patient will notice an immediate improvement [69].

6.8 Complications of Dermal Fillers

Adverse reactions from temporary dermal fillers are generally classified as early onset (up to 1 week after treatment) or late onset (weeks to years after treatment). However, most delayed onset reactions are associated with the non-biodegradable fillers such as silicone, polyacrylamide, and polymethylmethacrylate [41]. Early onset adverse reactions include injection site reactions, nodules, Tyndall effect (hyaluronic acid fillers), infection, hypersensitivity, and vascular compromise leading to tissue necrosis [41, 70]. Late or delayed onset adverse reactions include infection, biofilm formation, and granuloma formation; however, any or all of these can occur in temporary or non-biodegradable filler types as well [41]. There are steps practitioners can take to avoid several of these complications such as obtaining a thorough patient medical history, properly preparing the skin for the procedure by cleansing and disinfecting the treatment area, using aseptic technique during the procedure, using appropriate amounts of product, and utilizing vessel visualization using technology. Laser emitting diode (LED) or near infrared (NIR) devices that use targeted light to illuminate superficial blood vessels under the skin surface are helpful in avoiding bruising (see earlier discussion).

There are other technologies, such as ultrasound, that are useful in locating deeper anatomic structures and relationships. Ultrasound has been used in a variety of medical settings including cardiology, critical care, obstetrics and gynecology, and more recently, aesthetics. Using an ultrasound device can assist the aesthetic practitioner in locating deeper facial structures such as glands and, more importantly, vessels [71, 72]. Facial mapping of this extent offers an extra layer of patient safety and practitioner confidence. More detail is discussed in the Facial Danger Zones chapter.

6.9 Conclusion

Dermal filler and BoNT/A treatments are the two most popular aesthetic procedures in the world and have proven to be effective for skin improvement, volume replacement, and overall appearance. Understanding product mechanisms of action, proper placement and technique, use of imaging devices when appropriate, and awareness and management of potential complications are crucial to success and will ensure the best outcome for the patient.

References

1. Vigliante CE. Anatomy and functions of the muscles of facial expression. Oral Maxillofac Surg Clin North Am. 2005;17(1):1–15. v
2. Tamura BM. In: Issa BT, editor. Facial anatomy view for aesthetic fillers injections. Berlin: Springer International; 2018.
3. Rizo J, Sudhof TC. The membrane fusion enigma: SNAREs, Sec1/Munc18 proteins, and their accomplices—guilty as charged? Annu Rev Cell Dev Biol. 2012;28:279–308.
4. Frevert J. Pharmaceutical, biological, and clinical properties of botulinum neurotoxin type a products. Drugs R D. 2015;15(1):1–9.
5. Aoki KR, Guyer B. Botulinum toxin type a and other botulinum toxin serotypes: a comparative review of biochemical and pharmacological actions. Eur J Neurol. 2001;8(Suppl 5):21–9.
6. Daxxify medication guide. Revance Aesthetics. 2022. https://revance.com/wp-content/themes/allen-larson-theme/files/daxi-pi-andmed-guide.pdf.
7. Alam M, Tung R. Injection technique in neurotoxins and fillers: planning and basic technique. J Am Acad Dermatol. 2018;79(3):407–19.
8. Allergan. Botox cosmetic prescribing information. Package insert. 2017.
9. LLC MP. Xeomin Full Prescribing Information. 2018.
10. Carruthers J, Carruthers A. The use of botulinum toxin type a in the upper face. Facial Plast Surg Clin North Am. 2006;14(3):253–60.
11. Patil S, Willett O, Thompkins T, Hermann R, Ramanathan S, Cornett EM, et al. Botulinum toxin: pharmacology and therapeutic roles in pain states. Curr Pain Headache Rep. 2016;20(3):15.
12. Inc. IB. Dysport Full Prescribing Information. 2017.
13. Mohindru A, Bulloch S, Kronfeld N, et al. Analysis of clinical and non-clinical, peer reviewed, published studies investigating the use of commercially available botulinum toxins: an online literature review. In: Poster presented at: Second International Congress on Treatment of Dystonia (ICTD).
14. Shahzad A, Saad MN, Walter N, Malik AS, Meriaudeau F. Hyperspectral venous image quality assessment for optimum illumination range selection based on skin tone characteristics. Biomed Eng Online. 2014;13:109.
15. Thom CS, Dickson CF, Gell DA, Weiss MJ. Hemoglobin variants: biochemical properties and clinical correlates. Cold Spring Harb Perspect Med. 2013;3(3):a011858.

16. Lorenc ZP, Smith S, Nestor M, Nelson D, Moradi A. Understanding the functional anatomy of the frontalis and glabellar complex for optimal aesthetic botulinum toxin type a therapy. Aesthetic Plast Surg. 2013;37(5):975–83.
17. Carruthers A, Carruthers J. In: Dover JS, editor. Procedures in cosmetic dermatology: botulinum toxin. Philadelphia, PA: Elsevier Saunders; 2005. p. 141.
18. Upneeq prescribing information. Upneeq.com. 2023. https://www.upneeq.com/wp-content/uploads/2022/10/Upneeq-PI-IFU.pdf.
19. Wijemanne S, Vijayakumar D, Jankovic J. Apraclonidine in the treatment of ptosis. J Neurol Sci. 2017;376:129–32.
20. Carruthers A, Carruthers J. Eyebrow height after botulinum toxin type a to the glabella. Dermatol Surg. 2007;33(1):S26–31.
21. Kordestani R, Small KH, Rohrich RJ. Advancements and refinement in facial neuromodulators. Plast Reconstr Surg. 2016;138(4):803–6.
22. Carruthers J, Carruthers A. Aesthetic botulinum a toxin in the mid and lower face and neck. Dermatol Surg. 2003;29(5):468–76.
23. Carruthers J, Carruthers A. Botulinum toxin a in the mid and lower face and neck. Dermatol Clin. 2004;22(2):151–8.
24. Goodman GJ. The use of botulinum toxin as primary or adjunctive treatment for post acne and traumatic scarring. J Cutan Aesthet Surg. 2010;3(2):90–2.
25. Gassner HG, Sherris DA, Otley CC. Treatment of facial wounds with botulinum toxin a improves cosmetic outcome in primates. Plast Reconstr Surg. 2000;105(6):1948–53; discussion 54–5.
26. Baumeister JC, Papa G, Foroni F. Deeper than skin deep—the effect of botulinum toxin-a on emotion processing. Toxicon. 2016;118:86–90.
27. Magid M, Keeling BH, Reichenberg JS. Neurotoxins: expanding uses of neuromodulators in medicine—major depressive disorder. Plast Reconstr Surg. 2015;136(5 Suppl):111S–9S.
28. Rosen R, Stewart T. Results of a 10-year follow-up study of botulinum toxin a therapy for primary axillary hyperhidrosis in Australia. Intern Med J. 2018;48(3):343–7.
29. Rzany B, Bechara FG, Feise K, Heckmann M, Rapprich S, Worle B. Update of the S1 guidelines on the definition and treatment of primary hyperhidrosis. J Dtsch Dermatol Ges. 2018;16(7):945–52.
30. Pirazzini M, Rossetto O, Eleopra R, Montecucco C. Botulinum neurotoxins: biology, pharmacology, and toxicology. Pharmacol Rev. 2017;69(2):200–35.
31. Wade R, Llewellyn A, Jones-Diette J, Wright K, Rice S, Layton AM, et al. Interventional management of hyperhidrosis in secondary care: a systematic review. Br J Dermatol. 2018;179(3):599–608.
32. Shuo L, Ting Y, KeLun W, Rui Z, Rui Z, Hang W. Efficacy and possible mechanisms of botulinum toxin treatment of oily skin. J Cosmet Dermatol. 2019;18(2):451–7.
33. Habif TP. Clinical dermatology: a color guide to diagnosis and therapy. 6th ed. Amsterdam: Elsevier; 2016.
34. Li ZJ, Park SB, Sohn KC, Lee Y, Seo YJ, Kim CD, et al. Regulation of lipid production by acetylcholine signalling in human sebaceous glands. J Dermatol Sci. 2013;72(2):116–22.
35. Hanna E, Xing L, Taylor JH, Bertucci V. Role of botulinum toxin A in improving facial erythema and skin quality. Arch Dermatol Res. 2022;314(8):729–38. https://doi.org/10.1007/s00403-021-02277-0.
36. Schlessinger J, Gilbert E, Cohen JL, Kaufman J. New uses of Abobotulinumtoxin A in aesthetics. Aesthet Surg J. 2017;37(suppl_1):S45–58.
37. Sherris DA, Gassner HG. Botulinum toxin to minimize facial scarring. Facial Plast Surg. 2002;18(1):35–9.
38. Ziade M, Domergue S, Batifol D, Jreige R, Sebbane M, Goudot P, et al. Use of botulinum toxin type a to improve treatment of facial wounds: a prospective randomised study. J Plast Reconstr Aesthet Surg. 2013;66(2):209–14.
39. Gassner HG, Sherris DA. Addition of an anesthetic agent to enhance the predictability of the effects of botulinum toxin type a injections: a randomized controlled study. Mayo Clin Proc. 2000;75(7):701–4.
40. Surgery ISoAP. ISAPS International Survey on Aesthetic/Cosmetic Procedures. 2021.
41. Carruthers JC. In: Dover J, editor. Soft tissue augmentation. 3rd ed. Amsterdam: Elsevier; 2013.
42. Bogdan Allemann I, Baumann L. Hyaluronic acid gel (Juvéderm™) preparations in the treatment of facial wrinkles and folds. Clin Interv Aging. 2008;3(4):629–34.
43. Bray D, Hopkins C, Roberts DN. A review of dermal fillers in facial plastic surgery. Curr Opin Otolaryngol Head Neck Surg. 2010;18(4):295–302.
44. Duranti F, Salti G, Bovani B, Calandra M, Rosati ML. Injectable hyaluronic acid gel for soft tissue augmentation. A clinical and histological study. Dermatol Surg. 1998;24(12):1317–25.
45. Reed RK, Laurent UB, Fraser JR, Laurent TC. Removal rate of [3H]hyaluronan injected subcutaneously in rabbits. Am J Physiol. 1990;259(2 Pt 2):H532–5.
46. Laurent UB, Dahl LB, Reed RK. Catabolism of hyaluronan in rabbit skin takes place locally, in lymph nodes and liver. Exp Physiol. 1991;76(5):695–703.
47. Tezel A, Fredrickson GH. The science of hyaluronic acid dermal fillers. J Cosmet Laser Ther. 2008;10(1):35–42.
48. Allergan. Juvederm Voluma XC package insert. Dublin: Allergan; 2013.
49. Galderma. Restylane Lyft with Lidocaine Package Insert. 2018.
50. Flynn TC, Thompson DH, Hyun SH. Molecular weight analyses and enzymatic degradation profiles of the soft-tissue fillers Belotero balance, Restylane,

and Juvederm ultra. Plast Reconstr Surg. 2013;132(4 Suppl 2):22S–32S.
51. Muti GF. Midface 3D restoration with an innovative high G' filler. J Cosmet Dermatol. 2021;20(Suppl 2):7–11.
52. da Costa A, Biccigo DGZ, de Souza Weimann ET, Mercadante LM, Oliveira PRG, Prebianchi SB, et al. Durability of three different types of hyaluronic acid fillers in skin: are there differences among biphasic, monophasic monodensified, and monophasic polydensified products? Aesthet Surg J. 2017;37(5):573–81.
53. Allergan. Juvederm XC product insert. 2016.
54. Galderma. Restylane Refyne PI. 2016.
55. Galderma. Restylane Defyne PI. 2016.
56. Greene JJ, Sidle DM. The hyaluronic acid fillers: current understanding of the tissue device Interface. Facial Plast Surg Clin North Am. 2015;23(4):423–32.
57. Ridenour B, Kontis TC. Injectable calcium hydroxylapatite microspheres (Radiesse). Facial Plast Surg. 2009;25(2):100–5.
58. Lee JC, Lorenc ZP. Synthetic fillers for facial rejuvenation. Clin Plast Surg. 2016;43(3):497–503.
59. Carruthers A, Liebeskind M, Carruthers J, Forster BB. Radiographic and computed tomographic studies of calcium hydroxylapatite for treatment of HIV-associated facial lipoatrophy and correction of nasolabial folds. Dermatol Surg. 2008;34(Suppl 1):S78–84.
60. Belafsky PC, Postma GN. Vocal fold augmentation with calcium hydroxylapatite. Otolaryngol Head Neck Surg. 2004;131(4):351–4.
61. Rees CJ, Mouadeb DA, Belafsky PC. Thyrohyoid vocal fold augmentation with calcium hydroxyapatite. Otolaryngol Head Neck Surg. 2008;138(6):743–6.
62. Mevorach RA, Hulbert WC, Rabinowitz R, Kennedy WA, Kogan BA, Kryger JV, et al. Results of a 2-year multicenter trial of endoscopic treatment of vesicoureteral reflux with synthetic calcium hydroxyapatite. J Urol. 2006;175(1):288–91.
63. Aesthetics M. Radiesse lidocaine injectable implant. Frankfurt am Main: Merz North America; 2016.
64. Engelhard P, Humble G, Mest D. Safety of Sculptra: a review of clinical trial data. J Cosmet Laser Ther. 2005;7(3–4):201–5.
65. Humble G, Mest D. Soft tissue augmentation using sculptra. Facial Plast Surg. 2004;20(2):157–63.
66. Galderma. Sculptra Aesthetic Prescribing Information. 2016.
67. Schierle CF, Casas LA. Nonsurgical rejuvenation of the aging face with injectable poly-L-lactic acid for restoration of soft tissue volume. Aesthet Surg J. 2011;31(1):95.
68. Narins RS. Minimizing adverse events associated with poly-L-lactic acid injection. Dermatol Surg. 2008;34(Suppl 1):S100–4.
69. Attenello NH, Maas CS. Injectable fillers: review of material and properties. Facial Plast Surg. 2015;31(1):29–34.
70. DeLorenzi C. Complications of injectable fillers, part 2: vascular complications. Aesthet Surg J. 2014;34(4):584–600.
71. Safran T, Gorsky K, Viezel-Mathieu A, Kanevsky J, Gilardino MS. The role of ultrasound technology in plastic surgery. J Plast Reconstr Aesthet Surg. 2018;71(3):416–24.
72. Cral WG. Ultrasonography and facial aesthetics. Aesthetic Plast Surg. 2021;46:999.

Dermal Fillers for Facial Rejuvenation

7

Arun K. Garg

Abstract

The term *facial rejuvenation* refers to several different categories of treatments designed to improve the appearance of the face: plastic surgery such as rhinoplasty, blepharoplasty, and rhytidectomy; less invasive procedures such as dermal abrasions and chemical peels; and the growing list of minimally invasive therapies, including laser skin resurfacing, microdermabrasion, neurotoxin injections, and dermal filler injections. Dermal fillers are administered in a very short timeframe and have immediate results. This chapter explores the benefits of using dermal fillers and different methods regarding facial rejuvenation that support aesthetic procedures and correlate with positive results.

Keywords

Wrinkles · Anesthesia · Fillers · Microneedling · Chin augmentation · Scars · Frown lines · Nasolabial folds · Mental crease

A. K. Garg (✉)
University of Miami School of Medicine, Miami, FL, USA

7.1 Introduction

In 2019, the American Society of Plastic Surgeons reported that from 2000 to 2018, the number of facelift surgeries declined 9%, while the number of neurotoxin injections increased by a whopping 845%. Similarly, dermal filler treatments have increased 244% since 2006, the first year for which data were collected (Table 7.1) [1]. As these numbers demonstrate, neurotoxins and dermal fillers have radically changed the market for facial rejuvenation procedures in the United States, and this upward trend is expected to continue for at least the next several years.

Some of the reasons for this are obvious. Neurotoxins such as Botox Cosmetic (Allergan) and Dysport (Galderma) and dermal fillers can usually be administered in less than an hour; they produce effects that are apparent immediately or within days; and they require little or no downtime. Moreover, these aesthetic enhancements are subtle enough not to attract attention and thus can be undertaken discreetly, which many people appreciate. Indeed, the intent of these procedures is not to make a person look 20 years younger but rather for them to appear more radiant and refreshed at their present age (Fig. 7.1).

Unlike surgical procedures, neurotoxin and dermal filler treatments are luxuries that fit many budgets. At an average cost of $397 and $682 per site for neurotoxin and dermal filler (e.g., Juvéderm, Allergan) injections, respectively,

R. L. Bard (ed.), *Image-Guided Aesthetic Treatments*, https://doi.org/10.1007/978-3-031-36266-8_7

Table 7.1 Facial cosmetic procedure trends in the United States since 2000

Procedure	2018	2000	Change
Facelift (rhytidectomy)	121,531	133,856	−9%
Nose reshaping (rhinoplasty)	213,780	389,155	−45%
Eyelid surgery (blepharoplasty)	206,529	327,514	−37%
Botulinum toxin type A[a] injection	7,437,378	786,911	+845%
Soft tissue fillers[b] injection	2,676,970	778,000[c]	+244%

Data reported by the American Society of Plastic Surgeons (https://www.plasticsurgery.org/documents/News/Statistics/2018/cosmetic-procedure-trends-2018.pdf)
[a] Includes Botox, Dysport, and Xeomin
[b] Includes all commercial dermal fillers as well as platelet-rich plasma and acellular dermal matrix
[c] Number of procedures in 2006, the year data was first reported

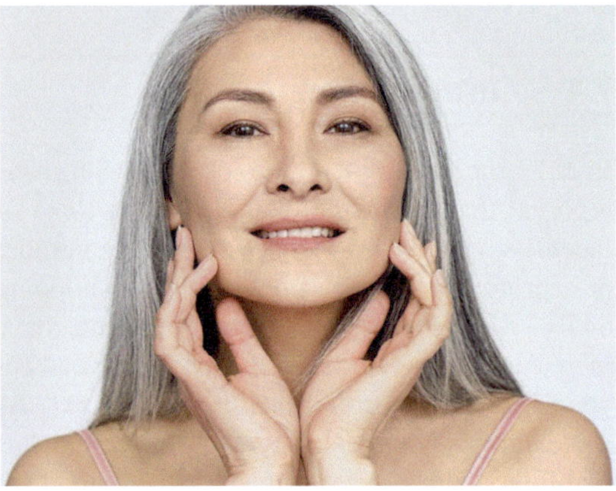

Fig. 7.1 The effects of neurotoxin and dermal filler treatments are subtle and appear natural, unlike plastic surgery procedures

these treatments are comparable to the cost of a day at the spa. Compare those numbers to the average cost of a simple rhinoplasty ($5350) or dermabrasion ($1250) [1].

The relative affordability of minimally invasive procedures makes them appealing to people at all income levels, including those who likely would never consider seeking surgical treatment to address their age-related aesthetic concerns. The popular stereotype that middle-aged women are the ones primarily driving this trend is not at play here. The so-called daddy do-over has been quietly gaining in popularity for several years, and the average age of patients skews younger all the time as more 20- and 30-somethings seek dermal filler treatment for acne scars, nose recontouring, lip augmentation, and other cosmetic enhancements. In 2018, individuals aged 20–39 made up 18% of all neurotoxin injections and 11% of dermal filler treatments [1].

7.2 Neurotoxins and Dermal Fillers: Understanding the Differences

Currently, there are approximately three neurotoxin procedures for every dermal filler procedure performed in the United States (7.4 million vs. 2.6 million) [1]. Botox, the first commercially available neurotoxin, was initially developed and gained FDA approval in 1989 as a therapeutic agent for the treatment of strabismus, an eye muscle disorder. Today, Botox is used to treat neck spasms (cervical dystonia), excessive sweating (hyperhidrosis), and an overactive bladder, among many other conditions. Botox Cosmetic was not FDA approved until 2002, just shortly before the approval of the first hyaluronic acid dermal filler in 2003.

7.3 Dynamic Versus Static Wrinkles

Although the aim of these injectable agents is the same—to smooth facial wrinkles—they achieve it through very different mechanisms of action. Cosmetic neurotoxin targets the dynamic lines of expression that result from repetitive facial movement (Fig. 7.2). It is injected directly into the muscles that animate these types of wrinkles, including frown lines, crow's feet, and forehead creases. The muscles become para-

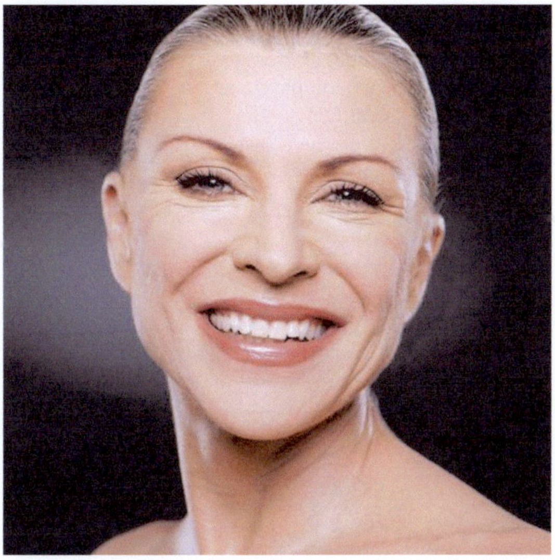

Fig. 7.2 Neurotoxins target the dynamic lines and folds of facial expression

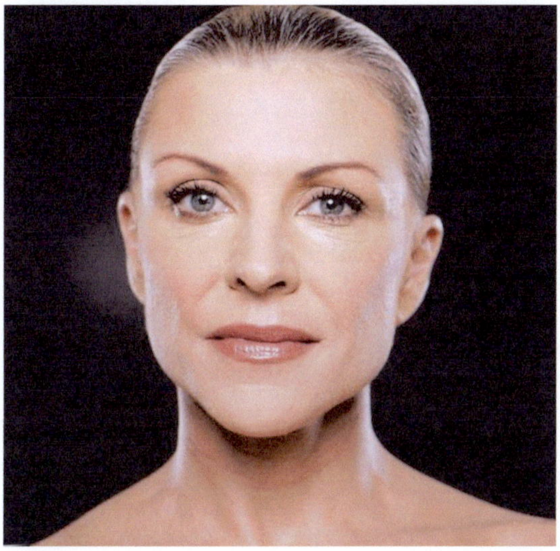

Fig. 7.3 Dermal fillers target the static lines and wrinkles that are manifestations of aging on skin

lyzed, and within 2 to 3 days, the lines and wrinkles disappear. These effects last an average of 3 to 4 months. Unlike neurotoxins, dermal fillers target static wrinkles, the ones we develop over time as we age (Fig. 7.3). These static wrinkles are present regardless of facial expression and usually accompany other visible effects of aging, such as hollowed cheeks and eye sockets, irregular or blotchy pigmentation, skin laxity, and dryness. These facial manifestations of intrinsic aging are a result of reduced collagen production and slower cell turnover rates. (Their appearance can, however, be accelerated by extrinsic factors such as chronic sun exposure and smoking.) Intrinsic aging is a natural consequence of physiologic changes over time that occur at variable yet genetically determined rates. In some lucky people, these lines, wrinkles, and folds do not make an appearance until they reach 55 or 60 years old, whereas others begin to see them in their late 30 s and 40 s, but for all of us they are an inevitable effect of aging.

Nevertheless, our society spends billions of dollars each year on expensive elixirs and procedures in our never-ending quest to prevent and diminish the visible signs of aging on our skin. Moreover, every year, the industry expands with new agents and modalities added to the long list of topical medical products (vitamin A acid, α-hydroxy acids, antioxidants, and moisturizers) and procedures (glycolic acid peels, deep peels, dermabrasion, laser resurfacing, and plastic surgery) already available (Table 7.2).

This chapter focuses exclusively on the treatment of a subset of static wrinkles and defects associated with aging: nasolabial folds, marionette lines, mental crease, malar and chin recession, frown lines, and scars. Based on his experience as an educator, the author has found that these conditions are relatively easy for novice practitioners to treat, and the outcomes are generally good. Coincidentally, the areas targeted by these procedures exhibit some of the earliest signs of aging, so patient demand for them is usually high.

Step-by-step instructions for treating these areas are preceded by a discussion of anesthesia techniques, a guide to choosing dermal filler products, and a complete how-to on performing facial microneedling. The latter is a simple yet effective procedure that provides all-over skin rejuvenation and perfectly complements the targeted dermal filler injections that are the main subject of this chapter.

Table 7.2 Costs and total expenditures of the multibillion-dollar industry to combat aging[a]

Procedure	National average surgeon/physician fee	Total expenditure
Cosmetic surgical procedures		
Cheek implant (malar augmentation)	$3015	$43,322,535
Chin augmentation (mentoplasty)	$2364	$38,769,600
Dermabrasion	$1249	$100,790,553
Ear surgery (otoplasty)	$3163	$72,382,092
Eyelid surgery (blepharoplasty)	$3156	$651,805,524
Facelift (rhytidectomy)	$7655	$930,319,805
Forehead lift	$3623	$140,554,285
Lip augmentation (other than injectable materials)	$1767	$54,527,853
Lip reduction	$2009	$2,147,621
Neck lift	$5424	$280,819,182
Nose reshaping	$5350	$1,143,723,000
Cosmetic minimally invasive procedures		
Botulinum toxin type A (Botox, Dysport, Xeomin)	$397	$2,952,639,066
Chemical peel	$669	$926,114,763
Injection lipolysis (e.g., Kybella [Allergan])	$1054	$67,448,622
Intense pulsed light (IPL) treatment	$391	$264,140,832
Laser hair removal	$285	$307,084,650
Laser skin resurfacing		
Ablative	$2071	$332,878,043
Nonablative (Frazxel [Solta Medical], etc.)	$1144	$495,961,752
Microdermabrasion	$131	$92,933,103
Nonsurgical skin tightening (Pelleve [Cynosure], Thermage [Solta Medical], Ultherapy [Ulthera])	$2059	$690,362,110
Soft tissue fillers		
Acellular dermal matrix	$2065	$17,707,375
Calcium hydroxyapatite (Radiesse [Merz North America])	$691	$157,018,694
Fat—face	$2126	$96,435,360
Hyaluronic acid (e.g., Juvéderm Ultra, Ultra Plus, Voluma, Volbella, and Vollure, Restylane Lyft and Silk [Galderma], Belotero [Merz North America])	$682	$1,451,925,486
Platelet-rich plasma (PRP)	$683	$87,010,102
Polylactic acid (Sculptra [Garderma])	$915	$111,556,800
Polymethyl-methacrylate microspheres (Bellafill [Suneva Medical])	$889	$15,614,396
Total 2018 expenditures		**$16,507,440,034**

[a] Data from the American Society of Plastic Surgeons [1]

7.4 Anesthesia for Dermal Fillers

In facial aesthetics, patients often assess the quality and success of treatment based not on the outcome, but on the process. Pain control is an integral part of the process.

7.4.1 Noninvasive Anesthesia Techniques

7.4.1.1 Cooling Therapy and Vibration

There are many different forms of cooling therapy that offer safe, simple, and effective pain

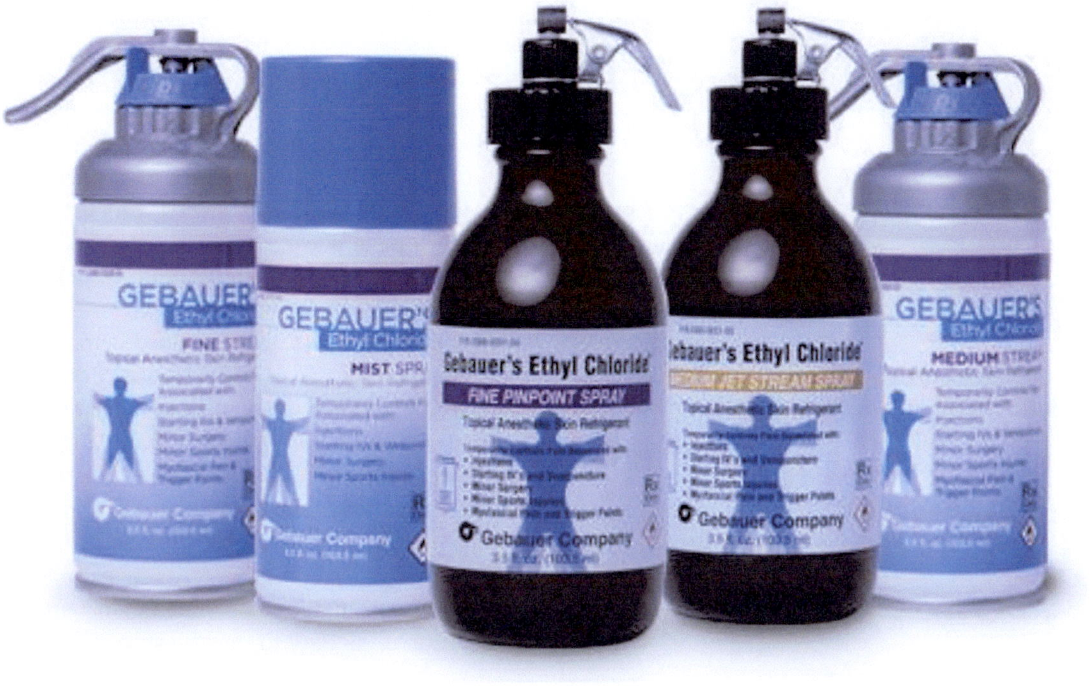

Fig. 7.4 Topical ethyl chloride (Gebauer) can be used to numb the injection site prior to injection of dermal fillers

control at the site of the injection. Ice packs, vapocoolants, and contact cooling devices can be used alone or in conjunction with topical anesthetics as a pretreatment for pain. Covered ice can be applied to the skin for about 1 to 2 min to numb injection sites [2, 3]. While this method will only blunt the pain at best, it is safe, inexpensive, and easy. Spraying the injection site with a vapocoolant, such as topical ethyl chloride (Fig. 7.4) or dichlorotetrafluoroethane skin refrigerant, desensitizes topical nerves immediately upon application. This method is less cumbersome than ice packs, fast-acting, and cost-effective. However, the spray should only be used in the cheek and nasolabial folds area, and caution should be exercised for those at risk for reactive hyperpigmentation [2]. Alternatively, contact cooling devices (Fig. 7.5), again applied to the injection site for only 1 to 3 min until the skin is erythematous, not only anesthetize the treatment area, but can also reduce post-treatment ecchymosis and swelling at the site due to the vasoconstrictive effects of the cold. However, prolonged contact at one site can result in injury to the epidermis.

Vibration (Fig. 7.6) has also been shown to be an effective method to minimize the pain of dermal filler injections [2]. The application of a vibration device to an area adjacent to the injection site is thought to reduce pain through stimulation-induced analgesia – a concept associated with the gate control theory of pain – and by relaxing facial muscles [3, 4]. The vibration is applied concurrently with the injection (Fig. 7.7) or just before it is administered, depending on the model used, and it is completely safe.

7.4.1.2 Topical Anesthesia

Topical anesthetics offer the same nerve-blocking qualities as injectables and can increase patient comfort when used separately or in conjunction with injectable anesthetics [5]. Lidocaine, alone or in combination with another anesthetic, is the most widely used topical anesthetic [6]. Today, many commercially prepared dermal fillers add lidocaine to the product, allowing patients with high resistance to pain the option to receive topi-

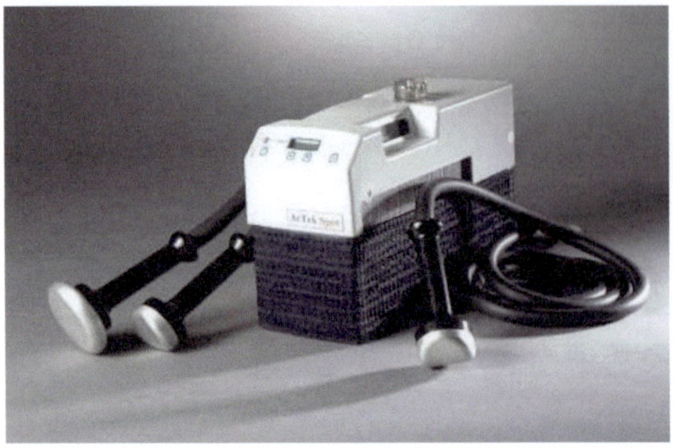

Fig. 7.5 A contact dermal cooling device (ArTek Spot, ThermoTek) not only numbs the skin but reduces post-treatment bruising and swelling as well

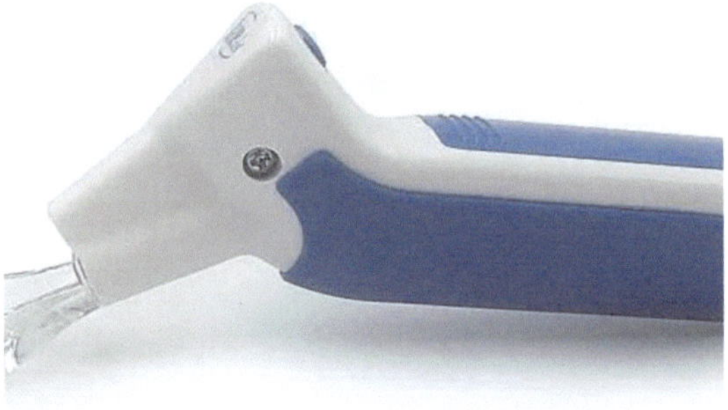

Fig. 7.6 A vibration anesthesia device (Blaine Labs) achieves its effect through stimulation-induced analgesia and muscle relaxation

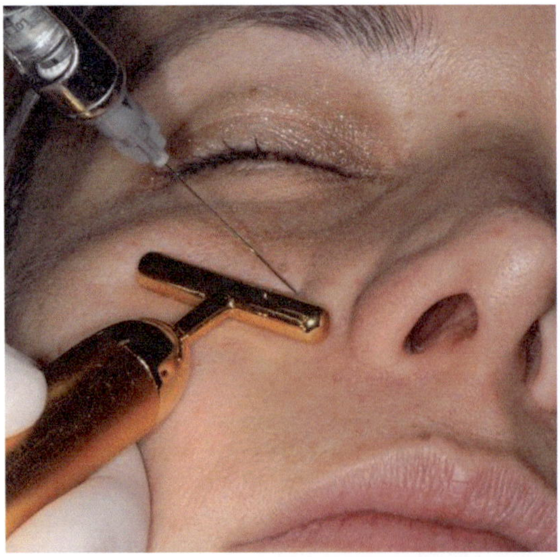

Fig. 7.7 Vibration anesthesia device applied concurrently with anesthesia injection

cal anesthetics alone in lieu of injectable anesthetics.

The effectiveness of a topical anesthetic depends on the depth of skin penetration, the location of the skin surface, the length of exposure time, and the concentration of the ingredients [6]. Table 7.3 lists several properties of different topical anesthetic types [7]. Most topical anesthetics take effect within 15 min of administration of a 0.5-mg dose.

Few complications are associated with the use of topical anesthesia (Table 7.4) [6]. For facial dermal filler procedures, topical anesthetic is applied on a relatively small surface area, and therefore the risk of toxicity is minor. The risk of this complication increases when these agents are used on larger surface areas, such as in certain laser treatments [6].

Topical anesthetic procedures begin with the application of alcohol to remove skin oils and to

Table 7.3 Properties of topical anesthetics

Topical anesthetic	Maximum dose	Onset (min)	Duration of effect (min)
Lidocaine	500 mg	<2	30–45
Lidocaine with prilocaine	60 mg	<60	60–120
Tetracaine	20 mg	3	45

Table 7.4 Complications associated with topical anesthesia

Adverse event	Signs and symptoms
Allergic reaction	Pruritis and papules locally, and the remote possibility of urticaria, angioedema, and anaphylaxis
Lidocaine toxicity of the central nervous system	Dizziness, tongue numbness, tinnitus, diplopia, nystagmus, slurred speech, seizures, respiratory distress
Lidocaine toxicity of the cardiovascular system	Arrhythmias, hypotension, cardiac arrest
Tetracaine toxicity of the central nervous system	Restlessness, agitation, seizure activity
Lidocaine, tetracaine, or prilocaine can cause methemoglobinemia	Cyanosis, acidosis

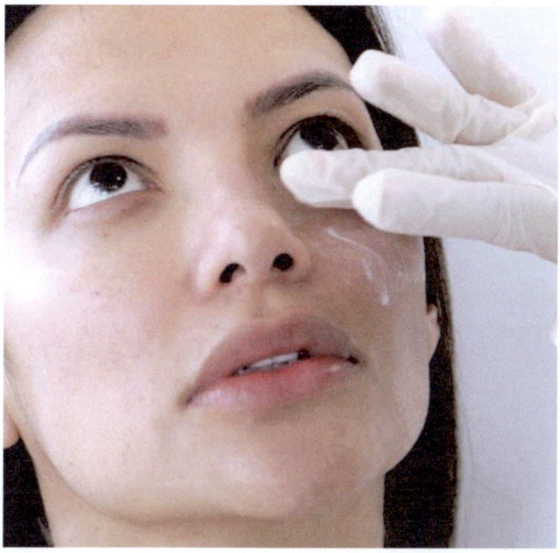

Fig. 7.8 A topical anesthetic cream will generally take effect within about 5 min and last at least 30 min, depending on the formulation

boost the penetration of the anesthetic. The anesthetic can then be rubbed directly on the skin either with gloved hands or a cotton applicator (Fig. 7.8). Alcohol is used again to remove the anesthetic once the nerve-blocking effect has been achieved.

7.4.2 Injectable Anesthesia

Local infiltration and ring blocks are the two most common methods of administering injectable lidocaine in small doses (0.5 to 6.0 mL). Local infiltration of a solution of 0.1-mL buffered lidocaine with epinephrine is used for most of the procedures covered in this chapter (Figs. 7.9 and 7.10). It usually requires a series of 3 to 6 subcutaneous injection sites, which should raise the skin slightly but not dimple it. Table 7.5 lists the maximum dose that should be given to an adult according to body weight [7]. Patients who are especially anxious or who have a low pain threshold for needle injections can be preemptively treated with any of the noninvasive anesthetic techniques described earlier. Alternatively, the clinician can apply a topical anesthetic about 15 min prior to treatment.

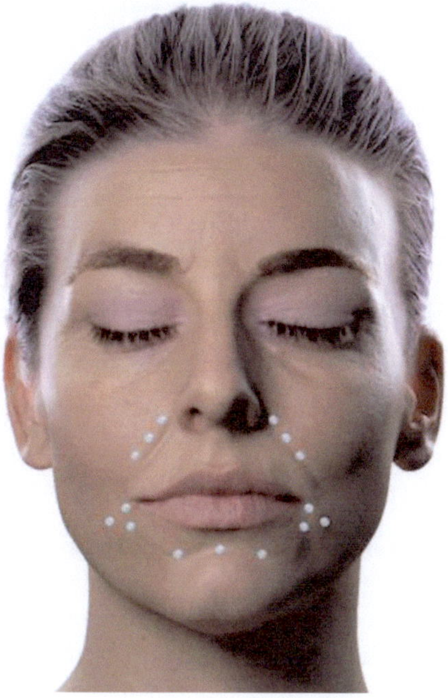

Fig. 7.9 Locations for local anesthetic infiltration in preparation for basic dermal filler treatment

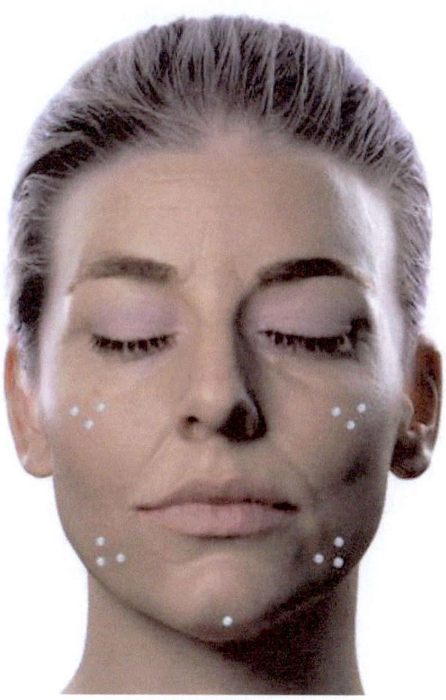

Fig. 7.10 Locations for local anesthetic infiltration in preparation for advanced dermal filler treatment

Table 7.5 Maximum dose of 2% lidocaine (20 mg/mL)

Lidocaine solution	Max adult dose by body weight	Max injection volume for 140 lb (64 kg) adult
2% lidocaine without epinephrine	4.5 mg/kg	13 mL
2% lidocaine with epinephrine	7 mg/kg	22 mL

Table 7.6 Properties of the ideal dermal filler

Safety	Efficacy	Practicality
Nonimmunogenic	Long-term benefit	Cost-effective
Noncarcinogenic	Natural feeling	Easy to use
Nonteratogenic	Nonmigratory	FDA-cleared
Noninfectious	Reproducible results	Removable or reversible
		Long shelf life

7.4.2.1 Local Infiltration Method

An 18-gauge, 1.5-in. needle is used to draw 1.0-mL buffered 2% lidocaine-epinephrine into a 1.0-mL syringe; the needle is then removed and replaced with a 30-gauge, 0.5-in. needle (unless otherwise directed). After the injection site has been cleaned with alcohol, 0.1 mL of the solution is injected at a time. Subsequent injections are administered on both sides of the face in accordance with the complexity of the site. Compression of the injected solution away from the treatment site can help reduce edema.

7.5 Dermal Filler Selection

A one-size-fits-all approach to facial augmentation will not yield optimal results. As dermal filling options continue to expand and evolve, the clinician must understand the unique properties and characteristics of each product and apply that knowledge to developing an individual treatment plan for each patient. Table 7.6 lists the qualities of an ideal filler product in terms of its safety, effectiveness, and convenience [8–10].

Dermal fillers can be classified in terms of *longevity*, *biodegradability*, and *mechanism of action*. In terms of longevity, facial dermal fillers are usually described as short-acting, long-acting, or "permanent," but there is wide latitude in how these terms are defined. Generally speaking, a short-acting filler can be expected to last up to 1 year, a long-acting filler up to 2 years, and a filler labeled as permanent (an obvious misnomer) for 5 years or more [11, 12]. In most discussions, duration of effect of a given product is a relative concept that makes reference to other products as the standard of comparison.

Biodegradability, which has a major impact on a product's longevity, is another classification that strays into gray territory [13, 14]. A product or agent can be labeled as (*1*) a biodegradable filler, (*2*) a filler with biodegradable particles, or (*3*) a nondegradable filler. Biodegradable fillers are fully reabsorbed by the body and are consequently short-lived. Fillers with biodegradable particles act by stimulating a response in the body to produce its own collagen before resorbing, which results in a longer-lasting effect. Nondegradable fillers are dual-acting: They induce a foreign-body reaction that stimulates the deposition of new collagen, but the nondegradable particles ultimately become permanently integrated into the connective tissue of the skin.

As the discussion of biocompatibility suggests, fillers can also be classified according to their mechanism of action [15, 16]. In this category, a distinction is made between a *volumizer*, which is a filler that achieves its effect by taking up space (giving added importance to the amount of product injected), and a *stimulator*, one that in some way induces the body to produce new collagen. Again, some products fit neatly into one of these two categories, while others fall somewhere in between.

Many products are used off-label by experienced dermatologists; the present discussion is restricted to those that have been cleared by the US Food and Drug Administration (FDA) for specific facial cosmetic indications.

7.5.1 Short-Acting Fillers

The two materials in this category are collagen and hyaluronic acid, both of which are natural components of human tissue. Although it was once the gold standard, collagen has been shown to resorb too rapidly and is no longer being used for dermal fillers.

7.5.1.1 Hyaluronic Acid

Hyaluronic acid (HA) is the most popular class of filler in the United States [17]. Produced naturally by the body and found in high concentrations in the skin, HA binds collagen and water together to provide hydration and augmentation. It is naturally biocompatible and resorbs at a slow rate. Because of its excellent moisture-retention capacity, HA is a key ingredient in many high-end skin care products on the market today. HA fillers are easy to handle and provide natural-looking results with little downtime. They also boast an important safety advantage over other types of fillers in that they can be immediately and safely reversed with hyaluronidase, making them especially favored by inexperienced clinicians.

HA filler products differ in terms of their rheologic and physicochemical properties (e.g., degree of HA concentration, particle size, consistency, viscosity, hardness, degree of water solubility, cross-linking technology), which play an important role in HA filler selection, location and plane of injection, and clinical outcomes. Juvéderm (Allergan), which is available in several different formulations, is the undisputed market leader, followed by Restylane (Galderma) and Belotero Balance (Merz North America). In general, more concentrated products with a greater degree of cross-linking (a manufacturing process used to slow resorption rate) provide increased longevity, but they have on occasion been associated with a higher risk for inflammation and nodule formation [18–20]. In addition, a higher G' (elasticity) means a stiffer gel and a deeper injection plane, and conversely a lower G' indicates a softer gel and a more superficial plane of injection [13]. Skin quality, degree of skin laxity, and anatomical location are some of the clinical factors that must be considered when selecting a product. Understanding the rheologic properties of the various HA products can make esthetic enhancement safer and more predictable.

7.5.2 Long-Acting Fillers

This category includes commercial products made of calcium hydroxyapatite and poly-L-lactic acid as well as cells harvested from the patient's own fat and blood tissues.

7.5.2.1 Calcium Hydroxyapatite

Calcium hydroxyapatite (CaHA) fillers provide immediate volume replacement while also stimulating a response in the body to produce its own collagen, resulting in a longer-lasting effect. CaHA is nonallergenic and inherently biocompatible, and it has a well-established safety profile. When used as a dermal filler, CaHA usually lasts for a minimum of 1 year before it is fully resorbed by the body.

Currently, only one CaHA dermal filler product is FDA cleared for use in the United States. Radiesse (Merz North America) consists of 30% synthetic CaHA microspheres suspended in a 70% aqueous carboxymethylcellulose gel carrier. The soluble carrier distributes the CaHA microspheres and gradually dissipates, while the microspheres induce neocollagenesis via fibroblast activation. Radiesse has a high G' and is highly viscous compared to other dermal fillers, a property that allows it to remain in place when it is injected and not migrate [15]. In 2009, a protocol for mixing Radiesse with lidocaine was approved by the FDA. This formulation significantly increases patient comfort during the injection process.

7.5.2.2 Poly-L-Lactic Acid

Poly-L-lactic acid (PLLA) is a synthetic polymer that is probably familiar to most readers as a key component of Vicryl sutures (Ethicon). PLLA is not a volumizer in the technical sense because it does not achieve its effect by taking up space. Its singular mechanism of action is the stimulation of neocollagenesis, which means that it restores but does not replace lost volume. Consequently, its full effects are gradual, requiring 3 to 4 injections performed at least 4 to 6 weeks apart. However, many patients continue to see improvement 2 years after the initial injection.

The injection protocol for PLLA is less convenient and more technique-sensitive than that of other fillers. The freeze-dried PLLA powder must be reconstituted in sterile water at least 24 h before the scheduled injection in order to form a suspension. To ensure a uniform concentration, PLLA should be injected at room temperature to avoid the risk of an uneven response. Also, because the effects of the filler are delayed, it is essential not to overcorrect, which puts patients at increased risk of developing minute palpable nodules at the injection site that can last as long as 1 year [21]. Over time, the PLLA microparticles are metabolized by the body and expelled as carbon dioxide. Sculptra Aesthetic (Galderma) is the only PLLA dermal filler available in the United States. It is primarily indicated for broad dermal correction rather than smoothing individual rhytids and is contraindicated in and around the lips. With regard to the procedures described in this chapter, Sculptra is ideal for augmentation of the malar areas and the chin.

7.5.2.3 Autologous Fat

Autologous fat transfer (AFT), also known as *lipofilling*, is a low-risk procedure that offers a number of advantages that many patients find attractive. First, fat grafts not only have an immediate volumizing effect on grooves and wrinkles, but stem cells that exist in the fat tissue are a rich source of growth factors that stimulate new collagen production. Second, most patients are delighted to be relieved of the extra fat around their abdomen or thighs. Third, because the filler consists of the patient's own cells, the risk of an allergic reaction is nonexistent. So far, however, most studies report disappointing long-term outcomes, primarily because of unpredictable resorption of up to 70% of the volume of the fat graft [22, 23]. Furthermore, there is strong disagreement among clinicians as to the ideal method for harvesting and handling the fat grafts [23]. Therefore, its long-term results are variable and unpredictable.

7.5.2.4 Platelet-Rich Plasma

Another autologous dermal filler option, platelet-rich plasma (PRP) offers all the benefits of lipofilling but without the drawbacks associated with fat graft harvesting [24]. Commonly used in orthopedics, cardiovascular surgery, plastic surgery, oral/maxillofacial surgery, and other surgical procedures to promote healing, PRP is inherently biocompatible and delivers an abundance of stem cells and other growth factors. Because it requires only a simple venipuncture procedure, it is significantly less painful, less invasive, and less expensive to harvest than autologous fat (Fig. 7.11). Adding PRP to facial lipofilling can reduce recovery time and improve the overall esthetic outcome.

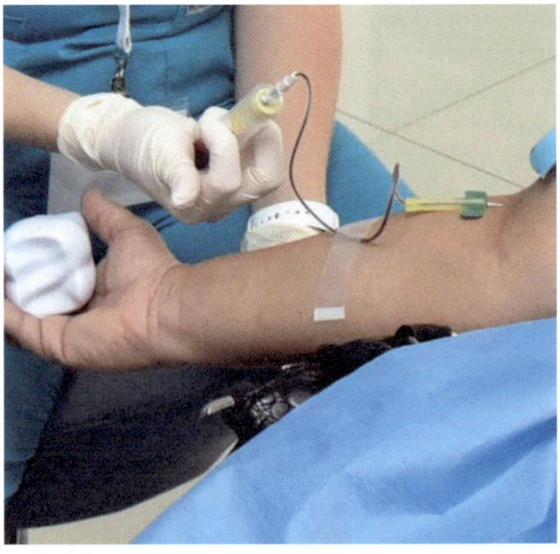

Fig. 7.11 PRP requires a venipuncture to draw the patient's blood but eliminates the cost of using a commercial product

7.5.3 Permanent Fillers

The "holy grail" among dermal filler manufacturers is a product that boasts the safety profile of HAs but without resorption and promises a permanent (5+ years) improvement in facial appearance. Today, only one agent has been shown to approach that ideal.

7.5.3.1 Polymethylmethacrylate

To date, the only "permanent" filler material approved by the FDA is composed of polymethylmethacrylate (PMMA), a nonbiodegradable, biocompatible, synthetic polymer that is also used in various medical materials and devices. A PMMA dermal filler is made of tiny microspheres carried in a collagen gel. When injected, it initiates a foreign body reaction that eventually leads to the production of new collagen. The collagen carrier provides immediate volume and lift in the short term, while the nonbiodegradable PMMA microspheres have a long-term "bulking" effect [25].

Bellafill (Suneva Medical) was the first (and so far only) PMMA dermal filler to be FDA-cleared (under a different trade name) for the correction of folds and wrinkles. It consists of 20- to 50-μm microspheres of PMMA suspended in a bovine collagen gel carrier, which acts as a glue, preventing the microspheres from clumping and allowing for new tissue ingrowth. Because the collagen is derived from an animal source, skin allergy testing is required 4 weeks prior to treatment. The collagen carrier is absorbed within 1 month of injection and replaced by the patient's connective tissue within 3 months [2]. The inherent downside to a "permanent" filler is that it is less forgiving when mistakes are made or complications arise.

7.6 Dermal Microneedling

As noted earlier, dermal filler injections and microneedling are complementary aesthetic treatments: Whereas dermal fillers target specific age-related wrinkles and volume deficits, dermal microneedling restores firmness and elasticity to the entire face.

Microneedling, also known as *collagen induction therapy*, delivers hundreds of tiny, invisible punctures to the top layer of facial skin. These micro injuries stimulate the body's natural wound-healing processes, leading to cell turnover and the production of new collagen and elastin. In addition, when topical serums such as PRP or HA are applied to the skin immediately after microneedling, nutrients fill the channels created by the microneedling to enhance the production of healthy new skin.

When performed correctly, microneedling creates approximately 200 punctures per square centimeter of facial skin. The microneedles penetrate 1.5 mm to 2 mm into the dermis (Fig. 7.12); at this depth, the needles cut through the epidermis but do not destroy it. Although the epidermis is only about 0.2 mm thick, it serves as the body's sole protection from the environment. Therefore, the epidermis, and particularly the stratum corneum, must remain intact.

Microneedling causes minimal bleeding because the needle penetrates for just a few fractions of a second and only capillaries are punctured. Nonetheless, this brief trauma elicits a mild inflammatory response, probably due to the release of histamine by mast cells. Researchers believe that each time the roller movement is repeated, the cells in the microchannels respond anew, temporarily putting them in an activated state. This leads to enhanced motility of epithelial and endothelial cells in the wounded area and subsequently stimulates gene expression of growth factors that facilitate healing [26]. Skin improvement is evident 3 to 4 weeks after a microneedling treatment.

7.6.1 Choosing a Microneedling Device

As the popularity of microneedling has increased over the past 5 years, the number of microneedling vendors and devices has also proliferated, making the process of selecting an appropriate

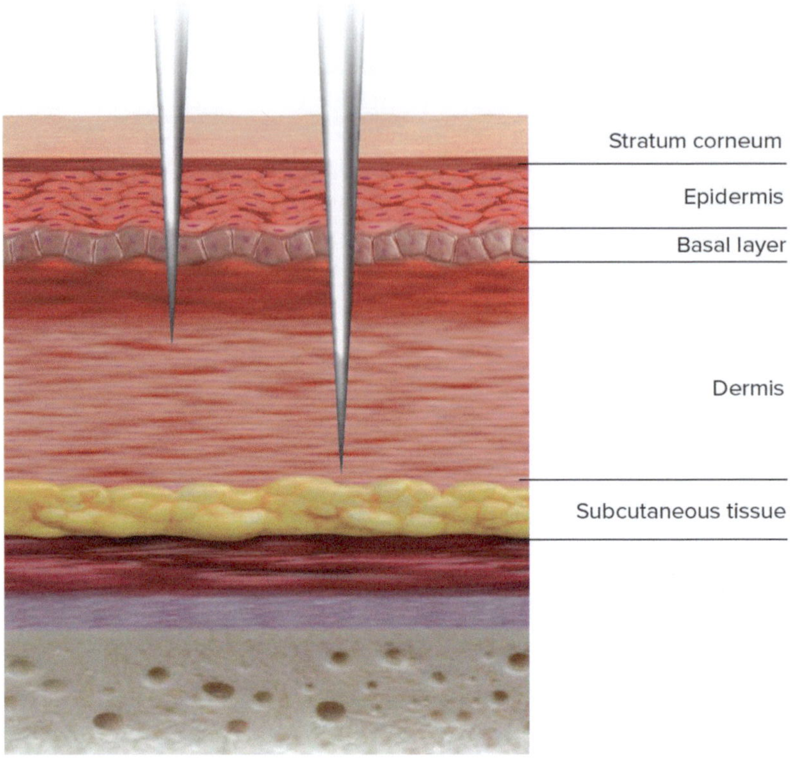

Fig. 7.12 Dermal fillers are injected into different layers according to the desired outcome. Injections in the mid to deep dermis (**a**) are generally administered using the linear thread technique, whereas those in the hypodermis (**b**) are made with the depot technique

device confusing and difficult. The following guidelines should help.

A majority of the products advertised on the Internet are intended for consumer use. The key difference in these devices is the length of the needles. Medical-grade dermal needling devices have needles ranging from 0.2 mm up to 3.0 mm. Longer needles are not considered safe for consumer use because of concerns about infection risk and potential contraindications, among other factors. Most consumer models have needles of 0.2 to 0.3 mm in length. Readers will want a professional model that is designed for single use to eliminate any risk of patient cross-contamination, but they should choose one with needles made of high-quality surgical steel or titanium and a comfortable grip.

Dermal rollers come in all sizes and shapes, with needles ranging from a single-row cluster of 24 to a multi-row cluster of 540. The number of rows is mostly a matter of personal preference, but keep in mind that some patients have very small facial features that will be challenging to navigate with a broad microneedling roller. However, the most important factor to consider is the length of the needles (Fig. 7.13). As noted previously, a variety of needle lengths are available. Figure 7.13 illustrates how deeply each standard needle length penetrates into the epidermis and dermis. For the average patient who presents for general anti-aging treatment of the face, choose a needle length no shorter than 0.5 mm and no longer than 1.5 mm to avoid reaching the dermis.

7.6.2 Topical Adjuncts

To amplify the regenerative effects of microneedling, PRP or HA is applied topically immediately after the procedure, where it is absorbed through the created microchannels to reach the epidermal and dermal layers of the skin.

PRP works by stimulating the proliferation of mesenchymal stem cells and fibroblasts, which secrete HA and type I collagen. When applied

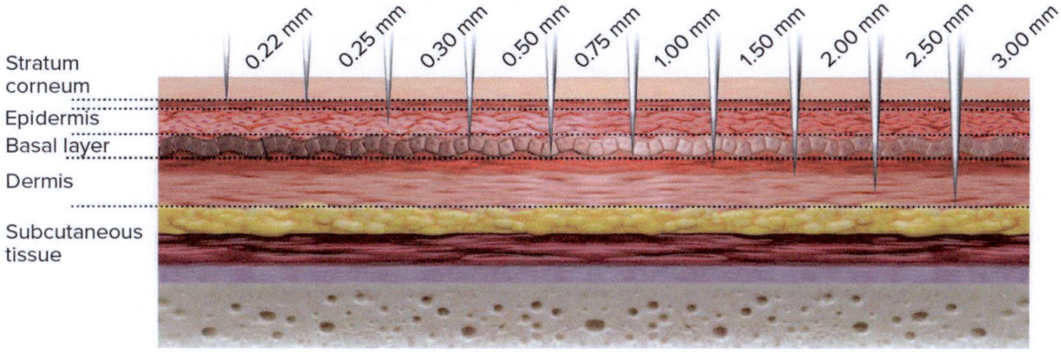

Fig. 7.13 The three basic layers of skin and microneedling

topically following microneedling treatment, PRP has been shown to improve skin texture, color homogeneity, elasticity, and firmness [27]. The adjunctive use of PRP with microneedling is low-cost, minimally invasive, and low-risk. For best results, the procedure should be repeated two to three times at intervals of 8 to 10 weeks. PRP is created by drawing the patient's blood, centrifuging it, and concentrating the blood's rich assortment of growth factors. This simple procedure is performed chairside and requires minimal investment by the clinician.

HA is a natural component of skin and the principal molecule involved in skin moisture. A key cause of aging in skin is the marked disappearance of epidermal HA, which results in dehydration, atrophy, and a gradual loss of elasticity [18]. Commercially available as both a topical and a dermal filler, hyaluronic acid has virtually no risk for allergic reaction. Topical HA serum can replenish moisture to the skin following microneedling to improve the appearance of fine lines and wrinkles.

7.6.3 Anesthesia

Microneedling treatment with needles of 2 mm or shorter is associated with minimal pain, and the procedure can be carried out under topical anesthesia, two key factors in its popularity among patients [28]. A variety of anesthetic creams are readily available for this purpose. Most patients who undergo microneedling under topical anesthesia report experiencing little to no pain during the procedure [29].

Treatments involving the use of needles that are longer than 2 mm require careful consideration of the most effective type of anesthesia to use, particularly in sensitive facial areas such as near the eyebrows, nose, and upper lip. Generally, dental blocks should be used in the perioral region and any other extremely sensitive areas. Patients should be instructed not to take any nonsteroidal anti-inflammatory drugs (NSAIDs) before a treatment procedure due to their coagulating effect. The use of an oral analgesic 1 h before the procedure is permitted, however. Valtrex (GlaxoSmithKline) can be used prophylactically by patients who are subject to getting cold sores as a result of microneedling.

7.6.4 Microneedling Procedure

7.6.4.1 Clinical Preparation

Before the procedure, make sure the patient has signed a consent for treatment and a complete set of patient photographs has been taken.

To begin, the patient's hair should be pulled back with a hair band or covered with a cloth cap. The patient's face should be thoroughly cleaned with an antiseptic cleanser and then wiped with alcohol. Do not use povidone. Next, a thin layer of topical anesthetic cream is applied over the treatment areas, keeping it away from the eyes. Although the onset of the anesthesia is typically less than 1 min, it is important to wait 15 min for a complete numbing effect, which should then last for 30 to 60 min. After 15 min, the anesthetic cream should be wiped away, and the skin should be cleaned once more.

The clinician should use eye protection during the treatment and when cleaning the needling device to prevent any contamination by the patient's blood.

7.6.4.2 Microneedling Technique

To use the dermal roller, place it on the skin and gently move it back and forth in one pattern (vertical, horizontal, or diagonal) in short strokes. For example, place the roller at the top of the forehead and move it down and then up three or four times in a vertical direction. When you finish, lift it off the skin (dragging may leave tracks), set it down in an adjacent area of the face, and move it up and down again three or four more times in a vertical direction.

As noted earlier, the goal is to create as many microchannels as possible. To accomplish this without leaving any gaps, mentally divide the face into regions and then treat each region in a logical sequence. The author recommends beginning treatment in the forehead area and moving clockwise to the patient's left cheek, followed by the chin, and ending with the right cheek area. The nose and philtrum areas are completed last. For each circuit, roll the device back and forth in only one pattern, as follows:

1. Vertical: Fig. 7.14. Move the micro roller forward and back in a vertical pattern, beginning at the right side of the forehead (on the clinician's left when facing the patient) and ending at the left side of the forehead. When you have finished the forehead, continue the vertical pattern on the patient's left cheek, then move to the chin, and end with the right cheek area.
2. Horizontal: Fig. 7.15. Move the micro roller from side to side in a horizontal pattern, beginning at the right side of the forehead and ending at the left side of the forehead. When you have finished the forehead, continue the horizontal pattern on the patient's left cheek, then move to the chin, and end with the right cheek area.

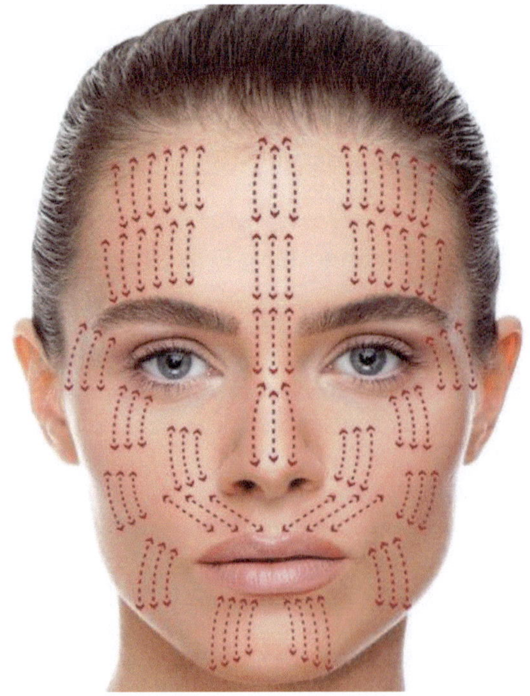

Fig. 7.14 Vertical

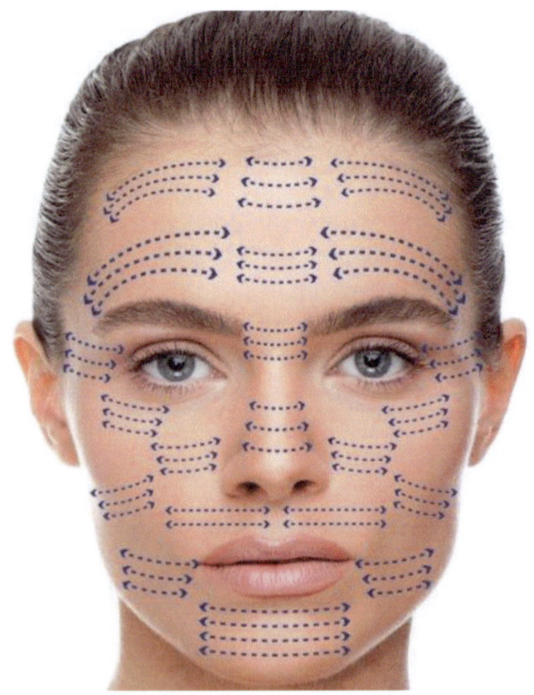

Fig. 7.15 Horizontal

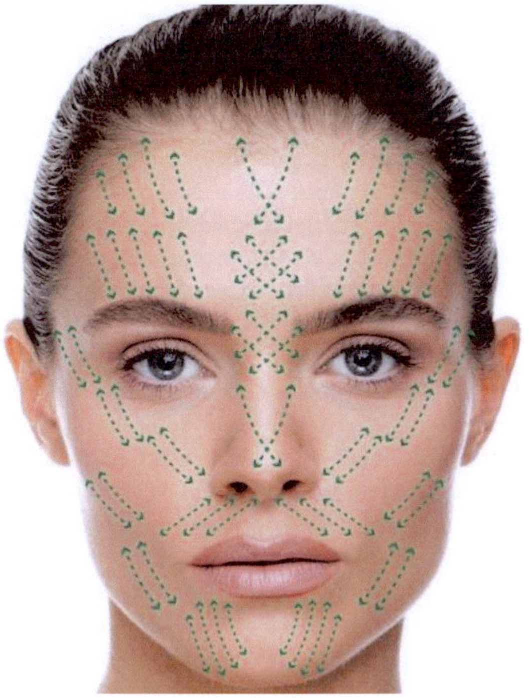

Fig. 7.16 Diagonal

3. Diagonal (left to right): Fig. 7.16. Move the micro roller in a diagonal pattern, from top left to bottom right from the clinician's point of view, beginning on the top right side of the forehead (the clinician's left when facing the patient) and ending on the bottom left side of the forehead (the clinician's right). When you have finished the forehead, continue the vertical pattern on the patient's left cheek, then move to the chin, and end with the right cheek area.
4. Diagonal (right to left): Fig. 7.16. Move the micro roller in a diagonal pattern, from top right to bottom left, beginning on the top right side of the forehead and ending on the bottom left side of the forehead. When you have finished the forehead, continue the vertical pattern on the patient's left cheek, then move to the chin, and end with the right cheek area.
5. Nose/philtrum areas. Treat these areas in the same manner, beginning with a vertical pattern and ending with a diagonal pattern.

   Deep-line wrinkles can be laid flat by stretching the skin with the thumb and fingers before roller application. These areas should be treated more deliberately to reflect the patient's desired outcomes. On completion of the entire face, one final circuit should be made, moving the roller in the direction away from the inner face to encourage lymph drainage. Similarly, these final strokes should move away from the nose when treating that area.

Always roll with a controlled motion and gentle pressure. When firm pressure is put on the skin during application of rolling devices, histamines are released. This histamine response often results in increased superficial reddening of the skin that may be present for several hours after the treatment. The use of a vibrating roller is not recommended because it can cause this condition to be much more severe.

Normal saline should be used to wash away the flow of blood in the needling area. Dried blood prevents nutrients from entering the skin and inhibits timely healing. During the procedure, the clinician can stop to clean the roller as necessary, taking care not to damage the needles. Because the needling channels remain open for no more than 15 min, a topical adjunct (HA or PRP) should be applied to the treated areas immediately after microneedling is completed.

7.6.5 Posttreatment Procedures

Although serum may ooze from the skin for up to 20 min after the procedure, bleeding should cease almost immediately. Bruising may persist. Once home, the patient should shower with tepid water for about 20 min, gently massaging and rinsing the treatment area to remove any fluids collected there. Bathing, which could cause contamination, is prohibited.

Erythema is the most noticeable side effect of the treatment, along with puffiness in the sensitive areas around the eyes, which may increase a day or two after treatment. Nevertheless, many patients feel comfortable and confident enough the day after a microneedling procedure to resume their normal public activities. If necessary, mineral makeup can be applied, but regular skin care products should not be used for the first

48 h after treatment. Sunscreen with a minimum SPF of 30 can be used beginning 1 day after the treatment but not earlier to prevent any potentially harmful ingredients from entering the exposed skin.

The patient should avoid direct sunlight for up to 1 month after microneedling treatment. After 3 to 5 days, the patient's skin will most likely feel dry and tight. This feeling can be relieved with moisturizers that contain ceramides. Vitamin A and topical omega-3 cream can be helpful in reducing inflammation, but toners with alcohol should be avoided. After several days, swelling will have disappeared along with most noticeable bruising, though flaky skin may persist. After 1 week, virtually no signs of the microneedling should remain. As early as several days after medical microneedling—once inflammation has decreased and based on the patient's comfort level—at-home rolling may be performed by patients who have vascular rosacea. For all other patients, the timing of additional clinical and/or at-home treatments should be based on the progression of natural healing that takes place after treatment. At least 1 month should pass before any more clinical microneedling is performed.

7.7 Dermal Filler Procedures

Dermal filler procedures require the clinician to master two basic skill sets. The first involves learning the various injection techniques and when to apply them. The second and more challenging skill involves learning how to recognize when you have reached the appropriate tissue plane to dispense the filler. This is very much an acquired skill, but there are some digital and visual cues that can help.

7.7.1 Basic Anatomy of Facial Skin

Briefly, human skin consists of three layers. The outermost layer is the epidermis, which protects the body from the external environment. It is composed mainly of cells and sensory nerves and relies on the dermis for both vascular and structural support. Averaging just 0.2 mm on the face, it is the thinnest of the three layers of the skin.

The dermis is located beneath the epidermis and accounts for about 90% of the skin's total thickness. The dermis houses all of the major structures, including blood vessels, hair follicles, and sweat glands, and stores most of the body's water supply. It is held together by collagen and elastin and provides blood-borne nutrients to the epidermis.

The hypodermis (or subcutaneous tissue), the innermost layer of the skin, consists of a network of collagen cells and fat, which insulates and protects the body. Blood vessels, nerves, and hair follicles also cross through the hypodermis, and it connects the dermis to the underlying fascia of the bones and muscles. Recently, a group of researchers used 3D scanning technology to measure the depth of the dermis and the superficial fat in various areas of the face. The results showed that the average dermal thickness is 1.51 mm in the thinnest regions and 1.97 mm in the thickest ones. Average thickness was determined to be 1.70 mm in the forehead, 1.85 mm in the malar area, and 1.82 in the perioral region. The average facial superficial fat thickness ranged from 1.61 mm in the dorsum to 5.14 mm in the perioral region, where it was thickest [30].

Male skin is characteristically thicker than female skin, but at about age 50 years, facial skin begins to thin as it loses elasticity, mostly because of reduced collagen production. Figure 7.17 displays the approximate depth of the dermis in various areas of the face in a middle-aged woman. Dermal fillers are injected at various depths, from the superficial dermis to just above the periosteum, depending on the desired outcome. The mid to deep dermis is the target for all of the dermal filler treatments covered in this chapter except malar and chin augmentation, which call for supraperiosteal placement. The step-by-step instructions for each procedure that follow include guidelines on how deeply to inject. Until they gain a certain amount of experience, readers should follow the recommenda-

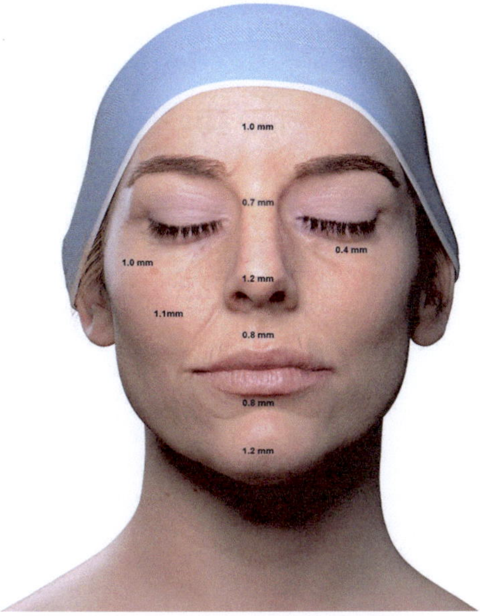

Fig. 7.17 By age 50 years, facial skin becomes noticeably thinner

tions of product manufacturers and experts. With practice and careful observation of how the tissue responds, the process will quickly become intuitive.

Depths can be determined during the injection process via digital sensitivity to the needle passing through the skin tissue, plunger pushback of the needle, and visibility of the needle tip and the response of the skin and subcutaneous tissues. Here are some clues:

- When the gray tip of the needle is visible and the skin blanches, it is too superficial and needs to be repositioned at a lower depth.
- The shape of the needle can still be discerned when it has reached the mid to deep dermis but not when it is in the subcutaneous plane.
- A palpable tap can be felt when the tip of the needle reaches the periosteum and bone.
- More resistance to plunger pressure is felt in the superficial to deep dermis than in the subcutaneous and supraperiosteal planes.
- When injecting into the dermis, placing downward pressure on the needle should cause the skin to dimple slightly.

7.7.2 Dermal Filler Injection Techniques

The choice of injection technique depends on the site being treated. Employing the appropriate technique is necessary to obtain uniform coverage of the site and is critical to achieving an optimal outcome. Important: Always prime the needle before inserting it into the skin by extruding a small amount from the tip to make sure the material is flowing properly.

7.7.2.1 Linear Threading

Linear threading is the most basic of all the injection patterns used for filler product placement (Fig. 7.18). In this technique, the full length of the needle is inserted at a 30° angle until it reaches the appropriate depth. As the needle is being withdrawn, firm and constant pressure is applied to the plunger to dispense filler product smoothly and evenly. The pressure on the plunger is not released until just before the needle is withdrawn from the skin. Immediately after the injection, the area is gently massaged to prevent any nodule formation.

This retrograde deposition technique creates a microchannel of filler material that is ideal for filling a nasolabial fold or smoothing a marionette line, and it serves as the basis for many of the other techniques.

7.7.2.2 Fanning

To visualize the fanning technique (Fig. 7.19), imagine making a series of linear thread injections from a single central insertion point. Now think of this insertion point as the base of the "fan."

To perform this technique, the full length of the needle is inserted at the center of the site being treated. As the needle is being withdrawn, a micro-channel of filler material is deposited (i.e., a linear thread injection is made). At the end of the "thread," however, the needle is only partially withdrawn. Next, the syringe is rotated in a slight arc and then fully reinserted, and a second linear thread of material is deposited adjacent to the first one. This pattern is repeated once more, with the syringe rotated again in the same direc-

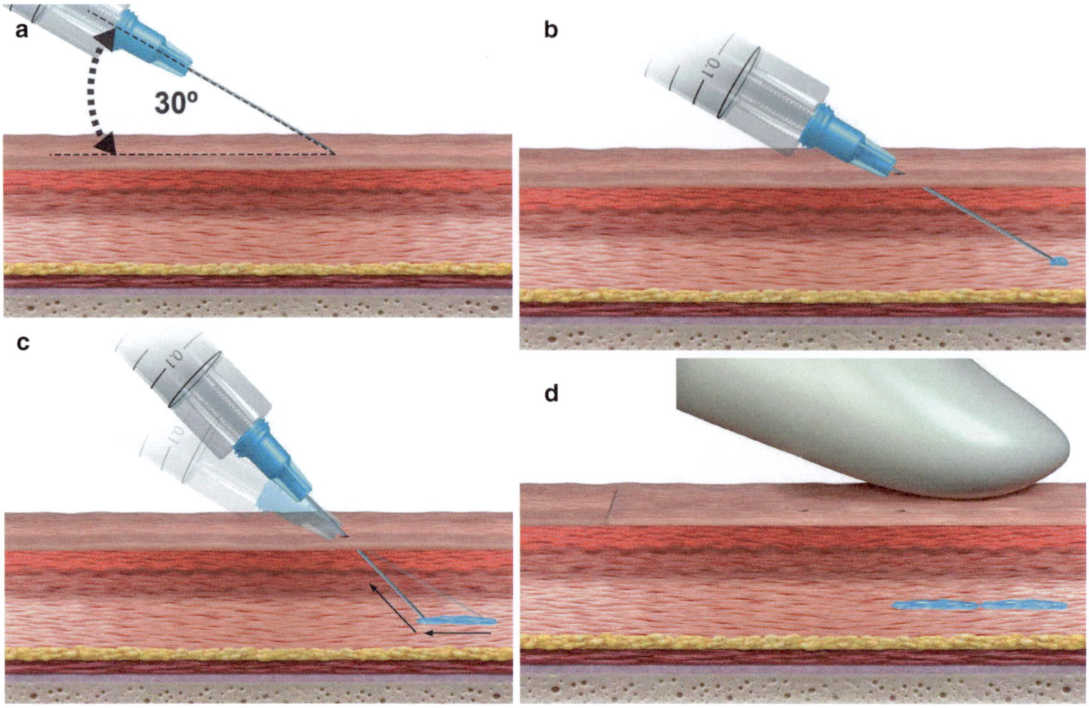

Fig. 7.18 Linear thread technique. (**a**) The needle is inserted at a 30° angle to the appropriate depth. (**b** and **c**) The needle is slowly withdrawn as pressure is applied to the plunger. Filler product is dispensed in a smooth line. (**d**) The area should be massaged immediately after the injection

tion. After the third linear thread injection has been made, the syringe is rotated (again without fully withdrawing it) in the opposite direction (i.e., medial to the first linear thread), and two more linear threads of filler material are injected. Again, once the injection is completed, the area is massaged to ensure that the filler is spread evenly and that there are no clumps.

This triangular fan pattern calls for a single insertion point to improve patient comfort and allows contiguous coverage of the site. However, to prevent buildup of product at the single point of entry, it is important to stop injecting before the needle is partially withdrawn after each linear thread has been made.

7.7.2.3 Depot

Unlike the linear thread technique, which is designed to fill in or "lift" a visible wrinkle or fold, the depot injection (Fig. 7.20) is used to modify the contour or to plump the tissue in an area such as the chin. Therefore, instead of injecting into the mid to deep dermis, the filler is injected into the supraperiosteal plane.

For this technique, the needle is slowly inserted all the way through the dermis and muscle until it gently touches the bone. When that tap is felt, the needle is withdrawn approximately 1 mm, and a bolus of filler is injected. The needle is then withdrawn. Additional depot injections are made accordingly until the desired volume enhancement has been achieved. Afterward, the injection site is gently compressed against the bone to smooth out any clumps. When administering a depot injection, it is important to deposit the filler below the muscle. When filler is inadvertently injected into the muscle, it can become displaced as a result of normal movement of the facial musculature and compromise the esthetic outcome.

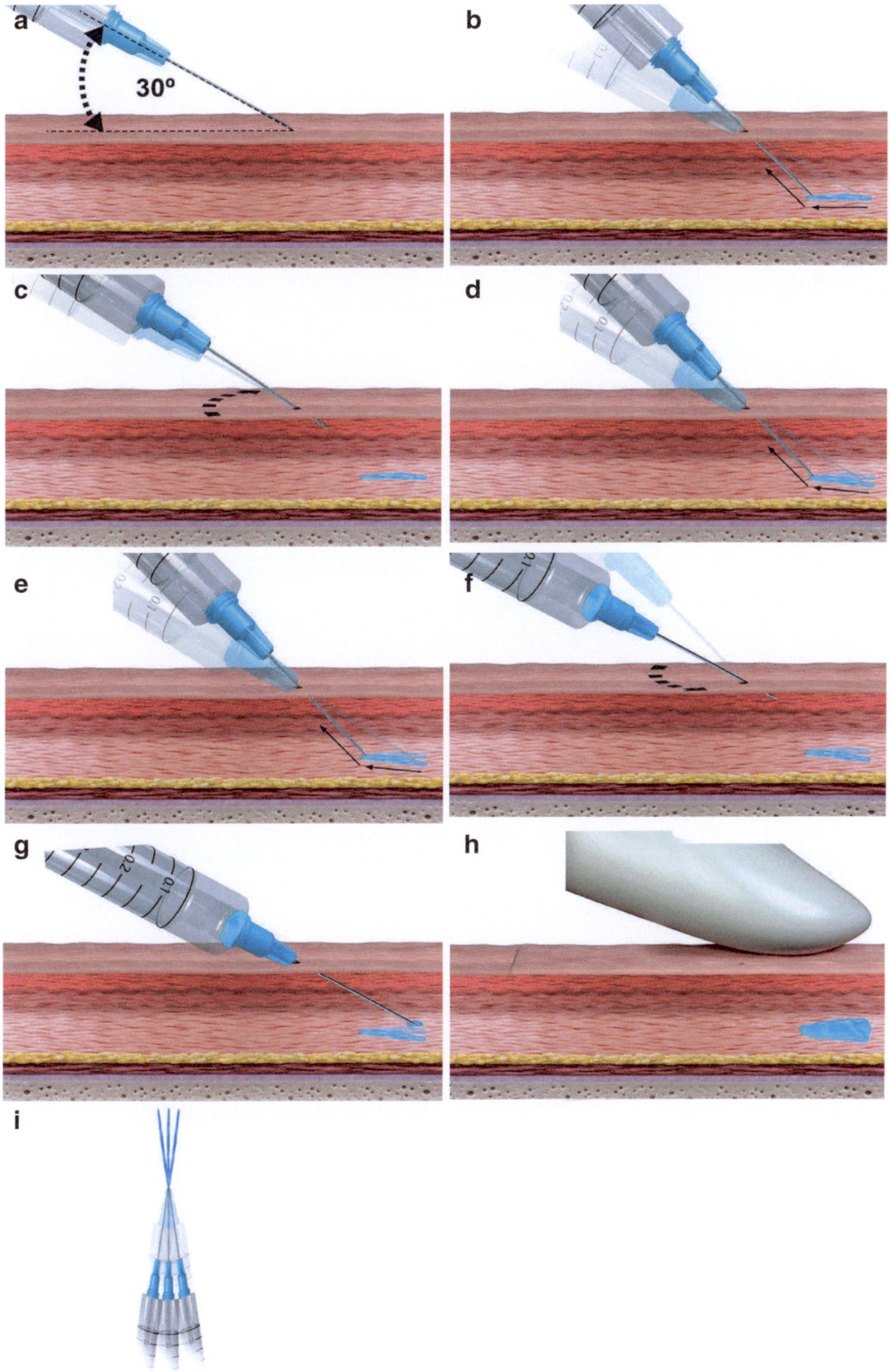

Fig. 7.19 Fanning technique. (**a**) Insert the needle at a 30° angle to the desired depth. (**b**) Inject a linear thread of filler product, but do not fully withdraw the needle. (**c**) Redirect the needle inferiorly and medially at a small angle. (**d** and **e**) Inject a linear thread of dermal filler adjacent to the previous thread. (**f**) Redirect the needle inferiorly and medially at a small angle, this time in the opposite direction. (**g**) Inject dermal filler adjacent to the first thread. (**h**) Firmly massage the area to ensure even distribution of the filler product. (**i**) With this technique, a single insertion point allows for contiguous coverage in a triangular or fan-shaped pattern

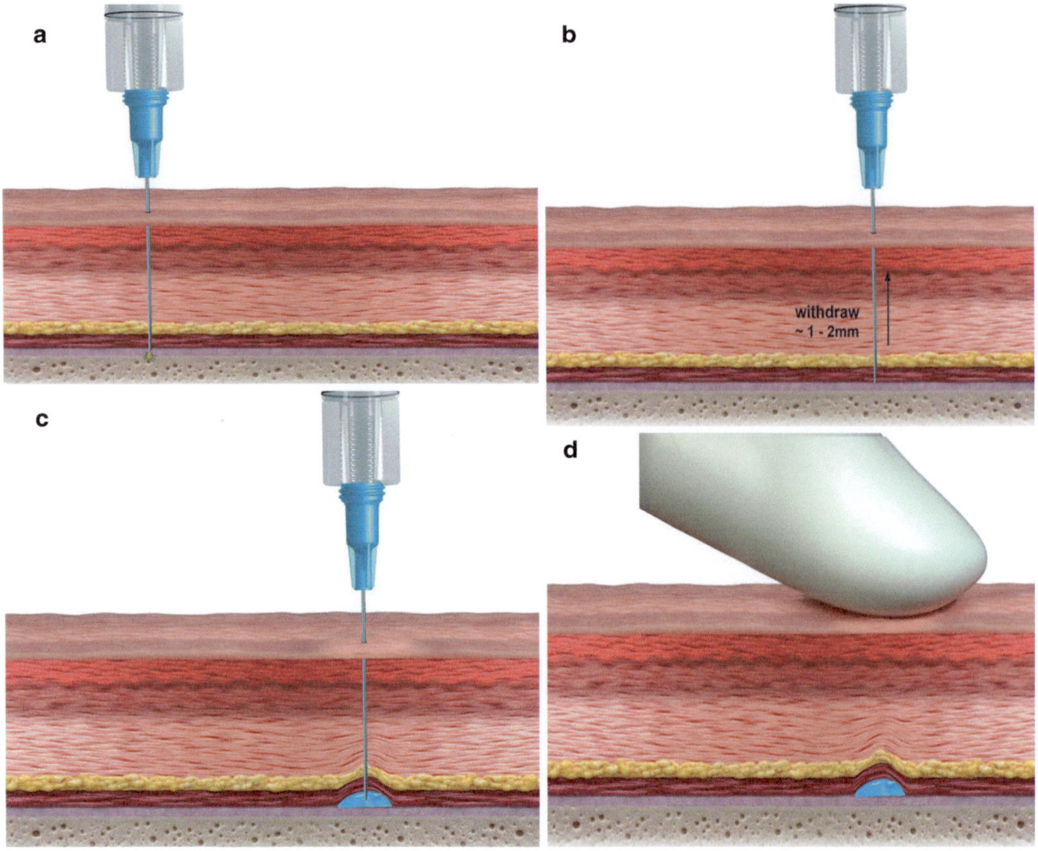

Fig. 7.20 Depot technique. (**a**) The needle is inserted at a 90° angle until it touches the bone. (**b**) Once the bone is felt, the needle is withdrawn about 1 mm. (**c**) Filler is then injected until the volume enhancement is achieved. (**d**) The injection site is compressed

7.7.3 Step By Step Dermal Filler Procedures

Step-by-step procedures for dermal filler treatment are presented below for eight conditions in the order of increasing complexity: nasolabial folds, marionette lines, mental crease, chin augmentation, extended mental crease, malar augmentation, frown lines, and scars. Each procedure begins with a description of the condition, indications, and contraindication for treatment, a list of the anesthesia and filler supplies needed, precautions to take under advisement, and the expected duration of treatment results. Each step in the procedure is then presented in the form of concrete instructions on the execution of each step in the procedure.

On completion of this chapter, readers will have the knowledge and confidence needed to begin offering dermal filler treatment for nasolabial folds and marionette lines to friends and family members and then to their patients. As their confidence grows, they can gradually expand their services to include the other treatment procedures presented in this chapter.

Box 7.1 lists the general contraindications for dermal filler treatment, and Box 7.2 lists the general medical supplies needed for the procedures discussed in this chapter.

Box 7.1 General Contraindications

- History of anaphylactic reaction
- Severe allergies
- Sensitivity or allergic reaction to dermal filler products
- Use of isotretinoin (Accutane, Roche) within the preceding 6 months
- Skin atrophy
- Poor healing
- Treatment area dermatosis
- An uncontrolled systemic condition
- Treatment area infection
- Hypertrophic or keloidal scarring
- Abnormal bleeding
- Pregnancy or nursing
- Body dysmorphic disorder
- Highly unrealistic expectations

Box 7.2 Basic Supplies Needed

- Alcohol pads
- Cotton-tipped applicators
- Handheld mirror
- Nonsterile gloves
- Nonwoven 3 × 3–in. gauze
- Surgical marker or white eyeliner pencil

7.7.3.1 Nasolabial Folds

Stretching from the nasal ala to the lip corners, nasolabial (or melolabial) folds are caused by loss of skin elasticity and soft tissue volume. Other causes include dermal atrophy, fat descending from the malar region, and hyperdynamic action of muscles in the midfacial region.

Indications and Contraindications

- In some patients, deep nasolabial folds are the result of excessive contraction of lip levator muscles in smiling and may require concomitant botulinum toxin treatment of the levator labii superioris alaeque nasi muscle for optimal results.
- If malar augmentation is also indicated in a patient scheduled for nasolabial fold treatment, the former should be performed first because the restoration of midface volume can reduce the severity of nasolabial folds.
- Moderate to severe nasolabial folds can be treated using two types of filler in a layering technique: Deep volume loss is addressed by a filler designed for structural support, while surface wrinkles are diminished via a more fluid and supple filler.
- Hanging or extremely lax skin is a contraindication for dermal filler treatment and should be corrected with surgery.

Anesthesia and Filler Supplies

- Buffered 2% lidocaine-epinephrine (total volume of 0.6 mL).
- 30-gauge, 0.5-in. needle.
- A topical anesthetic cream, such as a compounded formula of 10% benzocaine, 20% lidocaine, 10% tetracaine, and 10% dimethyl sulfoxide (DMSO) in a Lipoderm (Professional Compounding Centers of America) base (optional).

Suggested Dermal Fillers

- Juvéderm (Allergan).
- Belotero (Merz North America).
- Restylane (Galderma).
- Radiesse (Merz North America).
- Juvéderm Vollure (Allergan).
- Sculptra Aesthetic (Galderma).
- Bellafill (Suneva Medical).
- Platelet-rich plasma (PRP).

Suggested Quantity of Fillers

- Mild folds: 0.8 mL.
- Moderate folds: 1.6 mL.
- Severe folds: 2.4 mL.

Precautions

- Pain sensitivity increases as the nose is approached.
- Reduction, not full effacement, is the goal of dermal filler treatment of nasolabial folds.
- All injections must avoid the lateral nasal artery, which supplies blood to the nose and is located 2 to 3 mm above the alar groove.
- Caution: Immediate or delayed white blanching or a violaceous reticular pattern on the nose or nasolabial folds is a serious sign of occlusion (ischemia) from an intravascular injection and requires immediate attention to prevent tissue necrosis.

Dermal Filler Injection Technique

The patient is reclined at a 60° angle, and the folds are cleaned with alcohol. A 30-gauge, 0.5-in. needle is firmly attached to a prefilled dermal filler syringe to withstand plunger pressure. The clinician primes the needle by extruding a small amount of filler from its tip. Standing on one side of the patient, the clinician injects filler inferior and medial to the fold by inserting the needle at a 30° angle to the hub, toward the ala. The needle is then slowly withdrawn as the clinician injects a linear thread of filler in the mid to deep dermis with steady plunger pressure. The second injection is administered in the same manner, about 1 cm superior to the first. A third injection, 1 cm above the second, uses the fanning technique to distribute filler evenly by redirecting the needle inferiorly and medially before being fully withdrawn. The fanning can be repeated if more filler is needed. After moistening the skin with water, the clinician applies intraoral skin compression and/or stretches the skin between finger and thumb to even out the injected filler product. This often results in additional swelling/bruising. The clinician then moves to the other side of the patient and repeats the procedure on the contralateral fold.

Expected Duration of Results

- An additional dermal filler treatment (0.4 to 0.8 mL) may be required for static nasolabial folds.
- For dynamic folds, the additional treatment may be combined with botulinum toxin injections, particularly in cases of deep nasolabial folds.
- The longevity of the treatment results for nasolabial folds depends on the filler agent used, but averages approximately 6 to 9 months.

7.7.3.2 Marionette Lines

Marionette lines descend toward the jaw from the oral commissures or corners of the mouth, where the upper and lower lips meet. They are caused by dermal atrophy and reduction in skin elasticity, soft tissue volume, and mandibular bone volume (through resorption). Other causes include descent of fat from the mid-cheek area and hyperdynamic action of the muscles in the lower facial region.

Indications and Contraindications

- Excessive contraction of the depressor anguli oris muscles facilitates development of marionette lines in some patients. In such cases, botulinum toxin treatment of the depressor anguli oris muscles may be indicated to complement dermal filler treatment for wrinkle reduction.
- Restoring the volume deficit of an extended mental crease can help to reduce marionette lines in patients requiring both procedures.
- Moderate to severe volume deficits can be treated using two types of filler via layering: Deep volume loss is addressed by a filler designed for structural support, while surface wrinkles are diminished via a more fluid and supple filler.
- Associated esthetic challenges of the lower face include not only marionette lines but also

oral commissures, both of which can be treated effectively with dermal fillers.
- The look of sorrow associated with marionette lines makes the lateral lower lip a common target for dermal filler rejuvenation. As a result, the clinician must understand filler volume requirements and needle injection techniques for both areas.

Anesthesia and Filler Supplies

- Buffered 2% lidocaine-epinephrine (total volume of 0.6 mL).
- 30-gauge, 0.5-in. needle
- A topical anesthetic cream, such as a compounded formula of 10% benzocaine, 20% lidocaine, 10% tetracaine, and 10% DMSO in a Lipoderm base (optional).

Suggested Dermal Fillers

- Juvéderm Ultra.
- Juvéderm Volbella.
- PRP.
- Autologous fat transfer (AFT).

Suggested Quantity of Fillers

- Mild lines: 0.8 mL.
- Moderate lines: 1.6 mL.
- Severe lines: 2.4 mL.

Precautions

- Sensitivity to pain increases as the lip is approached.
- Dermal over treating or overfilling can cause unwanted contour changes for the lateral upper lip, vascular damage, or necrosis.

Dermal Filler Injection Technique

The patient is reclined at a 60° angle, and the marionette line area is cleaned with alcohol. A 30-gauge, 0.5-in. needle is firmly attached to a prefilled dermal filler syringe. Standing on one side of the patient, the clinician primes the needle by extruding a small amount of filler from its tip. The point of needle insertion is located by laying it atop the skin parallel and medial to the marionette line, with the tip of the needle 1 mm inferior to the lower lip. The needle hub marks the needle insertion point. The clinician inserts the needle superiorly toward the lower lip at a 30° angle to the skin and slowly advances it all the way to the needle hub. The needle is then slowly withdrawn as the clinician injects a linear thread of filler, mid to deep dermis, with steady plunger pressure. Before the needle is fully withdrawn, additional filler is delivered using the medial fanning technique. For this technique, the clinician redirects the needle medially several times with slight changes in angle, advancing to the hub each time to place dermal filler evenly. This process is repeated as needed to address line volume deficits, with two to three medial fanning injections made inferiorly at 1-cm distances.

Expected Duration of Results

- An additional dermal filler treatment may be required for static marionette lines.
- For dynamic lines, the additional treatment may be combined with botulinum toxin injections, particularly in cases of deep marionette lines.
- The duration of treatment results for marionette lines depends on the filler agent used, but averages approximately 6 to 9 months.

7.7.3.3 Mental Crease

The mental or labiomental crease appears as a line just above the chin. It is caused by hyperdynamic action of muscles in the lower facial region, dermal atrophy, and diminished skin elasticity. Other contributors are loss of soft tissue volume as well as mandibular bone and alveolar process resorption.

Indications and Contraindications

- Excessive contraction of the mentalis muscle facilitates development of a deep mental crease in some patients. In these cases, botulinum toxin treatment of the mentalis muscle is

indicated to complement dermal filler treatment for crease reduction.
- Restoring the volume deficit of a chin area can help to reduce mental crease deficits in patients requiring simultaneous procedures.
- Moderate to severe volume deficits can be treated using two types of filler via layering: Deep volume loss is addressed by a filler designed for structural support, while surface wrinkles are diminished via a more fluid and supple filler.
- Reduction of the mental crease is the aim of dermal filler treatment because the prominence of the crease intensifies with age.

Anesthesia and Filler Supplies

- Buffered 2% lidocaine-epinephrine (total volume of 0.6 mL) 30-gauge, 0.5-in. needle.
- A topical anesthetic cream, such as a compounded formula of 10% benzocaine, 20% lidocaine, 10% tetracaine, and 10% DMSO in a Lipoderm base (optional).

Suggested Dermal Fillers

- Belotero.
- Radiesse.
- Juvéderm.
- Restylane.
- PRP.

Suggested Quantity of Fillers

- Mild crease: 0.8 mL.
- Moderate crease: 1.6 mL.
- Severe crease: 2.4 mL.

Precaution

- Sensitivity to pain in the chin area increases as injections move from the most lateral to the medial region.

Dermal Filler Injection Technique

The patient is reclined at a 60° angle, and the crease area is cleaned with alcohol. A 30-gauge, 0.5-in. needle is firmly attached to a prefilled dermal filler syringe. Standing on one side of the patient, the clinician primes the needle by extruding a small amount of filler from its tip.

The initial injection point is the inferior/lateral section of the crease. It can be located by setting the needle atop the skin with the needle tip at the end of the crease; the needle hub marks the injection point. The clinician inserts the needle at a 30° angle to the skin and follows the outline of the crease superiorly and medially, all the way up to the needle hub. The needle is then slowly withdrawn as the clinician injects a linear thread of filler, mid to deep dermis, with steady plunger pressure. Next, the center of the crease is treated in the same fashion, beginning with a second injection immediately adjacent to the first.

The clinician moves to the other side of the patient to place the next injection on the opposite side of the patient's mental crease, beginning at the inferior lateral section and proceeding in the same fashion as the initial injection described above.

After moistening the skin with water, the clinician uses intraoral skin compression and/or stretches the skin between finger and thumb to even out the injected filler product. This often results in additional swelling/bruising.

Expected Duration of Results

- For static creases, an additional dermal filler treatment may be required.
- For dynamic creases, the additional treatment may be combined with botulinum toxin injections, particularly in cases of a deep mental crease resulting from hyperdynamic mentalis muscles.
- Ice or topical anesthesia should be used to help prevent distortion of tissue caused by lidocaine infiltration.
- The duration of treatment results for a mental crease depends on the filler agent used, but averages approximately 6 to 9 months.

7.7.3.4 Chin Augmentation

Chin augmentation is necessitated by contours of the chin that have become recessed or flattened, whether the chin is triangular (usually in women) or square (usually in men).

Indications and Contraindications

- Anterior and lateral views of the patient's chin profile should be used to assess how dermal fillers might be used for chin augmentation. For example, the lower lip projection should be slightly beyond the most anterior projection of the rounded (not flat) chin.
- Dermal fillers can help to restore soft tissue reduction that has led to recession or flattening not only of the chin but also of the malar regions.
- Note that anesthesia consists of topical cream in addition to buffered 2% lidocaine-epinephrine solution.

Anesthesia and Filler Supplies

- Buffered 2% lidocaine-epinephrine (total volume of 0.1–0.2 mL).
- 30-gauge, 0.5-in. needle.
- A topical anesthetic cream, such as a compounded formula of 10% benzocaine, 20% lidocaine, 10% tetracaine, and 10% DMSO in a Lipoderm base.
- Triangular chins should receive one 0.1-mL injection of anesthesia; square chins require two 0.1-mL injections.
- 27-gauge, 1.25-in. needle.

Suggested Dermal Fillers

- Juvéderm Voluma.
- Restylane Lyft.
- PRP.

Suggested Quantity of Dermal Fillers

- Mild recession and flattening of the chin typically requires a 0.6 to 0.8 mL volume of dermal filler.
- Moderate to severe chin recession and flattening requires a 1.3 to 1.5 mL volume of dermal filler.

Precautions

- Chin augmentation with dermal fillers should be avoided in patients whose chins are particularly small or recessed, as is often the case with micrognathia (mandibular hypoplasia), severe malocclusion, and craniofacial anomalies.
- Triangular chins should receive two fanning injections of filler in the deep dermis.
- Because excessive contraction of the mentalis muscle facilitates development of not only a deep mental crease but also chin flattening, botulinum toxin treatment of the mentalis muscle can complement dermal filler treatment for crease reduction and chin flattening.
- Restoring the volume deficit of a mental crease or an extended mental crease can help improve chin flattening conditions in patients requiring simultaneous procedures.
- Ice or topical anesthesia should be used to help prevent distortion of tissue caused by lidocaine infiltration.

Dermal Filler Injection Technique

The patient is reclined at a 45° angle, and the chin is cleaned with alcohol wipes. A 27-gauge, 1.25-in. needle is firmly attached to the dermal filler syringe. The clinician extrudes a small amount of filler via plunger pressure to prime the needle. The injection point is at the midline, which can be located by positioning the needle hub slightly below the midpoint of the jaw with the needle lying over the skin and pointing toward the lower lip. The needle tip should reach the upper boundary of the chin. The injection point is at the hub of the needle. The needle is inserted at a 90° angle all the way through the dermis and muscle until it touches the bone. When that tap is felt, the needle is withdrawn approximately 1 mm, and a bolus of filler is injected.

Once the first bolus of filler has been injected, the needle is partially withdrawn and re-angled distally. A second bolus of filler is deposited at the same depth as the first injection using the depot technique. The needle is again partially withdrawn and re-angled medially, and a third bolus of filler is injected subperiosteally using the depot technique. If necessary to achieve esthetic balance, the needle can be re-angled again superolaterally and/or inferolaterally and additional boluses of filler injected subperiosteally using the depot technique.

The clinician then applies pressure with the thumbs—medially, laterally, and around the outer boundaries of the chin—to even out any filler product beneath the skin that shows signs of poor, bumpy distribution. Areas that have not received any (or enough) filler product can be re-treated to achieve esthetic balance, but this time with simple linear threads via the same (or, if needed, an alternate) injection point, followed by additional thumb compression to ensure balanced product distribution.

Expected Duration of Results

- For chin augmentation asymmetries, follow-up treatment can include 0.2 to 0.3 mL of dermal filler injections.
- Mild recession and flattening of the chin typically requires a 0.6 to 0.8 mL volume of filler, whereas a moderate to severe chin recession and flattening requires a 1.3 to 1.5 mL volume of filler.
- Chin implants have been the typical treatment option for a recessed chin; however, a less invasive approach that uses dermal fillers with more structural support than those described in this chapter can achieve excellent results.

7.7.3.5 Extended Mental Crease

The triangular-shaped extended mental crease exhibits a loss of volume below the corners of the mouth and above the chin and is circumscribed by marionette lines. As the lower face ages, the extended mental crease can become more noticeable, often creating a facial affect of obstinacy or sorrow.

Indications and Contraindications

- Restoring the volume deficit in the chin and/or marionette line areas can help improve extended mental crease conditions in patients requiring simultaneous procedures.
- Dermal fillers that provide greater relative structural support can help address the substantive loss of volume in this area of the lower face.

Anesthesia and Dermal Filler Supplies

- Buffered 2% lidocaine-epinephrine (total volume of 0.6 mL).
- 30-gauge, 0.5-in. needle.
- 27-gauge, 0.25-in. needle.
- A topical anesthetic cream, such as a compounded formula of 10% benzocaine, 20% lidocaine, 10% tetracaine, and 10% dimethyl sulfoxide (DMSO) in a Lipoderm (Professional Compounding Centers of America) base.

Suggested Dermal Fillers

- Juvéderm Voluma (Allergan).
- Restylane Lyft (Galderma).
- Platelet-rich plasma (PRP).

Suggested Dermal Filler Quantities

- Mild extended mental crease: 0.8 mL.
- Moderate to severe extended mental crease: 1.6 mL.

Precautions

- Ice or topical anesthesia should be used to help avoid distortion of tissue caused by lidocaine infiltration.

Dermal Filler Injection Technique

The patient is reclined at a 60° angle, and the extended mental crease is cleaned with alcohol. A 30-gauge, 0.5-in. needle is firmly attached to a prefilled dermal filler syringe. The clinician primes the needle by extruding a small amount of filler from its tip. Standing on one side of the patient, the clinician lays the needle on the skin so that the hub rests at the medial-to-lateral portion of the crease; the needle hub marks the first insertion point. The clinician inserts the needle at a 30° angle to the skin and, moving toward the marionette line, advances the needle to its hub.

As the needle is slowly (but not fully) extracted, an inferior-advancing fanning technique is used to evenly deposit a linear thread of filler in the deep dermis in small increments. Shallow placement of dermal filler will result in noticeable unevenness on the surface of the skin. The injection is repeated as needed for adequate volumizing.

The clinician then moves to the opposite side of the patient and repeats the procedure on the contralateral side of the extended mental crease. The clinician then uses both thumbs to massage the treatment areas from the center outward to even out any poorly distributed filler.

Expected Duration of Results

- The longevity of the treatment results for extended mental crease depends on the filler agent used, but averages approximately 6 to 9 months.
- For persistent extended mental crease, follow-up treatment is required.

7.7.3.6 Malar Augmentation

A shallow, recessed appearance in the malar region can give the impression of premature aging perhaps more than any other facial area.

Indications and Contraindications

If patients require treatment of the nasolabial folds as well as malar augmentation, the latter should be performed first as volume restoration in the midface can reduce the need for reduction of nasolabial folds.

Anesthesia and Dermal Filler Supplies

- Buffered 2% lidocaine-epinephrine (total volume of 0.6 mL).
- 30-gauge, 0.5-in. needle.
- 28-gauge, 0.75-in. needle.
- A topical anesthetic cream, such as a compounded formula of 10% benzocaine, 20% lidocaine, 10% tetracaine, and 10% DMSO in a Lipoderm base.

Suggested Dermal Fillers

- Juvéderm Voluma.
- Belotero Balance (Merz North America).
- Radiesse (Merz North America).
- Restylane Lyft.
- Sculptra (Galderma).
- PRP.

Suggested Quantity of Dermal Filler

- 2.0 to 2.6 mL for malar augmentation.

Precaution

- Ice or topical anesthesia should be used to help prevent distortion of tissue caused by lidocaine infiltration.

Dermal Filler Injection Technique

The patient is reclined at a 60° angle, and the malar region is again cleaned with alcohol. A 28-gauge, 0.75-in. needle is firmly attached to the prefilled dermal filler syringe. Standing on one side of the patient, the clinician extrudes a small amount of filler from the needle to prime it.

Where the malar groove line intersects with the inferior margin of the zygoma bone, the clinician first inserts the needle at a 45° angle to the skin until it softly taps the zygoma bone and then withdraws it 1–2 cm. Dermal filler is then injected via the depot technique: 0.2–0.3 mL at full depth or 0.1 mL at half depth or less. The needle is removed when deposited filler volume is sufficient. Any filler that tracks in the dermis as a result of being injected during needle withdrawal must be expressed from the skin.

A second injection and deposit is made about 1 cm superolateral to the first injection, along the inferior zygoma. A third and final injection or deposit in this set of injections is made about 1 cm superolateral to the second. A second round of injections is then performed like the first round: The fourth injection is made about 1 cm superomedial to the original injection point, and the fifth about 1 cm superolateral to the fourth.

Nonpalpable filler areas in the malar region can be treated with boluses of sufficient size to even out the filler placement using the same injection protocols. Firmly smoothing the treated malar areas with the thumbs, mediolaterally, can provide additional filler balance.

The clinician then moves to the other side of the patient to treat the opposite malar region.

Expected Duration of Results

- The longevity of the treatment results for malar augmentation depends on the filler agent used, but averages approximately 6 to 9 months.
- For asymmetries in malar augmentation results, follow-up treatment is required.

7.7.3.7 Frown Lines

Frown lines (also known as *glabellar rhytids*) stretch vertically between the eyebrows and are produced dynamically when patients smile, laugh, or frown. Dynamic frown lines can evolve into static lines and be present when the face is at rest. Patients with frown lines often complain of projecting an effect of obduracy and annoyance.

Indications and Contraindications

- If the lines are a result of hyperdynamic muscle action, then botulinum toxin is the treatment of choice. Dermal filler treatments can often more effectively treat static frown lines.
- A topical anesthetic or ice is used to anesthetize the glabella.
- Linear thread filler injections are placed into the mid dermis for each line, beginning superiorly and proceeding inferiorly, with the need for additional injections determined by the length of the needle and of the frown lines.
- Because excessive contraction of the glabellar complex muscles facilitates development of dynamic frown lines, botulinum toxin treatment of the complex can not only reduce the lines but also provides a flatter plane for optimal filler application. Botulinum toxin treatment can be performed simultaneously with or even subsequent to the procedure, but the optimal time is 2 weeks prior to dermal filler treatment. Dermal filler reduction of surface static frown lines can be performed after patient recovery from more aggressive skin resurfacing and collagen stimulation (via ablative/non ablative lasers, dermabrasions, and chemical peels) or simultaneously with (or prior to) less aggressive versions of those procedures.

Precautions

- The thinnest dermal fillers should be administered via a 30-gauge, 0.5-in. needle to treat frown lines, where ischemia and vascular occlusion could develop in the glabella.
- To avoid the high risk of ischemia, tissue necrosis, and even blindness from arterial damage (retinal artery embolization) from tissue overfilling and vascular occlusion, the clinician should slowly inject thin filler products, intradermally, in low volumes with rearward needle movement and minimal plunger pressure.

Anesthesia and Filler Supplies

- Anesthetic: 0.5 g topical cream, such as a compounded formula of 10% benzocaine, 20% lidocaine, 10% tetracaine, and 10% DMSO in a Lipoderm base.
- 30-gauge, 0.5-in. needle.

Suggested Dermal Fillers

- Juvéderm.
- Teosyal RHA 2 (Teoxane).

Suggested Quantity of Dermal Filler

- 0.2 to 0.3 mL.

Dermal Filler Injection Technique

With the patient reclined at a 45° angle, the clinician stands behind the patient and applies alcohol to the frown line area. A 30-gauge, 0.5-in. needle is firmly attached to the prefilled dermal filler syringe. The clinician primes the needle by extruding a small amount of filler from the needle tip.

The injection begins at the most superior point of the frown line, at a 30° angle to the skin, directed inferiorly, mid-dermis, up to the hub of the needle and then slowly withdrawn to insert a linear thread of filler, following the natural lateral angle of the frown line. If the injection volume is insufficient, the clinician can inject filler once again in the same manner, approximately 0.5 in. below the first injection site. The clinician then uses both thumbs on the sides of the frown line to smooth the product evenly in the area. Any ischemia resulting from the procedure must be treated promptly and appropriately.

Expected Duration of Results

- The results of dermal filler treatment of frown lines typically last for 9 to 12 months.
- Persistent frown lines and scars could result from volume deficits, which can be addressed by additional small volumes of filler.
- In the case of dynamic frown lines, additional treatment may be accompanied by botulinum toxin injections.
- For superficial static frown lines that do not dissipate over several months, botulinum toxin and dermal filler treatments are in order, along with resurfacing procedures and collagen stimulation.

7.7.3.8 Scars

Composed of fibrotic tissue (often secured to subcutaneous tissue), atrophic scars can appear anywhere in the facial region as deep and narrow depressions—so-called ice pick scars—or they can have soft, round borders.

Indications and Contraindications

- Dermal filler treatment can effectively treat soft, distensible atrophic depression scars with round, soft edges resulting from acne, trauma, skin excisions, or chickenpox.
- Dermal fillers are inappropriate for treating ice pick and nondistensible scars.
- Dermal filler reduction of superficial depression scars can be performed after the patient recovers from more aggressive skin resurfacing and collagen stimulation (via ablative/non ablative lasers, dermabrasions, and chemical peels) or simultaneously with (or prior to) less aggressive versions of those procedures.
- Subcutaneous incisional surgery of barely distensible scars can be followed by dermal filler treatment.

Anesthesia and Filler Supplies

- Anesthetic: 0.5 g topical cream, such as a compounded formula of 10% benzocaine, 20% lidocaine, 10% tetracaine, and 10% DMSO in a Lipoderm base.
- 30-gauge, 0.5-in. needle.

Suggested Dermal Fillers

- Bellafill (Suneva Medical).
- Restylane.
- Juvéderm.
- PRP.

Suggested Dermal Filler Quantity

- 0.3 to 0.4 mL.

Precautions

- The thinnest dermal fillers should be administered via a 30-gauge, 0.5-in. needle to treat depression scars.
- To avoid tissue overfill or vascular occlusion (which can cause ischemia and necrosis), the clinician should slowly inject thin filler products, intradermally, in low volumes with rearward needle movement and minimal plunger pressure.

Dermal Filler Injection Technique

With the patient reclined at a 60° angle, the clinician stands on the side of the patient where the scar treatment area is located and cleans the area with alcohol. A 30-gauge, 0.5-in. needle is firmly attached to the prefilled dermal filler syringe. One side of the scar is chosen for the initial injection point, which begins slightly beyond the scar perimeter. Needle entry is made at a 15° angle to the skin, and the needle tip is advanced to the center of the scar. As the needle is withdrawn, a linear thread of filler is smoothly and evenly injected, superficial to mid-dermis. If the needle tip becomes visible, the clinician should redirect it deeper to avoid making the injection too shallow. Before it is withdrawn, the needle is fanned clockwise in small increments for even filler distribution. The injection should be discontinued if filler pools in the scar margins.

This injection procedure can be repeated to ensure proper filler volume before a second injection site is chosen opposite the first, which repeats the fanning injection treatment. Depending on the size of the treatment area, two similar opposing fanning injections can be made at quarter intervals from the first two injections. Finally, the skin of the treated area can be gently palpated via an intraoral finger and extraoral cotton-tipped instrument to smooth the filler distribution. Any ischemia resulting from the procedure must be treated promptly and appropriately.

Expected Duration of Results

- Treatment results for scars usually last approximately 6 to 9 months.
- Smoothing scars manually after the procedure can help prevent bumps.
- Compression of persistent bumps during follow-up visits can also help.

References

1. American Society of Plastic Surgeons. 2018 Plastic Surgery Statistics Report. https://www.plasticsurgery.org/documents/News/Statistics/2018/cosmetic-procedure-trends-2018.pdf. Accessed 21 Apr 2020.
2. Dayan SH, Bassichis BA. Facial dermal fillers: selection of appropriate products and techniques. Aesthet Surg J. 2008;28:335–47.
3. Smith KC, Comite SL, Balasubramanian S, Carver A, Liu JF. Vibration anesthesia: a noninvasive method of reducing discomfort prior to dermatologic procedures. Dermatol Online J. 2004;10:1.
4. Mally P, Czyz CN, Chan NJ, Wulc AE. Vibration anesthesia for the reduction of pain with facial dermal filler injections. Aesthetic Plast Surg. 2014;38:413–8.
5. Shapiro FE. Anesthesia for outpatient cosmetic surgery. Curr Opin Anaesthesiol. 2008;21:704–10.
6. Sobanko JF, Miller CJ, Alster TS. Topical anesthetics for dermatologic procedures: a review. Dermatol Surg. 2012;38:709–21.
7. Kouba DJ, LoPiccolo MC, Alam M, et al. Guidelines for the use of local anesthesia in office-based dermatologic surgery. J Am Acad Dermatol. 2016;74:1201–19.
8. Dastoor SF, Misch CE, Wang H-L. Dermal fillers for facial soft tissue augmentation. J Oral Implantol. 2007;33:191–204.
9. Urdiales-Gálvez F, Delgado NE, Figueiredo V, et al. Treatment of soft tissue filler complications: expert consensus recommendations. Aesthetic Plast Surg. 2018;42:498–510.
10. Bacigalupi R, Clark J, Lupo MP. An overview of injectable fillers with special consideration to the periorbital area. Cosmet Dermatol. 2012;25:421–6.
11. Cheng L-Y, Sun X-M, Tang M-Y, Jin R, Cui W-G, Zhang Y-G. An update review on recent skin fillers. Plast Aesthet Res. 2016;3:92–9.
12. Day DJ, Littler C, Swift RW, Gottlieb S. The wrinkle severity rating scale: a validation study. Am J Clin Dermatol. 2004;5:49–52.
13. Funt D, Pavicic T. Dermal fillers in aesthetics: an overview of adverse events and treatment approaches. Clin Cosmet Investig Derm. 2013;6:295–316.
14. Lin ZY, Shah V, Dhinakar A, Yildirimer L, Cui W-G, Zhao X. Intradermal fillers for minimally invasive treatment of facial aging. Plast Aesthet Res. 2016;3:72–82.
15. Van Loghem J, Yutskovskaya YA, Werschler WP. Calcium hydroxylapatite: over a decade of clinical experience. J Clin Aesthet Dermatol. 2015;8:38–49.
16. Werschler WP, Narurkar VN. Facial volume restoration: selecting and applying appropriate treatments. Technique poster. Cosmet Dermatol. 2006;19(suppl 2):S1.
17. Glogau RG. Fillers: from the past to the future. Semin Cutan Med Surg. 2012;31:78–87.
18. Mansouri Y, Goldenberg G. Update on hyaluronic acid fillers for facial rejuvenation. Cutis. 2015;96:85–8.
19. Fagien S, Bertucci V, von Grote E, Mashburn JH. Rheologic and physicochemical properties used to differentiate injectable hyaluronic acid filler products. Plast Reconstr Surg. 2019;143:707e–20e.
20. Obi G, International Society of Plastic and Aesthetic Nurses. How to choose a filler or neuromodulator to treat your patients' aesthetic concerns.

https://ispan.org/meeting/multimedia /files/2018/Presentations/1130-Obi.pdf. Accessed 21 Apr 2020.
21. Vleggaar D, Fitzgerald R, Lorenc ZP, et al. Consensus recommendations on the use of injectable poly-L-lactic acid for facial and nonfacial volumization. J Drugs Dermatol. 2014;13(suppl 4):s44–51.
22. Fontes T, Brandão I, Negrão R, Martins MJ, Monteiro R. Autologous fat grafting: harvesting techniques. Ann Med Surg (Lond). 2018;36:212–8.
23. Simonacci F, Bertozzi N, Grieco MP, Grignaffini E, Raposio E. Procedure, applications, and outcomes of autologous fat grafting. Ann Med Surg (Lond). 2017;20:49–60.
24. Cho K-H, Uthaman S, Park I-K, Cho C-S. Injectable biomaterials in plastic and reconstructive surgery: a review of the current status. Tissue Eng Regen Med. 2018;15:559–74.
25. Lemperle G, Knapp TR, Sadick NS, Lemperle SM. Artefill permanent injectable for soft tissue augmentation: I. Mechanism of action and injection techniques. Aesthetic Plast Surg. 2010;34:264–72.
26. Liebl H, Kloth LC. Skin cell proliferation stimulated by microneedles. J Am Coll Clin Wound Spec. 2012;4:2–6.
27. Strazzulla LC, Avila L, Lo Sicco K, Shapiro J. An overview of the biology of platelet-rich plasma and microneedling as potential treatments for alopecia areata. J Investig Dermatol Symp Proc. 2018;19:S21–4.
28. Hashim PW, Nia JK, Taliercio M, Goldenberg G. Local anesthetics in cosmetic dermatology. Cutis. 2017;99:393–7.
29. Alster TS, Graham PM. Microneedling: a review and practical guide. Dermatol Surg. 2018;44:397–404.
30. Kim YS, Lee KW, Kim JS, et al. Regional thickness of facial skin and superficial fat: application to the minimally invasive procedures. Clin Anat. 2019;32:1008–18.

Into the World of Laser Resurfacing

8

Robert L. Bard and Cameron Rokhsar

Abstract

Multiple laser outlets exist that rejuvenate and replenish the skin through resurfacing capabilities in its superficial layers. In varying degrees and technologies, these lasers improve the appearance of rhytides, lentigines, photodamage, scarring, and treat uneven pigmentation. The four major classes of dermatologic lasers being discussed in this chapter are ablative and nonablative lasers in both their fractionated and unfractionated forms. The milder nonablative lasers allow for briefer healing, whereas intense ablative lasers tend to be more effective but require longer downtimes and increased side effects. Then fractionating causes the laser to distribute the resurfacing effect leading to increased number of treatments but decreases risk of complications and recovery time.

Keywords

Laser resurfacing · Fractional · Ablative · Microscopic treatment zones (MTZs)

8.1 Introduction

Laser skin resurfacing uses different wavelengths of light to remove thin layers of the skin by contacting the epidermis and heating the dermis to shrink collagen fibers and increase cell reproduction. The formation of new skin cells creates a smoother and tighter surface over time [1]. Although laser resurfacing is not a substitute for surgical procedures, the appropriate laser can tighten the skin and improve the appearance of skin texture, rhytides, lentigines, vascularity, and a wide variety of scars.

R. L. Bard (✉)
The Angio Foundation and Bard Diagnostics, New York, NY, USA
e-mail: rbard@cancerscan.com

C. Rokhsar
Mount Sinai Hospital, Miami, FL, USA
e-mail: drrokhsar@cosmeticlaserskinsurgery.com

R. L. Bard (ed.), *Image-Guided Aesthetic Treatments*, https://doi.org/10.1007/978-3-031-36266-8_8

This chapter will be discussing and comparing the four types of lasers: ablative, nonablative, fractional ablative, and fractional nonablative. During ablative laser resurfacing, an intense beam of light energy destroys the epidermis and heats the dermis to stimulate collagen production. There are no zones of spared epidermal tissue remaining. Ablative lasers are more aggressive because they vaporize skin tissue while nonablative lasers are gentler, leaving the skin intact. There is far more downtime involved with ablative lasers with a difficult recovery process, but they produce the most impressive results.

Ablative laser is ideal for pigmentation issues, more severe facial wrinkles, and creating better skin texture. Nonablative lasers provide a more moderate degree of skin rejuvenation. They heat the water in deeper layers to tighten existing collagen and increase elastin production [2]. The nonfractionated lasers perform on the whole target area of the skin, whereas the fractionated laser leaves minuscule spaces between each beam of light that distributes on the skin [3]. For example, when seeing pixels on a computer screen, a nonfractional laser would hit every pixel, while a fractional laser will treat a percentage of the pixels on the screen. Moreover, the Fitzpatrick scale is numerically based from I to IV going from the lightest skin tone (I) to the darkest (VI) and is an important tool for deciphering what kind of laser treatment is appropriate for a patient.

8.2 Laser History

Lasers are a fairly new technology for the cosmetic dermatology community. They were initially introduced for treating vascular lesions while the carbon dioxide laser for skin resurfacing rapidly began replacing dermabrasion and chemical peels in the mid-1990s. At first, machines lacked pattern generators, were low-powered, needed multiple passes, and had greater treatment time to achieve deeper depths of ablation [4].

The carbon dioxide laser was used to vaporize tissue by absorbing chromophores of water with a wavelength of 10,600 nm. Continuous mode lasers were first used, but due to thermal damage and excessive depths of ablation, there were complications. This led to advances in laser systems to decrease complexities by delivering short laser pulses to the skin or by an opto-mechanical flash scanner used to scan a continuous laser beam in a spiral pattern. Tissue exposure time was minimized to 1 ms to allow minimal tissue ablation and thermal damage of 75 to 100 μm. However, long-term results showed pigmentary complications which led to the full-field carbon dioxide resurfacing laser. Around 2000, the laser industry was introduced with erbium-doped yttrium aluminum garnet (Er:YAG) lasers at 2940 nm targeting superficial resurfacing. These are 10 times more efficient with thermal damage of 5 to 10 μm. Combination of beams being delivered sequentially or simultaneously from systems of carbon dioxide and Er:YAG lasers also became popular for a brief period of time. Wavelengths of 2780 and 2790 nm for skin resurfacing were also introduced but have not had significant commercial success.

Additionally, lasers began to use nitrogen plasma energy to coagulate a very controlled depth of skin with results and healing times being similar to Er:YAG lasers. In 2004, Manstein et al. launched the idea of fractional photothermolysis, first performed commercially using fluences at 1550 nm at Solta Medical in Mountain View, California [4]. The latest wavelength lies with the thulium at 1927 nm by Solta Medical, another fractional laser especially effective in treating actinic keratosis and removing superficial pigment. The most recent fractional laser on the market is a hybrid fractional laser that in the same tunnel combines a 1470-nm nonablative pulse and coincident delivery of the Er:YAG fractional laser.

8.2.1 Ablative Nonfractional Lasers

As mentioned previously, ablative skin resurfacing removes the superficial epidermal layer of skin to produce one of the more dramatic outcomes from the rest of the lasers. The main mechanism in this laser works to superheat water molecules in the cells of skin tissue. Then as the water turns into vapor, the skin produces peeling layers of these dehydrated cells. As a result, collagen formation is increased, and retraction between the dermis and epidermis is condensed to make the skin firmer. These lasers are used to treat wrinkles, photodamaged skin, and deep acne scars [3]. The first ablative nonfractional device had complicated side effects including further scarring and difficulty healing. Recent technology has made these lasers to reduce trauma and decrease downtime with lasting efficacy but still pose a risk for infections, scarring, and discoloration.

Since the carbon dioxide laser was one of the first laser resurfacing technologies for facial rejuvenation, the side effect of scarring was high using continuous waves (CW). Short-pulse carbon dioxide lasers were produced to control the type and amount of tissue removed following a 2-week recovery period. Modern carbon dioxide lasers emit light at 10,600 nm with pulses less than 1 ms where the tissue vaporizes up to 20 to 30 μm per pulse to limit thermal damage to a 100 to 150 μm layer of tissue. Beams larger than 2 mm incite nonvaporization to increase the risk of serious thermal damage; therefore, beams are limited to 100 to 200 μm [3]. Existing old collagen is ablated and contracted immediately to stimulate new collagen production even long after the procedure is done. This is best suited for wrinkles around the mouth and eyes [5] as well as acne and atrophic scars [6]. Atrophic scars are most commonly caused by collagen damage from inflammatory skin diseases such as varicella or cystic acne that creates dermal depressions. Downtime includes oozing, bleeding, and crusting, but facial wrinkles are improved by 45% in successful patients. The most common side effect is hypopigmentation from this laser amounting to the injury caused by the treatment. Other side effects include infection, acne, and temporary hyperpigmentation which does not occur as often and only persists for a few months. About 55% of patients experience these side effects [7].

The other nonablative fractional laser is called the erbium-doped yttrium aluminum garnet (Er:YAG) laser. Its absorption coefficient is 16 times greater than the carbon dioxide laser because the light emitted in the infrared range is at 2940 nm, a frequency that is closer to the peak absorption range of water [3]. Greater absorption leads to a decrease in in-depth penetration and damage of the epidermis and surrounding tissue with more precise ablation. The linear relationship of Er:YAG laser was between the energy delivered and depth of ablation, with 3 to 4 μm ablated per joule fluence delivered [4]. Although this laser does not have as great of a tissue tightening effect, the side effects are less severe than the carbon dioxide laser with less postoperative edema. Physicians hoped to synergize the wavelengths of the two lasers and found that using the Er:YAG laser succeeding the carbon dioxide laser decreased the intensity of the side effects without having to change the amount of collagen and elastin production in the skin [8].

8.2.2 Nonablative Nonfractional Lasers

Nonablative fractional lasers produce a moderate treatment on the skin. It creates an environment for controlled tissue injury in the dermis to stimulate collagen production and dermal remodeling. Since it is a gentle treatment, the results are milder in comparison to ablative lasers. Patients who choose this laser seek gradual improvement with minimal downtime and side effects. The prospective impairs associated with these lasers are exceptionally lower compared to carbon dioxide/erbium lasers. Only a few hours of erythema is experienced with little to no peeling of the skin. Nonablative lasers are much less intense; therefore, four to six treatments are necessary to notice improvements in acne scars or uneven skin texture using varying wavelengths [9]. This would not be an ideal laser to combat wrinkles because of its mild nature to target overall skin rejuvenation. Patients who have darker skin tones (Fitzpatrick scale III–VI) are good candidates as well for nonablative use because it does not induce any lasting abnormal pigmentation [10]. With the help of nonablative technologies congruent with milder improvements, proper patient selection is important to the success of the procedure. The best candidates are between 35 and 55 years of age with moderately photodamaged facial skin, exhibiting as early rhytides, increased fragility and pore size, decreased elasticity, and coarser texture. Clinically noticeable epidermis irregularities in younger patients like the ones described may be too minimal, making any improvement difficult to detect. However, older patients tend to have severe textural mutations and much deeper rhytides so the subject may not be adequately satisfied with the outcome of the procedure, even after multiple sessions. These results are the outcome of epidermal melanin acting as a competing chromophore in the skin which becomes inversely related to wavelength. This means as wavelengths increase, the absorption of melanin progressively decreases and develops a nearly negligible result in the infrared portion of the electromagnetic spectrum. Therefore, patients with darker skin tones or patients with tans can safely benefit from longer wavelengths. Of course, excessive fluency and prolonged exposure to cryogen can and will add to dyschromia in these subjects.

From being in the mid-infrared laser class, the 1319 nm pulsed energy laser is effective at improving the appearance of fine lines, acne, acne scarring, skin tone, and overall texture [11]. It is safe to treat all skin types and colors but is not ideal for treating abnormal pigmentation or vascularity. This wavelength efficiently targets fibroblasts in the dermal layer used to stimulate collagen production with large-area pattern generators (LAPG). LAPG employs technology designed to non-sequentially distribute the laser path evenly. Side effects of this technology include overheating the skin and creating permanent damage. Otherwise, the LAPG allows the skin to be treated proportionately and completely.Additionally, the 1320 nm Nd:YAG long-pulsed laser was one of the first nonablative lasers available for commercial use. This laser stimulates collagen growth by specifically avoiding destruction to the epidermis layer and instead heats up the dermis. Water in the cells of the dermis perfectly absorbs a 1320 nm wavelength. Hemoglobin and melanin are not affected by this wavelength either and can be used to treat all skin shades from I to VI without having to observe pigmentation issues. The 1320 nm Nd:YAG laser promotes two major growth factors, basic fibroblast growth factor (bFGF) and inhibiting transforming growth factor β1 (TGF-β1) necessary to accelerate the vitality and volume of fibroblasts [12]. Then, tropoelastin production is intensified while collagen types I, III, and VII are stimulated from the promotion of these growth factors. The laser most effectively treats acne-related skin issues by minimizing sebum secretion by targeting sebaceous glands. It also reduces the appearance of scarring from past acne by resurfacing the tissue in the area, creating less depression in affected zones [13].

Inflammatory facial acne is also safely treated by the 1450-diode laser by causing damage to the sebaceous glands. This laser is a better option for treating acne scars specifically, as seen in Fig. 8.1, than the nonablative 1320-nm Nd:YAG laser because the water in the upper dermis is heated and thermally damaged [13]. One study in 2011 showed this laser producing a systemic effect with inflammatory acne vulgaris being resolved on both sides of the face when only one side was treated [14]. Downtime is limited significantly, similar to the other nonablative lasers in comparison to the ablative counterpart with side effects including temporary edema, erythema, and hyperpigmentation. All skin types can safely use this laser with mild to moderate improvement [15]. However, this laser is not ideal for patients looking to resolve facial wrinkling as that requires more ablative technology.

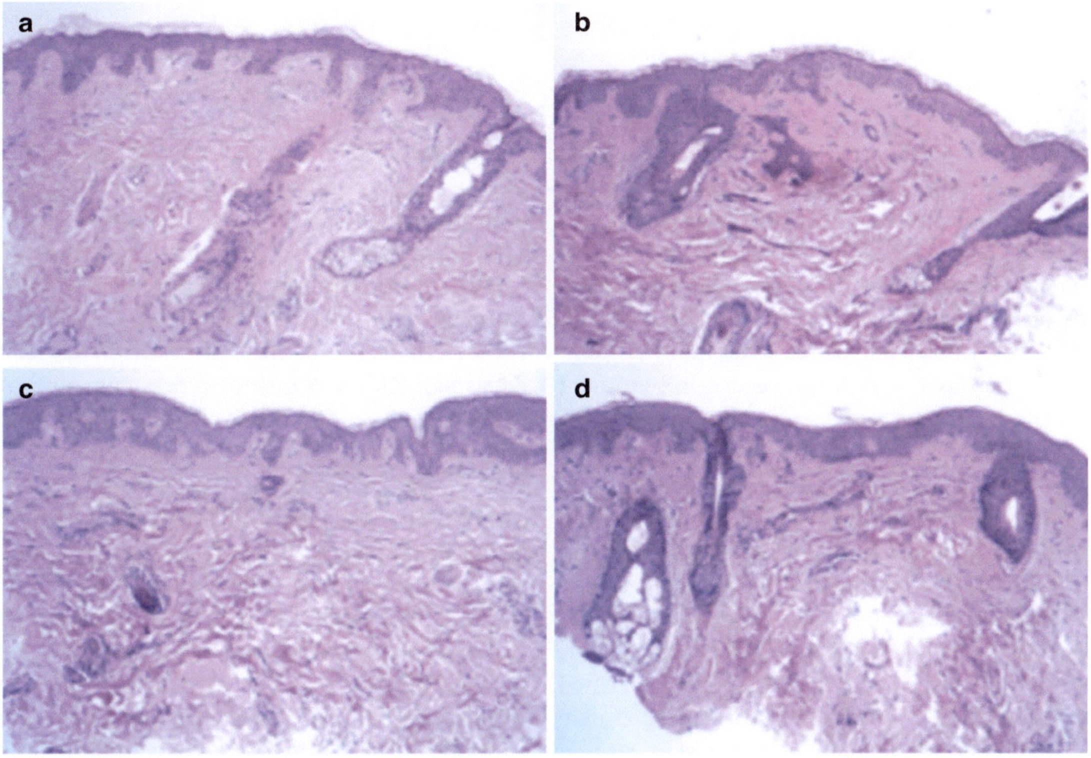

Fig. 8.1 All four images are histologic specimens of facial skin dyed with hematoxylin and eosin at ×10 magnification. (**a**) Facial skin before treatment with 1320-nm Nd:YAG laser. (**b**) Specimen 6 months after 31,320-nm Nd:YAG laser treatments demonstrates increased dermal collagen. (**c**) Facial skin before treatment with 1450-nm diode laser. (**d**) Facial skin 6 months after 31,450-nm diode laser treatments demonstrates increased dermal collagen [13]

8.2.3 Nonablative Fractional Lasers

Entering the market in 2005, nonablative fractional lasers are the most gentle and safest options out of the four laser types discussed in this chapter. The main focus of these lasers is to improve skin texture, fine lines, atrophic acne scars, and epidermal pigmentation in lighter skin types due to sun damage. Because of its gentle nature, this laser is available for use in other areas of the body such as the neck and chest, but the results are more moderate requiring multiple treatments. The fractional pattern of the laser results in faster healing profiles and less downtime. Nonablative fractional lasers can also be safe to use in darker skin types effectively without causing permanent pigmentation complications since they induce limited temporary melanocyte stimulation and tissue damage. These treatments tend to use topical anesthetics to decrease patient discomfort during the sessions. Treatment columns are delivered about 300–1200 μm deep with fractional nonablative technologies, in contrast to the typical 200–300 μm deep of a multi-pass CO_2 laser [16]. Since a zone of ordinary skin surrounds each microscopic treatment column, it allows the barrier function of the epidermis to be intact without any lasting visible wounding and the stratum corneum remains unimpaired during and after laser therapy. The normal intervening tissue permits rapid re-epithelialization into the treatment column through keratinocyte migration and division of transient amplifying cells. The surfaces of wounded areas are shed as microscopic epidermal and dermal necrotic debris (MENDs) after 2–3 days [17].

Significant post-inflammatory hyperpigmentation was observed, and pain in darker skin tones was more severe [18]. A key benefit of the fractional nonablative laser is that it can be securely applied to the neck, chest, and limbs, including hands and feet. Previously, these anatomic areas were at a high risk of acquiring side effects and complications from ablative and nonablative modalities. Aging of the neck includes poikiloderma of Civatte, skin laxity, and wrinkles. In Fig. 8.2, a nonablative fractional 1540 erbium-glass fiber laser was shown successfully to treat poikiloderma of Civatte and reduce the appearance of aging.

The first nonablative fractional laser had a fluence of 1410 nm and was very versatile on a broad range of patients because it is safe to use on Fitzpatrick skin types I to VI. The laser required about 3–5 treatments with 3–5 days of downtime due to its gentle ablation of the skin layers. Microscopic treatment zones (MTZs) are created by fractional photothermolysis. These are columns dispersed throughout the skin heating minuscule zones about one-tenth the size of a hair follicle to penetrate collagen in the dermis. The epidermis is not compromised; therefore, it maintains a rapid recovery after each treatment allowing some deep penetration, leaving healthy tissue to aid in repairing the zones of damage. Additionally, the 1440 Nd:YAG laser uses microcolumns of uniform heating to improve the appearance of rhytides [20]. Precise and regular patterns of tissue injury are achieved with the fractional component of lasers to retain healing in the epidermis while targeting the dermis as well. More treatments are required after 2–4 weeks from the previous treatment for the optimal outcome [21].

Studies on fractional photothermolysis for the treatment of periorbital rhytides 1 month after four treatments exposed mild improvement in 12% of patients, noticeable improvement in 30%, and moderate to significant improvement in 54%. Rokhsar and Fitzpatrick used fractional photothermolysis to treat 10 cases of resistant melasma. After 4–6 treatment sessions, 60% of patients achieved 75–100% clearing of melasma and 30% had less than 25% correction [22]. Furthermore, patient satisfaction has demonstrated fractional photothermolysis to be useful in the treatment of dilated pores, overall skin texture, and solar lentigines following a series of at least 3–5 treatment sessions spaced 2–4 weeks apart. This resurfacing laser appears to work better on fine to moderate rhytides in comparison to deeper lines and wrinkles with perioral vertical rhytides being particularly resistant to any serious improvement. Rhytides unfortunately are not improved to the same degree with lower recovery time procedures as they are with fractional ablative resurfacing. Moreover, fractional nonablative techniques have also been studied in treating acne scars. Rahman et al. assessed 53 atrophic scars which included acne scars, traumatic scars, striae, and surgical scars treated at both high and low energies. Results showed 92% of participants exhibited at least some clinical improvement and 66% of

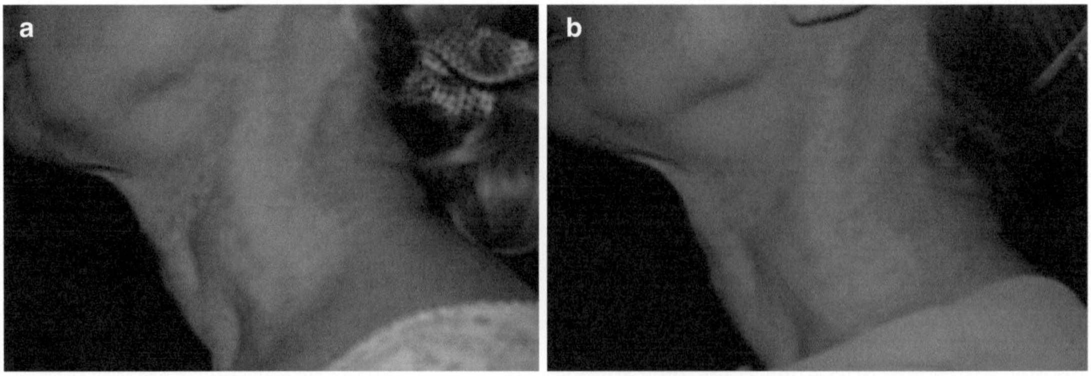

Fig. 8.2 A patient with poikiloderma of Civatte before (**a**) and 3 months after the last laser session (**b**) [19]

participants showed 50–100% improvement in their atrophic scarring [23].

8.2.4 Ablative Fractional Lasers

The most current generation of ablative lasers is the fractional ablative lasers starting in 2007. Ablative fractionated lasers are significantly safer than their nonablative counterparts while achieving mild skin tightening, photodamage, strophic scars, and pigmentation including hypopigmented scars. However, these lasers do pose a higher risk of scarring, discoloration, and skin infection than nonablative lasers [24]. Instead of MTZs, microscopic columns of ablated tissue are generated, extending from the epidermis into the dermis. Overall, moderate downtime and risk of complications are expected. Concerning rhytides, patients with fine or moderate wrinkling and periorbital rhytides reasonably respond better to nonablative technology than those with excessive laxity and deeper lines around the perioral area. Nevertheless, subjects with deeper lines are still eligible to be treated but should expect a limit to the amount of improvement seen, particularly with a single treatment. Success with the nonablative procedure is most readily only seen with the middle-aged population. Patients living in highly sun-exposed areas have greater photodamaged skin for their age, making it more difficult for them to receive the target "rejuvenated" goal. Patients desiring a greater elimination of rhytides should consider ablative laser procedures or surgical procedures. Fully ablative technology has been restricted to Fitzpatrick skin types I–II but is available to use on darker skin tones with caution to avoid post-inflammatory hyperpigmentation or hyperpigmentation [25].

There is 10,600 nm emitted by the CO_2 laser, 2940 nm emitted by the Er:YAG laser, and 2790 nm emitted by the yttrium scandium gallium garnet (YSGG) laser. The use of CO_2 lasers introduced fractional technology to the industry to reduce fine lines and wrinkles with one study showing 72% of participants with some improvement and 80% with a satisfactory reduction [26]. In order to maximize efficacy, CO_2 laser treatments have been pushed to higher coverages which can increase the chances of scarring and hypopigmentation. Only a single treatment is necessary to achieve anti-aging goals and needs aftercare to prevent infection and enhance the healing profile. The 2940 nm is absorbed with a high coefficient for water without thermal injury that the cells vaporize instantly, failing to achieve hemostasis during treatment. The CO_2 laser wavelength has a lower absorption coefficient for water; therefore, a significant amount of thermal damage transpires. Here, the advantage is exceptional hemostasis, but the disadvantage is an increased risk of causing excessive thermal injury and scarring. The YSGG laser wavelength's intermediate absorption coefficient for water created enough thermal damage to maintain adequate hemostasis without having the degree of thermal injury from a CO_2 laser.

There are four key parameters for the effectiveness and recovery of the fractional ablative laser. These are power, pitch, dwell time, and micro spot diameter. Manipulating these parameters can determine the healing profile of a patient, the extent of surface area treated, penetration depth, and degree of thermal injury. The power is energy delivered per microbeam varying from 5 to 100 mJ/microbeam per device. Additionally, as the pitch or spacing is decreased, the surface area is increased of the skin being treated. Dwell time is pulse duration, and this correlates with the degree of thermal damage, while microbeam diameter is important for penetration depth (Fig. 8.3).

Rahman et al. [27] described a study containing two parts, the first phase treating 24 patients with a prototype of an ablative device (what is now the Fraxel re:pair) at 5–40 mJ per pulse and 400 microthermal zones (MTZ) per cm^2 on the forearm with clinical and histologic evaluation at 1 month and 3 months post-treatment. These studies specified erythema and edema did not persevere as judged by the 3-month follow-up visit. Following this initial study, 30 patients were treated once or twice with the same prototype device, 5–40 mJ per pulse, and 400–1200 MTZ/cm^2. Investigators rated results from these settings as 26–50% improved in laxity and

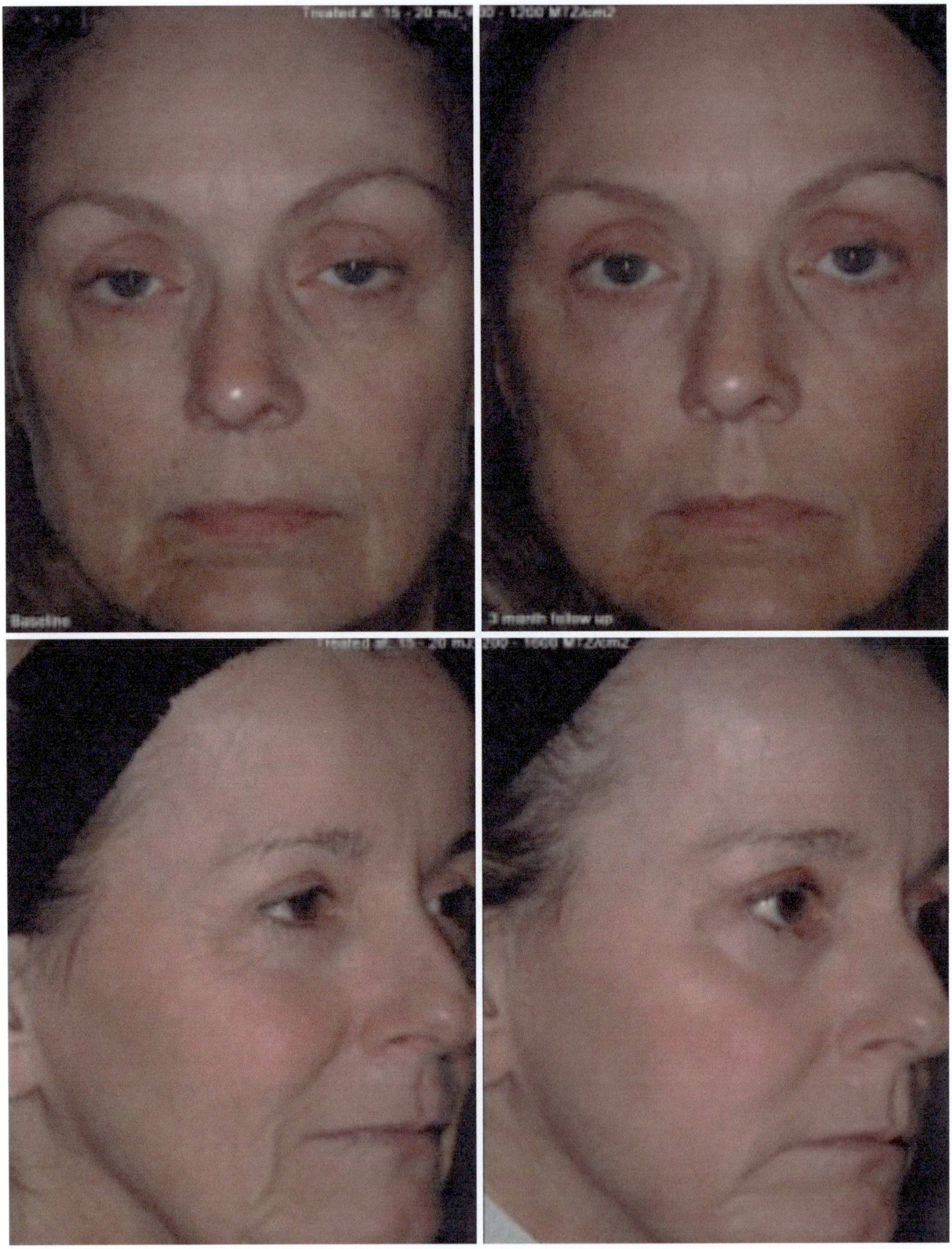

Fig. 8.3 Results of the ablative fractional laser before and after 3 months of the treatment

greater than 50% in texture, rhytides, vascular lesions, and pigmentation. The average improvement in the Fitzpatrick wrinkle scale was 1.47 (Fig. 8.4), showing fine textural changes with subtly accentuated skin lines. Additionally, six patients exhibited post-inflammatory hyperpigmentation after 3 months. Erythema was seen postoperatively in all patients as expected, persisting in 10 patients at 1 month and in 2 patients at 3 months. There were not any cases of delayed-onset hypopigmentation observed. Furthermore, Clementoni et al. investigated 55 patients and evaluated them again at 1 and 3 months [28]. Patients received a single-pass treatment with 100 mJ pulses with approximately 80-μm ablation and 200 μm of further thermal injury. Significant improvement was seen with fine lines, sallowness, mottled pigment, texture, but not telangiectasia or coarse wrinkles. The mean for healing time was 3.3 days, and erythema continued for a mean of 13.6 days. In addition, Berlin et al. reported a trial of ten patients ranging from 40 to 69 in age with skin type I–III, treated with one single pass on the full face [29]. Improvements in rhytides, texture, and elastosis on a five-point scale on blinded investigator analysis averaged 1.8 at 1 month and 1.6 at 3 months, with a slightly higher patient satisfaction rating. Histology displayed decreased solar elastosis, and electron microscopy displayed decreased diameter of collagen fibril, consistent with increased type III collagen destruction. No delayed hypopigmentation was observed in this experiment.

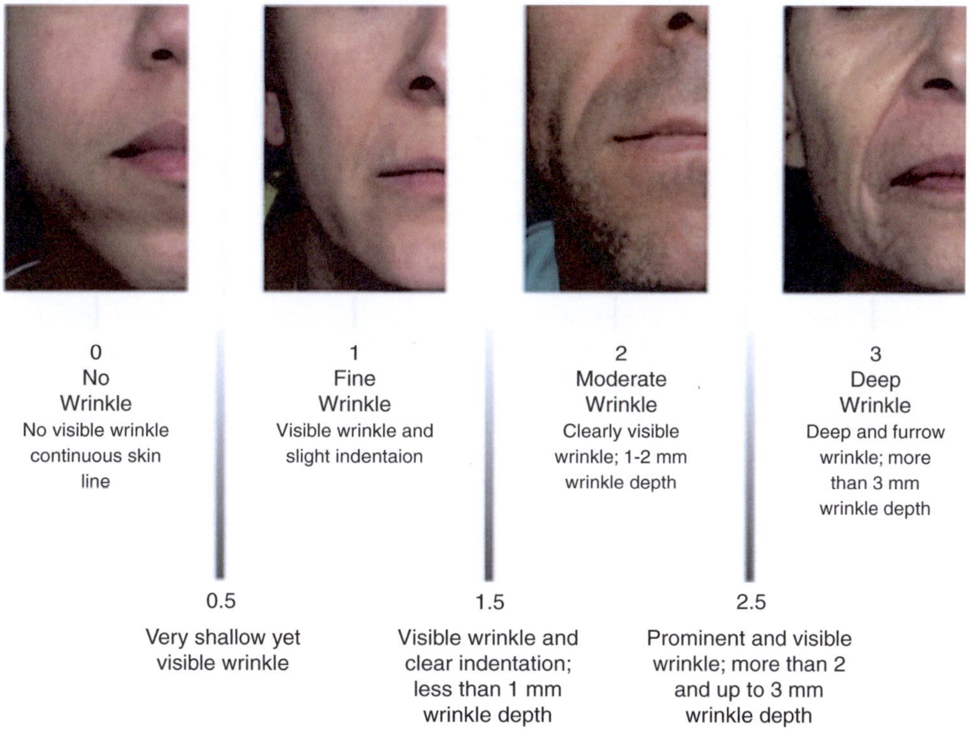

Fig. 8.4 Presented is the Modified Fitzpatrick Wrinkle Scale (MFWS). The MFWS comprises three main classes, in which definitions are based on a set of reference photographs and descriptions, and three inter-classes, in which definitions are based only on descriptions. Assessors were trained to apply this scale to volunteers and study patients by using photographs of nasolabial wrinkles either alone or with descriptions. Inter- and intra-assessment reliability coefficients were calculated using weighted kappa statistics [30]

8.3 Laser Complications

Erythema is superficial reddening of the skin and is regularly observed in the inflammatory healing process lasting up to 3 months from the CO_2 laser [31]. The level of erythema is dependent on how much thermal injury is done, the depth of the laser, and the skin type. This is typically self-resolving or patients are able to treat with mild topical corticosteroids or vascular laser. This same laser can treat telangiectasias which are dilated or broken blood vessels near the surface of the skin or mucous membranes that can arise after a resurfacing treatment creating transparency of the skin. Other skin eruptions can occur in the form of acne, milia, and contact dermatitis usually due to the over occlusion of topical products or overactivation of glands. Milia are extracted through a comedone extractor, and acne is treated with discontinuing occlusive agents and antibiotics. The skin is thin and highly sensitive; therefore, the access of topical agents to the Langerhans cells in the dermis is greatly increased. This means regular skin products are not well tolerated, and skin regimens with retinoids or other active ingredients should be discontinued.

Moreover, infection after laser resurfacing can be bacterial, fungal, or viral. The most well-known side effect of lasers is due to herpes simplex virus (HSV), especially in patients who are already prone to cold sores. Figure 8.5 shows herpes eruptions around the mouth to be painful and may prolong healing by 6 to 8 weeks and could possibly result in scarring if trauma is induced to the skin. The current recommendation is for all patients to be prophylaxed against HSV [32]. Some patients may avoid taking antiviral medications, whereas others may experience infections. The treatment is early recognition of the infection and treatment with oral antiviral agents. For very severe infections with herpes simplex or zoster, intravenous antiviral medication may be needed. For patients prone to this infection, the use of valacyclovir in a 10- or 14-day course is recommended as a preventative measure following facial laser resurfacing.

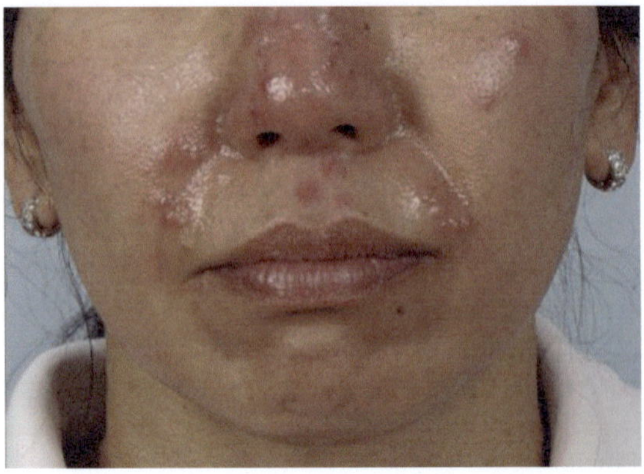

Fig. 8.5 This patient has experienced a herpes simplex virus breakout after receiving laser resurfacing treatment. The patient failed to take antiviral medication then was treated with valacyclovir 1000 mg 3 times a day and responded with no scarring [4]

Bacterial infection after laser resurfacing using an open treatment-like ablative technologies is uncommon, but with increasing methicillin-resistant *Staphylococcus aureus* (MRSA), patients have experienced infections after laser resurfacing treatment. Infection typically occurs 2–10 days after the procedure in post resurfacing patients [33]. Treatment usually follows the administration of broad-spectrum prophylactic antibiotics like cephalexin along with a culture of the skin for targeted antibiotic treatment after obtaining culture results from Gram and fungal stains. Like HSV, it is better for preventative action to be taken by prescribing patients a course of antibiotics to take after their procedure and providing the patient with instructions on meticulous wound care. Furthermore, fungal infections are not as common but infection with a yeast called *Candida albicans* can happen (Fig. 8.6). Symptoms show patients with an extremely red face after showing improvement in healing. Topical or oral antifungal medication should be given to the patient such as fluconazole.

Changes in skin pigmentation are a large side effect, especially in patients with darker skin tones depending on the laser. Hypopigmentation has been seen with the CO_2 and Er:YAG treatments and may not be apparent until 6 to 10 months post-treatment. This occurs when

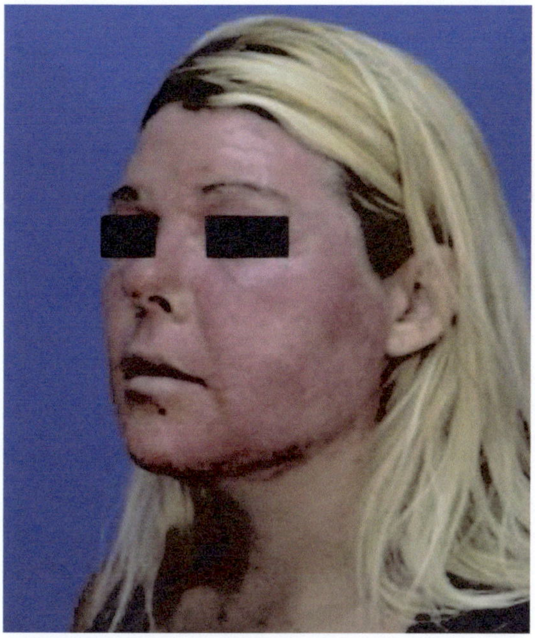

Fig. 8.6 Patient shown with a fungal infection after laser resurfacing treatment affecting the face [4]

aggressive and repeated resurfacing is undertaken for severe acne scarring or deep wrinkles and is more noticeable in IV–V skin types [34]. Not many effective treatments exist for hypopigmentation other than excimer laser therapy. The appearance is minimized by blending the margins of the resurfaced spaces with a zone of reduced energy density by lowering the millijoules or density setting on the instrument. On the other hand, post-inflammatory hyperpigmentation (Fig. 8.7) occurs often and again more commonly in darker skin types or patients who have had sun exposure. It is a self-resolving issue, but bleaching products and retinoids can accelerate the process to be cleared in 2 to 6 weeks. It is mostly observed in the perioral and malar area or if spot treated, in that targeted area [34].

Scarring is also an unpleasant and permanent side effect and can be due to an overly aggressive full-field or fractional treatment, infection, or trauma-induced by the patient dur-

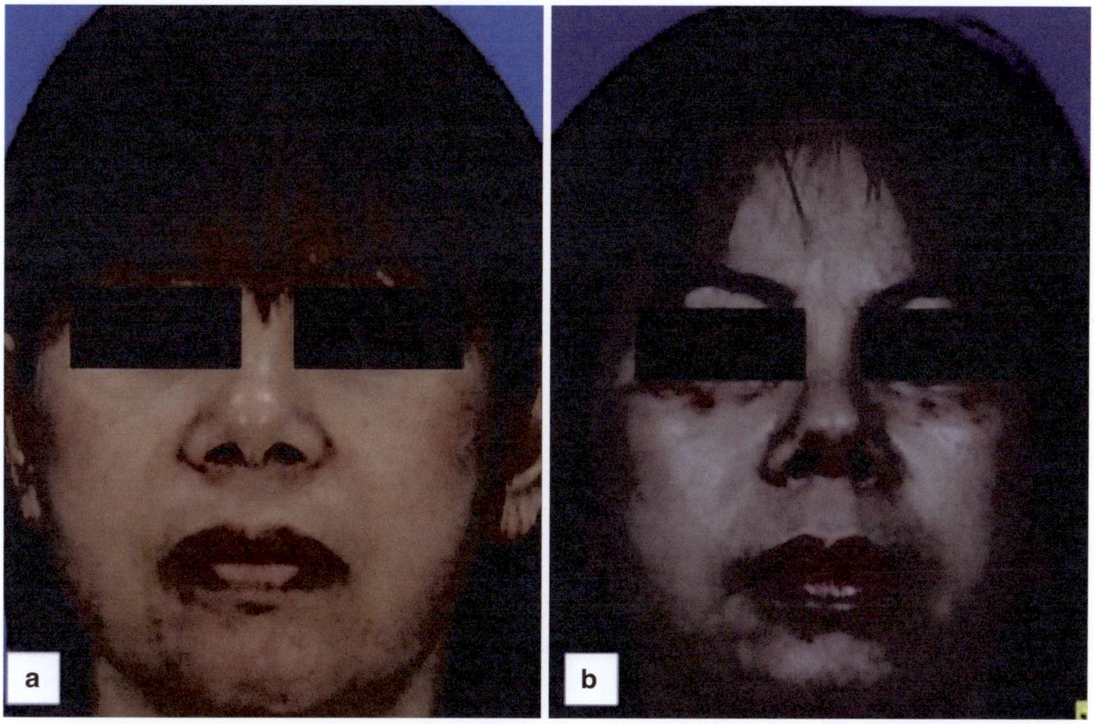

Fig. 8.7 A 49-year-old Asian woman who developed hyperpigmentation under the eyes following Er:YAG resurfacing [4]

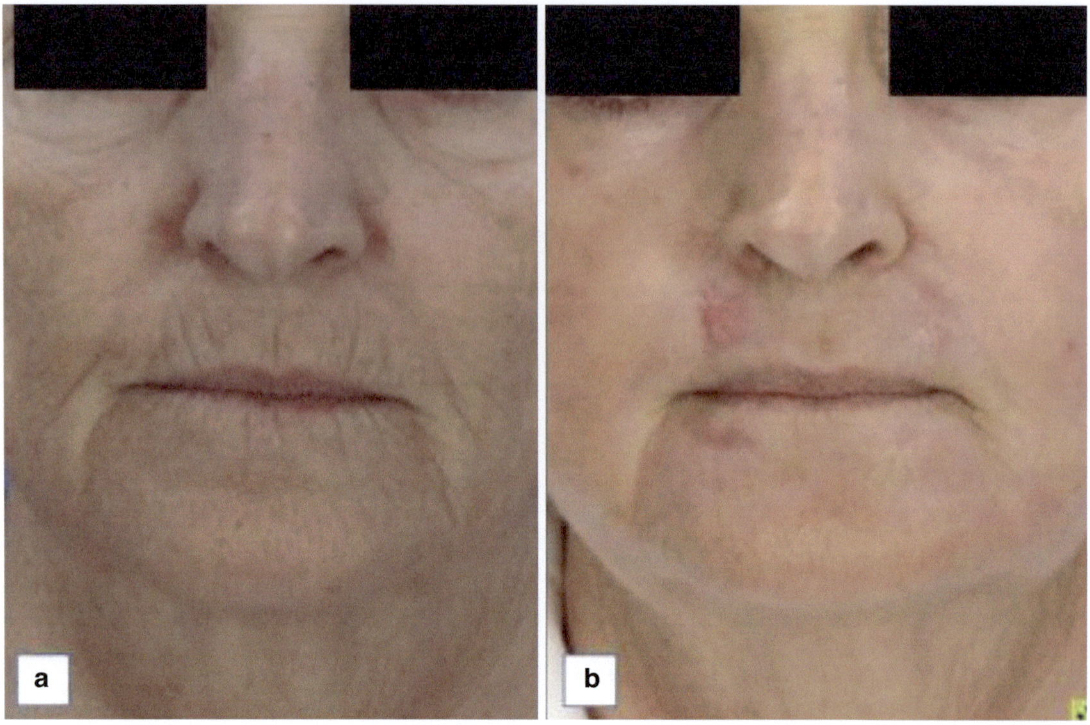

Fig. 8.8 A 64-year-old woman who developed a hypertrophic scar after laser resurfacing: (**a**) before and (**b**) after treatment with intralesional corticosteroids and IPL treatments [4]

ing healing. Infection can turn a second-degree burn caused by the laser into a third-degree burn with scarring. These infections are the most common cause of scarring in patients or from excessive fluence of density, multiple passes, or pulse stacking [35]. If the skin is heated beyond its ability to heal promptly without excessive fibrosis, scarring will be a side effect. The neck and chest are also more susceptible to scarring than the face due to having thinner skin in the dermis [36]. It is important to know whether a patient has been or is on isotretinoin as it totally suppresses sebaceous glands and can result in hypertrophic scarring. One must wait several months to years after isotretinoin use when they return back to normal skin oiliness and moisture before considering conservative laser treatment. Slow healing is also a major sign of incoming hypertrophic scarring, as seen in Fig. 8.8, which may be treated with intralesional corticosteroids and intralesional 5-fluorouracil.

8.4 Conclusion

Laser resurfacing has already changed the world of cosmetic procedures, and technology will only improve to work towards facing fewer consequences and greater benefits while being inclusive towards all skin types. Most ablative lasers offer great results but at the cost of long recovery times and the potential for more serious side effects. In contrast, nonablative technologies offer moderate results with much less downtime and side effects. Then, fractionated machinery combines the best aspects of both departments. Overall, many lasers have been made unique to the concern of each patient; therefore, it is important for physicians to provide the appropriate care.

References

1. Mayo Clinic Health System. How does fractional CO2 laser resurfacing erase signs of aging? YouTube. 2019. https://www.youtube.com/watch?v=oDGCjIuYDU4&ab_channel=MayoClinicHealthSystem. Accessed 4 Feb 2022.
2. Russell H. Non-ablative laser resurfacing Hannah. Glowday, Dr Sophie Shotter. https://www.glowday.com/laser-skin-treatments/non-ablative-laser-resurfacing/guide.
3. Jason P, et al. Current laser resurfacing technologies: a review that delves beneath the surface. Semin Plast Surg. 2012;26(3):109–16. https://doi.org/10.1055/s-0032-1329413.
4. Hruza GJ, Tanzi EL. Chapter 7: laser resurfacing. In: Lasers and lights. Edinburgh: Elsevier; 2018. p. 83–94.
5. Alexiades-Armenakas MR, Dover JS, Arndt KA. The spectrum of laser skin resurfacing: nonablative, fractional, and ablative laser resurfacing. J Am Acad Dermatol. 2008;58(5):719–37; quiz 738-40.
6. Alster TS, West TB. Resurfacing of atrophic facial acne scars with a high-energy, pulsed carbon dioxide laser. Dermatol Surg. 1996;22(2):151–4; discussion 154-5.
7. Ward PD, Baker SR. Long-term results of carbon dioxide laser resurfacing of the face. Arch Facial Plast Surg. 2008;10(4):238–43; discussion 244-5.
8. Goldman MP, Manuskiatti W. Combined laser resurfacing with the 950-microsec pulsed CO2 + Er:YAG lasers. Dermatol Surg. 1999;25(3):160–3.
9. Hantash BM, Gladstone HBG. Current role of resurfacing lasers. Ital Dermatol Venereol. 2009;144(3):229–41.
10. DeHoratius DM, Dover JS. Clin Dermatol. 2007;25(5):474–9.
11. Bogle MA. Fractionated mid-infrared resurfacing. Semin Cutan Med Surg. 2008;27(4):252–8.
12. Zhenxiao Z, Aie X, Yuzhi J, Xiaodong W, Xianqiang J, Jing S, Han Z, Junhui Z, Xiaojun Z, Yanjun Z. Skin Res Technol. 2011;17(4):505–9.
13. Yaghmai D, Garden JM, Bakus AD, Massa MC. Comparison of a 1,064 nm laser and a 1,320 nm laser for the nonablative treatment of acne scars. Dermatol Surg. 2005;31(8 Pt 1):903–9.
14. Darné S, Hiscutt EL, Seukeran DC. Evaluation of the clinical efficacy of the 1,450 nm laser in acne vulgaris: a randomized split-face, investigator-blinded clinical trial. Br J Dermatol. 2011;165(6):1256–62.
15. Chua SH, Ang P, Khoo LS, Goh CL. Nonablative 1450-nm diode laser in the treatment of facial atrophic acne scars in type IV to V Asian skin: a prospective clinical study. Dermatol Surg. 2004;30(10):1287–91.
16. Laubach H, Tannous Z, Anderson RR, Manstein D. A histological evaluation of the dermal effects after fractional photothermolysis treatment. Lasers Surg Med. 2005;36(Suppl 17):86.
17. Tannous Z, Laubach HJ, Anderson RR, Manstein D. Changes of epidermal pigment distribution after fractional resurfacing: a clinicopathologic correlation. Lasers Surg Med. 2005;36(Suppl 17):32.
18. Mahmoud BH, Srivastava D, Janiga JJ, Yang JJ, Lim HW, Ozog DM. Safety and effficacy of erbium-doped yttrium aluminum garnet fractionated laser for treatment of acne scars in type IV to VI skin. Dermatol Surg. 2010;36(5):602–9.
19. Tierney EP, Hanke CW. Treatment of Poikiloderma of Civatte with ablative fractional laser resurfacing: prospective study and review of the literature. J Drugs Dermatol. 2009;8:527–34.
20. Weiss RA, Gold M, Bene N, Biron JA, Munavalli G, Weiss M, Beasley K. Prospective clinical evaluation of 1440-nm laser delivered by microarray for treatment of photoaging and scars. J Drugs Dermatol. 2006;5(8):740–4.
21. Tanzi EL, Wanitphakdeedecha R, Alster TS. Fraxel laser indications and long-term follow-up. Aesthet Surg J. 2008;28(6):675–8, discussion 679–680.
22. Rokhsar CK, Fitzpatrick RE. The treatment of melasma with fractional photothermolysis: a pilot study. Dermatol Surg. 2005;31:1645–50.
23. Rahman Z, Tanner H, Jiang K. Treatment of atrophic scars with the 1550 nm erbium fiber fractional laser. Lasers Surg Med. 2006;38(Suppl 18):24.
24. Karsai S, Czarnecka A, Jünger M, Raulin C. Ablative fractional lasers (CO(2) and Er:YAG): a randomized controlled double-blind split-face trial of the treatment of peri-orbital rhytides. Lasers Surg Med. 2010;42(2):160–7.
25. Alster T, Hirsch R. Single-pass CO2 laser skin resurfacing of light and dark skin: extended experience with 52 patients. J Cosmet Laser Ther. 2003;5:39–42.
26. Christiansen K, Bjerring P. Low density, non-ablative fractional CO2 laser rejuvenation. Lasers Surg Med. 2008;40(7):454–60.
27. Rahman Z, MacFalls H, Jiang K, et al. Fractional deep dermal ablation induces tissue tightening. Lasers Surg Med. 2009;41:78–86.
28. Clementoni MT, Gilardino P, Muti GF, Beretta D, Schianchi R. Non-sequential fractional ultrapulsed CO2 resurfacing of photoaged facial skin: preliminary clinical report. J Cosmet Laser Ther. 2007;9:218–25.
29. Berlin AL, Hussain M, Phelps R, Goldberg DJ. A prospective study of fractional scanned nonsequential carbon dioxide laser resurfacing: a clinical and histopathologic evaluation. Dermatol Surg. 2009;35:222–8.
30. Shoshani D, Markovitz E, Monstrey SJ, Narins DJ. The modified Fitzpatrick Wrinkle Scale: a clinical validated measurement tool for nasolabial wrinkle severity assessment. Dermatol Surg. 2008;34(Suppl 1):S85–91; discussion S91. PMID: 18547187. https://doi.org/10.1111/j.1524-4725.2008.34248.x.
31. Trelles MA, Mordon S, Svaasand LO, Mellor TK, Rigau J, Garcia L. The origin and role of erythema after carbon dioxide laser resurfacing. A clinical and

histological study. Dermatol Surg. 1998;24(1):25–9. https://doi.org/10.1111/j.1524-4725.1998.tb04047.x.
32. Beeson WH, Rachel JD. Valacyclovir prophylaxis for Herpes simplex virus infection or infection recurrence following laser skin resurfacing. Dermatol Surg. 2002;28(4):331–6. https://doi.org/10.1046/j.1524-4725.2002.01155.x.
33. Christian MM, et al. Delayed infections following full.—Researchgate.net. https://www.researchgate.net/publication/227538114_Delayed_Infections_Following_Full-Face_CO2_Laser_Resurfacing_and_Occlusive_Dressing_Use.
34. Gregory RO, Seckel BR, Mayl N, Alster TS. Complications in laser resurfacing. Aesthet Surg J. 2000;20(3):231–7. https://doi.org/10.1016/S1090-820X(00)70022-7.
35. Ramsdell WM. Fractional CO2 laser resurfacing complications. Semin Plast Surg. 2012;26(3):137–40. https://doi.org/10.1055/s-0032-1329415.
36. Avram MM, Tope WD, Yu T, Szachowicz E, Nelson JS. Hypertrophic scarring of the neck following ablative fractional carbon dioxide laser resurfacing. Lasers Surg Med. 2009;41(3):185–8.

Low-Level Light Therapy with LEDs

9

Cari Green and Gabriel Borden

Abstract

Low-level light therapy (LLLT) employs athermal and atraumatic levels of illumination, typically in the visible or near-infrared (NIR) regions of the electromagnetic spectrum, to target tissue and stimulate a clinically useful local or systemic effect. LLLT has demonstrated beneficial applications in the areas of wound healing, pain management, and various musculoskeletal conditions as well as skin rejuvenation. This chapter dives into the benefits of using LED-based devices in aesthetic applications, resulting in a safer and more convenient approach to benefit patients.

Keywords

LEDs · LLLT · Photoprotection · Photoaging · Hyperpigmentation · Ultrasound · Cellular effects

C. Green (✉) · G. Borden
Forever Healthy Foundation,
Baden-Wurttemberg, Karlsruhe, Germany
e-mail: cg@forever-healthy.org; gb@forever-healthy.org

9.1 Introduction

The acronym LLLT originally denoted low-level *laser* therapy and was only later conveniently generalized to any suitable light source. In recent decades, since the commercial availability of narrow bandwidth designs, light-emitting diodes (LEDs) have become an increasingly preferred choice due to their low cost, safety, small size, and the ease with which they can be incorporated into a wide range of devices. They can be mounted in arrays, a property which, in addition to their other characteristics, disposes them favorably to large target surfaces such as the skin [1].

While skin aging is a topic of ongoing research, current understanding posits that aging ensues from cycles of damage followed by inflammation and partial repair, which can be initiated by intrinsic factors such as the production of reactive oxygen species during normal metabolism and extrinsic insults such as smoking or ultraviolet light exposure. Cellular level changes include protein oxidation and mitochondrial and DNA damage, while at the tissue level there is a gradual loss of collagen, elastin and subcutaneous fat as well as moisture content, and an increase in cellular senescence. Aesthetically, aged skin typically appears thinner, drier, looser, and more wrinkled; while overall aged skin appears paler and more translucent, and age spots (lentigo) appear in sun-exposed

R. L. Bard (ed.), *Image-Guided Aesthetic Treatments*, https://doi.org/10.1007/978-3-031-36266-8_9

areas [2, 3]. This chapter focuses on therapy with red and near-infrared (R/NIR; frequency ranges approximately 625–700 nm and 700–2500 nm, respectively) emitting LEDs designed to counteract these changes associated with skin aging.

9.2 Mechanism of Action

Photons incident upon the skin undergo scattering, absorption, and/or reflection in a wavelength-dependent manner. Penetration depth is limited via photon interaction with abundant chromophores such as melanin, hemoglobin, and water, which all have different, partially overlapping absorption spectra. In the visible through NIR range, penetration depth increases with wavelength, up to approximately 1000 nm when absorption by water begins to dominate [4]. The inquisitive reader can verify this phenomenon with a simple demonstration: take a household cold white light source such as a penlight, cover it with a fingertip (in a darkened room for best effect), and observe the red wavelengths escaping from all sides. This variation in the depth of penetration is one of the variables thought to account for the differential effects of different wavelengths of light.

The physiological response stimulated by illumination is termed photobiomodulation (PBM). Supporting the clinical literature, many in vitro studies have been published documenting PBM effects such as increased proliferation of cultured cells, increased oxidative phosphorylation in isolated mitochondria, and increased generation of signaling molecules [5–7]. An explanatory framework for PBM was proposed by Karu, consisting of three steps: absorption of light by a suitable chromophore resulting in a primary response; a second stage of signal transduction and amplification; and finally, PBM, with ensuing clinically observed effects [8].

A leading candidate for the role of primary chromophore has been cytochrome c oxidase (CCO). Karu reported a correspondence between illumination wavelength, acceleration of DNA synthesis in cultured cells, and the absorption spectrum of CCO [8]. It is expected that any chromophore responsible for the initiation of PBM would likely be involved in cellular signaling and/or metabolism, an expectation well filled by CCO given its central role in mitochondrial energy production as the final membrane protein complex in the electron transport chain.

Doubts remain, however, as recent authors have not detected any change in isolated CCO kinetics upon illumination with R/NIR wavelengths [9], while others have noted a proliferative effect even in cells completely lacking CCO [10]. Other researchers have proposed primary roles for flavins or protoporphyrins (though more prominently for visible, as opposed to NIR wavelengths) [11], hemoglobin and myoglobin (as potential nitric oxide sources)[12], and the nanoscale behavior of water [13]. Quite possibly, the robust downstream effects of incident light may be mediated by multiple primary photon acceptors and a variety of intermediate signaling molecules such as adenosine triphosphate (ATP), nitric oxide (NO), and reactive oxygen species (ROS).

9.3 Rejuvenative Effects of Low-Level Light Therapy with LEDs

9.3.1 Summary

Despite differences in penetration depth and likely primary absorption routes, red and NIR light stimulate substantially similar photobiomodulation effects involving changes in cell proliferation, differentiation, migration, inflammatory mediators, and collagen and elastin production. These changes are in turn believed to lead to the observed downstream aesthetic benefits in skin firmness and tone and reduction in wrinkles and age spots.

Though treatment with R/NIR wavelengths is the principal focus of this chapter, some studies listed below report results regarding R/NIR light in conjunction with other wavelengths, or when combined with adjunctive modalities, such as glycolic peels or pre-application of photosensitizer. These sources were included in order to provide a more comprehensive review of the developing application of LLLT to skin rejuvenation.

Some of the foundational work in LLLT referenced below was performed with non-LED light sources. In general, PBM depends primarily on wavelength and dose rather than light source, thus prior results using other methods of light generation are predicted to inform therapy with LEDs equally well in most cases.

While many trials referenced below were single- or double-blinded, and/or reported objective measurements, others were open trials that relied heavily on patient impressions. Perhaps predictably, when reported side by side, patients generally reported stronger and more frequent benefits than blinded experts. While it is important for clinicians to be aware that patients may often have a somewhat inflated perception of their treatment response, this is not necessarily a disadvantage; patient satisfaction is important in any specialty, but it carries heightened relative importance in aesthetic medicine.

9.3.1.1 Cellular-Level Effects

Many of the aesthetic benefits of LLLT are believed to follow from quantifiable effects on fibroblasts, the principal extracellular matrix (ECM) fibrous proteins collagen and elastin, and increased water content.

Following treatment with red and/or NIR light, fibroblasts from skin biopsies are observed to increase both in number and activity as evidenced by overall cell enlargement, increases in vimentin and number of mitochondria, and dilated endoplasmic reticula [14, 15].

Skin aging is associated with a downregulation in collagen synthesis and an elevation in expression of matrix metalloproteinases (MMPs) and enzymes responsible for the degradation of extracellular matrix collagen. MMP activity is in turn regulated by tissue inhibitors of matrix metalloproteinase (TIMP; there are four human isoforms). Multiple studies have reported an increase in collagen following LLLT therapy, as assessed through ultrasonography and biopsy followed by histology, immunofluorescence studies, and ultrastructural analysis of transmission electron micrographs [15–19]. Supporting the reported benefits to ECM collagen content, researchers have also documented decreases in MMPs and/or increases in TIMP-1 and TIMP-2 associated with LLLT [15, 16, 20].

In addition to collagen, two studies described increases in the elastin content of the dermis subsequent to therapy with R/NIR wavelengths, as judged by histology and ultrastructural analysis. A benefit to elastin denaturation and distribution, and mitigation of solar elastosis was also noted [15, 21]. Both patient impressions and more objective assessments using a Cutometer support improvements in the mechanical elasticity of the skin [15, 22, 23].

Finally, one report measured an approximately 15% increase in stratum corneum hydration and a 30% decrease in transepidermal water loss (TEWL) with a Corneometer and a TEWLmeter, respectively, following LED treatment [21].

9.3.1.2 ECM-Related Clinical Benefits

The thinning and laxity that derive from the diminished collagen, elastin, and water content of physiologically aging skin result in a loss of firmness and youthful texture and underlie many common undesired aesthetic features such as wrinkles, under-eye bags, increased pore size, and increased prominence of the nasolabial fold. There is considerable evidence that these frequent patient concerns regarding appearance can be at least partially remediated with LLLT.

A majority of participants in four trials employing red wavelengths alone or a combination of R/NIR sources reported increased skin firmness; results persisted at the 12-week follow-up [19, 22, 24, 25].

A benefit to skin texture has been reported according to several criteria: subjective assessments of patients or physicians [21, 23, 24, 26, 27], blinded image grading [16, 17, 20, 22, 28], and profilometry measurements [16–19]. Skin texture either continued to improve or was maintained for at least 12 weeks post-treatment in several studies.

Stirling and Haslam, in a small (*n*=27)) double-blind, randomized controlled trial (DB-RCT) of NIR-emitting LED therapy which included a split-face group, reported that 41% of subjects perceived an improvement of their under-eye bags, and of these, all but one correctly identified the eye that had received the treatment [29].

Baez and Reilly, using alternating therapy with red and NIR wavelengths from LED light sources, reported significant softening of the nasolabial fold as assessed by patients and unblinded observers [30]. The effect peaked at the 9-week follow-up (Fig. 9.1).

Amelioration of fine lines and wrinkles is one of the most common aesthetic LLLT treatment goals, and is frequently highlighted in the literature. Typically, 90% of patients perceive an improvement, and where quantitative measurements have been reported, an approximate 30% reduction is most often described.

Most studies used red and NIR wavelengths [15, 17, 22, 24, 28], while others employed yel-

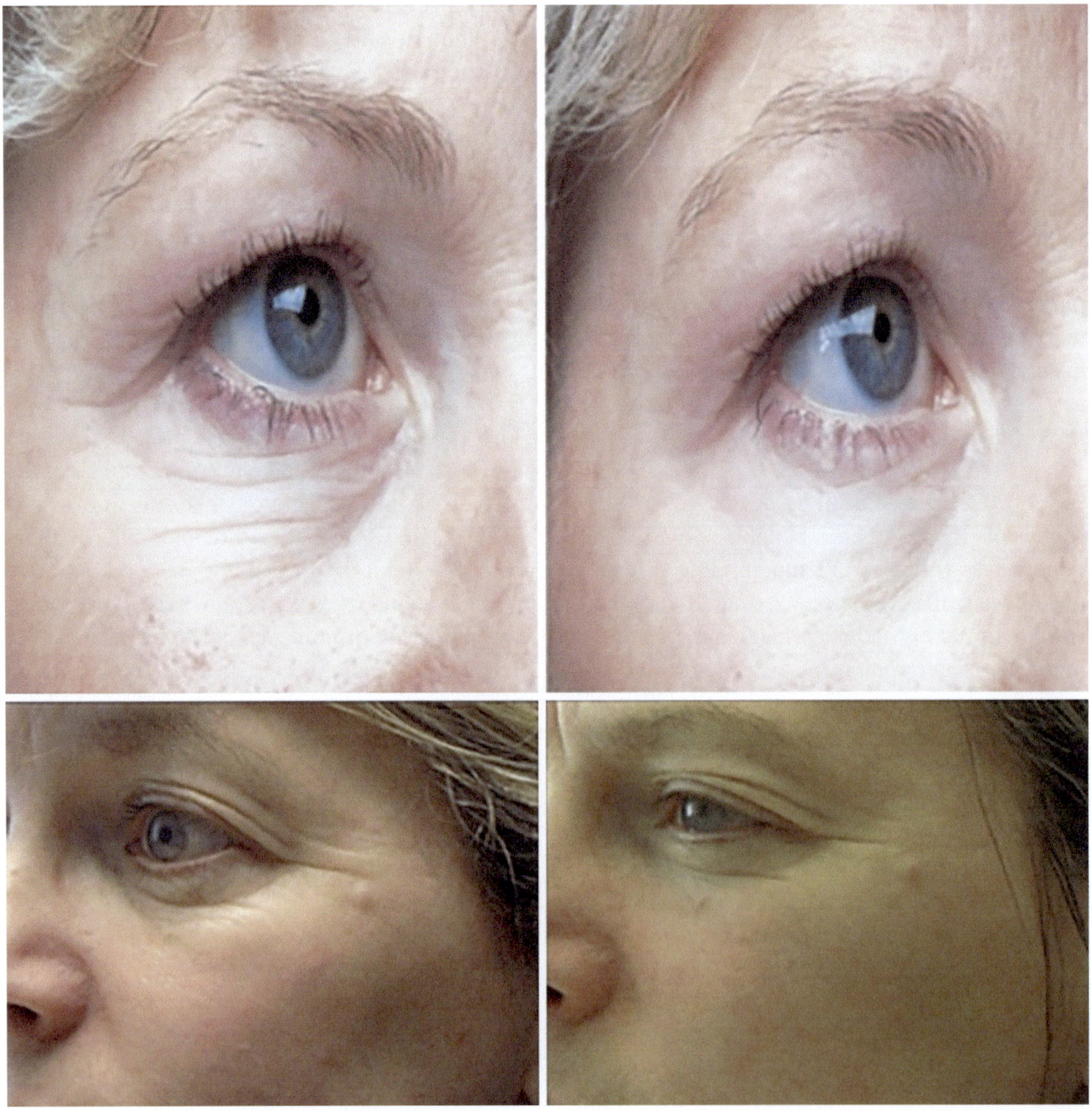

Fig. 9.1 Periorbital wrinkles before (left) and after (right) LLLT treatment (Photo courtesy of GlobalMed Technologies Co., Glen Ellen, California USA)

low light [26], blue light [18], or combined LLLT with glycolic peels [31]. In studies in which follow-up time points were included, at least a partial positive effect remained at 12 weeks post-treatment.

Effects on periocular wrinkles were specifically reported in four trials. A large majority of participants in all trials noticed an improvement; of the three trials reporting impressions of blinded observers, two trials reported a benefit [16, 19, 32, 33].

9.3.1.3 Photoprotection

In vitro, it has been shown that non-coherent, NIR radiation protects human dermal fibroblasts from solar UV toxicity [34]. A study in humans pretreated one of a given subject's thighs with 660 nm LED light, with the opposite thigh serving as a control. Additionally, some thighs were covered with a standardized film of SPF 15 sunscreen to function as positive controls. Exposed windows of subjects' thighs were then exposed to graduated UV-B doses sufficient to cause mild erythema. Pretreatment with red light was found to confer protection comparable to the SPF 15 sunscreen according to blinded evaluators [35].

9.3.1.4 Background Erythema

Two studies that used a 590 nm pulsed LED device as a light source reported improvements in background erythema [16, 26]. Redness was improved 1-week post-treatment in about 25% of subjects. This improvement continued to increase over time and peaked at the 4-month post-treatment follow-up when >40% of patients showed more than a 25% improvement. The benefits began to decline thereafter, and by 12 months, only about 12% of patients continued to exhibit a >25% improvement.

9.3.1.5 Reduction in Pore Size

Two studies showed significantly reduced pore size after 8 treatments over 4 weeks, an improvement that lasted at least 3 months. Treatments were conducted with LED or metal halide lamp sources using a combination of blue and NIR light, and concomitant glycolic peels and vitamin C cream; a control group receiving only peels and cream saw no change. Ninety percent of patients perceived an improvement in one study [36], while another reported that approximately 70% of blinded observers noted an improvement, dropping to roughly 60% at the 4-month follow-up [31].

9.3.1.6 Skin Complexion

Several trials of LLLT have described improvements in skin tone/complexion, using LED or gas discharge lamp light sources, with most employing a combination of wavelengths ranging from 415 to 890 nm. A majority of participants experienced improvements which persisted through 5- and 12-week post-treatment follow-ups. Results according to blinded assessors were reported in some studies [17, 22, 31], while other studies included only impressions of patients or unblinded physicians [23, 27].

9.3.1.7 Global Photoaging Scores

Four trials using LED light sources with yellow, red, and/or NIR wavelengths reported a decrease in "global photoaging" as evaluated by blinded assessment.

In two articles reporting results from the same trial, photoaging assessment scores were significantly improved at all follow-ups with 51.6% of the population experiencing a 25–50% improvement and 12.9% experiencing a 50–75% improvement at 3 months post-treatment [19, 32] (Fig. 9.2).

A trial that used a yellow light LED system found that more than 85% of patients showed at least a 25% improvement in the global photoaging score at 4 months post-treatment. This effect was reduced at 12 months but still significantly above the baseline [16].

The light-only arm of a trial comparing 2 sessions of photodynamic therapy (PDT) with LED red light therapy (3 treatments per week for 4 weeks) applied to forearm skin found that both therapies significantly reduced photoaging [21]. Dermoscopic evaluation 2 weeks after treatment showed marked improvement in skin appearance and reduction of photodamage in both groups (although it was more prominent in the PDT group).

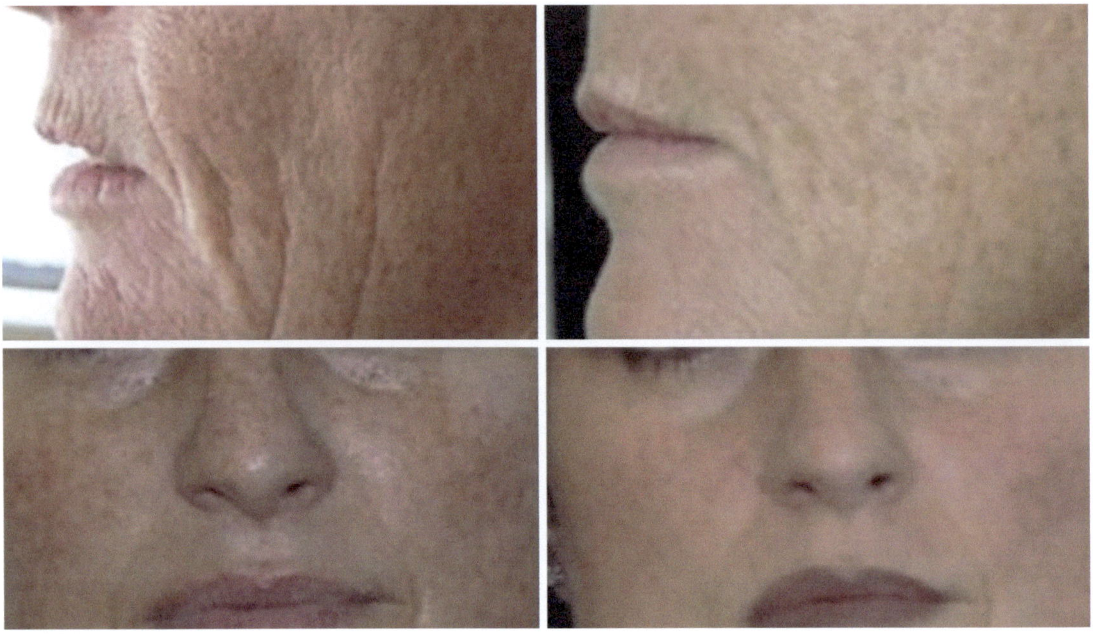

Fig. 9.2 Skin rejuvenation with LLLT, before treatment (left) and after (right) (Photo courtesy of GlobalMed Technologies Co., Glen Ellen, California USA)

9.4 Adverse Effects

9.4.1 Adverse Effects Occurring in Clinical Trials

9.4.1.1 Erythema

Erythema is one of the most common side effects of treatment with LLLT, occurring in several studies [18, 19, 23, 27, 28, 37–44]. It has occurred with several types of light sources, using many different devices, at all tested wavelengths including blue, yellow, red, and NIR. Depending on the trial, an incidence from 3 to 40% was reported; however, the effect was most often mild, and all cases of erythema were transient, resolving within hours to a couple of days.

9.4.1.2 Hyperpigmentation

Hyperpigmentation is one of the more serious potential side effects of LLLT, occurring with a variety of light sources and different devices, though more often in trials that included blue wavelengths as part of the treatment [27, 42, 45–54]. The hyperpigmentation was mild and affected from 8 to 80% of subjects within a given study. The duration was moderate, resolving over weeks to months.

9.4.1.3 Ocular Glare, Blurred Vision, and Ocular Floaters

One noted six cases of ocular glare appeared with both blue and red light, while a single study subject treated with red light alone reported blurred vision and ocular floaters [33]. Symptoms were more frequent in the group treated with red light, possibly due to the relatively higher lux of the red light. Ocular glare and blurred vision are resolved without treatment, while the participant who experienced floaters dropped out of the study. The floaters resolved over a period of 3 weeks without treatment. Difficulties with the use of eye protection were observed during the initial period of study in the subjects who eventually developed ocular symptoms. Complete eye protection and comprehensive instructions for using LED devices are necessary to mitigate this risk.

9.4.1.4 Other Adverse Effects

Acne trials, generally using blue wavelengths as a component of treatment, have reported several adverse effects not generally seen elsewhere in the literature, including dryness, pruritus, rash, and desquamation, though all were mild, brief, and resolved without intervention [38, 40, 42, 44, 55, 56].

Other trials (using blue and R/NIR wavelengths) have described reactions including pain, burning sensation, edema, and vesiculation, but again all mild (pain 1 out of 10 on visual analog scale) and self-limited [41, 43, 53, 57].

Two individual patients, with telangiectasia and a scar, respectively, reported a temporary increased prominence of those blemishes following treatment [17].

9.4.2 Risks for Preclinical Trials

9.4.2.1 Interactions with Malignancy

LLLT has been shown to stimulate growth and progression of cancer cells in vitro [58, 59] and in vivo [60, 61]. The effect may be biphasic and dose-dependent. In an LLLT study on melanoma in mice (660 nm), low-dose treatment reduced tumor size, while high-dose treatment increased the tumor size [60]. LLLT (660 nm, 424 mW/cm^2) every other day for 4 weeks in hamsters has been shown to increase the progression and negatively influence the histology of existing tumors [61].

IR radiation has also been shown to cause a condition called erythema ab igne that leads to an elevated risk of various types of skin cancer. However, the irradiances and cumulative dose in all cases were very high [62].

While the above are theoretical concerns, it should also be noted that R/NIR light is used as part of photodynamic therapy to treat cancers as well, in particular, actinic keratosis and basal cell carcinoma [63].

9.4.2.2 Photoaging

One study demonstrated that, following exposure to a high fluence of IR-A light (360 or 720 J/cm^2; 760–1440 nm), intact human skin exhibited upregulation of MMP-1 and downregulation of TIMP-1 [64]. Both of these effects would be expected to contribute to collagen and elastin degradation, in contrast to the beneficial effects described above reported by multiple authors using lower doses. In the same report, high fluence IR-A irradiation provoked a decrease in the antioxidant content of the skin.

IR radiation was shown to increase the actinic damage caused by UVA in guinea pigs [65]. While the study employed dosages similar to those used clinically (or encountered from natural solar radiation), the epidermis of the epilated guinea pig skin model used is several times thinner than human epidermis.

Acute exposure of human skin to an IR fluence over 1300 J/cm^2 has been shown to alter the balance between angiogenesis factor VEGF and its inhibitor TSP-2 [66] as well as increase mast cell number and tryptase expression in human skin in vivo [67].

9.4.3 Summary

More side effects are associated with blue light treatment than other wavelengths and were reported in disease treatment trials rather than in skin rejuvenation trials. Most studies showing negative effects of near-infrared radiation used artificial light sources far above the solar irradiance threshold, whereas those resulting from treatment with R/NIR wavelengths with dosing commonly used for skin rejuvenation were mostly mild and of a transient, self-resolving nature [62]. With LLLT, more is generally not better.

The most frequently reported adverse effects in R/NIR skin rejuvenation trials are erythema (resolving in hours or days), hyperpigmentation (resolving within weeks to months), and ocular symptoms (resolving within weeks and also linked with imperfect participant compliance with eye protection instructions). The potential risks that have appeared in preclinical trials, photoaging and carcinogenesis, arose in the context of much higher doses than are used in human LLLT trials, where they have been absent in the literature. Thus, in the event a troublesome adverse event arises during the course of therapy, it is straightforward for the practitioner and patient to simply pause treatment and then reassess.

9.4.4 Treatment Protocols

9.4.4.1 Contraindications and Risk Mitigation

Risk mitigation strategies for LLLT are to monitor for developing side effects and discontinue if they arise and to minimize the number of sessions. Eye protection, ideally of the "blackout" variety (as opposed to filtering or dimming), manufactured for use with LLLT should be used. LED sources are much safer than lasers, and momentary accidental eye exposure is unlikely to cause damage. Indeed, many LLLT devices have been commercialized without FDA or other medical regulatory approval because the light output is below a nominal hazard level. Nevertheless, it is imperative to always use proper precautions and follow manufacturers' safety guidelines.

Contraindications to R/NIR LLLT are few and, in general, are relative, not absolute. Many arise more from an abundance of caution rather than direct evidence of harm. Device manufacturers may provide their own guidance and patient screening recommendations. The following is a list of some of the most common clinical scenarios of concern for LLLT therapy and recommended mitigation approaches:

1. Cancer (over tumors or cancerous areas): see preclinical risks above for theoretical concerns in the context of local neoplasms. No convincing human in vivo studies clearly demonstrate harm; indeed, as noted above, light therapy in combination with topical photosensitizer is used to treat some cancers. Many practitioners and device manufacturers avoid or recommend against LLLT in the setting of cancer due to medicolegal concerns. LLLT treatment should be considered with caution in the presence of malignancy and only in consultation with the treating oncologist.
2. Direct irradiation of the eyes: most device manufacturers offer or recommend approved eye protection.
3. Photophobia or abnormally high sensitivity to light.
4. Concomitant use of photosensitizing medication.
5. Epilepsy, porphyria, and lupus erythematosus are listed as absolute contraindications for Omnilux devices.
6. Pregnancy: no studies showing harm or safety exist. Many practitioners and device manufacturers avoid or recommend against LLLT during pregnancy due to medicolegal concerns. Consider only in consultation with the patient's obstetrician.
7. Avoid direct irradiation over the thyroid gland: this is another theoretical concern, as yet unsubstantiated by human studies or clinical reports. One study reported a potent restorative effect to T3 following LLLT in Hashimoto thyroiditis; the possibility of unwanted changes in euthyroid individuals therefore warrants some caution [68]. Simply covering the thyroid area during treatment is a straightforward mitigation.
8. Individuals with very dark skin, or with dark tattoos or scars: dark pigments absorb more light than fair skin. Reducing exposure time or intensity accordingly, with heightened monitoring, is a reasonable approach. Similar flexibility may be applied to irradiation of scarred tissue.
9. Symptoms of unknown cause: common sense dictates avoiding adding non-mandatory variables such as LLLT in the presence of a pre-existing clinical mystery.

9.4.5 Dosing

LLLT is characterized by a biphasic dose-response in which lower doses are often more beneficial than higher ones [69]. Too low a dose can result in reduced effectiveness and too high a dose can lead to tissue damage. Many studies include negative results that could stem from inappropriate dosing rather than a defect in the treatment itself.

The dose imparted during a particular LLLT session corresponds to the fluence, the light energy incident upon tissue per unit area. Skin reflects just a few percent of incident photons in the visible and infrared bands [70]. The majority is therefore ultimately absorbed within tissue, often after scattering. Consequently, the absorbed dose is well approximated by the incident dose, calculated by taking the product of the incident power density and the treatment time. While this is conceptually straightforward, there are important considerations, chiefly safety, patient convenience, and device geometry and specifications.

LEDs are manufactured such that their output subtends a specified solid angle, forming a cone. In LLLT devices constructed with LED arrays, the output cones of individual LED components overlap, or even converge, at a particular distance according to the device geometry. Thus, intensity does not necessarily strictly decrease with distance, and it is possible for a more distant target to receive more intense illumination than a closer one. Proper relative positioning of source and target according to manufacturers' information is therefore imperative to ensure optimal beam intensity at the target and achieve desired effects.

Power delivery to tissue as a function of depth is another consideration. For R/NIR wavelengths, subsurface scattering and tissue structure and composition results in potentially greater energy deposition per unit volume within tissue than at the surface; peak energy deposition depth varies with wavelength, skin type, and condition and is challenging to measure empirically. As with penetration depth, peak energy deposition depth increases with wavelength within the commonly used therapeutic range [1, 71–73].

For LLLT to remain safely athermal, the power density of the incident beam must remain low relative to the dissipative capacity of the target tissue. On the other hand, clinical feasibility demands that treatment sessions be manageably brief. Fortunately, effective fluences described in the literature correspond to treatment times under half an hour with incident power density in the 100 mW/cm^2range, which perhaps not coincidentally is roughly equivalent to the incident power density of sunlight at noon on a clear summer day in mid-latitudes.

9.4.6 State of Target Cells and Tissues

Compromised cells have been shown to respond much more to LLLT than normal cells do [1]. Therefore, the magnitude of PBM depends on the condition of the cell at the moment of irradiation. For example, light stimulates cell proliferation only if cells are growing poorly at the time [74].

9.4.7 Pulsed Wave Vs. Continuous Wave Mode

Theoretically, pulsed bursts of light may travel deeper into tissues than continuous-wave radiation because the first part of a powerful pulse may contain enough photons to briefly saturate all chromophores in the upper tissue layers, leaving the remainder of the pulse to pass further into the tissue. However, the influence of continuous wave versus pulsed wave mode as well as precise pulsing parameters (i.e., duration, interval, pulse per train, pulse train interval) on cellular response has not been fully studied, and comparative studies have shown conflicting results [74]. Guidance on this variable must therefore await future research.

9.4.8 Treatment Frequency and Duration

While the optimal frequency and number of treatment sessions have not been rigorously determined, some practical rules of thumb can be reasonably formulated from the literature. Repeated exposure to large doses of incident IR power densities sufficient to cause heating reproduces a pattern of connective tissue damage similar to photoaging [69, 75]. Even with thermal power densities and low fluence dosing, it is advisable to minimize treatment sessions to avoid any possible photoaging or theoretical risk of carcinogenesis. However, many benefits reported in the literature peaked only after several weeks into the treatment regimen, suggesting that repeated sessions are necessary for maximum benefit. While the highest number of treatments described among the trials cited herein was 60, most studies utilized a total of 8–12 sessions and reported few adverse effects; this represents a sensible treatment guideline.

9.4.9 Sample Treatment Protocols

9.4.9.1 Summary

There are relatively few trials comparing different treatment protocols head-to-head, with Lee et al. [15] being perhaps the best exemplar. The protocols below are adapted from trials using Omnilux devices and the manufacturer's recommendations. They could be adapted for use with other devices emitting similar wavelengths, with care taken to reproduce the described fluence and dose by varying the distance between patient and device and, if necessary, treatment time.

Session Protocol

ï Cleanse and exfoliate the skin using a choice of polyethylene-based scrub, microdermabrasion or a mild peel with AHAs and BHAs.Ï 9 treatments over a 5-week period (IR 6 times + red 3 times).

ï 20 min per treatment.

ï 2–5 cm distance.

ï IR (830 nm, 55 mW/cm^2, 60 J/cm^2) on days 1, 3, 5, 15, 22, and 29.

ï Red (633 nm, 105 mW/cm^2, 126 J/cm^2) on days 8, 10, 12.

Session Protocol

ï Cleanse and exfoliate the skin using a choice of; polyethylene-based scrub, microdermabrasion or a mild peel with AHAs and BHAs.

ï 8 alternating treatments over a 4-week period (IR 4 times + red 4 times). ï 20 min per treatment.ï Allow at least 48 h rest-time between treatments.

ï 2_5 cm distance.

ï IR (830 nm, 55 mW/cm^2, 66 J/cm^2 per treatment).

ï Red (633 nm, 105 mW/cm^2, 126 J/cm^2 per treatment).

9.4.9.2 Maintenance Therapy

Monthly maintenance sessions (one with red light, one with NIR) are recommended after completing an initial series.

9.4.10 Evaluation of Treatment

9.4.10.1 Ultrasound

Wunsch and Matuschka used a DermaLab Combo ultrasound unit (Cortex Technology, Hadsund, Denmark) to generate a collagen intensity score, effectively measuring intradermal collagen density noninvasively [17]. This appears to be an under-utilized method of obtaining an objective measure of treatment response readily available to the clinician. In this imaging modality, a 20 MHz, rotating single element probe operating in B mode is used to scan to a depth of approximately 3 mm and instantly assess collagen level and dermal thickness. Besides the study cited above, other authors have monitored response to various treatments by measuring dermal collagen intensity with the DermaLab system [76, 77]. Beyond the specific collagen intensity score offered by the DermaLab system, there are other parameters and observations that may be gleaned from any suitable (≥20 MHz probe recommended) ultrasound platform [78]. For example, collagen loss and matrix degradation typical of skin aging in photoexposed regions is readily visualized by high-frequency ultrasound as a subepidermal hypoechogenic band [79, 80].

9.4.10.2 Profilometry

Profilometry, the study of surface features, is another modality available to the clinician to potentially guide and evaluate treatment. Historically as applied to the skin, profilometry involved first making a negative mold of the region of interest, typically of low viscosity silicone; variations in the thickness of this impression could then be measured by optical transmission to generate objective data reflecting surface characteristics [81]. Current state of the art devices employ contactless fringe projection to map multiple parameters over large areas, such as the entire face, in a single acquisition [80]. To some extent, roughness parameters derived from profilometry correlate with ultrasonographic dermal measurements [82], but overall, profilometry and ultrasound yield complementary information regarding surface and subsurface features, respectively.

9.5 Conclusion

Low level light therapy, using LED-based devices working in the red and near-infrared ranges, is a promising treatment modality for aesthetic medicine applications. It represents a relatively safe, convenient, and economically accessible approach with many potential benefits to the patient.

While imaging has long been part of LLLT research, it is increasingly possible, and indeed recommended, to employ imaging as part of clinical practice to inform and monitor therapy. A basic, but not to be overlooked method is to take a careful series of pre- and post-treatment photographs under reproducible lighting conditions; this is a method accessible to most practitioners. As mentioned above, appropriate investments in equipment allow measurements by ultrasound and profilometry.

Future directions for research in LLLT may beneficially include standard reporting of treatment parameters such as power density, treatment area, and distance to light source. The field would also be aided by more frequent reporting of standard clinical scales as well as further inclusion of objective measures such as collagen density and profilometric data. Finally, different protocols, for example, the two included in this chapter, will ideally be tested head-to-head in future work, in order to better establish the optimum course of therapy.

References

1. Calderhead RG, Tanaka Y. Photobiological basics and clinical indications of phototherapy for skin rejuvenation. In: Tanaka Y, editor. Photomedicine—advances in clinical practice. Chicago, IL: InTech; 2017. http://www.intechopen.com/books/photomedicine-advances-in-clinical-practice/photobiological-basics-and-clinical-indications-of-phototherapy-for-skin-rejuvenation.
2. Farage MA, Miller KW, Maibach HI. Textbook of aging skin. Berlin: Springer; 2017. https://doi.org/10.1007/978-3-662-47398-6.
3. Yin R, Hamblin M. Photoaging Photonics. 2013. 12:95–110.
4. Zhao Z, Fairchild PW. Dependence of light transmission through human skin on incident beam diameter at different wavelengths. In: Laser-tissue interaction IX. International Society for Optics and Photonics; 1998. p. 354–60. https://doi.org/10.1117/12.308184.short.
5. Ghali L, Dyson M. The direct effect of light therapy on endothelial cell proliferation in vitro. In: Steiner R, Weisz PB, Langer R, editors. Angiogenesis: key principles—science—technology—medicine. Basel: Birkhäuser; 1992. p. 411–4. https://doi.org/10.1007/978-3-0348-7001-6_68.
6. Gordon SA, Surrey K. Red and far-red action on oxidative phosphorylation. Radiat Res. 1960;12:325–39.
7. Karu T, Tiphlova O, Lukpanova GG, Parkhomenko IM. Effect of irradiation with monochromatic visible light on cAMP content in Chinese hamster fibroblasts. Il Nuovo Cimento D. 1987;9:1245–51.
8. Karu T. Primary and secondary mechanisms of action of visible to near-IR radiation on cells. J Photochem Photobiol B. 1999;49(1):1–17. https://linkinghub.elsevier.com/retrieve/pii/S101113449800219X.
9. Quirk BJ, Whelan HT. Effect of red-to-near infrared light on the reaction of isolated cytochrome c oxidase with cytochrome c. Photomed Laser Surg. 2016;34(12):631–7.
10. Lima PLV, Pereira CV, Nissanka N, Arguello T, Gavini G, Da Maranduba CMC, et al. Photobiomodulation enhancement of cell proliferation at 660 nm does not require cytochrome c oxidase. J Photochem Photobiol B. 2019;194:71–5.
11. Kushibiki T, Ishihara M. Biological function of low reactive level laser therapy (LLLT). In: Photomedicine—advances in clinical practice. London: IntechOpen; 2017. https://www.intechopen.com/chapters/52884.
12. Quirk B, Whelan H. Effect of red-to-near infrared light and a nitric oxide donor on the oxygen consumption of isolated cytochrome c oxidase. Photobiomodul Photomed Laser Surg. 2021;39:469.
13. Sommer AP, Schemmer P, Pavláth AE, Försterling H-D, Mester ÁR, Trelles MA. Quantum biology in

low level light therapy: death of a dogma. Ann Transl Med. 2020;8(7):440.
14. Takezaki S, Omi T, Sato S, Kawana S. Ultrastructural observations of human skin following irradiation with visible red light-emitting diodes (leds): a preliminary in vivo report. LASER Ther. 2005;14(4):153–9. http://www.jstage.jst.go.jp/article/islsm/14/4/14_4_153/_article.
15. Lee SY, Park K-H, Choi J-W, Kwon J-K, Lee DR, Shin MS, et al. A prospective, randomized, placebo-controlled, double-blinded, and split-face clinical study on LED phototherapy for skin rejuvenation: clinical, profilometric, histologic, ultrastructural, and biochemical evaluations and comparison of three different treatment settings. J Photochem Photobiol B. 2007;88(1):51–67. https://linkinghub.elsevier.com/retrieve/pii/S1011134407000632.
16. Weiss RA, McDaniel DH, Geronemus RG, Weiss MA. Clinical trial of a novel non-thermal LED array for reversal of photoaging: clinical, histologic, and surface profilometric results. Lasers Surg Med. 2005;36(2):85–91. https://doi.org/10.1002/lsm.20107.
17. Wunsch A, Matuschka K. A controlled trial to determine the efficacy of red and near-infrared light treatment in patient satisfaction, reduction of fine lines, wrinkles, skin roughness, and intradermal collagen density increase. Photomed Laser Surg. 2014;32(2):93–100. https://doi.org/10.1089/pho.2013.3616.
18. Nikolis A, Bernstein S, Kinney B, Scuderi N, Rastogi S, Sampalis JS. A randomized, placebo-controlled, single-blinded, split-faced clinical trial evaluating the efficacy and safety of KLOX-001 gel formulation with KLOX light-emitting diode light on facial rejuvenation. Clin Cosmet Investig Dermatol. 2016;9:115–25.
19. Goldberg D, Amin SP, Russell BA, Phelps R, Kellett N, Reilly L. Combined 633-nm and 830-nm led treatment of photoaging skin. J Drugs Dermatol. 2006;5(8):748.
20. Barolet D, Roberge CJ, Auger FA, Boucher A, Germain L. Regulation of skin collagen metabolism in vitro using a pulsed 660nm LED light source: clinical correlation with a single-blinded study. J Invest Dermatol. 2009;129(12):2751–9. https://linkinghub.elsevier.com/retrieve/pii/S0022202X15341749
21. Ji J, Zhang L-L, Ding H-L, Wang H-W, Huang Z, Wang X-X, et al. Comparison of 5-aminolevulinic acid photodynamic therapy and red light for treatment of photoaging. Photodiagnosis Photodyn Ther. 2014;11(2):118–21. https://linkinghub.elsevier.com/retrieve/pii/S1572100014000143.
22. Bhat J, Birch J, Whitehurst C, Lanigan SW. A single-blinded randomised controlled study to determine the efficacy of omnilux revive facial treatment in skin rejuvenation. Lasers Med Sci. 2005;20(1):6–10. https://doi.org/10.1007/s10103-005-0330-5.
23. Sadick NS. A study to determine the efficacy of a novel handheld light-emitting diode device in the treatment of photoaged skin. J Cosmet Dermatol. 2008;7(4):263–7. https://doi.org/10.1111/j.1473-2165.2008.00404.x.
24. Migliardi R, Tofani F, Donati L. Non-invasive periorbital rejuvenation: radiofrequency dual radiowave energy source (RF) and light emission diode system (LED). Orbit. 2009;28(4):214–8. https://doi.org/10.1080/01676830903043959.
25. Sadick NS, Laver Z, Laver L. Treatment of mild-to-moderate acne vulgaris using a combined light and heat energy device: home-use clinical study. J Cosmet Laser Ther. 2010;12(6):276–83. https://doi.org/10.3109/14764172.2010.538409.
26. Weiss RA, McDaniel DH, Geronemus RG, Margaret AW, Karen LB, Munavalli GM, et al. Clinical experience with light-emitting diode (LED) photomodulation. Dermatol Surg. 2006;31:1199–205. https://doi.org/10.1111/j.1524-4725.2005.31926.
27. Lee SY, You CE, Park MY. Blue and red light combination LED phototherapy for acne vulgaris in patients with skin phototype IV. Lasers Surg Med. 2007;39(2):180–8. https://doi.org/10.1002/lsm.20412.
28. Shaoul J, Mulholland RS. Evaluation of the safety and efficacy of a novel home-use device with diode arrays and contact heating for facial skin rejuvenation. J Cosmet Dermatol Sci Appl. 2011;1:119–24.
29. Stirling RJ, Haslam JD. A self-reported clinical trial investigates the efficacy of 1072 nm light as an anti-ageing agent. J Cosmet Laser Ther. 2007;9(4):226–30. https://doi.org/10.1080/14764170701400085.
30. Baez F, Reilly LR. The use of light-emitting diode therapy in the treatment of photoaged skin. J Cosmet Dermatol. 2007;6(3):189–94. https://doi.org/10.1111/j.1473-2165.2007.00329.x.
31. Fournier N, Fritz K, Mordon S. Use of nonthermal blue (405- to 420-nm) and near-infrared light (850- to 900-nm) dual-wavelength system in combination with glycolic acid peels and topical vitamin C for skin photorejuvenation. Dermatol Surg. 2006;32(9):1140–6. https://doi.org/10.1111/j.1524-4725.2006.32251.x.
32. Russell BA, Kellett N, Reilly LR. A study to determine the efficacy of combination LED light therapy (633 nm and 830 nm) in facial skin rejuvenation. J Cosmet Laser Ther. 2005;7(3–4):196–200. https://doi.org/10.1080/14764170500370059.
33. Nam CH, Park BC, Kim MH, Choi EH, Hong SP. The efficacy and safety of 660 nm and 411 to 777 nm light-emitting devices for treating wrinkles. Dermatol Surg. 2017;43(3):371–80. https://journals.lww.com/00042728-201703000-00008.
34. Menezes S, Coulomb B, Lebreton C, Dubertret L. Non-coherent near infrared radiation protects Normal human dermal fibroblasts from solar ultraviolet toxicity. J Invest Dermatol. 1998;111(4):629–33. https://linkinghub.elsevier.com/retrieve/pii/S0022202X15402362.
35. Barolet D, Boucher A. LED photoprevention: reduced MED response following multiple LED exposures.

Lasers Surg Med. 2008;40(2):106–12. https://doi.org/10.1002/lsm.20615.
36. Lask G, Fournier N, Trelles M, Elman M, Scheflan M, Slatkine M, et al. The utilization of nonthermal blue (405–425 nm) and near infrared (850–890 nm) light in aesthetic dermatology and surgery—a multicenter study. J Cosmet Laser Ther. 2005;7(3–4):163–70. https://doi.org/10.1080/14764170500344302.
37. Tjioe M, Smits T, Blokx WAM, Van De Kerkhof PCM, Gerritsen M-JP. High-dose long wave visible light induces perinuclear vacuolization *in vivo* but does not result in early photoageing and apoptosis: high-dose long wave visible light. Exp Dermatol. 2003;12(5):610–4. https://doi.org/10.1034/j.1600-0625.2003.00050.x.
38. Morton CA, Scholefield RD, Whitehurst C, Birch J. An open study to determine the efficacy of blue light in the treatment of mild to moderate acne. J Dermatol Treat. 2005;16(4):219–23. https://doi.org/10.1080/09546630500283664.
39. Goldberg DJ, Russell BA. Combination blue (415 nm) and red (633 nm) LED phototherapy in the treatment of mild to severe acne vulgaris. J Cosmet Laser Ther. 2006;8(2):71–5. https://doi.org/10.1080/14764170600735912.
40. Akaraphanth R, Kanjanawanitchkul W, Gritiyarangsan P. Efficacy of ALA-PDT vs blue light in the treatment of acne. Photodermatol Photoimmunol Photomed. 2007;23(5):186–90. https://doi.org/10.1111/j.1600-0781.2007.00303.x.
41. Szeimies R-M, Matheson RT, Davis SA, Bhatia AC, Frambach Y, Klövekorn W, et al. Topical methyl aminolevulinate photodynamic therapy using red light-emitting diode light for multiple actinic keratoses: a randomized study. Dermatol Surg. 2009;35(4):586–92. https://journals.lww.com/00042728-200904000-00003.
42. Sanclemente G, Medina L, Villa J-F, Barrera L-M, Garcia H-I. A prospective split-face double-blind randomized placebo-controlled trial to assess the efficacy of methyl aminolevulinate + red-light in patients with facial photodamage: MAL + red-light vs. placebo + red-light in facial photodamage. J Eur Acad Dermatol Venereol. 2011;25(1):49–58. https://doi.org/10.1111/j.1468-3083.2010.03687.x.
43. Dirschka T, Radny P, Dominicus R, Mensing H, Brüning H, Jenne L, et al. Photodynamic therapy with BF-200 ALA for the treatment of actinic keratosis: results of a multicentre, randomized, observer-blind phase III study in comparison with a registered methyl-5-aminolaevulinate cream and placebo: PDT with BF-200 ALA for AK. Br J Dermatol. 2012;166(1):137–46. https://doi.org/10.1111/j.1365-2133.2011.10613.x.
44. Kwon HH, Lee JB, Yoon JY, Park SY, Ryu HH, Park BM, et al. The clinical and histological effect of home-use, combination blue-red LED phototherapy for mild-to-moderate acne vulgaris in Korean patients: a double-blind, randomized controlled trial: blue-red LED phototherapy in the treatment of acne. Br J Dermatol. 2013;168(5):1088–94. https://doi.org/10.1111/bjd.12186.
45. Pathak MA, Riley FC, Fitzpatrick TB. Melanogenesis in human skin following exposure to long-wave ultraviolet and visible light**from the research Laboratories of the Department of dermatology of the Harvard Medical School at the Massachusetts General Hospital, Boston 14, Massachusetts. J Invest Dermatol. 1962;39(5):435–43. https://linkinghub.elsevier.com/retrieve/pii/S0022202X15497738.
46. Kollias N, Baqer A. An experimental study of the changes in pigmentation in human skin in vivo with visible and near infrared light. Photochem Photobiol. 1984;39(5):651–9. https://doi.org/10.1111/j.1751-1097.1984.tb03905.x.
47. Porges SB, Kaidbey KH, Grove GL. Quantification of visible light-induced melanogenesis in human skin. Photo-Dermatology. 1988;5(5):197–200.
48. Rosen CF, Jacques SL, Stuart ME, Gange RW. Immediate pigment darkening: visual and reflectance spectrophotometric analysis of action spectrum. Photochem Photobiol. 1990;51(5):583–8. https://doi.org/10.1111/j.1751-1097.1990.tb01969.x.
49. Kleinpenning MM, Smits T, Frunt MHA, van Erp PEJ, van de Kerkhof PCM, Gerritsen RMJP. Clinical and histological effects of blue light on normal skin. Photodermatol Photoimmunol Photomed. 2010;26(1):16–21. https://doi.org/10.1111/j.1600-0781.2009.00474.x.
50. Mahmoud BH, Ruvolo E, Hexsel CL, Liu Y, Owen MR, Kollias N, et al. Impact of long-wavelength UVA and visible light on Melanocompetent skin. J Invest Dermatol. 2010;130(8):2092–7. https://linkinghub.elsevier.com/retrieve/pii/S0022202X15349307.
51. Ramasubramaniam R, Roy A, Sharma B, Nagalakshmi S. Are there mechanistic differences between ultraviolet and visible radiation induced skin pigmentation? Photochem Photobiol Sci. 2011;10(12):1887. http://xlink.rsc.org/?DOI=c1pp05202k.
52. Weinstabl A, Hoff-Lesch S, Merk HF, von Felbert V. Prospective randomized study on the efficacy of blue light in the treatment of psoriasis vulgaris. Dermatology. 2011;223(3):251–9. https://www.karger.com/Article/FullText/333364
53. Kleinpenning MM, Otero ME, van Erp PEJ, Gerritsen MJP, van de Kerkhof PCM. Efficacy of blue light vs. red light in the treatment of psoriasis: a double-blind, randomized comparative study: blue light versus red light in psoriasis. J Eur Acad Dermatol Venereol. 2012;26(2):219–25. https://doi.org/10.1111/j.1468-3083.2011.04039.x.
54. Pfaff S, Liebmann J, Born M, Merk HF, von Felbert V. Prospective randomized long-term study on the efficacy and safety of UV-free blue light for treating mild psoriasis vulgaris. Dermatology. 2015;231(1):24–34. https://www.karger.com/Article/FullText/430495.
55. Papageorgiou P, Katsambas A, Chu A. Phototherapy with blue (415 nm) and red (660 nm) light in the treat-

ment of acne vulgaris: blue-red light treatment of acne. Br J Dermatol. 2000;142(5):973–8. https://doi.org/10.1046/j.1365-2133.2000.03481.x.
56. Kawada A, Aragane Y, Kameyama H, Sangen Y, Tezuka T. Acne phototherapy with a high-intensity, enhanced, narrow-band, blue light source: an open study and in vitro investigation. J Dermatol Sci. 2002;30(2):129–35.
57. Reinhold U, Dirschka T, Ostendorf R, Aschoff R, Berking C, Philipp-Dormston WG, et al. A randomized, double-blind, phase III, multicentre study to evaluate the safety and efficacy of BF -200 ALA (Ameluz®) vs. placebo in the field-directed treatment of mild-to-moderate actinic keratosis with photodynamic therapy (PDT) when using the BF -Rhodo LED ®lamp. Br J Dermatol. 2016;175(4):696–705. https://doi.org/10.1111/bjd.14498.
58. Sroka R, Schaffer M, Fuchs C, Pongratz T, Schrader-Reichard U, Busch M, et al. Effects on the mitosis of normal and tumor cells induced by light treatment of different wavelengths. Lasers Surg Med. 1999;25(3):263–71.
59. Sperandio FF, Giudice FS, Corrêa L, Pinto DS, Hamblin MR, de Sousa SCOM. Low-level laser therapy can produce increased aggressiveness of dysplastic and oral cancer cell lines by modulation of Akt/mTOR signaling pathway. J Biophotonics. 2013;6(10):839. https://doi.org/10.1002/jbio.201300015.
60. Frigo L, Luppi JSS, Favero GM, Maria DA, Penna SC, Bjordal JM, et al. The effect of low-level laser irradiation (in-ga-Al-AsP—660 nm) on melanoma in vitro and in vivo. BMC Cancer. 2009;9:404.
61. De Monteiro CJS, Pinheiro ALB, De Oliveira SCPS, Aciole GTS, Sousa JAC, Cangussú MCT, et al. Influence of laser phototherapy (λ660 nm) on the outcome of oral chemical carcinogenesis on the hamster cheek pouch model: histological study. Photomed Laser Surg. 2011;29(11):741–5. https://doi.org/10.1089/pho.2010.2896.
62. Barolet D, Christiaens F, Hamblin MR. Infrared and skin: friend or foe. J Photochem Photobiol B. 2016;155:78–85.
63. Ericson MB, Wennberg A-M, Larkö O. Review of photodynamic therapy in actinic keratosis and basal cell carcinoma. Ther Clin Risk Manag. 2008;4(1):1–9. https://www.ncbi.nlm.nih.gov/pmc/articles/PMC2503644/
64. Schroeder P, Lademann J, Darvin ME, Stege H, Marks C, Bruhnke S, et al. Infrared radiation-induced matrix metalloproteinase in human skin: implications for protection. J Invest Dermatol. 2008;128(10):2491–7.
65. Kligman LH. Intensification of ultraviolet-induced dermal damage by infrared radiation. Arch Dermatol Res. 1982;272(3–4):229–38.
66. Kim M-S, Kim YK, Cho KH, Chung JH. Infrared exposure induces an angiogenic switch in human skin that is partially mediated by heat: IR induces angiogenesis in human skin in vivo. Br J Dermatol. 2006;155(6):1131–8. https://doi.org/10.1111/j.1365-2133.2006.07510.x.
67. Kim M-S, Kim YK, Lee DH, Seo JE, Cho KH, Eun HC, et al. Acute exposure of human skin to ultraviolet or infrared radiation or heat stimuli increases mast cell numbers and tryptase expression in human skin *in vivo*. Br J Dermatol. 2009;160(2):393–402. https://doi.org/10.1111/j.1365-2133.2008.08838.x.
68. Ercetin C, Sahbaz NA, Acar S, Tutal F, Erbil Y. Impact of photobiomodulation on T3/T4 ratio and quality of life in hashimoto thyroiditis. Photobiomodul Photomed Laser Surg. 2020;38(7):409–12. https://doi.org/10.1089/photob.2019.4740.
69. Chung H, Dai T, Sharma SK, Huang Y-Y, Carroll JD, Hamblin MR. The nuts and bolts of low-level laser (light) therapy. Ann Biomed Eng. 2012;40(2):516–33.
70. Lister T, Wright PA, Chappell PH. Optical properties of human skin. J Biomed Opt. 2012;17(9):–90901.
71. Douplik A, Saiko G, Schelkanova I, Tuchin VV. The response of tissue to laser light. In: Jelínková H, editor. Lasers for medical applications. Sawston: Woodhead Publishing; 2013. p. 47–109. (Woodhead Publishing Series in Electronic and Optical Materials). https://www.sciencedirect.com/science/article/pii/B9780857092373500035.
72. Milanic M, Majaron B. Energy deposition profile in human skin upon irradiation with a 1,342 nm Nd:YAP laser. Lasers Surg Med. 2013;28:45.
73. Shimojo Y, Nishimura T, Hazama H, Ozawa T, Awazu K. Measurement of absorption and reduced scattering coefficients in Asian human epidermis, dermis, and subcutaneous fat tissues in the 400- to 1100-nm wavelength range for optical penetration depth and energy deposition analysis. J Biomed Opt. 2020;25(4):045002. https://www.spiedigitallibrary.org/journals/journal-of-biomedical-optics/volume-25/issue-4/045002/Measurement-of-absorption-and-reduced-scattering-coefficients-in-Asian-human/10.1117/1.JBO.25.4.045002.short.
74. Barolet D. Light-emitting diodes (LEDs) in dermatology. Semin Cutan Med Surg. 2008;27(4):227–38.
75. Cho S, Shin MH, Kim YK, Seo J-E, Lee YM, Park C-H, et al. Effects of infrared radiation and heat on human skin aging in vivo. J Investig Dermatol Symp Proc. 2009;14(1):15–9.
76. Borumand M, Sibilla S. Daily consumption of the collagen supplement pure gold collagen® reduces visible signs of aging. Clin Interv Aging. 2014;9:1747–58. https://www.ncbi.nlm.nih.gov/pmc/articles/PMC4206255/.
77. Hsu T-F, Su Z-R, Hsieh Y-H, Wang M-F, Oe M, Matsuoka R, et al. Oral hyaluronan relieves wrinkles and improves dry skin: a 12-week double-blinded, placebo-controlled study. Nutrients. 2021;13(7):2220. https://www.mdpi.com/2072-6643/13/7/2220.
78. Vergilio MM, Vasques LI, Leonardi GR. Characterization of skin aging through high-frequency ultrasound imaging as a technique for

evaluating the effectiveness of anti-aging products and procedures: a review. Skin Res Technol. 2021;27(5):966–73. https://doi.org/10.1111/srt.13033.

79. Crisan D, Lupsor M, Boca A, Crisan M, Badea R. Ultrasonographic assessment of skin structure according to age. Indian J Dermatol Venereol Leprol. 2012;78(4):519.
80. Bielfeldt S, Springmann G, Seise M, Wilhelm K-P, Callaghan T. An updated review of clinical methods in the assessment of ageing skin—new perspectives and evaluation for claims support. Int J Cosmet Sci. 2018;40(4):348–55. https://doi.org/10.1111/ics.12484.
81. Grove GL, Grove MJ, Leyden JJ. Optical profilometry: an objective method for quantification of facial wrinkles. J Am Acad Dermatol. 1989;21(3):631–7. https://linkinghub.elsevier.com/retrieve/pii/S0190962289702309.
82. Lee HK, Seo YK, Baek JH, Koh JS. Comparison between ultrasonography (Dermascan C version 3) and transparency profilometry (Skin Visiometer SV600). Skin Res Technol. 2007;14(1):8–12. https://doi.org/10.1111/j.1600-0846.2007.00257.x.

Tips and Tricks for Intense Pulse Light Treatment

10

Lucian Fodor and Sergiu Samuila

Abstract

IPL represents a technology that uses electromagnetic radiation energy with a wavelength situated in the visible light spectrum. With the use of thermal relaxation time (TRT), nonspecific injury of unaffected tissue is induced. This chapter explores the benefits of IPL technology, noting energy sufficiency and the rapid recovery time of patients.

Keywords

IPL · TRT · Chromophores · Photorejuvenation · Lesions · Scars · Hair removal · Laser · Hyperpigmentation · Body dysmorphic disorder

10.1 Introduction

The effects of the IPL therapy are based on the light-tissue interaction. The light that reaches the skin is absorbed, reflected, scattered, or transmitted into the surrounding structures (Fig. 10.1a–d). Each of these processes depends on the patient's characteristics or technical settings.

Heating effect due to light absorption is responsible for various changes at the molecular level, resulting in coagulation and denaturation of different protein structures of the target tissues [1–3]. Selective photo thermolysis represents the principle of IPL function [4].

Chromophores are the structural components of the tissues that absorb the light photons. They are situated at different depths in the skin and have different wavelengths of absorption (Fig. 10.2). The main chromophores present at the skin level are melanin, hemoglobin, water, and foreign pigmented tattoos [5] melanin, which is located mainly at the epidermis level, and hemoglobin, found in the vascular network of the dermis, are the principal targets of pulsed light treatment [6, 7] (Fig. 10.3a, b).

In order to obtain selective photothermolysis on a target tissue and avoid thermal injury on the surrounding tissues, a matching of wavelength and duration of pulse must be obtained. Thermal relaxation time (TRT), which represents the time needed to cool a small tissue, is a variable that influences the non-specific thermal injury of unaffected tissue. TRT is proportional to the square of the size [6]. When pulse duration is longer than TRT, complications secondary to thermal injury of the healthy tissue can occur [4].

L. Fodor (✉)
Plastic Surgery, Interservisan, MedÁrt Clinic, Cluj Napoca, Romania
e-mail: office@drfodor.ro

S. Samuila
Plastic Surgery, Emergency District Hospital, Cluj-Napoca, Romania

R. L. Bard (ed.), *Image-Guided Aesthetic Treatments*, https://doi.org/10.1007/978-3-031-36266-8_10

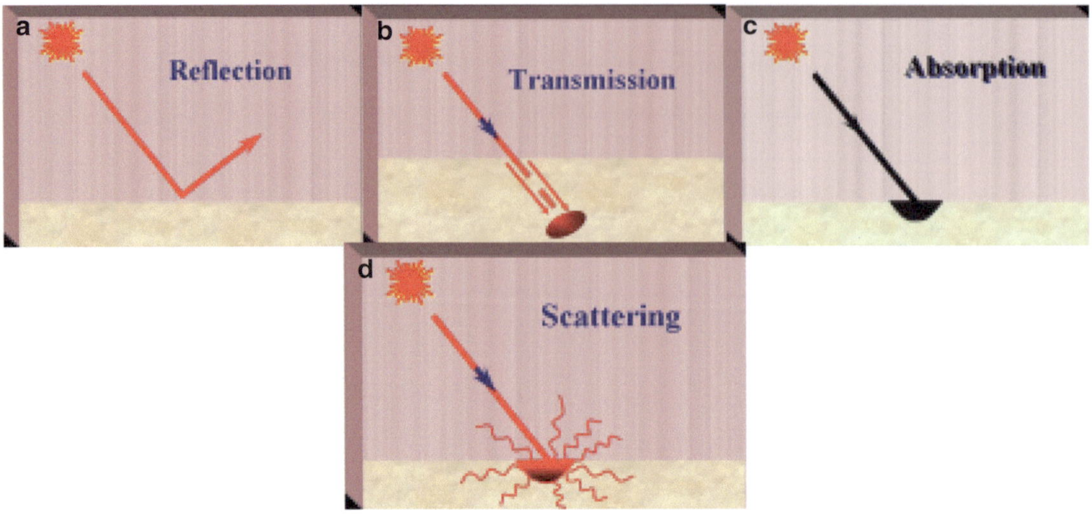

Fig. 10.1 (**a**) Scattering effect (photos from Fodor and Ullmann second edition). (**b**) Reflection of the light (photos from Fodor and Ullmann second edition). (**c**) Light transmission (photos from Fodor and Ullmann second edition). (**d**) Light absorption. (Photos from Fodor and Ullmann second edition)

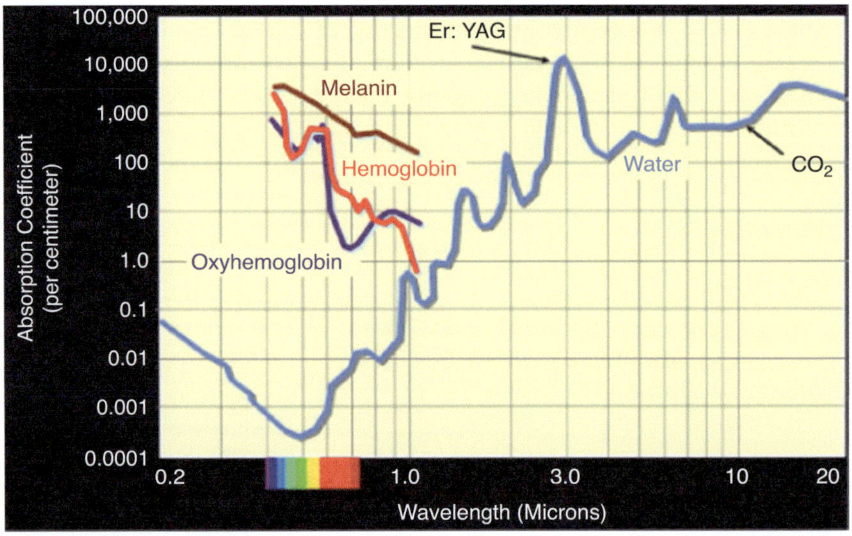

Fig. 10.2 Light absorption for different chromophores. (Photos from Fodor and Ullmann second edition)

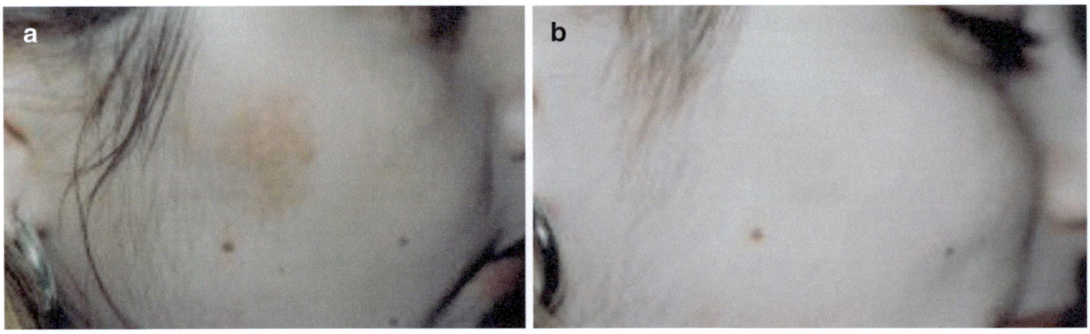

Fig. 10.3 (**a**) Café-au lait in a young person. The melanin is the main chromophore. (**b**) Good result after two IPL treatments. (Photos from Fodor and Ullmann second edition)

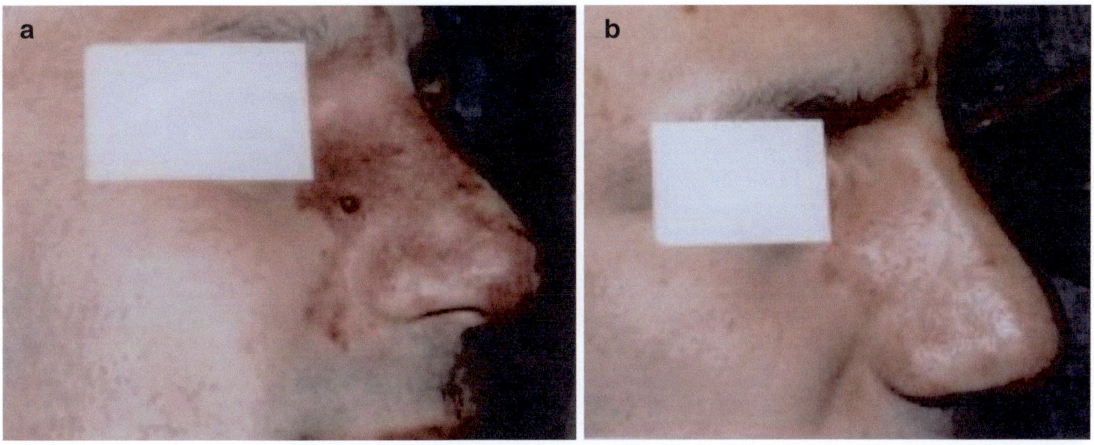

Fig. 10.4 (**a**) PWS—adult type over the nose. The chromophore is the hemoglobin. (**b**) Good result after ten IPL treatments. (Photos from Fodor and Ullmann second edition)

10.2 Indications

ILP devices utilize a light source to emit polychromatic light with wavelengths between 420 and 1200 nm and have the possibility to adjust numerous parameters of the devices, e.g., fluence, pulse duration and frequency, and filter type. This versatility allows for the treatment of a wide range of skin conditions, including telangiectasias, facial wrinkles, photorejuvenation, hyperpigmentation, ephelides, lentigines, melasma, rosacea, acne, poikiloderma of Civatte, port wine stains (PWS) (Fig. 10.4a, b), hemangiomas, superficial leg veins, and scars [8].

10.3 Vascular Lesions

In cases of vascular lesions, the target tissues are the blood vessels located in the dermal plexus of the skin. Using specific filters, the shorter and superficial penetrating wavelengths can be eliminated, and longer wavelengths can be delivered to the specific chromophores existing in the vascular lesions, e.g., oxyhemoglobin and deoxyhemoglobin. Secondary to light absorption by these chromophores, selective vascular destruction can be obtained with limited non-specific melanin absorption with unwanted results [9, 10] (Fig. 10.5a, b).

Chronic venous insufficiency is a condition with a height prevalence reported in Western countries of 17–40% [11]. Telangiectasias, dilated superficial small veins (<1 mm), and subcutaneous dilated veins (<3 mm) called reticular veins are manifestation of chronic venous insufficiency and one of the most common cutaneous lesions for which laser procedures are requested [9, 12–14]. Although numerous therapy options exist for this lesion, including sclerotherapy, electrodesiccation, and laser therapy, these procedures are associated with numerous side effects, such as scarring, hyperpigmentation, ulceration, purpura, and telangiectatic matting [10, 15]. ILP has grown in popularity as the treatment method for vascular lesions with rare and often mild side effects, most commonly including swelling and erythema [16] (Fig. 10.6a, b). Studies have demonstrated a high level of efficiency in the treatment of telangiectasias and reticular veins. Goldman et al. reported that 79% of patients achieved between 75% and 100% complete disappearance of the dilated vein located in the lower limb [17]. Moreover, for deeper located veins, IPL can be associated with traditional laser therapies [18, 19].

A study compared the results of IPL and Nd:YAG laser for vascular lesions represented by facial telangiectases, leg veins, or cherry angiomas. In this prospective study, 25 patients

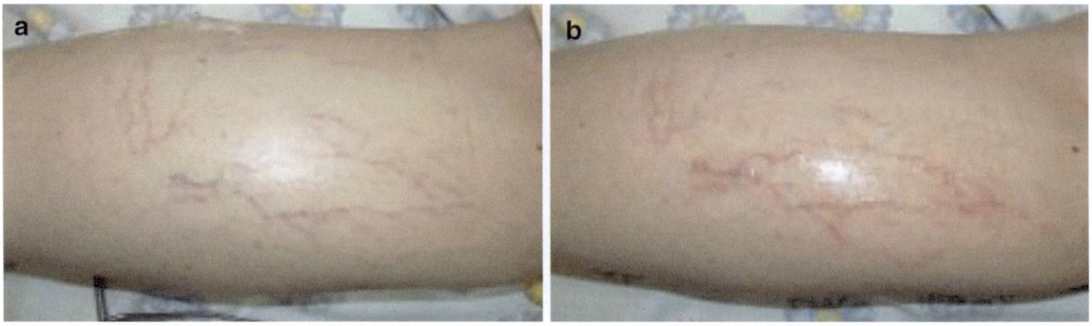

Fig. 10.5 Leg veins before (**a**) and after (**b**) three treatments. (Photos from Fodor and Ullmann second edition)

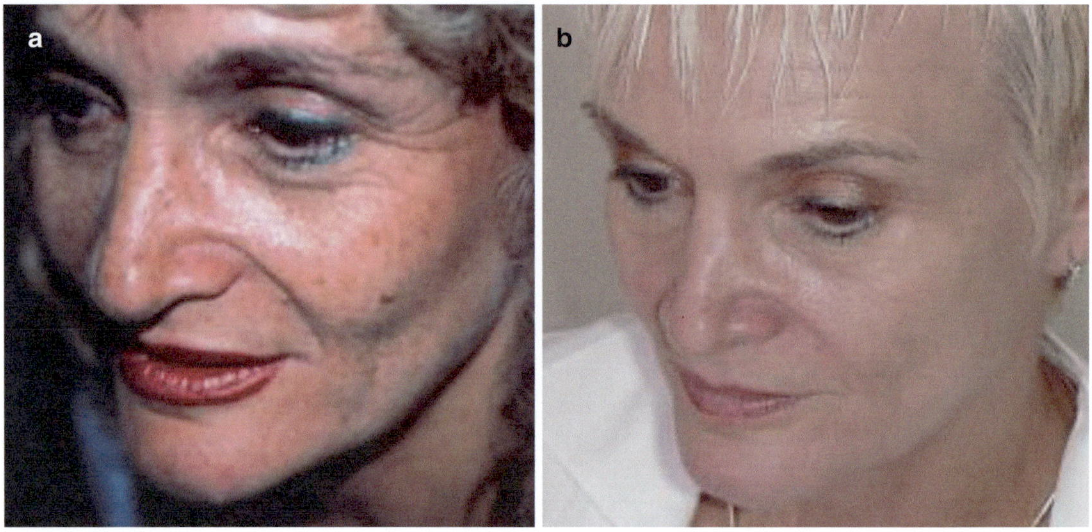

Fig. 10.6 (**a**) 56 years old woman with mainly pigmentation changes (photos from Fodor and Ullmann, first Edition). (**b**) 6 months after the third treatment. (Photos from Fodor and Ullmann, second Edition)

were enrolled and IPL and Nd:YAG laser were used side-by-side for the same lesions and with the same frequency. Eighty percent of patients in the IPL group and 56% of patients from the laser group had no complications. Comparison of satisfaction between the two groups showed a significantly higher level of satisfaction in Nd:Yag laser group. Subgroup analysis showed that, in the IPL treated group, more satisfaction was obtained in patients who presented with telangiectases, cherry angiomas, and leg veins <1 mm, while laser group patients with a high level of satisfaction were those with leg veins >1 mm [20].

10.4 Photorejuvenation

Photorejuvenation of the skin is another important applicability of IPL. Aged skin suffers numerous structural changes as a result of the action of numerous factors, including sun exposure, diseases, smoking, and hereditary factors [21]. These changes are represented by disruption of vascular endothelium, alteration of function and structure of the melanocyte, and degradation of the collagen with increased synthesis of elastin and fibrillin [22, 23]. The result is increased skin laxity, decreased volume, and the appearance of vascular and pigmented lesions, such as telangiectasis, lentigines, ephelides, melasma, and Poikiloderma de Civatte. The skin of the face, neck, chest, and hands is most exposed to the sun and most affected by these changes [21].

In addition to the cosmetic problem, some pigmentary changes increase the risk of skin cancer. By using different wavelengths, IPL therapy can target different chromophores present in these lesions, e.g., melanin, oxyhemoglobin, deoxygenated hemoglobin, and methemoglobin [24, 25].

Moreover, aged skin treated with IPL suffers histological modifications that improve the skin quality and thickness and ameliorates soft wrinkles [26]. Numerous mechanisms are responsible for these effects, including fibroblast activation, collagen remodeling, and increased synthesis of pro-collagen type III endothelial disruption and cytokine activation [27, 28].

An important advantage of IPL therapy compared to other more aggressive methods is that the skin is left intact, without disruption of the epidermis. This results in a low recovery time following the treatment and a decreased risk of complications compared with other ablative rejuvenation methods [25, 28, 29]. Numerous studies have reported excellent results regarding skin texture and pigmentary changes following IPL. Robert et al. reported improvement of skin texture in 83% of patients and 79% for pigmentation lesions with 4 years of follow-up [30]. Similarly, 75% of patients treated for ephelides and lentigines showed good and excellent result following 3–5 sessions [30].

Another advantage is that IPL can be utilized in association with other therapies with positive results. Ayse et al. evaluated the effect of Neodymium-doped Yttrium Aluminum Garnet (Nd:YAG) laser compared with IPL and Nd:YAG laser on photoaged skin located on the dorsal hands of 35 females. The results showed statistically significant improvement in scores of pigment, wrinkles, sallowness, and global score when IPL was combined with Nd:YAG laser [31].

10.5 Scars

Scars represent an important psychological and functional problem for patients. Pathological scars, e.g., keloids or hypertrophy, are still difficult to treat or prevent, despite increased knowledge of the wound healing process and various treatment options. The mechanism of IPL action on scar treatment is not fully understood, but the vascular component, which leads to collagen overgrowth and melanin, which is a scar component is probably a IPL target (Fig. 10.7). In a study that included 109 patients with hypertrophic scars following surgical incisions, traumatic cuts, acne, keloids, and burns, 92.5% showed clinical improvement with reductions in height, erythema, and hardness after an average of eight treatments sessions [32]. However, IPL for scars does not have as widespread an application as for other lesions.

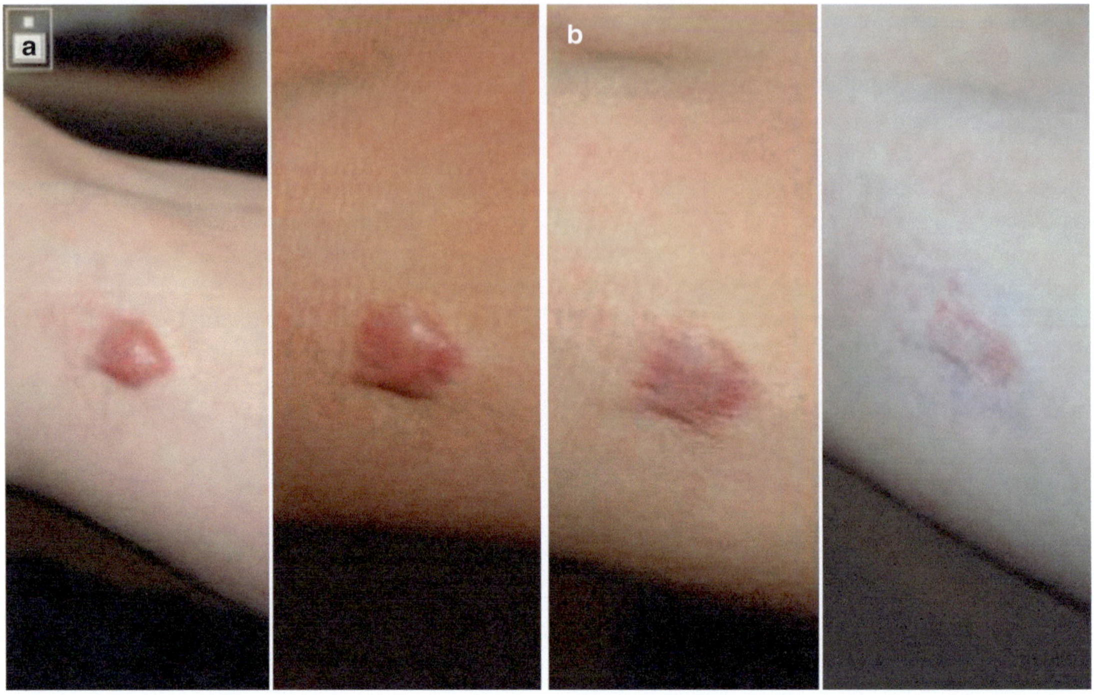

Fig. 10.7 (**a**) Hypertrophic scar: Significant reduction of vascular component in the thicker areas before and after three IPL treatments. (**b**) Keloid: Scar after three sessions of IPL. Dermoscopy performed immediately after the first treatment showed a variation of the color from red-blue to red. (Photos from Fodor and Ullmann, second Edition)

10.6 Hair Removal

Another important application of IPL is for hair removal. This effect can be used for patients suffering from excessive hair disorders, e.g., Hirsutism and Hypertrichosis, or for non-cosmetic conditions [33, 34]. For example, flaps from hair-bearing regions used to reconstruct different segments of the digestive or genital tract can produce significant disturbance of second hair growth, including dysphagia, halitosis, obstruction, and infection. Definitively removing hair without affecting the flap physiology represents an important advantage of IPL treatment [35–38]. (Fig. 10.8a, b). The mechanism of IPL for hair removal is the selective photothermolysis caused by light absorbed by melanin chromophores located in the hair structure [39]. Although numerous methods for hair removal exist, e.g., shaving, waxing, electrolysis, and topical creams, these are temporary methods associated with side effects, including pain, hyperpigmentation, scarring, and burns [40]. Laser and IPL are two methods of permanent hair loss [41]. Many studies have confirmed the efficacy of ILP regarding long-term effects. Because of its wide spectrum wavelength, IPL devices have a better penetration compared with laser devices, and using a short wavelength, red-brown hair can be removed. Bjerring et al. compared the result of IPL and Ruby laser after three treatments. 93.55% hair reduction was obtained after IPL compared with 54.8% after Ruby laser. Moreover, the pain level was 3.5 times higher in the laser group [42].

Two disadvantages can be mentioned when using IPL for hair removal. First, white-gray hair contains little melanin, and this makes it less susceptible to IPL treatment compared with dark hair [43]. Fitzpatrick skin type has a high quantity of melanin and is more susceptible to thermal damage of the surrounding skin due to absorption of IPL energy by these chromophores [44].

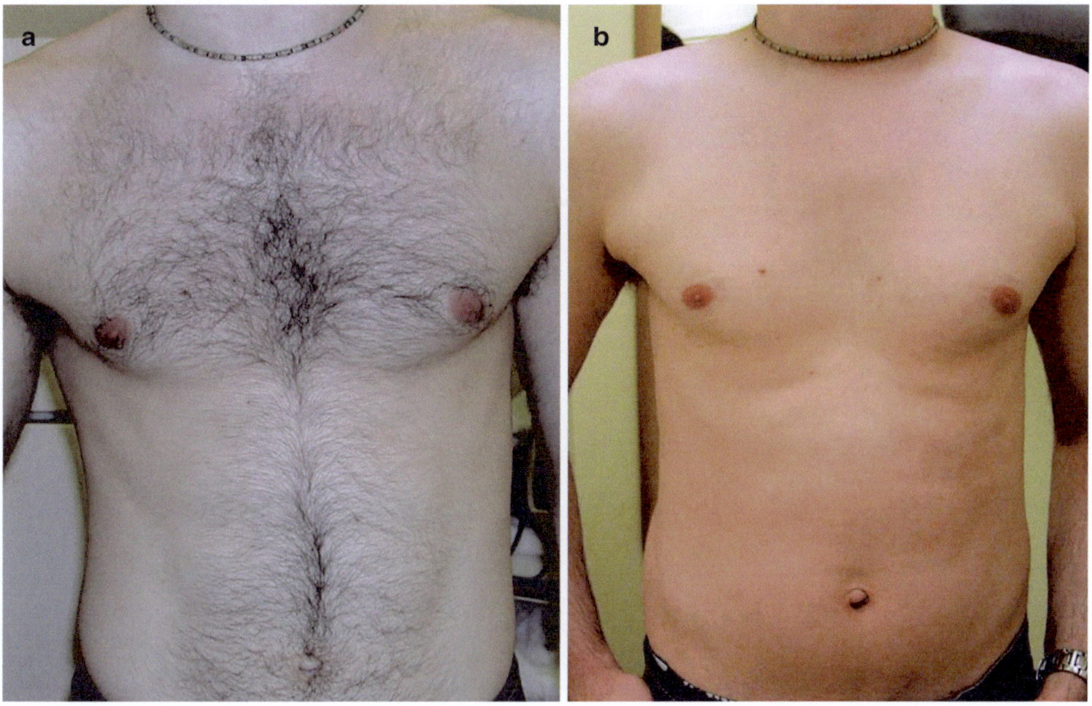

Fig. 10.8 Before (**a**) and after (**b**) six IPL treatments. (Photos from Fodor and Ullmann first edition)

10.7 Pigmented Lesions

Pigmented skin lesions represent a complex skin problem difficult to treat and frequently have a significant impact on the patient [45]. Some of these lesions associated with the photoaging process or other intrinsic factors can be adequately managed by using IPL. Despite the decrease of 10–20% of melanocytes with each decade, the density of melanocytes in chronically exposed skin remains twofold higher, leading to pigmented lesions. Ephelides are small brown macules resulting from hyperpigmentation of the basal cells and increased dimension and activity of the melanocytes. Lentigines are dark brown macules, varying in size from millimeters to 1 cm. They can have a mottled appearance second to varying degrees of pigmentation that can be found within one lesion, e.g., dark brown, light brown, yellow, or even black, and may confluence over time [46].

Pigmentary changes, e.g., lentigines, located over the dorsal hand represent the most frequent cause of aesthetic hand consultation [47] (Fig. 10.9a, b).

Numerous treatment methods are available for pigmentary changes. Topical depigmentation agents are the simplest, but they can only lighten the lesions without removal. More aggressive treatments represented by mechanical or chemical peels or cold therapy are more prone to side effects, such as scars and hypopigmentation [25].

For selective photothermal damage of the melanin chromophore, IPL can safely treat these hyperpigmented lesions, resulting in younger looking skin. Commonly, numerous sessions are needed to improve the aspects, but the effect of the therapy is seen even after the first session [46].

Based on the ability of the IPL device to target multiple chromophores, e.g., hemoglobin, melanin, and due to its broad band of wavelength, it can be used to treat some pigmented lesions in which both vascular and melanin components are present [48]. Melasma is an acquired condition with multifactorial ethology, including sun

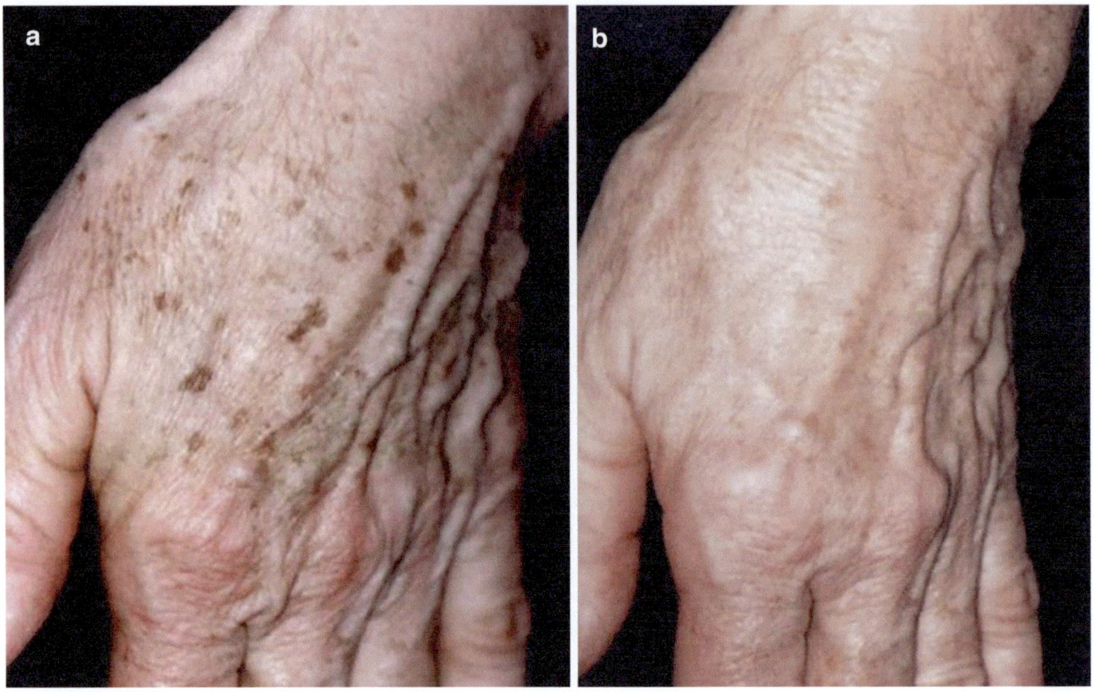

Fig. 10.9 (**a**) Lentigines located on the dorsum of the hand. (Photos from Fodor and Ullmann, second Edition). (**b**) Excellent result after two sessions. (Photos from Fodor and Ullmann, second Edition)

exposure, genetic predisposition, and hormonal balance. Clinically, it manifests as irregular, well-delineated, and intensely pigmented areas with variation regarding size and color from ochre-yellow to dark gray. Based on the location of the lesions, melasma can be classified as centrofacial (63%), malar (21%), and mandibular (16%). The results of 38 patient treated with 3–5 sessions of IPL show excellent and good effects in 47.37% and 28.95%, respectively, of patients [45].

Poikiloderma of Civatte represents a genetic disease with an autosomal dominant pattern morphologically characterized by atrophy, telangiectasia, and pigmentary abnormalities. The lateral neck and upper chest are the areas affected by these changes, while the submental region is spared. Topical or oral medications are inefficient on pigmentary and vascular changes present in the lesion, and more aggressive treatment is frequently associated with side effects, e.g., pitted white scars, scarring irregular hypopigmentation. IPL has demonstrated a good alternative to the oldest methods of treatment with a high rate of success and a low risk of complications [48].

A study conducted by Fodor et al. compared the results of IPL treatment in three groups of 30 consecutive patients treated for skin rejuvenation, hair removal, and small vascular lesions. There was no significant difference between the groups regarding the level of satisfaction and willingness to continue or to recommend the treatment. Most of the complications occurred in the rejuvenation group (86.6%), with erythema and blisters being the most frequently encountered complication. In the hair removal group, 67% of patients had no complication, as did 75% of the vascular lesion group [49]. Another study that compared data from 59 patients treated for skin rejuvenation reported very good results for the majority of patients, while the most common side effect was redness, followed by edema and crusts [50].

With a great area of applicability, IPL technology benefits from numerous other advantages. Compared to other laser treatments, patients have a rapid recovery time. Side effects are uncommon

Table 10.1 Advantages and disadvantages of IPL [8, 51]

Advantages	Disadvantages
Lower price	Contact of handpieces with the skin
Great versatility	Need for gel application on the skin
Large spot size	Risk for complications in dark-skinned patients
Rapid recovery time	Impossibility to focused the light

and, most frequently, are represented by erythema and pain. These reactions last between 2 and 48 h post-treatment and depend on various parameters that can be adjusted. Most of the procedures do not require topical anesthesia. Pain and skin irritation can be reduced by using cooling systems and applying topical gels [8].

The drawbacks of IPL include the risk of complications in dark-skinned patients, for whom special attention must be given in order to prevent unwanted effects. Using short wavelengths and special cooling technology incorporated in some IPL devices permits the use of this therapy even for this special category of individuals. For the untrained user, the large variety of settings can represent a disadvantage because of thermal injury that can occur secondary to inappropriate light administration. In the case of gel application, there is a risk of missing immediate skin reaction secondary to limited visibility. Direct skin contact and the heavy weight of the handpiece are other disadvantages of the IPL device [8]. Advantages and disadvantages of IPL are summarized in Table 10.1.

10.8 Tips and Tricks in IPL

There are some key points for IPL practitioners to avoid complications and patient dissatisfaction.

The first tip refers to the identification of the unsuitable patient for this procedure. There are some "red flags" that need to be identified at the first presentation. These are represented by patients who have great expectations, those with familial or marital disapproval, surgiholic individuals, or suffering from body dysmorphic disorder. Moreover, a person who wants an aesthetic procedure being pushed by others is not a good candidate [52]. We can include these persons in two main categories: those who are anatomically unsuited and those who are psychologically unsuited [53]. A well-motivated patient suffering from a major deformity with minimal concern about it is a good candidate, as any degree of improvement leads to great satisfaction [53, 54]. Persons with unrealistic and great expectations are those who expect a major and immediate change of their physical aspect and a positive improvement of their lives secondary to the procedure (Fig. 10.10a, b). They have difficulty in understanding the realistic aspects of the procedure and the fact that any procedure is associated with some risk of unpredictable complications [52]. Surgiholic individuals are those with multiple aesthetic interventions, who often search for a new young doctor, hoping for an innovative technique. They are up-to-date about the latest procedures and have an exact image of what the procedure will improve. These patients can represent a trap for the inexperienced doctor because of the false assumption that they can understand the risks and benefits of the intervention based on previous experience [52].

Body dysmorphic disorder represents a serious psychiatric problem encountered in aesthetic practice, the most common personality disorder seen by the plastic surgeon. These patients are characterized by obsessive concerns that affect their social life, about an anatomical irregularity that, in reality, is non-existent or imperceptible. These patients have unrealistic expectations from aesthetic intervention, and dissatisfaction occurs in most cases. Frequently, there exists a discrepancy in what these patients understood from the information provided by the practitioner before intervention and the information that was actually said. For this reason, complete and detailed documentation and photographs pre- and post-intervention are essential for any patient [52].

The first consultation is an important step in IPL therapy as well as in other aesthetic surgery procedures. Apart from identification of an unsuitable category of patients mentioned above, there are some steps that must be taken. Correct

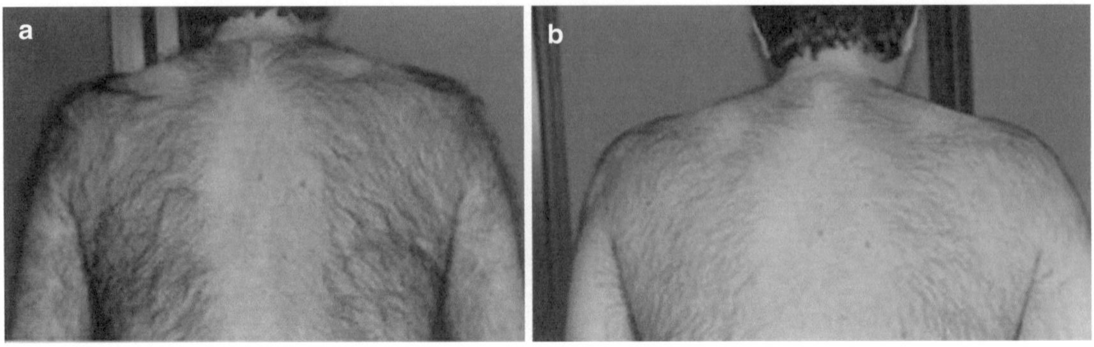

Fig. 10.10 (**a**) Hypertrichosis—before IPL treatment (photos from Fodor and Ullmann second edition). (**b**) Partial response after five IPL treatments. The patient was unhappy with the result and stopped the treatments. (Photos from Fodor and Ullmann second edition)

diagnosis of the pathology to be treated is essential. Pigmentary lesions that are suspected for skin malignancy must be avoided before a clear diagnosis is made. Dermatoscopy of a skin biopsy prior to IPL is necessary for a correct diagnosis. Many vascular lesions benefit from laser or IPL treatment, including acquired isolated lesions or lesions from a complex disease. A high energy device is used for these lesions, and serious side effects can occur. Because of misdiagnosis of a vascular birthmark, a significant number of patients receive inefficient and possibly dangerous treatment [55].

The complete health status of a patient must be evaluated to identify those patients suffering from conditions that contraindicate IPL therapy, e.g., pregnancy and severe venous insufficiency with dilated veins [56]. Comprehensive verbal and written information must be offered to the patients to exclude unrealistic expectations. This information includes the principles of IPL and the chances of success, alternative treatment, a comprehensive diagnosis, anesthesia type, recovery period, number of treatment sessions, and costs. Although rare, some side effects and complications may appear following the treatment, including erythema, pigmentary change, blistering, purpura, crusting, hypertrophic or keloid scars, and infections. All of these should be discussed with the patient. A signed informed consent is obtained after all important information is obtained from the patient and all the abovementioned information is clearly discussed [51, 56].

A method that increases the chance that patients fully understand the information offered by you at the first visit is to offer him the opportunity to take the informed consent home to sign it there and to avoid performing the procedure on the same day.

Most IPL treatments necessitate a various number of sessions which extend sometimes over long periods. Appropriate photo documentation should be performed at the beginning of the treatment and again periodically, for evaluation of the efficacy and guide to treatment [55].

Some patients suitable for IPL treatment require special care. These are patients with implants located in the treatment area, a heart pacemaker, or those suffering from diabetes, hemophilia, or other coagulopathies. A history of Herpes simplex requires the administration of antiviral prophylaxis following the treatment [51]. Fitzpatrick skin type IV–V needs special precaution. For these patients, an appropriate energy level and spacing between treatments must be selected to reduce the higher risk of hypo- or hyperpigmentation. The high amount of melanin present in darker skin types acts as a competing chromophore for the light delivered by the device. This results in reducing the effective light at the target tissue and diminishes the efficacy of the treatment. All of these aspects should be discussed and explained before treatment. By using high fluence and longer wavelengths, the light can penetrate deeper into the skin layers to reach the target lesion, e.g., vascular abnormality, but the risk of side effects is raised. An adequate cooling method is a safer trick to reduce the risk for these patients [55].

Another category of patient who requires special consideration are infants with hemangiomas or patients presenting with complex vascular malformations. For these, IPL or other laser procedures represent only a part of the treatment, and a multidisciplinary approach is mandatory prior to treatment. Identifying those patients who previously received other methods of treatment is important because the effect of therapy can be diminished. For example, vascular lesions treated with electrodesiccation, irradiation, or intralesional administration of corticosteroid or other sclerosant agents can develop fibrosus tissue. If the fibrosis is extended to the treatment area, it can diminish the effect of ILP [55].

Knowing the limitations of IPL is another essential aspect in practice because there are some conditions that contraindicate this therapy. These include pregnancy or breastfeeding and previous intake of drugs that cause photosensitization, e.g., retinoids or diseases associated with skin photosensitivity. Similarly, suntanned patients have a greater risk for complications if they are exposed to IPL therapy, especially for pigmentation changes and burns. For optimal results, the patient must use sun protection creams with an SPF of 50 for a few weeks prior to treatment during the summer months. No make-up should be in the treatment area because this can interfere with light transmission and absorption [51, 55].

At every initial treatment or when new parameters are introduced, performing a short test before the treatment helps to prevent unanticipated effects. The test should be representative for the entire treatment by placing it in the treatment area at an inconspicuous site. The skin reaction is observed and, if necessary, device parameters will be adjusted [51, 55]. In our practice, we invite patients for evaluation after 1 week. In the event of complications, we adjust the parameters, e.g., decrease the fluence, increase the pulse delay, and perform a second test on a different area.

If there are no local signs of complications and no complaints from the patient after the test, the entire area can be treated [51].

In our treatment protocol, following this step, the area that needs to be treated is cleaned using wet gauze, paying special attention to make-up removal. Pain during IPL treatment is a constant side effect but, for most patients, it is tolerable. Cooling and local anesthesia are methods for preventing or treating pain [51]. In our clinical practice, we have observed that procedures associated with longer wavelengths and higher fluences are more painful. Pain perception varies between individuals; we have encountered both patients who do not complain of pain without local anesthesia and patients who claim pain even when local anesthesia was used. An aspect regarding pain must be mentioned as a tip for avoiding other local complications. Even if the patient claims pain during treatment, this must always be at a supportable level. If the patient complains of severe pain, this must alert the practitioner because it appears as a consequence of side effects caused by heat destruction of the tissue [55].

The most widely used topical anesthetics are ELAM (Astra Pharmaceuticals) and ELA-MAX (Ferndale Laboratories) which have superior effects compared to Tetracaine and Betacaine-LA [57]. Under occlusive dressing, dermal anesthesia is obtained after 60 min by acting on free nerve endings located in the dermis [58–60]. The anesthetic ointment must be cleaned before treatment. An increase of the anesthetic effect was observed 15–30 min after its removal [59, 61]. Most common side effects of anesthetic creams are represented by local erythema, edema, and skin blanching [61]. In practice, it is important to distinguish these side reactions with the signs that indicate a positive response of the therapy, e.g., bluish appearance, perilesional erythema, blanching, or urticariform reaction (Fig. 10.11a, b). All of these aspects must be explained to the patients to avoid concern about a negative effect.

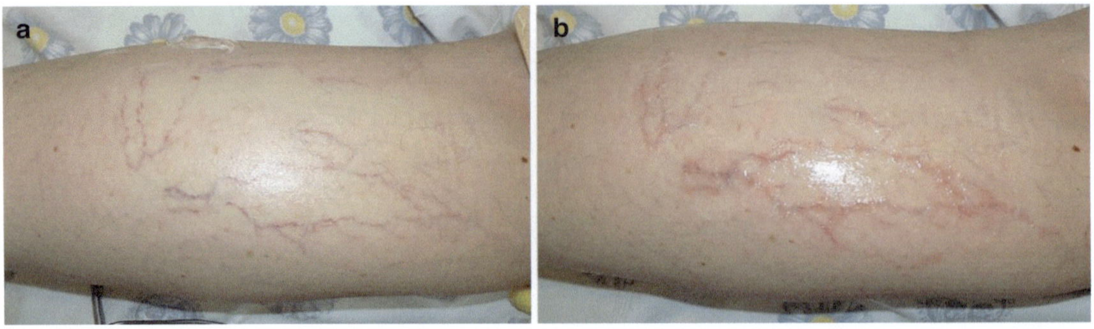

Fig. 10.11 (**a**) Small size leg veins before treatment. (Photos from Fodor and Ullmann second edition). (**b**) "Urticariform" reaction immediately after treatment. (Photos from Fodor and Ullmann seco edition)

More severe complications present in infants or patients who use inhibitor drugs of glucose-6-phosphate dehydrogenase or drugs that induce methemoglobinemia conversion of hemoglobin to methemoglobin which produces tissue hypoxia [62].

The cooling process represents an important part for most IPL treatments. Beside the effect of pain decrease during treatment, appropriate skin cooling is important for preventing epidermal damage. By decreasing the epidermal temperature while the chromophore temperature remains unchanged, the therapy remains effective and safer. This method allows for the use of higher fluencies without increasing the side effects. There are three methods of cooling: precooling, parallel cooling, and post cooling [55].

Spray and contact cooling are the most commonly used methods for most IPL devices. Both of these methods are associated with the risk of epidermal frost injuries if the pre-cooling time is not adequately controlled. The risk is higher when spray is used because of low control of precooling time. Fifty for 1 s is the ideal pre-cooling time [63, 64]. Though very rare, and mainly occurring in darker skin types, post-inflammatory hyperpigmentation due to spray or air cooling has been reported [55].

An important trick when the contact cooling method is used is not to apply pressure on the treated area, especially when vascular lesions are treated. When pressure is applied, the underlying small vessels will collapse, diminishing the energy absorbed by the target chromophore, e.g., hemoglobin, minimizing the desired effect. The same effect can be had if the handpiece of the device is applied with pressure on the skin [55] (Fig. 10.12).

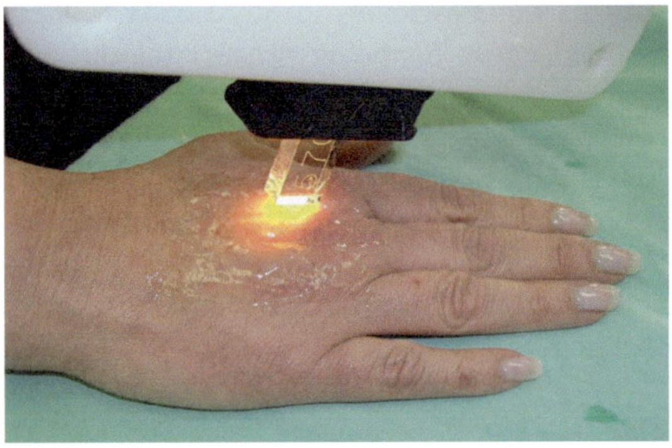

Fig. 10.12 Correct position of handpiece. (Photos from Fodor and Ullmann second edition)

Basic materials needed for IPL treatment include cold transparent gel which must be applied in a thin layer (2–3 mm) before the treatment to enhance the contact between the skin and the handpiece and protective eyeglasses. These must be used by the patient and the staff for the entire period of the treatment [65].

For most IPL procedures, many sessions are needed. Vascular lesions, such as telangiectasias or angiomas, require a few sessions, but for more severe lesions, e.g., rosacea, poikiloderma, and port wine stains, multiple treatment sessions are required. Monthly sessions for 3–4 months are recommended for dyschromias or redness. Multiple sessions must be repeated every 4–6 weeks for hair removal. The patient must be advised about this aspect at the beginning of treatment, because the desired effect may not be visible after the first treatment. Choosing the interval between sessions is very important because shortening the interval can lead to complications [16, 65].

Despite the high level of safety, IPL may be associated with complications. Some of these are related to patient skin reactivity. They are harder to be anticipated by the practitioner. For this reason, the patient must be informed about this aspect and the operator must be able to treat them.

Because IPL is operator-dependent, some professional errors can occur, leading to complications. These errors can be prevented with adequate training and knowledge. The source of errors must be known by any practitioner in order to adequately prevent them: deficit training or low documentation, incorrect diagnosis, and indication of incorrect handling of the device. Therefore, it is mandatory for any person who performs IPL procedures to be familiar with the specific performance and limitations of the device, because a confusing number of devices are available, including home use devices [55, 66]. These devices use less energy compared to professional ones and benefit from a safety system which limits their use to fair skin. Theoretically, because of low energy delivery to the tissue, adverse reactions will be less severe compared to professional devices [67]. However, keloid scars, which are considered to be extremely rare, and severe complications following IPL have been reported in one case using a home device to remove a tattoo [68].

A special training program offered by the manufacturer of the device or by an experienced user is our recommendation before using any IPL device. In contrast with some "money motivated cosmetic centers," where people with minimal training can use the device, there are some countries which provide that laser devices can be used only by physicians or by a delegated person under the supervision and full responsibility of a qualified physician [55].

Without specific dermatologic skills and training, in addition to laser-specific training, a laser operator is not fully prepared to understand the invasive nature of some IPL procedures. Moreover, he or she may not be capable of managing some of the complications that may be encountered, e.g., burns, skin infection, and skin wounds. An obvious example is when an inappropriately trained person utilizes IPL for photoaged skin. If their dermatologic knowledge is insufficient, a severe lesion such as basal cell carcinoma, squamous cell carcinoma, or lentigo maligna can be missed with severe consequences for the patient [55, 66]. Complications like zebra appearance second hair removal can be very disturbing for patients (Fig. 10.13a, b). This can be avoided easily by the proper use of the device. Avoiding overlapping of the footprint leads to untreated strips of skin in the area. The footprint should be adjusted and re-treating the area can improve the result. On the other hand, care should be taken to prevent scarring or textural changes when overlapping more than 10% [55].

There is a series of skin characteristics that can influence the susceptibility of one area of the body to IPL treatment. These include some intrinsic skin characteristics, such as thickness, blood perfusion, number of sebaceous glands, hair follicles, melanocytic nevi, or other individual related hallmarks, e.g., tattoo, suntan, and skin resistance. The anterior chest and neck are areas where the skin is fragile and the risk for scarring is greater. Reducing the radiant exposure of these regions by 10–20% limits the risk for complications [55].

Knowing these aspects, practitioners can reduce the risk of complications by accurately adjusting the parameters of the device.

As mentioned above, some side effects are harder to anticipate and may appear. The users must have the capability of understanding the causes and treating them correctly. Most commonly, these complications are minor and resolve within 1–48 h after treatment. Less frequently, they can last up to 7 days or, in cases of pigmentation disorders, up to 18 months. Using photodynamic therapy with

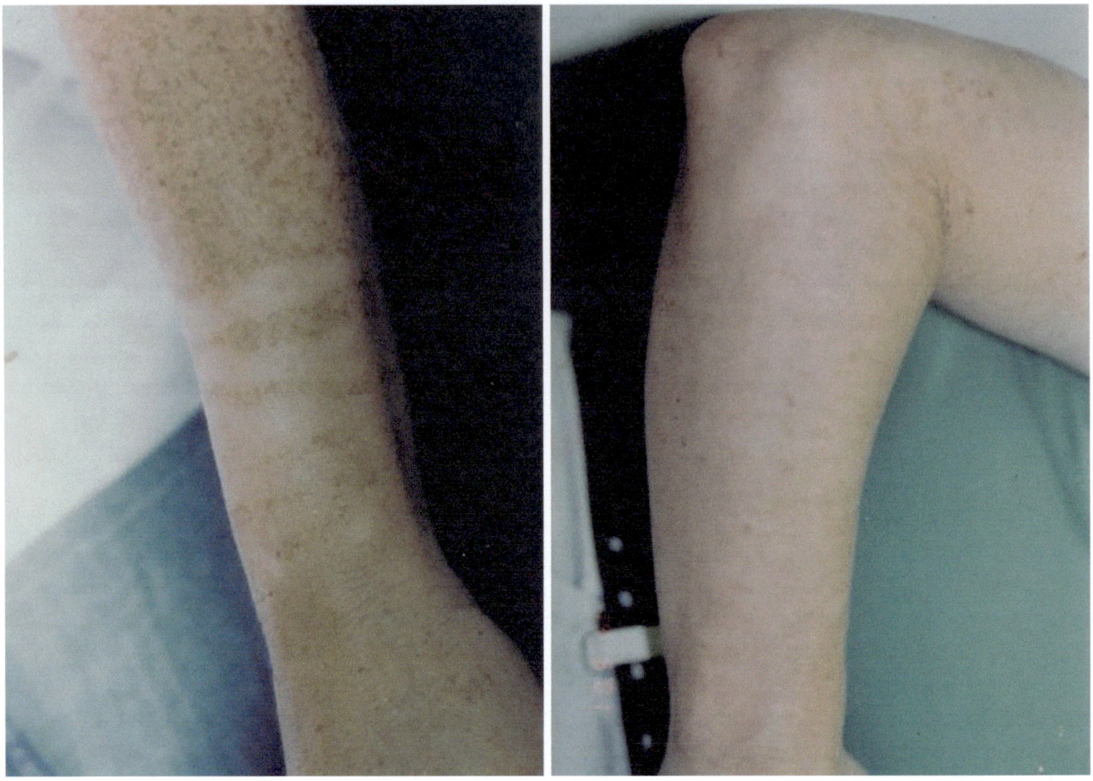

Fig. 10.13 "Zebra" appearance due to improper training and handling of the device. (Photos from Fodor and Ullmann second Edition)

5-aminolevulinic acid can cause the same adverse effects as after IPL, but more severe [69, 70].

Some of the most common side effects are represented by swelling and/or mild discomfort felt by the patient during treatment and immediately afterwards, such as erythema and edema, crust, and blistering [55]. More severe complications, such us permanent pigmentary changes, hair growth stimulation, leukotrichia, uveitis, iritis, scarring, ulceration, and reticulohistiocytoma, are more rarely encountered in practice. In order to manage the situation when a complication appears, we recommend the following steps:

First, stop the treatment immediately and, if possible, treat the complication. Cooling the area immediately may relieve the pain or discomfort related by the patient. Avoiding scratching in case of blisters and crust must be strictly recommended for preventing infections or scars [55].

Topical steroid creams can be used in patients with a history of prolonged edema for reducing the recovery time. Usually, there is no need for moisteners in case of crust or blisters because they tend to peel off. We recommend topical antibiotics only in the presence of erythema or oozing. Antiviral prophylaxis must be used in patients with a history of herpes. Shorter cutoff filters can be used to treat new growth hair which appears to be thicker and darker and more difficult to treat [71]. Scars following IPL tend to be hypopigmented and slightly depressed. Treatment of these lesions is not well defined, but CO_2 laser, dermabrasion, or chemical peeling can improve the aesthetic result [71].

Second, in order to allow skin recovery, the time intervals between treatments must be extended. There is no clear optimal time interval reported in the literature. We postpone the next session for a few weeks, and the fluence and pulse delay are adjusted to reduce the energy delivered to the skin.

Identify the cause of the complication. This can be poor handling of the device, e.g., high pressure, low contact, or some device settings. In this situation, the device settings, e.g., pulse duration, energy used or filters, or the technique, must be adjusted, and a test must be performed on a different area to evaluate the results. Another important cause of unwanted results can be poor compliance of the patient after therapy. There are some recommendations that must be followed. These include avoiding unprotected sun exposure and daily applications of UVA/UVB SPF30 or higher creams for at least 8 weeks [69, 70, 72]. The topical use of antioxidants can enhance IPL effects and reduce erythema and blistering [73]. Vitamin C can increase the whitening effect by reducing the melanin production and can be used for skin rejuvenation [74].

Other recommendations are to avoid photosensitizing medication, picking and scratching of the treatment area, prolonged bathing, or sauna. During the healing phase, e.g., 7–10 days, the skin is very delicate and must be handled with care.

It is very important to clarify that side effects are the result of lack of compliance. The practitioner should possess an adequate "technique" in discussion with the patient because some may refuse to recognize that the recommendations were not followed. A trick for avoiding these situations is to avoid direct questions and try to use indirect questions.

References

1. Jacques SL. Laser-tissue interactions. Photochemical, photothermal, and photomechanical. Surg Clin North Am. 1992;72(3):531–58. https://doi.org/10.1016/S0039-6109(16)45731-2.
2. Mignon C, Tobin DJ, Zeitouny M, et al. Shedding light on the variability of optical skin properties: finding a path towards more accurate prediction of light propagation in human cutaneous compartments. Biomed Opt Expr. 2018;9(2):852–72. https://doi.org/10.1364/BOE.9.000852.
3. Herd RM, Dover JS, Arndt KA. Basic laser principles. Dermatol Clin. 1997;15(3):355–72. https://doi.org/10.1016/S0733-8635(05)70446-0.
4. Piacquadio DJ, Chen DM, Farber HF, et al. Photodynamic therapy with aminolevulinic acid topical solution and visible blue light in the treatment of multiple actinic keratoses of the face and scalp: investigator-blinded, phase 3, multicenter trials. Arch Dermatol. 2004;140(1):41–6. https://doi.org/10.1001/ARCHDERM.140.1.41.
5. Mignon C, Tobin DJ, Zeitouny M, Uzunbajakava NE. Shedding light on the variability of optical skin properties: finding a path towards more accurate prediction of light propagation in human cutaneous compartments. Biomed Opt Expr. 2018;9(2):852. https://doi.org/10.1364/BOE.9.000852.
6. van Gemert MJC, Welch AJ. Time constants in thermal laser medicine. Lasers Surg Med. 1989;9(4):405–21. https://doi.org/10.1002/LSM.1900090414.
7. Fitzpatrick TB. The validity and practicality of sun-reactive skin types I through VI. Arch Dermatol. 1988;124(6):869–71. https://doi.org/10.1001/ARCHDERM.124.6.869.
8. Fischer DL, Han H, Gade A, Nestor MS. Intense pulsed light for the treatment of pigmented and vascular disorders and lesions: a review. Dermatol Rev. 2021;2(2):69–81. https://doi.org/10.1002/DER2.47.
9. Astner S, Anderson RR. Treating vascular lesions. Dermatol Ther. 2005;18(3):267–81. https://doi.org/10.1111/J.1529-8019.2005.05025.X.
10. Kauvar ANB, Lou WW. Pulsed alexandrite laser for the treatment of leg telangiectasia and reticular veins. Arch Dermatol. 2000;136(11):1371–5. https://doi.org/10.1001/ARCHDERM.136.11.1371.
11. Beebe-Dimmer JL, Pfeifer JR, Engle JS, Schottenfeld D. The epidemiology of chronic venous insufficiency and varicose veins. Ann Epidemiol. 2005;15(3):175–84. https://doi.org/10.1016/J.ANNEPIDEM.2004.05.015.
12. Nakano LCU, Cacione DG, Baptista-Silva JCC, Flumignan RLG. Treatment for telangiectasias and reticular veins. Cochrane Database Syst Rev. 2021;10(10):CD012723. https://doi.org/10.1002/14651858.CD012723.PUB2.
13. Hercogova J, Brazzini B, Hautmann G, Ghersetich I, Lotti T. Laser treatment of cutaneous vascular lesions: face and leg telangiectases. J Eur Acad Dermatol Venereol. 2002;16(1):12–8. https://doi.org/10.1046/J.1468-3083.2002.00355.X.
14. Porter JM, Moneta GL. An International Consensus Committee on Chronic Venous Disease. Reporting standards in venous disease: an update. International Consensus Committee on Chronic Venous Disease. J Vasc Surg. 1995;21(4):635–45. https://doi.org/10.1016/S0741-5214(95)70195-8.
15. West TB, Alster TS. Comparison of the long-pulse dye (590-595 nm) and KTP (532 nm) lasers in the treatment of facial and leg telangiectasias. Dermatol Surg. 1998;24(2):221–6. https://doi.org/10.1111/J.1524-4725.1998.TB04140.X.
16. DiBernardo BE, Pozner JN. Intense pulsed light therapy for skin rejuvenation. Clin Plast Surg.

2016;43(3):535–40. https://doi.org/10.1016/J.CPS.2016.03.008.
17. Goldman MP, Eckhouse S (1996) Photothermal sclerosis of leg veins. ESC Medical Systems, LTD Photoderm VL Cooperative Study Group. Dermatology Associates of San Diego County, Inc, California, La Jolla, USA. https://pubmed.ncbi.nlm.nih.gov/8624656/. Accessed 7 Dec 2021
18. Sadick NS. A dual wavelength approach for laser/intense pulsed light source treatment of lower extremity veins. J Am Acad Dermatol. 2002;46(1):66–72. https://doi.org/10.1067/MJD.2002.117851.
19. Colaiuda S, Colaiuda F, Gasparotti M. Treatment of deep underlying reticular veins by Nd:Yag laser and IPL source. Minerva Cardioangiol. 2000;48:329.
20. Fodor L, Ramon Y, Fodor A, Carmi N, Peled IJ, Ullmann Y. A side-by-side prospective study of intense pulsed light and Nd:YAG laser treatment for vascular lesions. Ann Plast Surg. 2006;56(2):164–70. https://doi.org/10.1097/01.SAP.0000196579.14954.D6.
21. Fisher GJ, Varani J, Voorhees JJ. Looking older: fibroblast collapse and therapeutic implications. Arch Dermatol. 2008;144(5):666–72. https://doi.org/10.1001/ARCHDERM.144.5.666.
22. Bernstein EF, Chen YQ, Tamai K, et al. Enhanced elastin and fibrillin gene expression in chronically photodamaged skin. J Investig Dermatol. 1994;103(2):182–6. https://doi.org/10.1111/1523-1747.EP12392693.
23. Ary G, Isher JF, Eng Z, et al. Pathophysiology of premature skin aging induced by ultraviolet light. N Engl J Med. 2009;337(20):1419–29. https://doi.org/10.1056/NEJM199711133372003.
24. Rox Anderson R, Parrish JA. Selective photothermolysis: precise microsurgery by selective absorption of pulsed radiation. Science (New York, NY). 1983;220(4596):524–7. https://doi.org/10.1126/SCIENCE.6836297.
25. Goldman A, Prati C, Rossato F. Hand rejuvenation using intense pulsed light. J Cutan Med Surg. 2008;12(3):107–13. https://doi.org/10.2310/7750.2008.07025.
26. Maruyama S. Hand rejuvenation using standard Intense Pulsed Light (IPL) in Asian patients. Laser Ther. 2016;25(1):43–54. https://doi.org/10.5978/ISLSM.16-OR-04.
27. Liu H, Dang Y, Wang Z, Chai X, Ren Q. Laser induced collagen remodeling: a comparative study in vivo on mouse model. Lasers Surg Med. 2008;40(1):13–9. https://doi.org/10.1002/LSM.20587.
28. Sadick NS. Update on non-ablative light therapy for rejuvenation: a review. Lasers Surg Med. 2003;32(2):120–8. https://doi.org/10.1002/LSM.10127.
29. Goldberg DJ. Current trends in intense pulsed light. J Clin Aesthet Dermatol. 2012;5(6):45. https://www.ncbi.nlm.nih.gov/pmc/articles/PMC3390232/. Accessed 7 Dec 2021.
30. Weiss RA, Weiss MA, Beasley KL. Rejuvenation of photoaged skin: 5 years results with intense pulsed light of the face, neck, and chest. Dermatol Surg. 2002;28(12):1115–9. https://doi.org/10.1046/J.1524-4725.2002.02113.X.
31. Oktem A, Kocyigit P. Comparison of effectiveness of 1,064-nm Nd:YAG laser and Nd:YAG laser–IPL combination treatments in hand skin rejuvenation. J Cosmet Laser Ther. 2016;18(5):270–4. https://doi.org/10.3109/14764172.2016.1157366.
32. Erol OO, Gurlek A, Agaoglu G, Topcuoglu E, Oz H. Treatment of hypertrophic scars and keloids using intense pulsed light (IPL). Aesthet Plast Surg. 2008;32(6):902–9. https://doi.org/10.1007/S00266-008-9161-7.
33. Vissing AC, Taudorf EH, Haak CS, Philipsen PA, Hædersdal M. Adjuvant eflornithine to maintain IPL-induced hair reduction in women with facial hirsutism: a randomized controlled trial. J Eur Acad Dermatol Venereol. 2016;30(2):314–9. https://doi.org/10.1111/JDV.13447.
34. Wendelin DS, Pope DN, Mallory SB. Hypertrichosis. J Am Acad Dermatol. 2003;48(2):161–82. https://doi.org/10.1067/MJD.2003.100.
35. Moreno-Arias GA, Vilalta-Solsona A, Serra-Renom JM, Benito-Ruiz J, Ferrando J. Intense pulsed light for hairy grafts and flaps. Dermatol Surg. 2002;28(5):402–4. https://doi.org/10.1046/J.1524-4725.2002.01211.X.
36. Kuriloff DB, Finn DG, Kimmelman CP. Pharyngoesophageal hair growth: the role of laser epilation. Otolaryngol Head Neck Surg. 1988;98(4):342–5. https://doi.org/10.1177/019459988809800414.
37. Gil-Vernet A, Arango O, Gil-Vernet J, Gelabert-Mas A, Gil-Vernet J. Scrotal flap epilation in urethroplasty: concepts and technique. J Urol. 1995;154(5):1723–6. https://doi.org/10.1016/S0022-5347(01)66766-1.
38. Giraldo F, Solano A, Mora MJ, Smith V. Hair growth in the vagina after reconstruction with pudendal thigh flaps in congenital vaginal agenesis. Plast Reconstr Surg. 1998;102(3):924–5. https://doi.org/10.1097/00006534-199809030-00066.
39. Vaidya T, Hohman MH, Kumar DD. Laser hair removal. Treasure Island, FL: StatPearls; 2021. https://www.ncbi.nlm.nih.gov/books/NBK507861/. Accessed 7 Dec 2021.
40. Warner J, Weiner M, Gutowski KA. Laser hair removal. Clin Obstet Gynecol. 2006;49(2):389–400. https://doi.org/10.1097/00003081-200606000-00020.
41. Görgü M, Aslan G, Aköz T, Erdoğan B. Comparison of alexandrite laser and electrolysis for hair removal. Dermatol Surg. 2000;26(1):37–41. https://doi.org/10.1046/J.1524-4725.2000.99104.X.
42. Bjerring P, Cramers M, Egekvist H, Christiansen K, Troilius A. Hair reduction using a new intense pulsed light irradiator and a normal mode ruby laser. J Cutan Laser Ther. 2000;2(2):63–71. https://doi.org/10.1080/14628830050516470.

43. Roosen GF, Westgate GE, Philpott M, Berretty PJM, Nuijs T, Bjerring P. Temporary hair removal by low fluence photoepilation: histological study on biopsies and cultured human hair follicles. Lasers Surg Med. 2008;40(8):520–8. https://doi.org/10.1002/LSM.20679.
44. Sadick NS, Shea CR, Burchette JL, Prieto VG. High-intensity flashlamp photoepilation: a clinical, histological, and mechanistic study in human skin. Arch Dermatol. 1999;135(6):668–76. https://doi.org/10.1001/ARCHDERM.135.6.668.
45. Zoccali G, Piccolo D, Allegra P, Giuliani M. Melasma treated with intense pulsed light. Aesthet Plast Surg. 2010;34(4):486–93. https://doi.org/10.1007/S00266-010-9485-Y.
46. Ortonne JP. Pigmentary changes of the ageing skin. Br J Dermatol. 1990;122(Suppl 35):21–8. https://doi.org/10.1111/J.1365-2133.1990.TB16121.X.
47. Briganti S, Camera E, Picardo M. Chemical and instrumental approaches to treat hyperpigmentation. Pigment Cell Res. 2003;16(2):101–10. https://doi.org/10.1034/J.1600-0749.2003.00029.X.
48. Weiss RA, Goldman MP, Weiss MA. Treatment of poikiloderma of Civatte with an intense pulsed light source. Dermatol Surg. 2000;26(9):823–8. https://doi.org/10.1046/J.1524-4725.2000.00060.X.
49. Fodor L, Carmi N, Fodor A, Ramon Y, Ullmann Y. Intense pulsed light for skin rejuvenation, hair removal, and vascular lesions: a patient satisfaction study and review of the literature. Ann Plast Surg. 2009;62(4):345–9. https://doi.org/10.1097/SAP.0B013E3181856D6A.
50. Fodor L, Peled IJ, Rissin Y, et al. Using intense pulsed light for cosmetic purposes: our experience. Plast Reconstr Surg. 2004;113(6):1789–95. https://doi.org/10.1097/01.PRS.0000117301.87544.6D.
51. Babilas P, Schreml S, Szeimies RM, Landthaler M. Intense pulsed light (IPL): a review. Lasers Surg Med. 2010;42(2):93–104. https://doi.org/10.1002/LSM.20877.
52. Gorney M. Recognition and management of the patient unsuitable for aesthetic surgery. Plast Reconstr Surg. 2010;126(6):2268–71. https://doi.org/10.1097/PRS.0B013E3181F619DA.
53. Martello J, Bailey J. Doctor-patient relationship. The consultation. Clin Plast Surg. 1999;26(1):53–5. https://doi.org/10.1016/s0278-2391(00)80035-x, vi.
54. Gorney M, Martello J. Patient selection criteria. Clin Plast Surg. 1999;26(1):37–40. https://doi.org/10.1016/s0278-2391(99)90744-9.
55. Adamič M, Pavlovic MD, Troilius Rubin A, Palmetun-Ekbäck M, Boixeda P. Guidelines of care for vascular lasers and intense pulse light sources from the European Society for Laser Dermatology. J Eur Acad Dermatol Venereol. 2015;29(9):1661–78. https://doi.org/10.1111/JDV.13177.
56. Webb MS. Failure in communication. Clin Plast Surg. 1999;26(1):41–51. https://doi.org/10.1016/S0094-1298(20)32317-8.
57. Friedman PM, Fogelman JP, Nouri K, Levine VJ, Ashinoff R. Comparative study of the efficacy of four topical anesthetics. Dermatol Surg. 1999;25(12):950–4. https://doi.org/10.1046/J.1524-4725.1999.99138.X.
58. Friedman PM, Mafong EA, Friedman ES, Geronemus RG. Topical anesthetics update: EMLA and beyond. Dermatol Surg. 2001;27(12):1019–26. https://doi.org/10.1046/J.1524-4725.2001.01855.X.
59. Evers H, von Dardel O, Juhlin L, Ohlsén L, Vinnars E. Dermal effects of compositions based on the eutectic mixture of lignocaine and prilocaine (EMLA). Studies in volunteers. Br J Anaesth. 1985;57(10):997–1005. https://doi.org/10.1093/BJA/57.10.997.
60. Greenbaum SS, Bernstein EF. Comparison of iontophoresis of lidocaine with a eutectic mixture of lidocaine and prilocaine (EMLA) for topically administered local anesthesia. J Dermatol Surg Oncol. 1994;20(9):579–83. https://doi.org/10.1111/J.1524-4725.1994.TB00150.X.
61. Langdon RJ, Yousefi PD, Relton CL, Suderman MJ. Laser-induced pain for evaluation of local analgesia: a comparison of topical application (EMLA) and local injection (Lidocaine). Anesth Analg. 1988;67(2):115–23.
62. Guardiano RA, Christopher WN. Direct comparison of EMLA versus lidocaine for pain control in Nd:YAG 1,064 nm laser hair removal. Dermatol Surg. 2005;31(4):396–8. https://doi.org/10.1111/J.1524-4725.2005.31104.
63. Zenzie HH, Altshuler GB, Smirnov MZ, Anderson RR. Evaluation of cooling methods for laser dermatology. Lasers Surg Med. 2000;26:130–44. https://doi.org/10.1002/(SICI)1096-9101(2000)26:2<130::AID-LSM4>3.0.CO;2-J.
64. Altshuler GB, Zenzie HH, Erofeev AV, Smirnov MZ, Anderson RR, Dierickx C. Contact cooling of the skin. Phys Med Biol. 1999;44(4):1003–23. https://doi.org/10.1088/0031-9155/44/4/014.
65. Arildsson M, Asker CL, Salerud EG, Strömberg T. Skin capillary appearance and skin microvascular perfusion due to topical application of analgesia cream. Microvasc Res. 2000;59(1):14–23. https://doi.org/10.1006/MVRE.1999.2206.
66. Greve B, Raulin C. Professional errors caused by lasers and intense pulsed light technology in dermatology and aesthetic medicine: preventive strategies and case studies. Dermatol Surg. 2002;28(2):156–61. https://doi.org/10.1046/J.1524-4725.2002.01087.X.
67. Town G, Botchkareva NV, Uzunbajakava NE, et al. Light-based home-use devices for hair removal: why do they work and how effective they are? Lasers Surg Med. 2019;51(6):481–90. https://doi.org/10.1002/LSM.23061.
68. Friedmann DP, Mishra V, Buckley S. Keloidal scarring from the at-home use of intense pulsed light for tattoo removal. Dermatol Surg. 2017;43(8):1112–4. https://doi.org/10.1097/DSS.0000000000001168.
69. Wat H, Wu DC, Rao J, Goldman MP. Application of intense pulsed light in the treatment of dermatologic disease: a systematic review. Dermatol

Surg. 2014;40(4):359–77. https://doi.org/10.1111/DSU.12424.
70. Kontoes PP, Vlachos SP, Marayiannis KV. Intense pulsed light for the treatment of lentigines in LEOPARD syndrome. Br J Plast Surg. 2003;56(6):607–10. https://doi.org/10.1016/S0007-1226(03)00218-2.
71. Moreno-Arias GA, Castelo-Branco C, Ferrando J. Side-effects after IPL photodepilation. Dermatol Surg. 2002;28(12):1131–4. https://doi.org/10.1046/J.1524-4725.2002.02117.X.
72. Feng YM, Zhou ZC, Gold MH. Hair removal using a new intense pulsed light source in Chinese patients. J Cosmet Laser Ther. 2009;11(2):94–7. https://doi.org/10.1080/14764170902883220.
73. Mohanan S, Basheerahmed P, Priyavathani R, Nellainayagam G. New intense pulse light device with square pulse technology for hirsutism in Indian patients: a pilot study. J Cosmet Laser Ther. 2012;14(1):14–7. https://doi.org/10.3109/14764172.2011.649764.
74. Thacker P, Kumar P. Near infrared pulsed light for permanent hair reduction in fitzpatrick skin types IV and V. J Cutan Aesthet Surg. 2016;9(4):249–53. https://doi.org/10.4103/0974-2077.197078.

Aesthetic Treatments with Focused Ultrasound

11

Mary Nielsen

Abstract

There are many treatments that are available for anti-aging, but Ultherapy®, a division of Merz, is a treatment that is approved by the US Food and Drug Administration to lift and tighten skin on the face and neck, including the eyes and brow area and the décolleté. This new method is not intended as a substitute for the dramatic results of surgery, but is offered as a non-surgical alternative for mild to moderate skin laxity. This chapter explores the benefits of Ultheraspy and Software. These new aesthetic therapy treatments and if they were to be incorporated in routine medical practice could positively shift non-invasive aesthetic procedures.

Keywords

Aesthetics · Skin of color · Focused ultrasound · HIFU · Ethnicity · Ultherapy · Sofwave

The original version of the chapter has been revised. A correction to this chapter can be found at https://doi.org/10.1007/978-3-031-36266-8_20

M. Nielsen (✉)
Spectrum Advanced Aesthetics Institute, Portland, OR, USA
e-mail: mary@spectrumlasertraining.com

11.1 Introduction

Aesthetic ultrasound using a transducer to visualize and treat the tissue beneath the surface of the skin in a non-invasive method was introduced in the early 2000s and is still being perfected today. We will review the first FDA devices registered for tissue lifting and look at some additional implications for use due to newer studies.

Ultherapy® treatments can work beyond the deepest layers of the skin, reaching into the SMAS, or Superficial Muscular Aponeurotic System. This is the layer of mesh-like tissue predominantly in the cheeks but connected to the superficial muscles in the lower face and neck (Fig. 11.1).

During a facelift, the SMAS is repositioned, along with the skin. Jowling is eliminated, the neck is tighter, and cheeks are elevated. An incision is made at the temple hairline, around the ears and ends at the scalp behind the ears. To tighten the neck area, an incision may be made under the chin as well. Then fat is redistributed on the face, jowls, and neck. Muscles are lifted and repositioned. Skin is redraped and excess skin trimmed away.

Ultherapy® sound waves send energy into the body and receive the echoing waves back. The ultrasound is used in two ways: to see beneath the surface of the skin and to create a specific treatment plan for each patient by treating with high-focused energy (HIFU) at predetermined depths

R. L. Bard (ed.), *Image-Guided Aesthetic Treatments*, https://doi.org/10.1007/978-3-031-36266-8_11

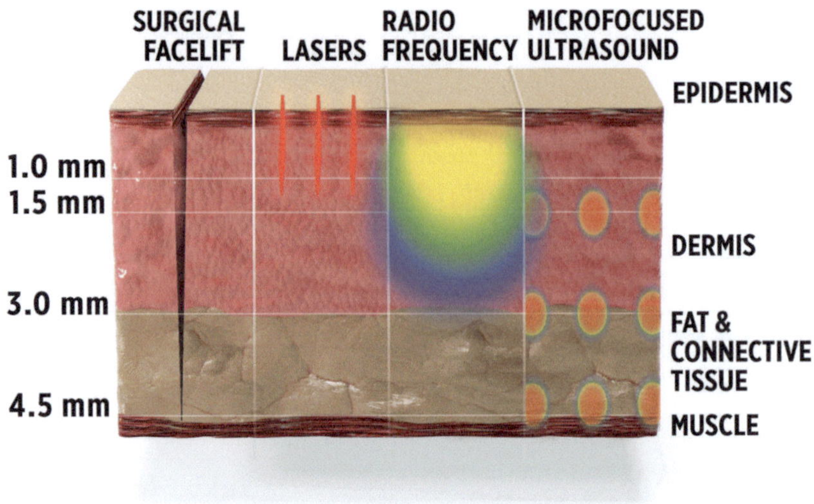

Fig. 11.1 Orange circles on the (R) indicate depth of the Ultherapy pulses. The deepest orange circle is the SMAS

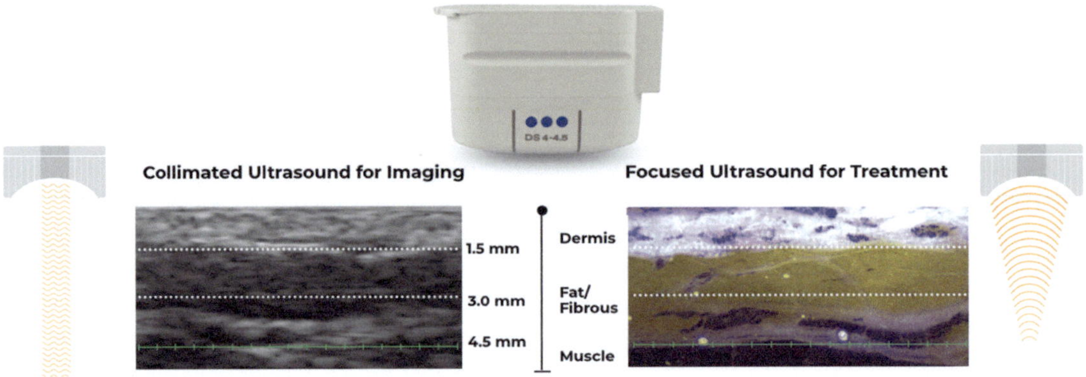

Fig. 11.2 Green indicates depth of focused ultrasound energy to tissue

in the tissue, while bypassing the surface of the skin.

Transducers pulse high-focused ultrasound energy precisely and consistently heating tissues to between 60 and 70 °C or over 140 °F at specific depths. This induces collagen denaturation and some minor tissue contraction. Additional tissue contraction happens over the course of 3–6 months as the body's wound healing process works to induce neocollagenesis and improve skin elasticity. Weak collagen is reorganized and strengthened. The final effect is improved skin tightness and actual tissue lifting (Fig. 11.2).

11.2 Ultherapy® Patient Consultation

The patient should have mild to moderate skin laxity. The older the patient, the lesser the collagen naturally available in the tissue, so results may be minimal. Ultherapy® is not a substitute for a facelift. Patient expectations should be realistic and the patient must understand that immediate results will not happen. Final results may take 6 months or longer. Multiple treatments may be necessary and often a series of three treatments spaced 3 months apart are recommended.

11.3 Ultherapy® Indications and Contraindications

The patient with mild to moderate skin laxity and an understanding that results will be gradual is an ideal candidate for an Ultherapy® treatment. It is intended for tissue lifting of the brow, submentum, and neck. It is also FDA cleared for improving lines and wrinkles on the décolleté. Ultherapy® is Fitzpatrick neutral so any skin color can be treated.

Ultherapy® is contraindicated for open lesions or wounds in the treatment area, or severe or cystic acne in the treatment area. A patient with a bleeding disorder, or who is on anticoagulant drugs, should not receive treatment. A patient with breast implants or a pacemaker should not be treated with Ultherapy® for décolleté lifting. Pregnancy, lactation, skin cancer, and emotional instability are all contraindications as well.

11.4 Ultherapy® Treatment

The consent form should be signed after the patient has had the opportunity to ask questions. Photos are very important. Since the results are visible months after the treatment, a visual record of the patient's skin and amount of laxity is needed for comparison down the road. The technician is gloved and topical numbing solution should be applied and allowed to work for at least 30 min. The numbing solution should be removed with a double cleanse.

Appropriately marking the treatment area is a critical step in the process. Ulthera should not be performed beyond the preauricular tragus to avoid the carotid arteries and jugular veins. The thyroid should be avoided as well as the mandibular nerve. If the mandibular nerve is treated, the patient may experience temporary facial drooping for several weeks as the nerve recovers. The treatment area should be marked with a while pencil with the templates provided according to the pattern provided in the treatment protocol (Fig. 11.3).

Ultrasound gel is applied. Treatments should be done on a minimum of two planes in the tissue, from deep to shallow. Typically, this is done at 4.5 and 3.0 mm, but a third pass at 1.5 mm can also be done and may offer additional lifting and tissue contraction. The operator must carefully position the transducer on the skin, being certain of complete contact. By observing the transducer

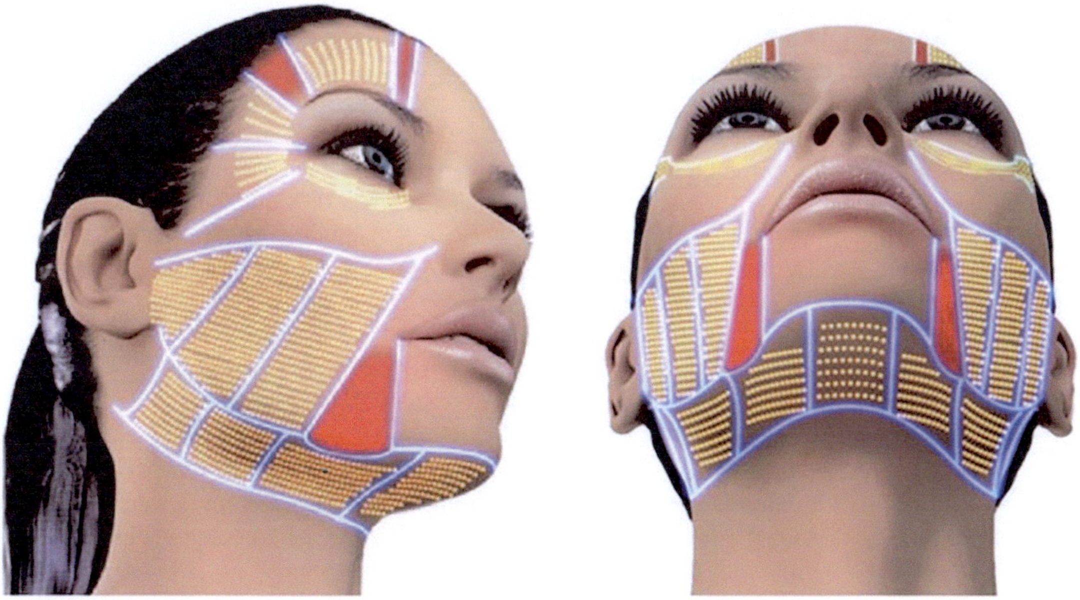

Fig. 11.3 Appropriate facial marking prior to Ulthera treatment

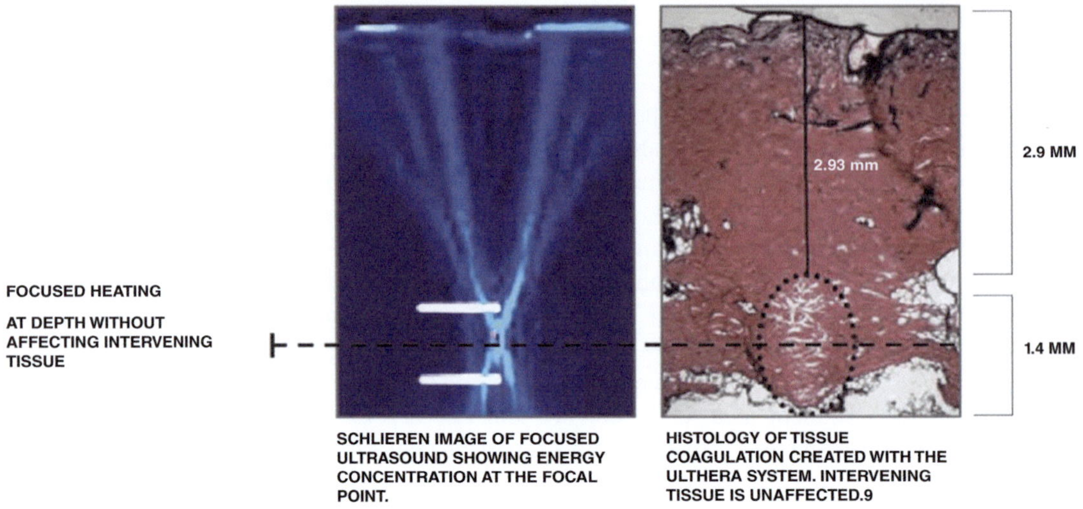

Fig. 11.4 Point of thermocoagulation

screen, the skincare specialist can avoid firing energy into the bone, which can be very uncomfortable for the patient. The transducer will deliver 20 tiny thermal coagulation points of ultrasound energy as deep as 8 mm below the surface of the skin with each firing of the handpiece. Additional ultrasound gel should be applied if the patient's skin absorbs it. The handpiece should not be fired on dry skin. The treatment area should be completed per the manufacturer's suggested guidelines, including multiple passes in specific areas. The micro-focused ultrasound pulse creates a point of thermocoagulation, leaving the tissue surrounding it intact (Fig. 11.4).

Do not overtreat. Treatment should not be done on the eyes or with a technique where the energy may reach the eyes.

Upon completion of the treatment, the gel should be removed. A hydrating antioxidant serum and SPF should be applied.

11.5 Ultherapy® Side Effects and Complications

Erythema and edema are common and usually resolved within several hours after treatment, although they may last several days. Discomfort will be based on each patient's pain tolerance and is most acute as the energy is being delivered. It should not be lasting or lingering.

Skin sensitivity may occur for several days after treatment. Bruising may occur occasionally. Transient numbness, tingling, or muscle weakness may be evident, but resolves within 2–6 weeks of treatment.

Complications can include fat loss and even greater skin laxity, if done too deeply for the specific treatment area.

11.6 Ultherapy® Post-treatment

The patient should be diligent with SPF and recommended home skincare regimen and return for photos in 3–4 months. Photos should be taken again at 6 months for comparison.

11.7 Ultherapy® Safety and Sanitation

The device and transducers should be sanitized according to the manufacturer's instructions and state infection control guidelines (Figs. 11.5 and 11.6).

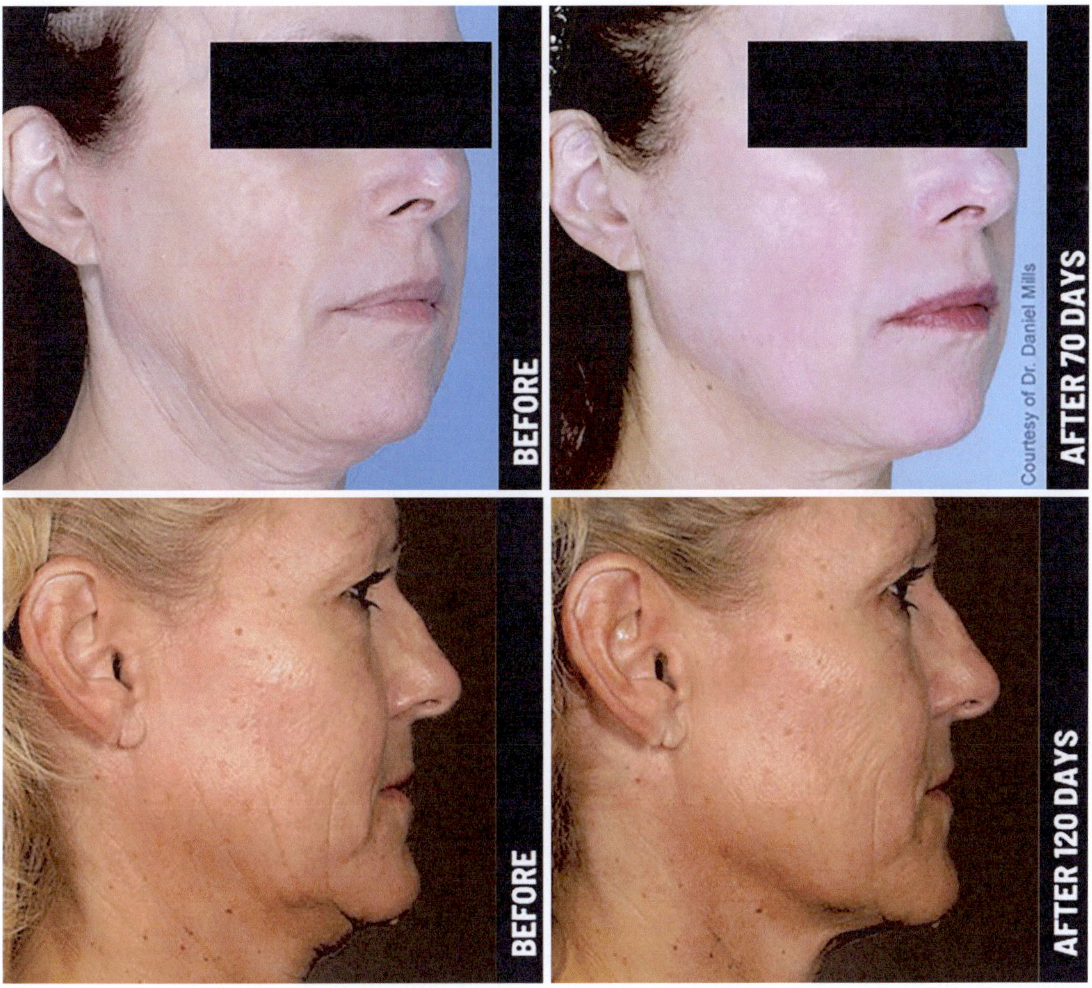

Figs. 11.5 and 11.6 Before and after examples

11.8 Sofwave

Sofwave® is another device approved by the FDA for improvement in fine lines and wrinkles. The results do not mimic a facelift but provide a non-surgical option for mild to moderate rhytids. Sofwave® sends intense ultrasound beam (IUB) energy into the body at a depth of 1.5–1.8 mm and provides contact cooling to protect the skin's surface. The proprietary technology emits an array of high intensity, high frequency, parallel ultrasound beams generated by multiple transducers which are in direct contact with the skin (Fig. 11.7).

Seven transducers pulse high-focused ultrasound energy precisely and consistently heating tissues to between 60 and 70 °C or over 140–158 °F at the depth of 1.5–1.8 mm with surface contact cooling. The body's wound healing process works to induce neocollagenesis and elastogenesis. This ultimately improves fine lines and wrinkles. Weak collagen is reorganized and strengthened.

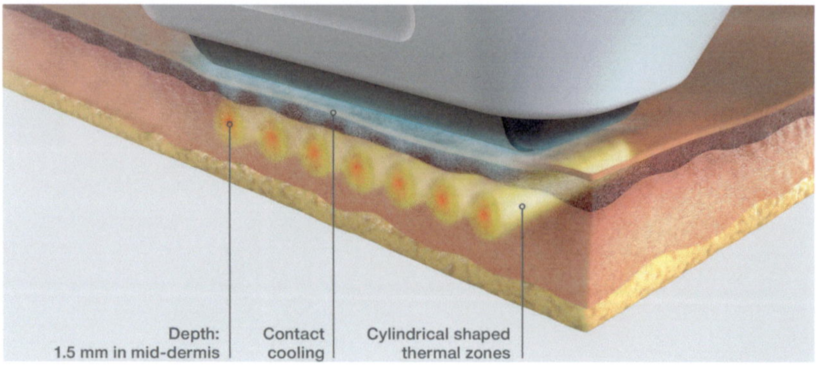

Fig. 11.7 Example of how Sofwave® works

11.9 Sofwave® Patient Consultation

The patient should have mild to moderate skin laxity. The ideal patient is one who is already familiar with neuromodulators and dermal fillers and is ready for another modality for reducing the effects of UV radiation and other forms of intrinsic and extrinsic aging. Patients over the age of 60, depending on their skin health, may not see dramatic results. The older the patient, the lesser the collagen naturally available in the tissue, so results may be minimal. Sofwave® is not a substitute for a facelift but is a good option for a patient who is not a surgical candidate. Patient expectations should be realistic, and the patient must understand that results could be evident within a week, but optimum results are seen at 12 weeks. Clients may need more than one treatment if they have deeper rhytids.

11.10 Sofwave® Indications and Contraindications

The patient with mild to moderate skin fine lines and wrinkles, mild to moderate laxity, and an understanding that results will be gradual is an ideal candidate for a Sofwave® treatment.

Ultrasound waves are not influenced by melanin so Sofwave® is safe for any Fitzpatrick skin type.

Sofwave® is contraindicated for open lesions, wounds, or significant scarring in the treatment area, or severe or cystic acne in the treatment area. Sofwave® is contraindicated for patients with pacemakers or other implanted cardiac devices. Pregnancy, lactation, skin cancer, and emotional instability are all contraindications as well. Treatment is not recommended directly over dermal fillers.

11.11 Sofwave® Treatment

Photos are very important. Since the results are optimized 12 weeks after the treatment, a visual record of the patient's skin and degree of rhytids is needed for comparison down the road. Patients often forget what they looked like. The consent form should be signed after the patient has had the opportunity to ask questions.

The technician is gloved and topical numbing solution should be applied and allowed to work for at least 30 min. The numbing solution should be removed with a double cleanse.

Sofwave® has a specific marking pattern for the treatment area to ensure all areas are effectively treated. The treatment area should be marked with a while pencil with the templates provided according to the pattern provided in the treatment protocol.

There is no technician visualization of the tissue beneath the transducer on a screen, as with Ultherapy®. The applicator's proprietary solid-state energizer module which holds the multiple ultrasound transducers allows for direct contact of the ultrasound transducers to the skin. This unique direct skin contact enables the integration of cooling and real-time temperature monitoring for excellent epidermal protection, accurate targeting of the thermal effect, and optimal pain management.

Do not overtreat. Treatment should not be done on the eyes or with a technique where the energy may reach the eyes. A hydrating antioxidant serum and SPF should be applied.

11.12 Sofwave® Side Effects and Complications

Erythema and edema are common and usually resolved within several hours after treatment, although they may last several days. Discomfort will be based on each patient's pain tolerance and is most acute as the energy is being delivered. It should not be lasting or lingering.

Skin sensitivity may occur for several days after treatment. Initial studies had zero negative complications.

11.13 Sofwave® Post-treatment

The patient should be diligent with SPF and recommended home skincare regimen and return for photos in 12 weeks. At this point, discussion about a second treatment may be considered based on comparisons between baseline and after photos (Figs. 11.8, 11.9, 11.10, and 11.11).

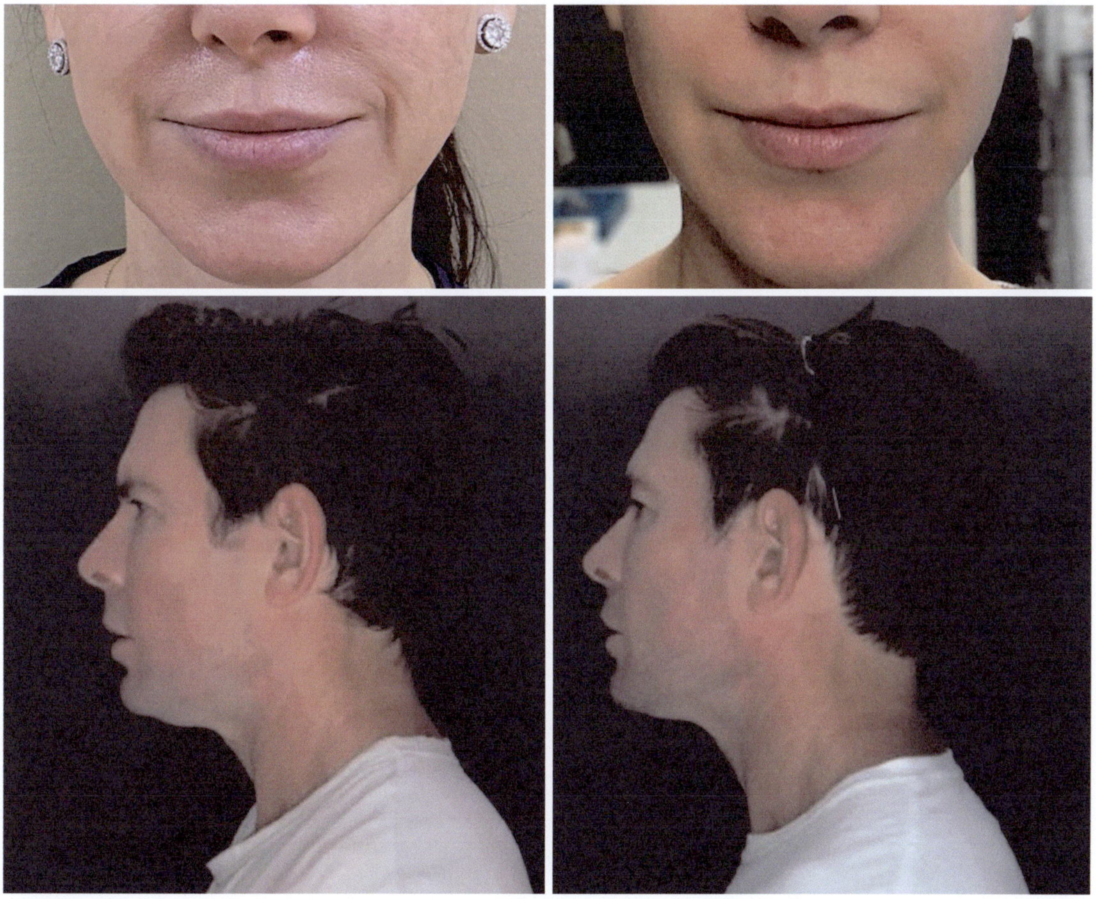

Figs. 11.8–11.11 Before and after

11.14 Sofwave® Safety and Sanitation

The device and transducer handpiece should be sanitized according to the manufacturer's instructions and state infection control guidelines.

It is important to distinguish IUB technology (Sofwave®) from HIFU (Ultherapy®). The IUB parallel ultrasound beam is less sensitive to scattering by differences in the skin structure's different absorption rates. The power density in IUB is generated by the transducer directly without the need for consideration of underlying tissue acoustic properties. The HIFU beam has a greater risk of injuring the epidermal tissue at 1.5 mm pulse because there is no direct contact cooling. Sofwave IUB transducers are in direct contact with the skin, measuring skin temperature and providing protection to the epidermis. HIFU transducers are extracorporeal to the skin, and the ultrasound gel that is essential does not allow for cooling or energy control mechanisms to be implemented.

11.15 Newer Studies on Aesthetic Multi-Focused Ultrasound Treatments

Several new studies show promise that high-focused ultrasound has unknown potential for skin treatment effectiveness. A pilot study by Joel Schlessinger, MD, revealed positive outcomes for patients diagnosed with erythematotelangiectatic rosacea, in the June 2021 issue of Journal of Drugs in Dermatology. Dr. Schlessinger's researchers treated 91 patients who had been positively diagnosed with erythematotelangiectatic rosacea. Diagnostic tools included a Clinician Erythema Assessment score greater than three and a Patient Self-Assessment score greater than 2. In this randomized study, subjects received one or two high-density micro-focused ultrasound treatments. Treatment success was determined to be a one-point change in erythema at the 90-day post-treatment interval.

All four treatment groups demonstrated success rates of 75–93%. The group that underwent one high-density micro-focused ultrasound treatment. Bruising, tenderness, and/or soreness and redness were the most commonly noted side effects. A larger randomized controlled study on the effectiveness of one high-density multi-focused ultrasound treatment is needed to validate this small study's results.

Patients' concerns about pore size could be managed if the study done by Vasanop Vachiramon, MD, proves to be effective on a larger scale. Dr. Vachiramon reported in Journal of Cosmetic Dermatology in August 5, 2021, that a randomized single-blinded split face study included 46 patients with enlarged facial pores. Each side of the face was randomly selected to a treatment of multi-focused ultrasound or multi-focused ultrasound plus the injections of calcium hydroxyapatite.

An Antera 3D system was used to measure pore volume objectively. A subjective assessment by a physician using a pore-grading system of 0–4 and patients ranked their own pore size improvements using the visual analog scale, 1–10.

The pore volume of both treated sides declined significantly compared with baseline. The lowest score was seen at 4 months. Patients preferred the dual modality option. Performing a combined technique of both modalities showed greater improvements at each follow-up visit, but at 4- and 6-month follow-ups, there were significant visual differences between the two sides of the face.

The combination treatment of micro-focused ultrasound and injections of calcium hydroxyapatite was successful in treating outer thigh cellulite in another study published in the Aesthetic Surgery Journal on December 19, 2020. Jesse R. Smith, MD; Michael Sheehan, PA-C; and Laurie A. Casas, MD, performed treatments on 60 women, ages 30–60 with body mass indexes less than 28 kg/m^2 who were concerned about outer thigh skin laxity.

Treatment included delivering 150 multi-focused ultrasound pulse lines at a focal depth of 3.0 and 4.5 mm per outer thigh. Immediately after delivering ultrasound energy, CaHA was injected into the subdermis with a dilution factor of 1.5 mL diluted 1:1 with 1.5 mL of 2% lidocaine solution per outer thigh.

Each woman used a subjective scale related to their body image, judgment about excess skin, and satisfaction with their hips and outer thighs, including psychosocial distress using Body-Q within 1 week of treatment. Body-Q is a patient-reported outcome instrument used for weightloss and body contouring treatments using 27 independently functioning scales, with no clinician input. Sixty days following treatment, women completed another Body-Q evaluation and reported statistically significant improvement in appearance and quality of life. The study originators believe this protocol may be expanded to treat other body areas beyond the outer thighs.

There are several points to success with a practice performing Ultherapy®. A skilled technician who can visualize internal structures and maximize placement of lines of multi-focused ultrasound energy at the appropriate depths and appropriate patient selection, including setting patient expectations for subtle results in tissue lifting that will not be immediately visible. The Ulthera® transducers are a consumable cost of over $2000, so return-on-investment must be carefully managed.

Sofwave® has no consumable cost for the practice so the price point for a treatment is typically 20–30% less than an Ultherapy® treatment, which is more attractive for the patient and ultimately provides a faster return-on-investment.

Ultrasound technology will continue to evolve and become more relevant in aesthetic medicine. Laser treatments offer increased risk of post-inflammatory hyperpigmentation if a negative side effect occurs. Ultrasound's ability to provide color-blind treatments, meaning it is applicable to all Fitzpatrick skin types, will make it a more attractive device as our country transitions to a population of blended ethnicities and skin of color becomes the majority [1–18].

References

1. Dermatology Times and Multimedia Medical, LLC. n.d.. http://dermatologytimes.modernmedicine.com/dermatology-times/news/user-defined-tags/dermatology/assessing-ultherapy-ultrasound-device-beingsma. Accessed 28 Feb 2017.
2. ClinicalTrials.gov. n.d.. https://clinicaltrials.gov/ct2/show/NCT01368874.
3. Araco A. Prospective study on clinical efficacy and safety of a single session of microfocused ultrasound with visualization for collagen regeneration. Aesthet Surg J. 2020;40:1124–32.
4. Dayan E, Burns AJ, Rohrich RJ, Theodorou S. The use of radiofrequency in aesthetic surgery. Plast Reconstr Surg Glob Open. 2020;8:e2861. https://journals.lww.com/plasreconsurg/Fulltext/2008/01000/Innovation.78.aspx.
5. Fabi SG. Noninvasive skin tightening: focus on new ultrasound techniques. Clin Cosmet Investig Dermatol. 2015;8:47–52. https://www.ncbi.nlm.nih.gov/pmc/articles/pmc4327394/.
6. Gutowski KA. Microfocused ultrasound for skin tightening. Clin Plast Surg. 2016;43:577–82. https://cdn.mdedge.com/files/s3fs-public/issues/articles/SCMS_Vol_32_No_1_Microfocused_Ultrasound.pdf.
7. Laubach HJ, Makin IR, Barthe PG, Slayton MH, Manstein D. Intense focused ultrasound: evaluation of a new treatment modality for precise microcoagulation within the skin. Dermatol Surg. 2008;34:727. https://onlinelibrary.wiley.com/doi/abs/10.1111/j.1524-4725.2008.34196.x.
8. Oni G, et al. Evaluation of a microfocused ultrasound system for improving skin laxity and tightening in the lower face. Aesthet Surg J. 2014;34(7):1099–110. https://academic.oup.com/asj/article/34/7/1099/2801381.
9. Lee HS, Jang WS, Cha Y-J, Choi Y-H, Tak Y, Hwang E, Kim BJ, Kim MN. Multiple pass ultrasound tightening of skin laxity of the lower face and neck. Dermatol Surg. 2012;38:20–7. https://onlinelibrary.wiley.com/doi/abs/10.1111/j.1524-4725.2011.02158.x?casa_token=7_OCddsOrS8AAAAA:AiXpjAJceBYh0LqD-vMY-jNiawOBdc-pW98K3nE_RRhbmjn7lgkbQH9Rx45cZBQDarR0fa4sRnNzZkCi.
10. Lu P-H, Yang C-H, Chang Y-C. Quantitative analysis of face and neck skin tightening by microfocused ultrasound with visualization in Asians. Dermatol Surg. 2017;43(11):1332–8. https://journals.lww.com/dermatologicsurgery/Abstract/2017/11000/Quantitative_Analysis_of_Face_and_Neck_Skin.3.aspx.
11. Lee HS, Jang WS, Cha YJ, et al. Multiple pass ultrasound tightening of skin lax-

ity of the lower face and neck. Dermatol Surg. 2012;38:20–7. https://onlinelibrary.wiley.com/doi/abs/10.1111/j.1524-4725.2011.02158.x?casa_token=7_OCddsOrS8AAAAA:AiXpjAJceBYh0LqD-vMY-jNiawOBdc-pW98K3nE_RRhbmjn7lgkbQH9Rx45cZBQDarR0fa4sRnNzZkCi.
12. ClinicalTrials.gov. n.d.. https://clinicaltrials.gov/ct2/show/NCT04829227.
13. Cision PR Newswire. n.d.. https://www.prnewswire.com/news-releases/arielle-kauvar-md-announces-new-technology-to-improve-fine-lines-and-wrinkles-on-the-face-and-neck-with-successful-clinical-study-pivotal-to-sofwaves-fda-510k-clearance-301088783.html.
14. Schlessinger J, Lupin M, McDaniel D, George R. Safety and effectiveness of microfocused ultrasound for treating Erythematotelangiectatic rosacea. J Drugs Dermatol. 2019;18(6):522. https://pubmed.ncbi.nlm.nih.gov/31251544/.
15. MedEsthetics. n.d.. https://www.medestheticsmag.com/news/article/21148583/microfocused-ultrasound-for-erythematotelangiectatic-rosacea.
16. MedEsthetics. n.d.. https://www.medestheticsmag.com/research/devices/news/21615238/merz-aesthetics-microfocused-ultrasound-reduces-pore-size.
17. Smith JR, et al. Using the BODY-Q to evaluate appearance and quality of life following treatment of skin laxity of the outer thigh with microfocused ultrasound and calcium hydroxylapatite. Aesthet Surg J. 2020;40(11):1219–31.
18. Sasaki GH, Tevez A. Clinical efficacy and safety of focused-image ultrasonography: a 2-year experience. Aesthet Surg J. 2012;32:601–12. https://academic.oup.com/asj/article-abstract/32/5/601/218440.

Nonsurgical Esthetics for Facial Rejuvenation and Hair Restoration Using Autologous PRP and Adipose Tissue Concentrate

12

Peter A. Everts

Abstract

Autologous biological preparations have emerged as a growing area of medical innovation in a variety of medical, interventional procedures. These cellular therapies are often referred to as autologous biologics. These preparations are derived from the patient's own tissues, including blood, bone marrow, and fat tissue to prepare platelet-rich plasma (PRP), bone marrow concentrate (BMC), and adipose tissue concentrate (ATC), respectively. Autologous biologics comprising signaling cells and molecules have the potential to play adjunctive roles in a variety of regenerative esthetic treatment plans, by stimulating and enhancing tissue repair.

Despite the progress in understanding biological technologies and improvements in clinical applications, definitive and accepted standards to prepare different biological bioformulations are still lacking. In this chapter, I will discuss recent developments regarding autologous biological PRP and adipose tissue preparations and compositions regarding platelet dosing, leukocyte activities concerning innate and adaptive immunomodulation, inflammation, angiogenesis, and provide some reported outcomes in facial rejuvenation and hair restoration.

Keywords

Autologous biologics · Platelet-rich plasma · Adipose tissue concentrate · Esthetics · Facial rejuvenation · Hair restoration · Platelet dosing · Leukocytes · Inflammation immunomodulation · Angiogenesis · Outcomes

12.1 Introduction

The human body has an endogenous system of tissue repair, regeneration, through growth factors, cytokines, stem- and progenitor cells, signaling cells, and other cell types, as they are found in almost every type of tissue. It is important to understand the terminology used in relation to tissue repair and regeneration.

12.2 Nonsurgical Esthetics and Regenerative Medicine

Nonsurgical esthetics, defined here as facial rejuvenation and hair restoration, employing a variety of injection techniques using autologous PRP and adipose tissue concentrate (ATC) can be safely executed by well-trained physicians at

P. A. Everts (✉)
Science and Clinical Research, Gulf Coast Biologics, Fort Myers, FL, USA
e-mail: peter@gulfcoastbiologics.com

R. L. Bard (ed.), *Image-Guided Aesthetic Treatments*, https://doi.org/10.1007/978-3-031-36266-8_12

point of care with dedicated devices. The objectives of nonsurgical autologous biological therapies are to support the body to form new functional tissues to replace degenerative or defective ones and to provide therapeutic treatment for conditions where conventional therapies are inadequate.

12.3 Autologous Biologics

The term biologics has been introduced for the treatment of a variety of medical disorders with autologous orthobiologic preparations such as PRP and ATC. Several of these autologous products are showing promising regenerative results, even though there is a magnitude of biological active cellular products commercially available. This chapter is not meant to be exhaustive, but to shed light on cell mechanisms following esthetic procedures with biologically prepared products from whole blood and adipose tissues.

12.4 Platelet-Rich Plasma

PRP therapies have been used for various indications for more than 30 years, resulting in considerable interest in the potential of PRP in esthetics and regenerative medicine applications. Autologous PRP is defined as the processed liquid fraction of autologous peripheral blood with a platelet concentration above the baseline [1]. Currently, PRP therapies are suitable treatment options with clinical benefits and encouraging patient outcomes reported [2–4]. However, new therapeutic insights and needs have challenged the practicality and effectiveness of PRP clinical applications as many different commercially available PRP and PRP-like systems are being used [5]. A profuse variability in final PRP cellular contents has been reported. Not surprising, different PRP devices contribute to distinctive PRP properties and bioformulations, which may explain inconsistencies in patient outcomes. In this chapter, the fundamentals of autologous PRP technology and its biological properties are comprehensively described as PRP applications in nonsurgical esthetics are used increasingly.

12.5 Adipose Tissue Concentrate

A source for autologous mesenchymal stem cells is adipose tissue (AT), which can be harvested via lipo-aspiration of subcutaneous fat, from various areas of the body, like the abdomen, thighs, flank, and perigluteal region [6]. Later in the chapter, I touch on some essentials regarding AT harvesting, stromal vascular fraction (SVF), cellular structures, and their immunomodulatory actions, and angiogenic effects.

12.6 The Rationale for PRP in Nonsurgical Esthetic Applications

The past decade has seen an exponentially growing interest in PRP applications in the medical arena, claiming tissue repair, regenerative, and restorative properties, treating many pathologies, including dermatologic, cosmetic, reconstructive, and oro-maxillofacial pathologies [7]. Due to a plethora of, alleged, indications for autologous biological therapies in esthetic and cosmetic conditions (Table 12.1), this chapter focuses only on the application of PRP growth factors and ATC in facial tissue rejuvenation and hair restoration.

Table 12.1 Overview of reported PRP treatment indications in esthetic and cosmetic medicine [8–10]

Acne (anthropic) scars
Actinic scarring
Alopecia variations
Breast augmentation
Burns
Facial aging
Facial folds
Hand rejuvenation
Hyperpigmentation
Lichen sclerosus
Lipodermatosis
Loss of tissue volume
Melasma
Photodamaged skin
Striae distensae
Traumatic scars
Ulcers
Vitiligo

12.7 Facial Tissue Rejuvenation

Rejuvenation of the aging facial skin by intradermally and/or subdermally PRP has been accepted as a common therapy. This is based on the premise of platelet growth factor (PGF) stimulation and the activation of dermal fibroblasts, myofibroblasts, and induction of collagen synthesis and subsequent tissue remodeling of the ECM. Significant improvements in skin texture, color, and reduced wrinkle depth have been reported.

Histologic and patient satisfaction scores show that this treatment has promise for the applications of periorbital wrinkles, periorbital hyperpigmentation, and skin photoaging [11]. The biological and biochemical processes that are involved in wound healing cascades are similar to the needed changes to reverse the effects of intrinsic and extrinsic skin aging [12]. After facial PRP injection, dermal fibroblast starts proliferating in the skin and activated platelets contribute to an increased production of collagen type I [13]. A diversity of PGFs, with their specific characteristics (Table 12.2), play pivotal roles in tissue regenerative processes. Like the mechanisms involved in wound healing, PRP acts on skin aging through collagen remodeling, stimulating a thickening of the superficial layer of the skin, and simultaneously improving cell regeneration [15]. The effectiveness of PRP injections in tissue repair, skin rejuvenation, and hair growth is determined by the biocellular activity of the PRP, including the growth factors present in the platelets that are applied. More specifically, platelet-derived growth factor (PDGF) recruits macrophages and fibroblasts and stimulates macrophages to secrete growth factors, such as transforming growth factor beta (TGF-β), to produce collagen to improve skin elasticity and wrinkles. Vascular endothelial growth factor (VEGF) promotes endothelial cell proliferation and blood vessel formation, and epidermal growth factor (EGF) promotes cell differentiation and re-epithelialization. Additionally, insulin-like growth factor-1 (IGF-1) is capable of augmenting skin barrier function. Therefore, specific PGFs, in combination with available platelet proteins, cytokines, and chemokines, regulate fundamental cellular activities. These include (neo)angiogenesis, formation of the ECM, mitogenesis, and chemotaxis [16].

Moreover, PRP can promote the proliferation and multiple differentiation of adipose derived mesenchymal stem cells (AD-MSCs), contributing to improve the loss of fat volume [17] Furthermore, it has been suggested that improvements in skin elasticity and cosmetic appearance are due to a variety of mechanisms, including changes in cell-cycle regulators, and increased expression of procollagen alpha, and elastin. In addition, MMP-1 and MMP-3 degrade and remove cells of the photodamaged tissue matrix [18]. In Fig. 12.1, multiple cellular effects of PRP injections in facial rejuvenation are shown that contribute to collagen production and ultimately an increase in facial tissue volume.

Table 12.2 PRP-based growth factors, angiogenetic factors, and platelet cytokines (Partial List)

		Function and effects
Growth factors	PDGF (AA-BB-AB)	Mitogenic for mesenchymal cells and osteoblasts; stimulates chemotaxis and mitogenesis in fibroblast/glial/smooth muscle cells; regulates collagenase secretion and collagen synthesis; stimulates macrophage and neutrophil chemotaxis
	TGF (α–β)	Stimulates undifferentiated mesenchymal cell proliferation; regulates endothelial, fibroblastic, and osteoblastic mitogenesis; regulates collagen synthesis and collagenase secretion; regulates mitogenic effects of other growth factors; stimulates endothelial chemotaxis and angiogenesis; inhibits macrophage and lymphocyte proliferation
	HGF	Regulates cell growth and motility in epithelial/endothelial cells, supporting epithelial repair and neovascularization during wound healing
	EGF	Proliferation of keratinocytes, fibroblasts, and stimulates mitogenesis for endothelial cells
	FGF (a-b)	Promotes growth and differentiation of chondrocytes and osteoblasts; mitogenic for mesenchymal cells, chondrocytes, and osteoblasts
	CTGF	Promotes angiogenesis, cartilage regeneration, fibrosis, and platelet adhesion
	IGF-1	Chemotactic for fibroblasts and stimulates protein synthesis. Enhances bone formation by proliferation and differentiation of osteoblasts
	KGF	Regulates epithelial migration and proliferation
Cytokines	IL-1	Promotes systemic inflammation
	IL-6	Pro inflammation—anti inflammation
	PF-4	Calls leucocytes and regulates their activation. Antiangiogenetic properties
	SDF-1α	Calls CD34+ cells, induces their homing, proliferation, and differentiation into endothelial progenitor cells stimulating angiogenesis. Calls mesenchymal stem cells and leucocytes
	TNF	Regulates monocyte migration, fibroblast proliferation, macrophage activation, and angiogenesis

PDGF: platelet-derived growth factors; TGF: transforming growth factor; VEGF: vascular endothelial growth factor; EGF: epidermal growth factor; FGF: fibroblast growth factor; CTCG: connective tissue growth factor; IGF: insulin-like growth factor; HGF: hepatocyte growth factor; KGF: keratinocyte growth factor; 5-HT: serotonin; Ang-1: angiopoietin-1; Endo: endostatin; IL-1: interleukin 1; IL-6: interleukin 6; IL-8: interleukin 8; PF4: platelet factor 4; SDF: stromal cell derived factor; TNF: tumor necrosis factor
Modified from Everts et al. [14]

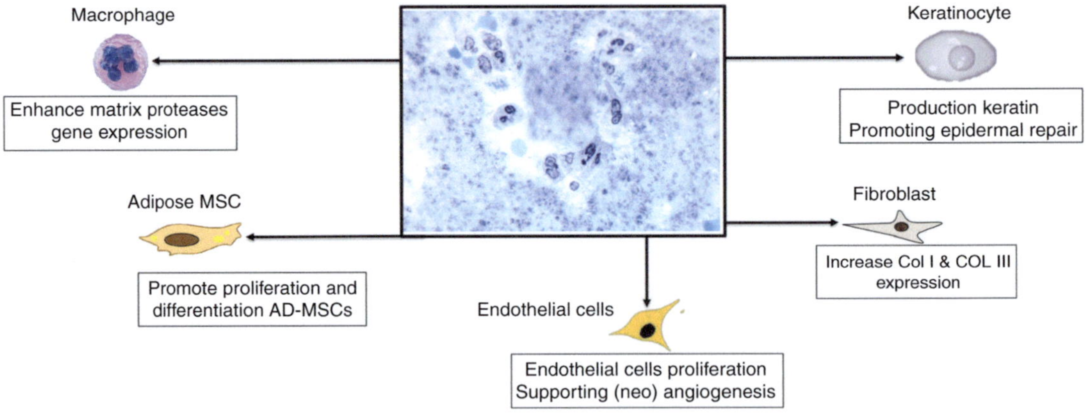

Fig. 12.1 The multiple cellular effects of PurePRP® injections in facial rejuvenation procedures. Following intradermal and subdermal PRP injections, platelets become activated and release their content. Platelet constituents contribute to a variety of cellular processes of macrophages, AD-MSCs, endothelial cells, keratinocytes, and fibroblasts. In response to the presence of an injected platelet dose, these cells demonstrate particular functions like proliferation, differentiation, (neo) angiogenesis, collagen, and gene expression. Ultimately, collagen is produced with epidermal and ECM repair, promoting facial rejuvenation. Cave: the PRP smear in this graphic had a platelet concentration of 2.1×10^9/mL

12.8 Hair Restoration

The precise mechanism of action of PRP in the promotion of hair growth is still not completely defined. The dermal papilla (DP) cells produce a variety of platelet growth factors, like VEGF, HGF, IGF, and FGF. Once platelets in PRP become activated, they induce the proliferation of DP cells by activating extracellular signal-related kinase and protein kinase B cell signaling [19, 20]. PRP platelet growth factors EGF and PDGF upregulate the cell signaling pathways and increase the transcription of genes involved in cellular proliferation and differentiation. Additionally, PGFs are responsible for maintaining the hair follicle in the anagen phase of the hair cycle, as demonstrated by Li et al. It can be assumed that activated PRP affects hair cycling by prolonging the length of the anagen phase and preventing apoptosis and the catagen phase [21]. Therefore, delivering PRP to DP cells to upregulate PGFs within these cells, aiming to lengthen the anagen phase, is very plausible with the objective to shorten the hair growth cycle [22]. Similarly, Takikawa et al. described that PGFs act indirectly on stem cells found in the bulge area of follicles, resulting in neovascularization and folliculogenesis [23]. Furthermore, Garg mentioned that PRP stimulated dormant hair follicles by normalizing the scalp milieu with reduced fibrosis and neovascularization, instigated by the activities of FGF and VEGF [24].

12.9 Fundamentals of Platelet-Rich Plasma (PRP)

The most well-known physiological role of platelets is the control of hemorrhage, where they accumulate at tissue injury sites and damaged blood vessels. These events are instigated by the expression of integrins and selectins that stimulate platelet adhesion and aggregation, leading to the formation of the platelet plug. However, during PRP preparation procedures, clothing should be always avoided as this will jeopardize the preparation of an adequate and viable autologous biological injectate. PRP can be characterized as a complex composition of autologous multicellular blood components in a small volume of plasma, acquired from a fraction of peripheral venous blood. Following a 2-spin, density gradient centrifugation procedure, blood cells are separated to form a buffy-coat layer. Finally, a PRP treatment vial containing platelets and some leukocytes can be retrieved from the concentration device, as shown in Fig. 12.2. Albeit, that specific PRP devices produce different PRP biologics, with different bio-cellular compositions.

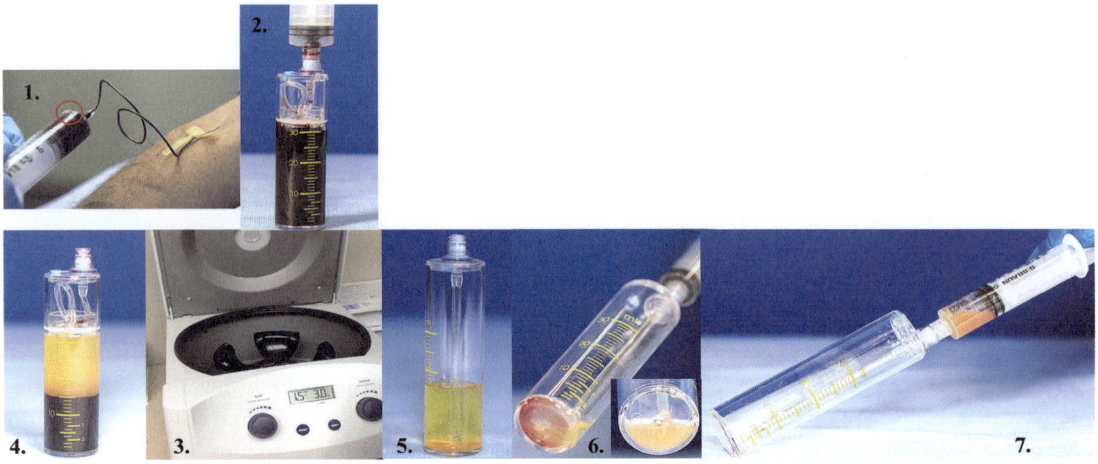

Fig. 12.2 Procedural steps of a 2-spin PRP preparation method to prepare autologous PRP (used with permission from EmCyte Corporation, Fort Myers FL USA, PurePRPII® device). (1) A volume of whole blood is drawn from the median antecubital vein, with anticoagulant in the syringe (red circle), the baseline platelet concentration was 215 × 10^3/μL. (2) The concentration device is loaded with anticoagulated whole blood, avoiding damaging the blood. (3) The concentration device is loaded in a dedicated centrifuge for the first spin. (4) The typical aspect after the first spin: plasma is the first layer, a small intermediate layer, and the RBCs. (5) After the second spin, platelets and other cells are layered in an organized fashion on the bottom of the device, below the platelet-poor plasma fraction. (6) The PPP fraction is removed, based on a specific treatment procedure, leaving the sticky cells (final PRP injectate) at the bottom of the device. The remaining plasma is used to resuspend the platelets and other cells. (7) After careful resuspension, the PRP volume is extracted from the device. In this graphic a 30 mL PurePRP® kit was used to produce 4 mL of PRP, with a platelet concentration of 2.1 × 10^9/mL

12.10 Different PRP Devices Use Different Preparation Methods

A clear consensus across treatment indications and type of PRP to use is nonexistent, making it difficult to compare PRP products and their related therapy outcomes. In the majority of reported cases, platelet concentrate therapies are all grouped under the term "PRP," even for the same clinical indication [25]. Therefore, this lack of a consensus in PRP preparation methods contributes to inconsistent PRP patient outcomes, based on enormous differences in PRP composition and formulation, specimen quality, including platelet concentrations. Nonetheless, for some medical fields (e.g., OA and tendinopathies), progress has been made in understanding the variations in the PRP formulations, delivery routes, platelet function, and other PRP constituents influencing tissue repair and tissue regeneration. Unfortunately, in facial and hair biological therapies, this progress is still absent. At present, more than 40 different "PRP" devices and methods are in the market, using single-spin and dual-spin technologies to prepare PRP. Noteworthy, most single spin device technologies consist of simple laboratory test tube (design), not capable of producing density separation layers, as shown in Fig. 12.3. After the first centrifugation procedure, the whole blood components are separated into two basic layers, the platelet (poor) plasma suspension and the RBC layer. After a second centrifugation step, the needed PRP volume can be extracted for patient application. In Fig. 12.2, at the bottom of the PRP device, an organized

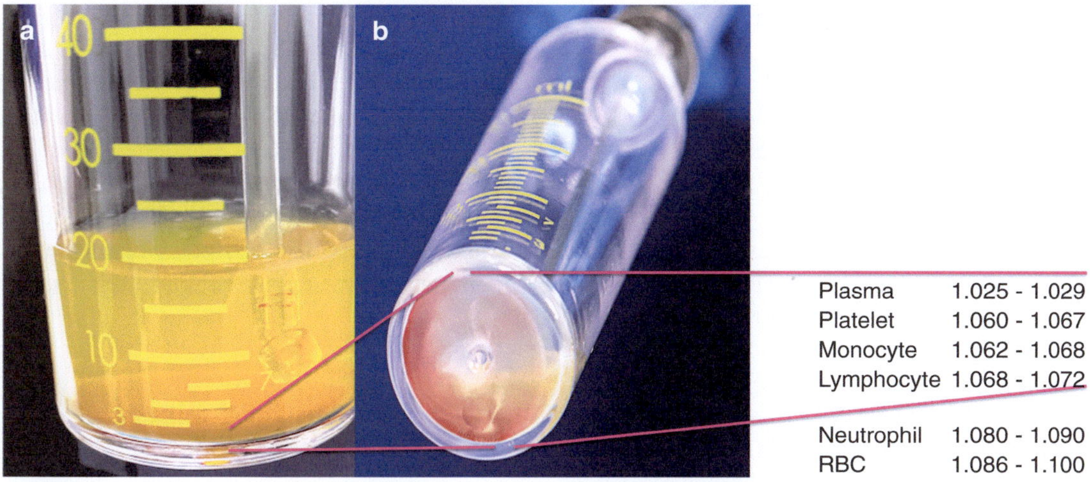

Fig. 12.3 (**a**, **b**) Two-spin PRP preparation procedures result in cellular density gravitational separation. Cells are organized according to their specific densities (used with permission from EmCyte Corporation, Fort Myers FL USA, PurePRPII® device). In this graphic, a 30-mL PRP kit was used to produce 4 mL of PRP, with a platelet concentration of 2.1×10^9/mL

multicomponent buffy coat layer (indicated between the blue lines) is visible, containing high concentrations of platelets, monocytes, and lymphocytes, based on the specific cellular densities. In this example a minimal percentage of neutrophils (<0.3%) and RBCs (<0.1%) was extracted, following a neutrophil poor PRP preparation protocol, modified from Everts et al. [26].

12.11 Platelet-Derived Constituents in PRP

PRP should meet the prerequisites (platelet dosage, minimal RBC contamination, addition, or removal of specific leukocytes) to produce significant clinical outcomes. These PRP qualifications, combined with elucidating the activities of different PGFs, platelet proteins, cytokines, and chemokines, contribute to the understanding of the fundamental tissue repair mechanisms involving various biological processes: mitogenesis, angiogenesis, chemotaxis, and extracellular matrix formation [27]. Figure 12.4 details the platelet structures and their specific functions. In early PRP applications, α-granules were the most cited intraplatelet structures because of the presence of many PGFs [28]. To a lesser degree, coagulation factors and regulators of angiogenesis were cited with PRP preparations. Additional factors include less famous chemokine and cytokine constituents, functioning to recruit and activate other immune cells, or induce endothelial cell inflammation [29].

The dense granule constituents like ADP, serotonin, polyphosphates, histamine, and epinephrine are more implicit as modifiers of platelet activation and thrombus formation [30]. Most importantly, many of these elements have immune cell-modifying effects. Other platelet dense granule constituents (e.g., glutamate and serotonin) induce T-cell migration and increase monocyte differentiation into dendritic cells, respectively [31]. In PRP, the dense granule-derived immune modifiers are highly enriched and have substantial immune functions. This indicates a relationship between the PRP and immunomodulatory potential.

12.12 Essentials of Clinical PRP Preparations

12.12.1 Platelet Activation and Tissue Repair Mechanisms

After PRP is applied in tissues to initiate tissue repair mechanisms, PRP platelets interact with a broad range of cells to induce regenerative tissue remodeling mechanisms, following the classic functions of platelets, platelet clot formation, growth factor, and cytokine release. More specifically, following PRP injection, platelets interact with leukocytes, endothelial cells, and resident or circulating cells that are involved in tissue reorganization, following the induction and regulation of hemostasis [32]. After controlled delivery of nonactivated PRP, the platelets will be activated by the interaction with platelet tissue factor (factor III), present in subendothelial tissues and leukocytes. Other activation pathways can be induced by the addition of $CaCl_2$ and/or thrombin to PRP preparations. Following platelet activation, the platelet α-, dense, lysosomal, and T-granules undergo regulated exocytosis and release their contents into the extracellular environment (Fig. 12.4) [33, 34]. As a result, a platelet plug will develop in the injected microenvironment, as the first step of the healing cascade with the release of signaling molecules, triggering the recruitment and activation of inflammatory cells through a broad range of cell membrane receptors and soluble mediators, which are released upon PRP platelet activation [35].

12.12.2 The Platelet Numbers in PRP are Critical

PRP treatment protocols have evolved immensely over the past 10 years. Through experimental and clinical research, we now have a better understanding of platelet and other cellular physiology. Systematic reviews, meta-analyses, and randomized controlled trials denote the effectiveness of PRP biological technologies in many medical fields, including dermatology [36], plastic surgery [37], sports medicine [38, 39], pain management [40], and orthopedic surgery [41]. The therapeutic actions of PRP and

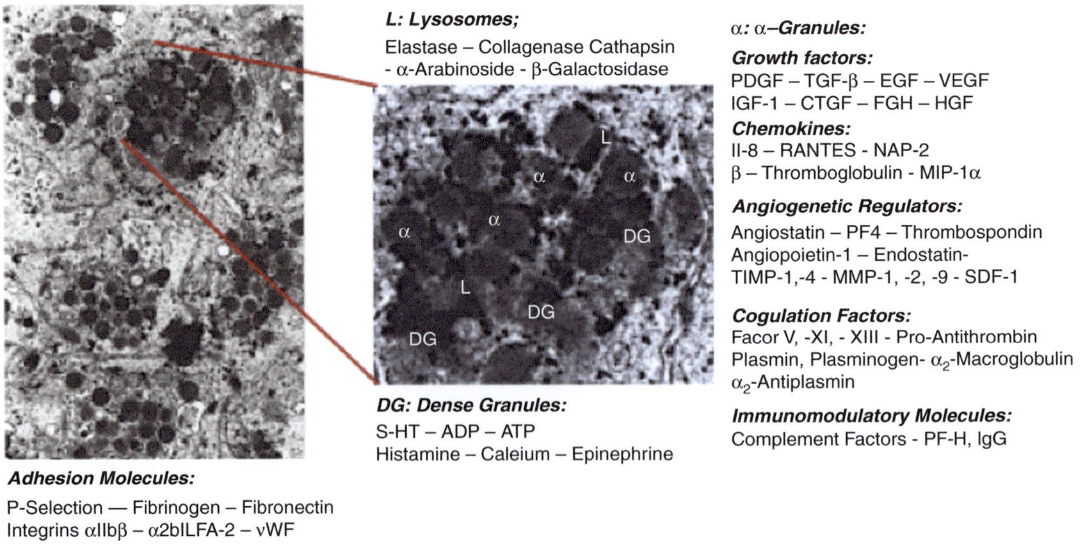

Fig. 12.4 Electron microscopic picture of a cluster of platelets after a PRP preparation showing the various intraplatelet structures form volunteer (PE), at magnification ×10,000. The three platelet cellular constituents are clearly visible: of α-granules, dense granules (DG), and lysosomes (L), including some platelet surface adhesion molecules. (Adapted and modified from Everts et al. [26])

other platelet concentrates stem from the release of a multitude of factors involved in tissue repair and regeneration. Following platelet activation, the formed platelet plug acts as a temporary extracellular matrix, allowing cells to proliferate and differentiate [1]. Therefore, it is fair to assume that higher platelet dosages will generate an elevated local concentration of released platelet bioactive factors. However, the correlation between platelet dose, concentration, and the concentration of released platelet bioactive growth factors and agents may not be precise because there are marked differences in baseline platelet counts between individual patients [42], and differences exist between PRP preparation methods [4, 43]. Likewise, several platelet growth factors involved in tissue repair mechanisms reside in the plasma fraction of PRP (e.g., hepatic growth factor and insulin-like growth factor 1). In research, study results are quickly obtained because the different parameters can be precisely controlled. Several in vitro PRP studies have demonstrated that cells respond to PRP in a dose-dependent manner. Nguyen and Pham [44] showed that very high concentrations of PGF are not necessarily advantageous for cell stimulatory processes and may be counterproductive. Some in vitro studies have indicated that high PGF concentrations may have detrimental effects [45]. One reason could be that the quantity of cell membrane receptors is limited. Thus, once the PGF levels are too high compared to the available receptors, they negatively affect cell function [46]. Although in vitro studies have many advantages, they also have some weaknesses.

12.12.3 Why Are Nonconsistent Outcomes Following PRP Applications Reported?

Unfortunately, a large variability in clinical outcomes has been reported following PRP applications in general, and these nonconsistent outcomes have led to confusion among practitioners [47, 48]. It has been suggested that this is due to significant variances in PRP preparation protocols and thus platelet properties [2, 49, 50]. The effectiveness of PRP injections is determined by which type of PRP is being used: plasma-type PRP or buffy coat PRP. Commercially available whole blood PRP systems are designed for the preparation of PRP; however, they produce major differences in cellular composition [51]. A buffy coat PRP product can enhance cell proliferation and differentiation, cell migration, and ECM buildup, producing a concentration of platelets meeting the definition outlined by Marx of >1 million cells/μL [1]. "PRP-like" products (single spin test-tube-based PRP devices) have a low to no platelet concentration in the final injectable product and consist mainly of plasma [5, 52]. These devices will demonstrate a less significant to no effect when compared to a buffy coat (double spin) PRP products, which are rich in platelets and specific leukocytes, capable of tissue repair such as monocytes [26]. Platelet-rich plasma preparations for nonsurgical esthetic procedures should be characterized as a small volume of plasma, with a substantial concentration of platelets (>1 million platelets/μL), with options for specific leukocytes, with minimal red blood cell contamination, since skin rejuvenation and tissue repair result from cell proliferation, angiogenesis, and cell migration aimed at remodeling the ECM [38]. Furthermore, several PRP technology systems are often based on antiquated devices and preparation protocols, using outdated science, as they were initially mainly used in surgical procedures and not in nonsurgical interventions. The intended use of surgically employed PRP devices was introduced as a regenerative supportive tool to stimulate surgical outcomes like bone growth, optimize surgical wound healing, and chronic wounds. The PRP characteristics of these outdated devices do not meet the current bioformulation criteria for interventional procedures and they have a too simplified view on the true regenerative capacities of all the constituents that can be present in PRP products.

12.12.4 Variations in PRP Preparation

Many papers have addressed the differences in PRP preparations protocols, producing different bio-formulations [39, 53]. In general, PRP device comparison studies should not support decision making, as they indicate a large variation in platelet concentrations among the large variety of available PRP devices [25]. Fadadu et al. demonstrated that there are substantial differences in commercially available PRP devices regarding bioformulations and PRP platelet concentration and therefore platelet dosing potential [5]. In their study, 33 PRP systems and protocols were evaluated. Some of these systems produced final PRP preparations with a PRP platelet factor increase as low as 0.52 (less than that of whole blood) with a single spin kit [54]. In contrast, the dual-spin device produced the highest platelet concentration (1.6 × 10^6/μL) [5]. Their study clearly suggested that PRP platelet concentrations positively correlate with an increased whole blood collection volume and centrifugal separation protocols. Magalon et al. performed and extensive technical and biological review of medical PRP producing devices [55]. Their review led to the documentation of 50 different PRP devices. The blood harvesting volume determined classification of the devices, and this was one of the most variable parameters as it varied between 6 and 180 mL. Interestingly, only 14 of these 50 devices have been sufficiently characterized in the literature to be classified in all variations of PRP classification (Table 12.3). The variance among PRP devices regarding the potential for platelet dosing ranged from 300 million to more than 12 billion platelets. It is without saying that the impact of such differences among PRP characteristics and the subsequent effects in tissue rejuvenation and tissue repair is meaningful in affecting patient outcomes.

Table 12.3 Description of PRP and Sub-PRP Classifications

Type of PRP	Components
Platelet-Rich Plasma (PRP)	Rich in platelets
	Leukocyte presence
	Normal plasma proteins ratio
Pure-PRP (P-PRP)	Rich in platelets
	No leukocytes
	Normal plasma protein ratio
Leukocyte-Rich PRP (LR-PRP)	Rich in platelets
	Rich in leukocytes, incl. neutrophils
	Normal plasma protein ratio
Leukocyte-Poor PRP (LP-PRP)	Rich in platelets
	Minimal leukocyte presence
Platelet-Rich Fibrin (PRF)	Poor in platelets
	No leukocyte presence
	Normal plasma protein ratio
Platelet-Rich Fibrin Matrix (PRFM)	Poor in platelets
	No leukocyte presence
	Normal plasma protein ratio
	Activated product

12.12.5 What PRP Platelet Concentrations Are Warranted?

It is important to understand the minimally required platelet concentration needed to induce an angiogenic response, stimulate cell proliferation, and cell migration. Currently, PRP is characterized by its absolute platelet concentration, thereby shifting from the initial definition of PRP consisting of a platelet concentration above baseline values [1] to a minimum platelet concentration of more than 1 × 10^6/μL or an approximately fivefold increase in platelets from baseline [56]. "Clinical PRP" should contain a critical dose of concentrated platelets to produce beneficial therapeutic effects. The platelets in clinical PRP should stimulate cell proliferation, synthesis of mesenchymal and neurotrophic factors, contribute to chemotactic cell migration, and stimulate immunomodulatory activities [57, 58]. Marx was the first to demonstrate the enhancement of bone and soft tissue healing with a minimum platelet count of $1 \times 10^6/\mu L$ [1]. These results were confirmed in a transforaminal lumbar fusion study that demonstrated significantly more fusion when the platelet dose was greater than 1.3×10^6 platelets/μL [59]. Moreover, Giusti et al. [60] revealed that a dose of 1.5×10^9 platelets/mL is needed for tissue repair mechanisms to induce a functional angiogenic response through endothelial cell activity. In Giusti's study, higher concentrations reduced the angiogenic potential of platelets in follicular and perifollicular angiogenesis. Furthermore, earlier data indicate that the PRP dose also affects the magnitude of the therapy outcome [61]. Therefore, to significantly induce an angiogenic response and stimulate cell proliferation and cell migration, clinical PRP should contain at least 7.5×10^9 deliverable platelets in a 5-mL PRP treatment vial.

12.12.6 Is There a Role for Leukocytes in PRP Preparations?

Leukocytes greatly influence the intrinsic biology of acute and chronic tissue conditions because of their immune and host-defense mechanisms. The presence of specific leukocytes in PRP preparations can cause significant cellular and tissue effects. More specifically, different PRP two-spin and buffy coat systems utilize different preparation protocols, thereby producing different concentrated neutrophil, lymphocyte, and monocyte cell counts with different cellular ratios [51, 62] Eosinophils and basophils do not withstand the centrifugal processing forces as their cell membranes are too fragile and will rupture, losing their integrity. Notably, the "PRP" of the so-called plasma/test tube-based single-spin devices do not contain any leukocytes. Further research is needed to develop a consensus regarding the role and magnitude of leukocytes in PRP bioformulations to treat certain pathologies and conditions adequately and safely.

12.13 Neutrophils

Neutrophils are essential leukocytes in numerous healing pathways that create dense barriers against invading pathogens [63] in conjunction with antimicrobial proteins present in platelets [64]. Neutrophils play an important role in the inflammatory process preceding tissue regeneration due to their release of both pro and anti-inflammatory molecules. Lana et al. found that the combination of neutrophils and activated platelets could have a more positive than detrimental effect during tissue repair in joint applications [65].

The presence of neutrophils in PRP preparations is mostly based on the treatment objectives. Exacerbated tissue inflammatory levels can be necessary in chronic wound care PRP biological treatments [14], or applications directed toward bone growth or healing [66]. The use of a full buffy coat PRP treatment vial is also frequently mentioned in chronic tendinopathy treatments [67, 68]. Importantly, additional neutrophil functions have been uncovered in several models, emphasizing their roles in angiogenesis and tissue restoration [69]. However, neutrophils can also cause harmful effects and, thus, are not indicated for some applications. Zhou and Wang demonstrated that the use of PRP rich in neutrophils could result in a higher collagen type III to collagen type I ratio, adding to fibrosis and decreased tendon strength [70]. Other neutrophil-mediated deleterious properties are the release of inflammatory cytokines and metalloproteinases (MMPs) that promote proinflammatory and catabolic effects when applied to tissues [71]. In nonsurgical esthetic procedures, the inclusion of leukocytes in PRP has been avoided [2, 36, 72].

12.14 Lymphocytes

In the buffy coat of PRP preparations, mononuclear T and B lymphocytes are more concentrated than any other leukocytes. They are critically involved in cell-mediated cytotoxic adaptive immunity. Lymphocytes can elicit a cell response to fight infection and adapt to intruders [73]. Furthermore, T lymphocyte-derived cytokines (interferon-γ [IFN-γ] and interleukin-4 [IL-4]) strengthen macrophage polarization [74]. Weirather et al. demonstrated that regular T lymphocytes indirectly contribute to tissue healing in a mouse model by modulating monocyte and macrophage differentiation [75].

12.15 Monocytes and Macrophages

Depending on the PRP preparation devices used, monocytes may be prominent or absent in prepared PRP. Unfortunately, their manifestation and regenerative capabilities are rarely discussed in the literature. Therefore, little attention is given to monocytes in preparation methods or final formulations. In the orthobiological literature, leukocyte differentiation is rarely addressed and the reporting of PRP preparation protocols has been highly inconsistent. Furthermore, most published studies do not present the PRP preparation methods needed for protocol reproducibility, even though PRP biological preparations containing specific leukocytes can significantly contribute to proinflammation, immune modulation, tissue repair, and regeneration. While monocytes and macrophages play key roles in immunomodulatory processes and tissue repair mechanisms [76].

Monocyte populations are heterogeneous and originate from progenitor cells in the bone marrow via hematopoietic stem cell pathways and traffic via the bloodstream to peripheral tissues depending on the microenvironmental stimuli. During homeostasis and inflammation, circulating monocytes leave the bloodstream and are recruited to injured or degenerated tissues. They can act either as effector cells or progenitors of macrophages (MΦs). Monocytes, macrophages, and dendritic cells represent the mononuclear phagocyte system (MPS) [77]. A typical feature of the MPS is the plasticity in their gene expression patterns and functional overlap between these cell types. In degenerated tissues, resident macrophages, local-acting growth factors, proinflammatory cytokines, apoptotic or necrotic cells, and microbial products initiate the differentiation of monocytes into MPS cell populations [78]. During the monocyte-to-MΦ transition, particular MΦ phenotypes are produced [76]. MΦ phenotype 1 (MΦ1) is characterized by inflammatory cytokine secretion and the production of both VEGF and FGF. The MΦ2 phenotype consists of anti-inflammatory cells, producing mainly extracellular matrix components and angiogenic factors [79]. From these data, it is reasonable to assume that C-PRP preparations containing a high concentration of monocytes and MΦs are likely to contribute to better tissue repair because of their anti-inflammatory tissue repair and cell signaling capabilities. Gupta et al. indicated in a hair restoration review that PRP should be rich in monocytes [36]. The importance of monocytes in PRP for facial rejuvenation was recently for the first time accurately investigated by Mercuri and associates [80].

12.16 Red Blood Cells

The role of RBCs in tissue regeneration has never been established. RBCs are responsible for transporting oxygen to tissues and removing carbon dioxide from tissues to the lungs [81]. They have no nucleus and are made of protein-bound heme molecules. Iron and heme components inside RBCs facilitate the binding of oxygen and carbon dioxide. Normally, the RBC life cycle is approximately 120 days. They are removed from circulation by macrophages by a process termed RBC senescence. Under conditions of shear forces (e.g., whole blood phlebotomy procedures, immune-mediated processes, oxidative stress, or inadequate PRP concentration protocols), RBCs in the PRP specimens could become damaged. As a consequence, the RBC cell membrane disintegrates and releases toxic hemoglobin (Hb), measured as plasma-free hemoglobin (PFH), hemin, and iron [82]. PFH and its degradation products (heme and iron) collectively lead to detrimental and cytotoxic effects to tissues, causing oxidative stress, loss of nitric oxide, activation of inflammatory pathways, and immunosuppression. These effects ultimately lead to microcirculatory dysfunction, local vasoconstriction with vascular damage, and significant tissue injury.

Most importantly, when PRP-containing RBCs is delivered to tissues, it causes a local response called eryptosis, which triggers the release of a potent cytokine, macrophage migration inhibitory factor [79]. This cytokine inhibits the migration of monocytes and macrophages. It exerts profound proinflammatory signals to surrounding tissues that inhibit the migration of stem cells and fibroblast proliferation and causes significant local cellular dysfunction. Based on the above explanation, limiting RBC contamination in PRP preparations is important.

12.17 Immunomodulatory Effects Following PRP Injections

The body can identify foreign bodies and injured tissues in acute or chronic conditions to initiate the wound-healing cascade and related inflammatory pathways. The innate and adaptive immune systems protect the host from infection, with essential roles for leukocytes overlapping between both systems, as displayed in Fig. 12.4. Specifically, monocytes, macrophages, neutrophils, and natural killer cells have pivotal roles in the innate system, whereas lymphocytes and their subsets play similar roles in the adaptive immune system [83].

12.18 Innate Immune System

The role of the innate immune system is to identify intruding microbes or tissue fragments and stimulate their clearance. Activation of the innate immune system occurs when certain molecular structures, termed surfaceexpressed pattern recognition receptors, bind to pathogen-associated molecular patterns and damage-associated molecular patterns. Interestingly, platelets also express several immunomodulatory receptor molecules on their surface, such as P-selectin, transmembrane protein CD40 ligand (CD40L), cytokines (e.g., IL-1β), and platelet-specific toll-like receptors (TLR), enabling them to interact with various immune cells [84]. Neutrophils, monocytes, and dendritic cells are the most common innate immune cells in the blood. Their recruitment is required for an adequate early-phase immune response. Platelet–leukocyte interactions regulate inflammation, wound healing, and tissue repair when PRP is used in regenerative medicine applications. More specifically, the platelet TLRs stimulate platelet–neutrophil interactions [85], which regulate the so-called leukocyte oxidative burst by modulating the release of reactive oxygen species (ROS) and myeloperoxidase (MPO) from neutrophils [86]. Furthermore, the platelet–neutrophil interaction with neutrophil degranulation results in the formation of neutrophil-extracellular traps (NETs). NETs comprises of the neutrophil nucleus and other neutrophil intracellular contents that trap bacteria and kill them by NETosis. The formation of NETs is an essential killing mechanism for neutrophils [87]. As a result of PRP platelet activation, monocytes can migrate to diseased and degenerative tissues where they perform adhesion activities while secreting inflammatory molecules that may alter chemotaxis and modify proteolytic properties [88]. Additionally, platelets can modulate the effector functions of monocytes by inducing the activation of monocyte NF-κb [89], a critical mediator of the inflammatory response and the activation and differentiation of immune cells.

Therefore, PRP preparation devices that can yield high concentrations of monocytes from whole blood have the advantage of this mechanism in tissue repair processes after application.

12.19 Adaptive Immune System

The adaptive immune system employs antigen-specific receptors and remembers previous pathogen encounters and destroys these pathogens during subsequent encounters with the host. However, these adaptive immune responses are slow to develop. Cognasse et al. [84] showed that platelet components contribute to danger sensing and tissue repair and suggested that the interaction of platelets with leukocytes facilitates the activation of the adaptive immune response.

During adaptive immune responses, platelets promote monocyte and macrophage responses. Thus, platelet granular constituents directly affect adaptive immunity by expressing CD40L [90], a molecule critical to the modulation of adaptive immune responses, as they promote T cell responses to inflammatory stimuli for robust pro and anti-inflammatory responses [91]. Moreover, platelets have an abundance of cell surface receptors that can prompt platelet activation, with the release of numerous inflammatory and bioactive molecules stored within different platelet granules, thus influencing both innate and adaptive immune responses [92].

12.20 Angiogenetic Effects Related to PRP Preparations

Ideally, the PRP preparations employed in non-surgical regenerative esthetic therapies allow for the delivery of biomolecules released by a high concentration of platelets, which are ultimately (passively) activated at the target tissue site. As a result, countless physiological cascades are initiated, resulting in on-site immunomodulatory and inflammatory processes, and angiogenesis stimulating healing and tissue repair activities [93]. Neo angiogenesis is a vibrant, multistep process involving the sprouting and organization of microvessels from preexisting blood vessels. Angiogenesis progresses due to multiple biological mechanisms, including endothelial cell migration, proliferation, differentiation, and division. These cellular processes are prerequisites to the formation of new blood vessels. They are essential for the outgrowth of preexisting blood vessels to restore blood flow and support the high metabolic activity of tissue repair and tissue regeneration. These new vessels allow the delivery of oxygen and nutrients and the removal of by-products from the treated tissues [94].

Within a degenerative microenvironment (including a low oxygen tension, low pH, and high lactate levels), local angiogenic factors try to restore angiogenic activities. It has been demonstrated that the overall PRP platelets effects on (neo) angiogenesis are pro-angiogenic and stimulatory [95]. Notably, Landsdown and Fortier [96] reported on the various outcome effects related to the PRP constituents, including intraplatelet sources of numerous angiogenic modulators.

The administration of PRP, more specifically the delivery of high concentrations of PGFs and other platelet cytokines, can induce angiogenesis, vasculogenesis, and arteriogenesis because stromal cell-derived factor-1a binds to the specific cytokine receptors on endothelial progenitor cells. Another important and essential factor in restoring angiogenic pathways is synergy between multiple PGFs. Richardson et al. [97] demonstrated that the synergistic activities of the angiogenic factors platelet-derived growth factor-bb (PDGF-BB) and VEGF results in the rapid formation of a mature vascular network compared to the individual growth factor activities. Most importantly, Giusti and co-workers concluded in a dose-defining study that the optimal platelet dose to promote angiogenesis was 1.5×10^6 platelets/μL [63]. Therefore, it is fair to assume that PRP preparations with high concentrations of platelets contain high concentrations of the stimulatory proangiogenic PGF VEGF, contributing to significant angiogenetic effects, when compared to PRP preparations with less than 1.5×10^6 platelets/μL. In facial regenerative rejuvenation procedures, PRP contributed to the proliferation of stem cells and promoted repair through neoangiogenesis and collagen production stimulatory processes [98].

In a review from Cervantes et al., PRP was a significant contributor in promoting neo angiogenesis in patients with androgenetic alopecia (AA) [99]. Investigators observed a significant increase in small blood vessel count around the hair follicles after PRP treatment compared with control-treated patients, supporting the notion that PRP promotes angiogenesis via the release of vascular growth factors, increasing the perifollicular vascular plexus through the increase of VEGF and PDGF levels [43].

12.21 The Use of Ultrasound Imaging (US) in Facial Esthetic Procedures

Several studies have used a variety of techniques to examine characteristic signs of photoaging in the epidermis and dermis, utilizing ultrasound imaging (US), histologic examination, and optical coherence tomography [11]. More recently, the US has been portrayed to guide facial injection procedures to avoid complications and precision delivery.

12.22 US to Objectively Measure PRP Effects on SLEB Evolution

US has been employed in facial esthetic procedures, following PRP injections to measure the cutaneous regenerative effects in dermal thickness [100]. In this study, a lineal 18 MHz probe was used, and US revealed that a single PRP dose induced the augmentation of soft tissue and promoted skin surface remodeling in terms of an increase in dermal thickness increase. We used a modified 20-MHz probe to measure thickness and density of the subepidermal low echogenic band (SLEB), with calculations of subcutaneous fat thickness, defined as the number of pixels/mm^2 [2]. In normal aging, this band between the epidermis and dermis becomes larger and less dense. Measuring the SLEB may be a sensitive marker for age-dependent photoaging (Fig. 12.5). US was used as an objective measuring tech-

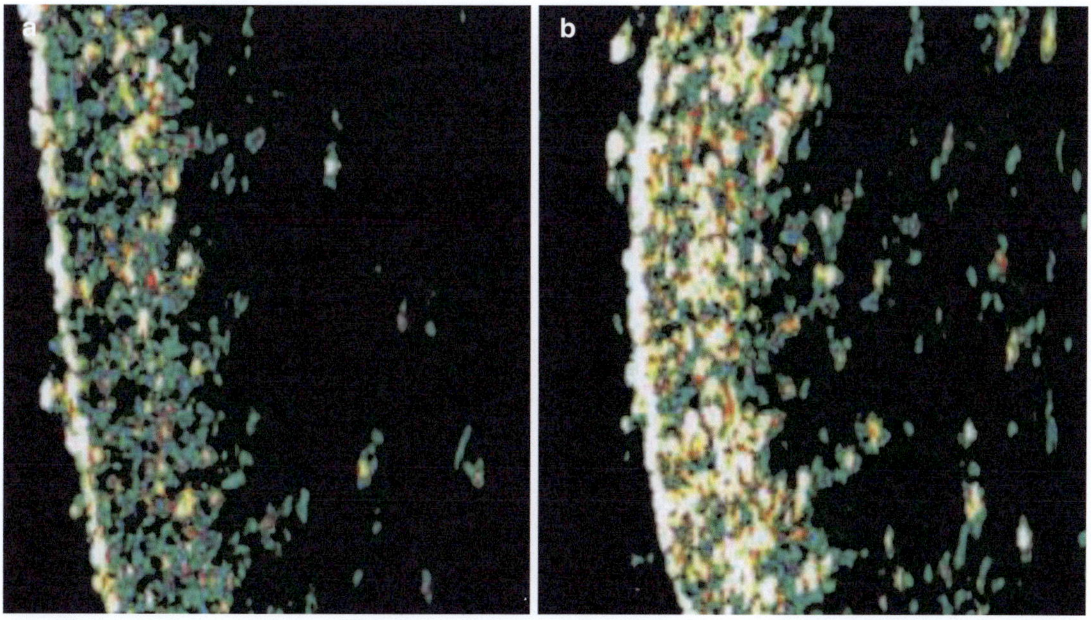

Fig. 12.5 Skin morphology effect was evaluated by ultrasonography parameters, using a 20-MHz probe to measure thickness and density of the subepidermal low echogenic band (SLEB). In (**a**), the skin morphology before PRP injection is shown. In (**b**), the same patient and an image of the same region is showing a dramatic decrease in thickness (23%, $p < 0.05$) with an increase in density (24%, $p < 0.001$), after a second PurePRP® injection

nique, and it revealed an increased density in SLEB and decrease in SLEB size, at 2- and 6-months post PRP treatment.

12.23 US for Precision-Guided PRP Delivery to Avoid Complications

Most cosmetic treatment procedures are performed safely. However, complications following nonautologous filler injections have been reported. Causative reasons were too strong cross-linking of the filler product and filler–host interactions. Furthermore, injection technique-related complications have been reported, with the accumulation or dislocation of the product due to muscle movement, intravascular injection, or vascular compression of filler material [101]. Potentially, this can lead to skin necrosis or, in rare cases, blindness [102]. Unfortunately, it has been suggested that the minor signs of vascular compression may be misapprehended as injection-related pain, swelling, and bruising [103].

US imaging has been used as a valuable tool in nonsurgical orthobiological therapies for many years to improve the safety of these procedures as the amount, location, and depth of the injected biological preparation can be identified. Recently, US-guided precision injections have been proposed for the delivery of intralesional hyaluronic acid. Vascular and nerve structures in the proposed treatment areas can be easily visualized by US mapping techniques (Fig. 12.6a–c), contributing to the prevention of complications, as blood vessels are not visible clinically [104]. Anatomical mapping of the face blood vessels and nerve structures is crucial, as individual variations in facial blood vessel anatomy have been described [105]. Noninvasive US allows for the visualization of facial arteries, veins, and nerves of the treatment sites.

12.24 PRP Employment in Esthetic Nonsurgical Procedures

PRP preparations have gained increasing popularity with widespread use in diverse medical fields and is as complex as blood itself and likely more complex than traditional pharmaceutical drugs. The underlying rationale for PRP therapy is that the application of concentrated platelets at tissue sites may initiate tissue repair via the release of many biologically active growth factors, cytokines, lysosomes, and adhesion proteins that are responsible for initiating the hemostatic cascade, synthesis of new connective tissue, and revascularization. PRP preparations are living biomaterials, and the outcomes of clinical PRP applications are dependent on the intrinsic, versatile, and adaptive characteristics of the patient's blood, including specific cell constituents that may be more present in PRP specimen [39]. Another important element that might affect treatment outcomes is the interaction of PRP constituents with the recipient local microenvironment. PRP concentrates can stimulate the supraphysiological release of growth factors to

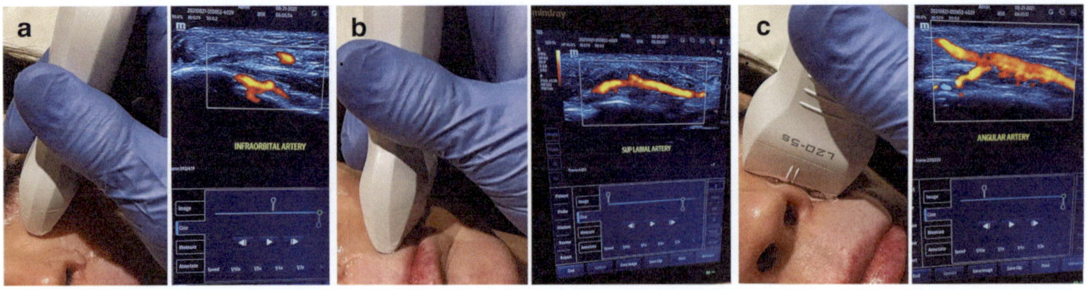

Fig. 12.6 (a–c) US can be used for precision-guided facial autologous biological injections locating critical arteries, veins, and nerves using duplex sonography

Table 12.4 Variances in PRP commercial products and specimen differences

	Angel®	GPSIII®	PurePRP-A®	Classic PRF	Regenkit®-A-PRP
PLT increase from BL	4.8	4.2	6.6	1.9	0.7
Platelets (×10⁶/mL)	856	754	1175	338	125
WBC (×10⁶/mL)	7.1	19.8	10.7	0.1	0.3
Monocyte %	33	15	72	0	0
RBC (×10⁹/mL)/HCT	0.3/2.8	1.1/8.1	0.1/1.1	0/0	0/0
PRP volume (mL)	3	6	7	2	5
T.D. PLTs (×10³/μL)	2568	4524	8225	677	623

Same donor laboratory study (N = 12, only male donors), with average baseline platelet count of 178 × 10^6/mL, unpublished data

PLT: platelet; BL: baseline; WBC: white blood cell; RBC: red blood cell; PRP: platelet-rich plasma; T.D. PLT: total deliverable platelets (platelet dose). Angel®: Arthrex, Naples FL, USA; GPS III®: Zimmer Biomet, Warsaw IN, USA; PurePRP®: EmCyte Corporation, Fort Myers FL, USA; Regenkit®-A-PRP: Mont-sur-Lausanne, Switzerland

jump-start healing in chronic degenerated and dormant tissues and accelerate repair processes [27, 106]. At all stages of the tissue repair process, a wide variety of growth factors, cytokines, and locally acting regulators contribute to most basic cell functions via endocrine, paracrine, autocrine, and intracrine mechanisms, as shown in Table 12.2.

The main advantages of most currently commercially PRP devices include its safety and their effective biological preparation techniques [107]. Most importantly, PRP is an autologous product with no known adverse effects, in contrast to the commonly used dermal fillers and other nonautologous biological products [108–110]. The enthusiasm to use PRP is often overshadowed as there are no clear regulations regarding the bioformulation and composition of an injectable PRP composition and PRP compositions vary greatly regarding cellular content and PGF concentrations [53, 111]. Furthermore, the vital roles of other cellular constituents present in these blood-derived products are partially understood, which was further aggravated by a lack of scientific data, mystical belief, commercial interests, and lack of standardization and classification [25]. In Table 12.4, an overview of the differences between some commercially available PRP and "PRP-like" devices is displayed, regarding platelet, leukocyte cell (WBC) content, RBC contamination, preparation volumes, and platelet dosing capabilities.

12.25 Facial Rejuvenation Procedures

Intradermal and/or subdermal autologous PRP injections for the treatment of photoaging skin, wrinkles, acne scars, and periorbital hyperpigmentation have gained popularity. Maisel-Campbell et al. conducted a review to systematically assess the evidence regarding the safety and effectiveness of PRP for reducing the visible signs of aging [112]. A literature search was performed including prospective trials and case series, assessing PRP for skin aging studies with ten or more patients. Twenty-four studies, representing 480 patients treated with PRP, were included. Sixteen studies mentioned mild and transient adverse events, with no reports of infection, scarring, or post-inflammatory hyperpigmentation. Post-injection pain, burning sensation, and erythema were reported in most of these mild events. If bruising/ecchymosis at injection sites was noted, it was resolved within 2 weeks. No serious adverse events were noted in their review. Although the reported degree of skin improvements was less than 50%, patients generally reported high satisfaction rates. The authors concluded that the results in outcomes were limited by the heterogeneity in PRP preparation and application techniques and lack of standardization in outcome measures. In a recent systematic review and meta-analysis by Evans et al., the rejuvenation potential of PRP in periorbital pathologies was analyzed [11]. PRP treatment of periorbital area pathologies resulted in histologic improvements of photoaging with increased subjective satisfaction scores and blind evaluator assessments of rejuvenated skin appearance.

12.26 Hair Restoration

In a recent systematic review from Roohaninasab et al., reviewing 564 articles, the efficacy and safety of PRP injections were evaluated in patients with various forms of alopecia [113]. In 62.5% of treated patients, an increase in hair growth, and thickness of hair was reported. Interestingly, the simultaneous use of PRP and Minoxidil demonstrated the highest rate of improvement and satisfaction. In patients suffering from alopecia errata (AE), PRP efficacy was higher (76%) compared to patients treated for AA show high efficacy of 42.75%. The main reported side effect was pain following PRP injection. The authors concluded that PRP applications had a relatively high efficiency, with low and tolerable side effects, combined with a low recurrence rate. Furthermore, they recommend optimization of dosing, injection techniques, and the number of sessions and intervals between sessions should be subject to further studies. Mercuri et al. performed a systematic review exclusively on female androgenetic alopecia (FAGA), affecting approximately 40% of women by the age 50. Eight ($n = 8$) clinical studies were identified with a total of 197 enrolled female subjects with a mean age of 38.9 years. In their review, patients well tolerated the PRP procedure, producing high levels of patient satisfaction with an improvement in the quality of life in patients affected by FAGA [80].

12.27 Basics of Adipose Tissue Concentrate (ATC) Preparation

Aside from PRP and BMC preparations, adipose tissue (AT) has been used as a cell-based therapy in orthobiological and regenerative medicine procedures to create an adipose tissue concentrate (ATC), harvested, and prepared at point-of-care in an office setting. Autologous AT is a heterogeneous biological source of various cellular tissue components. Furthermore, concentrated adipose tissue provides clinicians with a physiological 3D multicellular scaffold, including adipose stem cells (ASCs) and stromal cells. Both autologous or allogeneic ATC have been employed in clinical trials to treat conditions such as lipoatrophy, muscular dystrophy, myocardial infarction, stroke, and spinal cord injury [114]. ATCs have demonstrated to be effective in the treatment of plastic reconstructive surgical procedures, nonsurgical cosmetic interventions, and other regenerative applications, comparable to MSCs originating from BMCs. Like other MSCs, ASCs can differentiate into cells of mesodermal (osteoblasts, adipocytes, and chondrocytes), endodermal (hepatocytes, pancreatic cells), and ectodermal (neurons) primary layers [115].

12.28 Adipose Tissue Structure

Adipose tissue is a highly vascularized connective tissue, abundantly present throughout the human body. White AT (WAT) is responsible for energy storage and plays a pivotal physiological role in maintaining metabolic homeostasis in the body by releasing release of several adipocytokines, growth factors, and cytokines that may act in an endocrine or paracrine fashion [116]. Brown AT (BAT) plays a significant role in thermogenesis via the actions of uncoupling protein 1. BAT cells present the ability to disperse energy by producing heat to ensure body temperature regulation, rather than storing it as triglycerides [117].

12.29 Adipose Tissue as a Source of Stem Cells

In 2002, Zuk et al. performed the first characterization of adult stem cells, isolated from lipoaspirates, demonstrating that ASC derived from WAT lipoaspirate exhibits MSC properties, like plastic-adherent, multipotency, and differential capacity [118–120]. AT MSCs have a high proliferation capacity and multilineage cell differentiation potential, capable of differentiating into adipogenic, chondrogenic, myogenic, osteogenic, and neurogenic cells [121]. These AT-specific characteristics are combined with an abundance of MSCs when compared to MSCs derived from bone marrow [122, 123]. Therefore, AT preparations prepared from WAT have great potential in clinical orthobiological tissue repair applications [124, 125]. Furthermore, Yun et al. described the AT MSC-mediated effects on the reduction of proinflammatory cytokines, chemokines, cellular apoptosis, and collagenases [126]. Moreover, AD-MSCs have been shown to be immune-privileged [127].

During the last decade, AT has been one of the most studied tissues in the last decade [128–130] and increasingly popular among practitioners as they value the high MSC content in ATC and they consider harvesting of subcutaneous WAT beneath the skin as a relatively easy procedure. Consequently, physicians might consider that MSCs from ATC have distinct advantages over "conventional" BMC preparations for orthobiological applications.

12.30 Describing Stromal Vascular Fraction (SVF)

The use of AT in regenerative medicine is based on the separation of the vascular stroma contained in ATC, allowing for access to AD-MSCs [131, 132]. The isolation of AD-MSCs from WAT involves the separation of adipocytes from the remaining adipose cells of the SVF. SVF is a heterogeneous collection of cells contained within adipose tissue and can be isolated from fat using different disruption techniques, enzymatic digestion, or mechanical emulsification (ME). Various preparation techniques, including centrifugation (density gradient layer separation), exist to prepare a viable biological specimen to initiate SVF production. Centrifugation techniques have proven to be an effective means to safely wash, rinse, eliminate the infranatant-extracellular fluid, separate free lipids, and residual oil, to prepare concentrated adipose tissue. In Fig. 12.7, the final processed adipose tissue is shown.

AD-MSCs and SVF cells, both contained in the SVF, meet the four criteria for MSCs as defined by the International Society for Cellular Therapies (ISCT) [133]. The presence of these cells can be measured by laboratory techniques, including flow cytometry techniques, as each cell has their own unique cell surface marker [134]. In Table 12.5, the heterogenous SVF cellular distribution is shown.

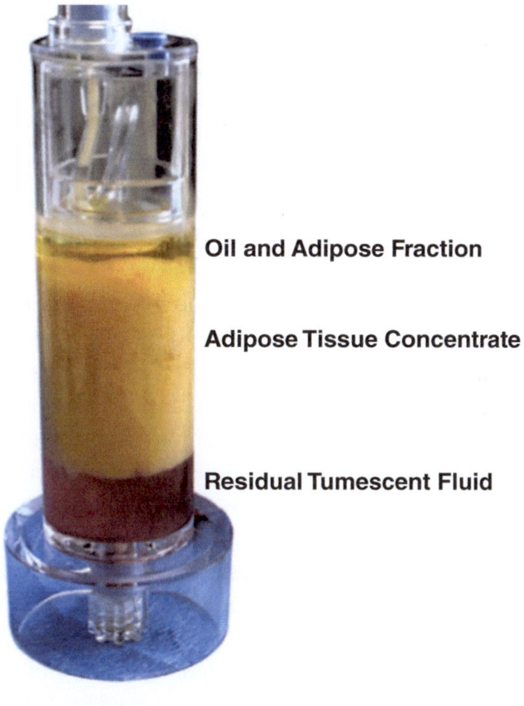

Fig. 12.7 Centrifuged density separation of adipose tissue, showing on top the adipose oil and adipose fraction. The middle layer is the ATC, and at the bottom of the concentration device (Progenikine® Adipose Concentration System, EmCyte Corporation, Fort Myers FL USA, with permission) is the residual tumescent fluid. In the syringe, the collected ATC after, first, removal of the oil from the top and then the infranatant fluid from the bottom

Table 12.5 SVF cellular distribution

15–30% Stromal cells:
AD-MSCs
Preadipocytes
Fibroblasts
35–45% Hematopoietic-lineage cells:
Erythrocytes
Platelets
Neutrophils
Lymphocytes
Monocytes/macrophages
1–15% Hematopoietic stem and endothelial progenitor cells
3–5% Pericytes
10–20% Endothelial cells
5–15% Smooth muscle cells

AD-MSCs adipose mesenchymal stem cells

12.31 Enzymatic Digestion Versus Mechanical Emulsification

Enzymatic digestion techniques use enzymes (collagenase) to isolate stromal and MSCs from adipose tissue by digesting the peptide bonds in the collagen of WAT with the destruction of extracellular structures. Centrifugation techniques are employed to separate the floating adipocytes from the pelleted SVF, following good manufacturing practices regarding closed, sterile, and safe isolation processes [135]. In these preparation protocols, a combination of enzymatic digestion and incubation/agitation has been identified, producing an adipose-derived cellular SVF (AD-cSVF).

Freshly isolated SVF can be directly applied, without the need for further cell separation or in vitro expansion. AT-MSCs constitute as much as 1% of SVF cells compared with the 0.001–0.002% of BM-MSCs in bone marrow [136] Furthermore, detrimental erythrocytes are usually removed using a lysis buffer with a standard enzymatic processing protocol, compared with a BMC product, which contains a significant number of erythrocytes [135]. In current FDA guidelines, enzymatic cellular prepared SVF products fall into the "more than manipulated" category and require specific clinical trials to examine and report the long-term safety and efficacy of such products in human clinical uses. Another method to produce SVF refers to the definition of adipose-derived tissue SVF (AD-tSVF). This method signifies to the adipose stromal cell population within a bioactive scaffold, or extra cellular matrix tissue, as described by Alexander [137]. AT, acquired via lipo-aspiration techniques, can be concentrated to an ATC by centrifugation and is thereafter subject to mechanical disruption by a process termed mechanical emulsification (ME). Hereafter, the final product is often termed micro fat or nano fat, since it is composed of both cellular and native structural fragments [138, 139]. Therefore, emulsified AD-tSVF does not produce a 100% concentrated cellular product, when compared to AD-cSVF (Fig. 12.8). Ultimately, after ME of ATC, the final AD-tSVF treatment specimen is injected into (degenerated) tissue structures enabling the AD-MSCs to repair damaged and diseased tissues. An advantage of this ME method is that the prepared AD-tSVF offers the ability to provide a bioactive cellular tissue matrix after tissue application. Additionally, anti-inflammatory or immunosuppressive factors are secreted, capable of exerting immunomodulatory effects [140]. Noteworthy, AD-tSVF preparations and their subsequent applications are approved by the FDA.

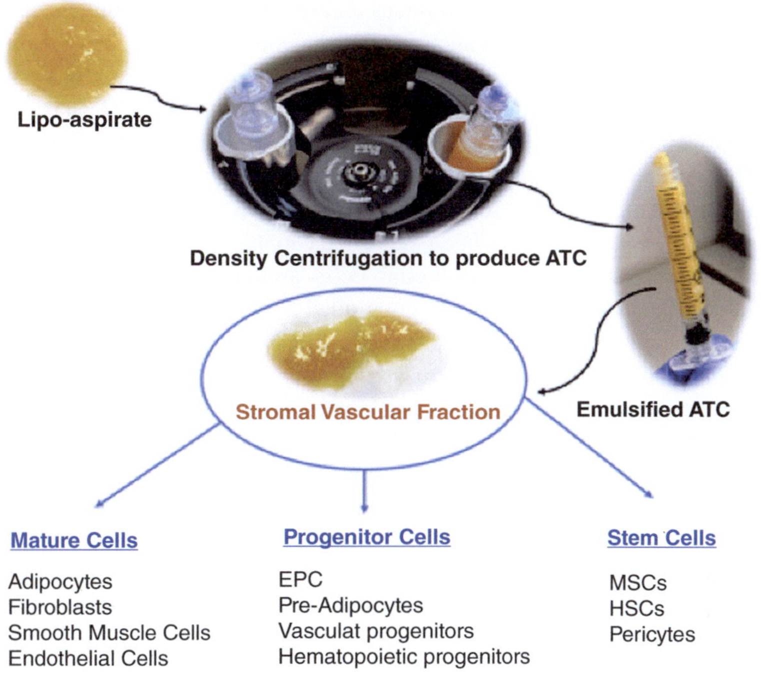

Fig. 12.8 Cellular SVF preparation method. Adipose tissue is harvested following lipo-aspiration and subsequently processed in a centrifuge for density cellular layering. After Centrifugation, the ATC can be ME before application as an orthobiological preparation. After EM, SVF cellular components will be liberated from the concentrated AT. This heterogenous mixture is grouped in mature, progenitor, and stem cells

12.32 Immunomodulatory Effects of Adipose Tissue

Several studies have compared the immunomodulatory abilities of AD-MSCs and BM-MSCs and have shown that they exhibit similar effects when used in autoimmune diseases and chronic inflammatory conditions [141–143]. AD-MSCs can regulate the immune system via direct cell–cell communication and indirectly through the secretion of soluble mediators, growth factors, and extravascular vesicles [144, 145]. In adipose tissue, AD-MSC interacts with numerous cell types, including immune cells, endothelial cells, preadipocytes, hematopoietic cells, nerve cells, endothelial cells, and pericytes surrounding the blood vessels. The AD-MSCs interact with immune cells because they can regulate and influence activity of T cells, B cells, and macrophages, in vitro and in vivo [146]. Indirect cell–cell communication is instigated by AD-MSCs when they secrete soluble mediators and extravascular vesicles (exosomes and microvesicles) that are known to have therapeutic effects in regenerative medicine [147]. The most cited soluble mediators are proinflammatory and anti-inflammatory cytokines, adipokines, antioxidative, proangiogenic, antiapoptotic, growth factors (like, VEGF, FGF, and TGF), and specific interleukins (IL-6 and IL-7). Currently, the clinical production of SVF to acquire AD-MSCs is subject to investigations addressing their immunomodulatory potential in regenerative medicine. Critical aspects in these studies are the ability to develop standardized preparation protocols to ensure effective and safe use in orthobiological procedures.

12.33 Angiogenetic Properties of Adipose Tissue

AT has been intensely studied for the treatment of multiple conditions as they have great potential in nonsurgical and surgical plastic and cosmetic procedures and other applications in regenerative medicine. AD-MSCs show paracrine activity and exhibit differentiation potential toward different cell lineages (adipogenic, osteogenic, chondrogenic, and myogenic lineages), while providing immunosuppressive properties and low immunogenicity [148]. AT produces and secretes various angiogenic factors such as angiopoietin-2 and VEGF, as well as adipokines such as leptin and adiponectin, which influence, modulate angiogenesis, and the vascular structure [149]. This suggests an autoregulatory function for angiogenesis in AT. Interestingly, precursor cells in blood vessel walls have been identified capable of differentiating into endothelial cells and/or adipocytes in WAT [150]. They concluded a high adipogenic potential, linking EC and adipocytes in terms of interchangeability based on cell–cell interactions, enabling them to participate in the formation of angiogenesis and neo-vascular structures. Therefore, AD-MSCs might affect the growth of capillary networks, which are required in adipose tissue enlargement [151]. Furthermore, by enhancing angiogenesis and vasculogenesis, AD-MSCs promote neovascularization, which is fundamental in the treatment of tissue repair and post (ischemic) injuries. These specialized characteristics of ATC were demonstrated by Miranville et al., revealing the expression of CD34 and CD133 of AD-MSCs, which can differentiate into endothelial cells, contributing to revascularization [124]. Not only do AD-MSCs stimulate angiogenesis through differentiation into epithelial cells but also through paracrine activity, releasing angiogenic factors. More specifically, the cellular components of SVF are rapidly restored to form new vessels in diseased tissue structures following orthobiological injections [152] Neovascularization is further stimulated by stromal cells through the release of VEGF, TGF-b, and hepatocyte growth factor (HGF) [153]. Macrophages have demonstrated to be important cells in SVF for the proper structural organization of new blood vessels [152].

12.34 ATC Contributes to Tissue Repair Processes

Tissue repair processes following ATC and AD-tSVF preparations for orthobiological indications are based on their stromal, multipotent, and hematopoietic cell populations. In addition, AD-tSVF can produce an assortment of angiogenic, hematopoietic, and antiapoptotic factors that further expedite tissue repair (regeneration) via autocrine and paracrine actions [1]. SVF has the capacity to attain positive treatment outcomes through multiple cell components and tissue scaffold interactions with the extracellular matrix (ECM). The ECM is known as a potent scaffold in many tissues and accelerates the capability of regenerative functions by nearby cells [131]. The ECM encompasses structural proteins excreted by fibroblast, such as collagen, fibronectin, and elastin. A typical ECM characteristic is its ability to interact dynamically with integrin proteins on adhesive cells, triggering signaling pathways and changes in cell activity [154]. Furthermore, the ECM contributes to the growth of vascular infrastructure during angiogenesis [155]. Since the SVF comprises of matrix-secreting fibroblasts and other stromal cells, the clinical application of ATC and SVF is possibly beneficial to various tissue types that benefit from a three-dimensional (3D) scaffold, like the ECM of tendons, which is composed of collagen and a smaller fraction of elastin embedded in a hydrated proteoglycan matrix [156].

ATC and AD-MSCs have been recognized as effective regenerative treatment modalities over the past decade. Aside from their capacity to differentiate into a variety of mature cell types, the stromal fraction within the SVF, including fibroblasts and stem cells, stimulates angiogenetic processes, and the ECM secretes, among others, collagen proteins [157]. It has been suggested that fibroblast-derived ECM components are essential for the development of blood vessels and that angiogenesis necessitates synergy between stromal and endothelial populations [158]. Therefore, regenerative mechanisms demand synergy between angiogenesis and the synthesis of ECM proteins, founding a suitable milieu for tissue healing. Another tissue repair process is mediated by the presence of monocytes and macrophages in SVF. Approximately 5–15% of these cells are anti-inflammatory macrophage phenotype M2, an important component in controlling the environment for regeneration [159].

Additionally, 10–15% of the SVF comprises of lymphocytes, including regulatory T cells contributing to tissue immune responses [159]. It appears that the heterogeneous composition of tissue SVF has distinct advantages. The interplay of controlled inflammation with immunomodulatory properties of AD-MSCs, as precursors to ECM formation and angiogenesis, provides the necessary constituents for cellular and musculotendinous repair processes and promotes the restoration of functional tissue. Recently, ATC has been used to support wound closure in patients with chronic and recalcitrant wounds. It is well known that chronic and diabetic wounds are mainly the result of lack of angiogenesis. To date, several clinical studies report the use of AT and AD-MSCs to increase dermal wound healing [160, 161]. The improved wound healing, at least partly, seems to relate to the enhanced angiogenetic activity in the wound by the administered ATC and AD-MSCs in the wound edges where angiogenesis is stimulated by the vasculature present in the cSVF. In Fig. 12.9, ATC is injected in the wound edges of a chronic lower extremity ulcer.

Since AT is a rich and easily harvestable source of AD-MSCs and various growth factors, it has been widely used hitherto for facial rejuvenation and volumization procedures. Increasing evidence shows that dermal adipocytes are tortuously associated with hair follicles (HFs) and may be necessary to drive follicular stem cell activation. Published data show encouraging preliminary results for the use of AT and ATC as a treatment option for hair growth (Fig. 12.10) [162, 163].

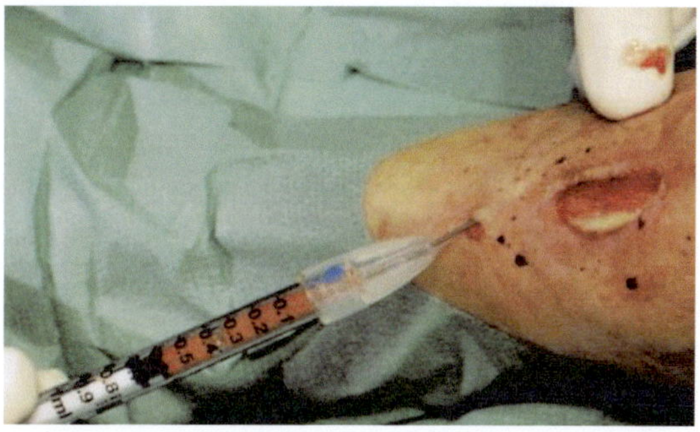

Fig. 12.9 ATC is injected in a fanning way with a blunt needle in the wound edges of a lower extremity ulcer, not responding to conventional therapies for more than 9 months, to induce wound (neo)angiogenesis to support in full wound closure

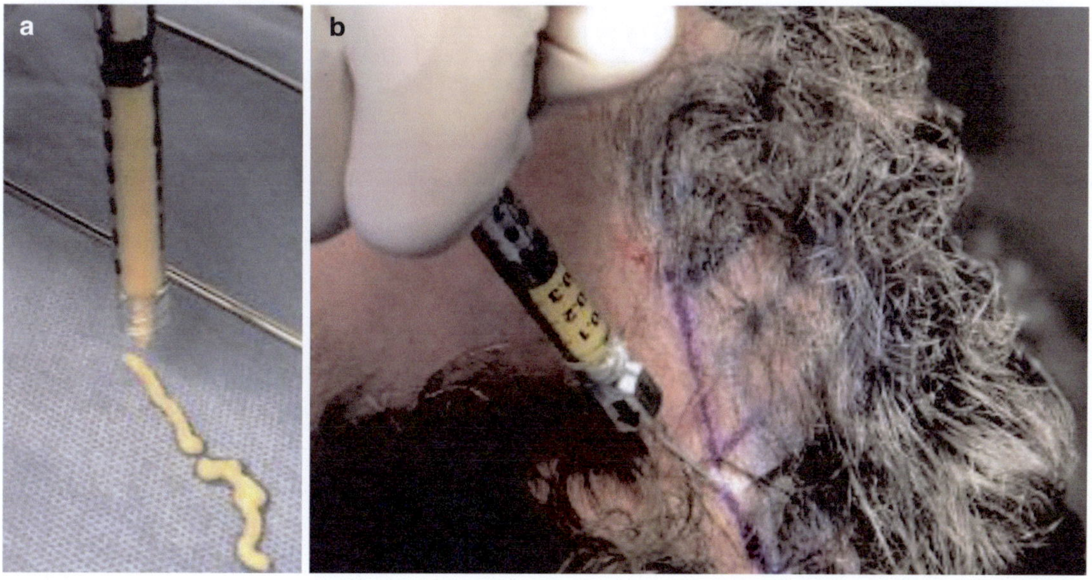

Fig. 12.10 In (**a**), AT was concentrated to ATC and successively mechanically emulsified. In (**b**), the emulsified adipose tissue is injected in the scalp, using a blunt 25 G cannula in a patient with androgenic alopecia for hair restoration

12.35 Adipose Tissue Harvesting Procedure

Liposuction is the removal of subcutaneous fat by which it is possible to obtain the adipose tissue for autologous fat transplantations and the preparation of ATC, for ASCs therapeutic treatments. The procedure is executed by means of aspiration cannulas, introduced through small skin incisions, assisted by suction. Its basic principles have been elaborated by Illouz, who was the first to introduce the modern, safe, and widespread method of liposuction with a blunt-tipped cannula as well as subcutaneous infiltration to facilitate adipose breakdown and aspiration [164, 165]. The procedure preserves neurovascular structures while maintaining fluid balance, with minimal patient discomfort [166]. In 1985, the tumescent liposuction technique was introduced by Klein [167]. Later, Coleman introduced a new three-step technique to decrease trauma to adipose tissue following liposuction: manual lipoaspiration under low pressure, centrifugation for 3 min at 3000 rpm, and 3D matrix reinjection [168]. In general, lipoaspiration techniques should not affect cell viability and consequently the yield of ASCs [133, 169].

Harvested WAT is transferred to a concentration device using minimal processing steps for autologous concentrated fat grafting preparations and ultimately ASC functionality. In Table 12.6, an overview of adipose harvesting and preparation phases is described, further illustrated in Fig. 12.11, using the Progenikine® adipose concentrating system (EmCyte Corporation, Fort Myers, FL USA).

Table 12.6 Summary of procedural steps and considerations for the preparation of ATC

A. *Tumescent fluid preparation:* a sterile NaCl solution consisting of anesthetics (lidocaine for pain relieve and epinephrine for blood vessels to constrict to minimize RBC contamination in fat tissue during harvesting).
B. *Tumescent injection:* via small skin cuts, a thin blunt injector needle is injected in the target adipose harvesting area.
C. *Waiting time:* reports indicate to wait at least 20 min before starting the fat harvesting procedure. This time is needed for the fluid to cause the injected area to swell and stiffen, supporting in easy in fat removal.
D. *Adipose harvesting:* with a dedicated harvester cannula, fat tissue is harvested using liposuction, by applying manually negative pressure to a collection syringe fat is removed from the area that was injected with tumescent fluid.
E. *Racking and decanting:* syringes filled with harvested fat are placed in a rack, with plunger in upward direction. After the adipose harvesting, leave all syringes in the rack for 10–15 min, with the luer connection of the syringe capped. Decant the supernatant (tumescent fluid) by removing the cap, until adipose tissue starts to block the luer.
F. *Transfer the decanted fat:* into a disposable processing device and place it in a dedicated centrifuge to concentrate the AT specimen.
G. *Centrifugation protocol*: density layer separation by centrifugation, producing ATC. Follow the instruction for use of the preparation device to extract ATC.
H. *Mechanical emulsification:* a method to emulsify the ATC, by moving the two syringes back and forward through a restraining device to size the ATC, making it suitable for tissue injection.

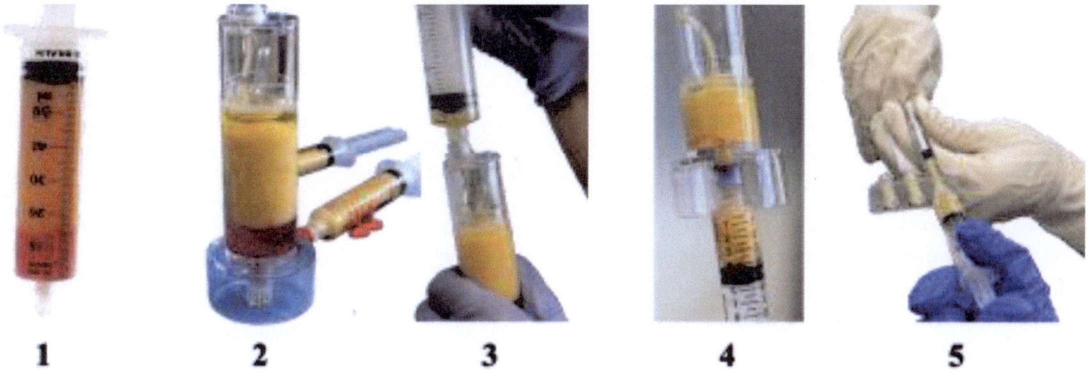

Fig. 12.11 Emulsified ATC preparation method. After harvesting of AT, the extracted AT is racked and decanted from the syringe (1). After density centrifugation (2), the oil (3), and tumescent fluid are removed from the concentration device. Subsequently, the ATC is collected in a syringe (4). Before applying the ATC, an emulsifier device (Adicen) is used to size the ATC (breaking down the adipocytes), jumpstarting the AD-cSVF preparation before injection (5)

12.36 Summary

PRP treatments and autologous adipose tissue cell-based therapies have emerged as alternative strategies in nonsurgical esthetic procedures to overcome the limitations and consequences of more invasive treatment procedures. These biological technologies have been used safely and effectively for decades to overcome post-surgical treatment morbidities like the risk of infection, wound healing disturbances, and hemorrhage [170].

PRP can be easily prepared from a fresh unit of whole blood, simple to administer, and can ultimately secrete multiple platelet growth factors and other cytokines, for regulating various physiological reparative cascades. Harvesting of adipose tissue has been referred to as a minimal invasive procedure to extract fat for the preparation of ATC and AD-cSVF, capable of stimulating the proliferation and differentiation of different cell types. The tissue repair and regenerative ability of PRP and adipose tissue preparations have been extensively documented in the literature in multiple areas within esthetic-cosmetic plastic nonsurgical procedures, including skin rejuvenation and alopecia. Current literature supports the use of PRP in nonsurgical esthetics in facial rejuvenation and hair restoration procedures.

Rejuvenation of the aging facial skin by intradermally and/or subdermally PRP has been accepted as a common therapy, as well as AT injections for facial volume restoration procedures. This is based on the premise of PGF stimulation and activities of AD-cSVF, activating dermal fibroblasts, myofibroblasts, inducing collagen synthesis, and the subsequent tissue remodeling of the ECM. Significant improvements in skin texture, color, and reduced wrinkle depth have been reported.

PRP and adipose treatments for androgenic alopecia hold some of the strongest and most convincing evidence for successful hair restoration. PRP increases proliferation rates of human DP cells that regulate hair follicle growth. Additionally, PGFs bind and interact with DP cells and local stem cells, activating the proliferative phase of the hair cycle, initiating hair follicle formation and maintenance. The anagen phase of the hair cycle is thus maintained, while delaying the catagen phase, ultimately increasing hair density. ATC has strong immunomodulatory capabilities and angiogenetic properties to stimulate hair follicle behavior.

Excellent results have been reported with these treatment modalities. However, variances in positive therapy outcomes have also been reported. A significant problem with biological cell-based therapies is the absence of consensus on the standardization of adequate and proven bioformulations and product validation, as parameters for quality control. In many presented studies, the description of the PRP injectate, cellular dosing, and preparation methods was inconsistent. A lack of standardization permits the use of less effective PRP and adipose tissue preparation devices, therefore jeopardizing clinical outcomes and patient satisfaction.

However, the high expectations of biological therapies in the many nonsurgical esthetic procedures, with consistent positive outcomes, can be accomplished after clarifying the scientific barriers, with consensus on pathology-specific bioformulations for PRP and ATC.

References

1. Marx RE. Platelet-rich plasma (PRP): what is PRP and what is not PRP? Implant Dent. 2001;10(4):225–8.
2. Everts PA, Pinto PC, Girão L. Autologous pure platelet-rich plasma injections for facial skin rejuvenation: biometric instrumental evaluations and patient-reported outcomes to support antiaging effects. J Cosmet Dermatol. 2019;18(4):985–95.
3. Liang Z-J, Lu X, Li D-Q, Liang Y-D, Zhu D-D, Wu F-X, et al. Precise intradermal injection of nanofat-derived stromal cells combined with platelet-rich fibrin improves the efficacy of facial skin rejuvenation. Cell Physiol Biochem. 2018;47(1):316–29.
4. Samadi P, Sheykhhasan M, Khoshinani HM. The use of platelet-rich plasma in aesthetic and regenerative medicine: a comprehensive review. Aesthet Plast Surg. 2019;43(3):803–14.
5. Fadadu PP, Mazzola AJ, Hunter CW, Davis TT. Review of concentration yields in commercially available platelet-rich plasma (PRP) systems: a call for PRP standardization. Reg Anesth Pain Med. 2019;44(6):652–9.
6. Mohamed-Ahmed S, Fristad I, Lie SA, Suliman S, Mustafa K, Vindenes H, et al. Adipose-derived and bone marrow mesenchymal stem cells: a donor-matched comparison. Stem Cell Res Ther. 2018;9(1):168.
7. Motosko CC, Khouri KS, Poudrier G, Sinno S, Hazen A. Evaluating platelet-rich therapy for facial aesthetics and alopecia: a critical review of the literature. Plast Reconstr Surg. 2018;141(5):1115–23.
8. Merchán WH, Gómez LA, Chasoy ME, Alfonso-Rodríguez CA, Muñoz AL. Platelet-rich plasma, a powerful tool in dermatology. J Tissue Eng Regen Med. 2019;13(5):892–901.
9. Xiao H, Xu D, Mao R, Xiao M, Fang Y, Liu Y. Platelet-rich plasma in facial rejuvenation: a systematic appraisal of the available clinical evidence. Clin Cosmet Investig Dermatol. 2021;14:1697–724.
10. Garg S, Bansal A. Platelet-rich plasma in interventional dermatology and trichology: how far have we come? Cosmoderma. 2021;1:12.
11. Evans AG, Ivanic MG, Botros MA, Pope RW, Halle BR, Glassman GE, et al. Rejuvenating the periorbital area using platelet-rich plasma: a systematic review and meta-analysis. Arch Dermatol Res. 2021;313(9):711–27.
12. Martin P. Wound healing–aiming for perfect skin regeneration. Science. 1997;276(5309):75–81.
13. Elghblawi E. Platelet-rich plasma, the ultimate secret for youthful skin elixir and hair growth triggering. J Cosmet Dermatol. 2018;17(3):423–30.
14. Everts PA. Autologous platelet-rich plasma and mesenchymal stem cells for the treatment of chronic wounds. In: Hakan Dogan K, editor. Wound healing - current perspectives. London: IntechOpen; 2019. https://www.intechopen.com/books/wound-healing-current-perspectives/autologous-platelet-rich-plasma-and-mesenchymal-stem-cells-for-the-treatment-of-chronic-wounds. Accessed 4 Oct 2019.
15. Yuksel EP, Sahin G, Aydin F, Senturk N, Turanli AY. Evaluation of effects of platelet-rich plasma on human facial skin. J Cosmet Laser Ther. 2014;16(5):206–8.
16. Everts P, Hoogbergen MM, Weber TA, Devilee RJJ, van Monftort G, de Hingh IHJT. Is the use of autologous platelet-rich plasma gels in gynecologic, cardiac, and general, reconstructive surgery beneficial? Curr Pharm Biotechnol. 2012;13(7):1163–72.
17. Li H, Han Z, Liu D, Zhao P, Liang S, Xu K. Autologous platelet-rich plasma promotes neurogenic differentiation of human adipose-derived stem cells in vitro. Int J Neurosci. 2013;123(3):184–90.
18. Cho EB, Park GS, Park SS, Jang YJ, Kim KH, Kim KJ, et al. Effect of platelet-rich plasma on proliferation and migration in human dermal fibroblasts. J Cosmet Dermatol. 2019;18(4):1105–12.
19. Alves R, Grimalt R. A review of platelet-rich plasma: history, biology, mechanism of action, and classification. Skin Appendage Disord. 2018;4(1):18–24.
20. Gentile P, Cole J, Cole M, Garcovich S, Bielli A, Scioli M, et al. Evaluation of not-activated and activated PRP in hair loss treatment: role of growth factor and cytokine concentrations obtained by different collection systems. Int J Mol Sci. 2017;18(2):408.
21. Li W, Enomoto M, Ukegawa M, Hirai T, Sotome S, Wakabayashi Y, et al. Subcutaneous injections of platelet-rich plasma into skin flaps modulate proangiogenic gene expression and improve survival rates. Plast Reconstr Surg. 2012;129(4):858–66.
22. Jain R, De-Eknamkul W. Potential targets in the discovery of new hair growth promoters for androgenic alopecia. Expert Opin Ther Targets. 2014;18(7):787–806.

23. Takikawa M, Nakamura S, Nakamura S, Ishirara M, Kishimoto S, Sasaki K, et al. Enhanced effect of platelet-rich plasma containing a new carrier on hair growth. Dermatol Surg. 2011;37(12):1721–9.
24. Garg S. Outcome of intra-operative injected platelet-rich plasma therapy during follicular unit extraction hair transplant: a prospective randomised study in forty patients. J Cutan Aesthet Surg. 2016;9(3):157.
25. Chahla J, Cinque ME, Piuzzi NS, Mannava S, Geeslin AG, Murray IR, et al. A call for standardization in platelet-rich plasma preparation protocols and composition reporting: a systematic review of the clinical orthopaedic literature. J Bone Jt Surg. 2017;99(20):1769–79.
26. Everts P, Onishi K, Jayaram P, Lana JF, Mautner K. Platelet-rich plasma: new performance understandings and therapeutic considerations in 2020. Int J Mol Sci. 2020;21(20):7794.
27. Everts PAM, Knape JTA, Weibrich G, Hoffmann J, Overdevest EP, Box HAM, et al. Platelet-rich plasma and platelet gel: a review. J Extra Corpor Technol. 2007;14:174.
28. Lubkowska A, Dołęgowska B, Banfi G. Growth factor content in PRP and their applicability in medicine. J Biol Regul Homeost Agents. 2012;26:3S.
29. Blair P, Flaumenhaft R. Platelet alpha-granules: basic biology and clinical correlates. Blood Rev. 2009;23(4):177–89.
30. Iberg CA, Hawiger D. Natural and induced tolerogenic dendritic cells. J Immunol. 2020;204(4):733–44.
31. Ganor Y, Besser M, Ben-Zakay N, Unger T, Levite M. Human T cells express a functional ionotropic glutamate receptor GluR3, and glutamate by itself triggers integrin-mediated adhesion to laminin and fibronectin and chemotactic migration. J Immunol. 2003;170(8):4362–72.
32. Koupenova M, Clancy L, Corkrey HA, Freedman JE. Circulating platelets as mediators of immunity, inflammation, and thrombosis. Circ Res. 2018;122(2):337–51.
33. Morrell CN, Aggrey AA, Chapman LM, Modjeski KL. Emerging roles for platelets as immune and inflammatory cells. Blood. 2014;123(18):2759–67.
34. Thon JN, Peters CG, Machlus KR, Aslam R, Rowley J, Macleod H, et al. T granules in human platelets function in TLR9 organization and signaling. J Cell Biol. 2012;198(4):561–74.
35. Everts PA, Brown Mahoney C, Hoffmann JJ, Schönberger JP, Box HA, van Zundert A, et al. Platelet-rich plasma preparation using three devices: implications for platelet activation and platelet growth factor release. Growth Factors. 2006;24(3):165–71.
36. Gupta AK, Cole J, Deutsch DP, Everts PA, Niedbalski RP, Panchaprateep R, et al. Platelet-rich plasma as a treatment for androgenetic alopecia. Dermatol Surg. 2019;45(10):1262–73.
37. Willemsen JCN, Van Dongen J, Spiekman M, Vermeulen KM, Harmsen MC, van der Lei B, et al. The addition of PRP to facial lipofilling: a double-blind placebo-controlled randomized trial. Plast Reconstr Surg. 2018;141:331.
38. Abuaf OK, Yildiz H, Baloglu H, Bilgili ME, Simsek HA, Dogan B. Histologic evidence of new collagen formulation using platelet rich plasma in skin rejuvenation: a prospective controlled clinical study. Ann Dermatol. 2016;28(6):718.
39. Everts PAM, Hoffmann J, Weibrich G, Mahoney CB, Schönberger JPAM, van Zundert A, et al. Differences in platelet growth factor release and leucocyte kinetics during autologous platelet gel formation. Transfus Med. 2006;16(5):363–8.
40. Cengiz IF, Pereira H, Espregueira-Mendes J, Reis RL, Oliveira JM. The clinical use of biologics in the knee lesions: does the patient benefit? Curr Rev Musculoskelet Med. 2019;12(3):406–14.
41. Muchedzi TA, Roberts SB. A systematic review of the effects of platelet rich plasma on outcomes for patients with knee osteoarthritis and following total knee arthroplasty. Surgeon. 2018;16(4):250–8.
42. Amable P, Carias RB, Teixeira MV, da Cruz PÍ, Corrêa do Amaral RJ, Granjeiro J, et al. Platelet-rich plasma preparation for regenerative medicine: optimization and quantification of cytokines and growth factors. Stem Cell Res Ther. 2013;4(3):67.
43. Gentile P, Calabrese C, De Angelis B, Dionisi L, Pizzicannella J, Kothari A, et al. Impact of the different preparation methods to obtain autologous non-activated platelet-rich plasma (A-PRP) and activated platelet-rich plasma (AA-PRP) in plastic surgery: wound healing and hair regrowth evaluation. Int J Mol Sci. 2020;21(2):431.
44. Nguyen PA, Pham TAV. Effects of platelet-rich plasma on human gingival fibroblast proliferation and migration in vitro. J Appl Oral Sci. 2018;26:e20180077. http://www.scielo.br/scielo.php?script=sci_arttext&pid=S1678-77572018000100480&lng=en&tlng=en. Accessed 5 Jul 2020.
45. Vahabi S, Yadegari Z, Mohammad-Rahimi H. Comparison of the effect of activated or non-activated PRP in various concentrations on osteoblast and fibroblast cell line proliferation. Cell Tissue Bank. 2017;18(3):347–53.
46. Miller EJ, Lappin SL. Physiology, cellular receptor. Treasure Island, FL: StatPearls Publishing; 2020. http://europepmc.org/books/NBK554403.
47. Frautschi RS, Hashem AM, Halasa B, Cakmakoglu C, Zins JE. Current evidence for clinical efficacy of platelet rich plasma in aesthetic surgery: a systematic review. Aesthet Surg J. 2017;37:353.
48. Gupta AK, Versteeg SG, Rapaport J, Hausauer AK, Shear NH, Piguet V. The efficacy of platelet-rich plasma in the field of hair restoration and facial aesthetics—a systematic review and meta-analysis. J Cutan Med Surg. 2019;23(2):185–203.
49. Atiyeh B, Oneisi A, Ghieh F. Platelet-rich plasma facial rejuvenation: myth or reality? Aesthet Plast Surg. 2021;45:2928. https://link.springer.

com/10.1007/s00266-021-02300-9. Accessed 21 Nov 2021.
50. Magalon J, Chateau AL, Bertrand B, Louis ML, Silvestre A, Giraudo L, et al. DEPA classification: a proposal for standardising PRP use and a retrospective application of available devices. BMJ Open Sport Exerc Med. 2016;2(1):e000060.
51. Fitzpatrick J, Bulsara MK, McCrory PR, Richardson MD, Zheng MH. Analysis of platelet-rich plasma extraction: variations in platelet and blood components between 4 common commercial kits. Orthop J Sports Med. 2017;5(1):232596711667527.
52. Degen RM, Bernard JA, Oliver KS, Dines JS. Commercial separation systems designed for preparation of platelet-rich plasma yield differences in cellular composition. HSS J. 2017;13(1):75–80.
53. Mazzucco L, Balbo V, Cattana E, Guaschino R, Borzini P. Not every PRP-gel is born equal Evaluation of growth factor availability for tissues through four PRP-gel preparations: Fibrinet®, RegenPRP-Kit®, Plateltex® and one manual procedure. Vox Sang. 2009;97(2):110–8.
54. Kushida S, Kakudo N, Morimoto N, Hara T, Ogawa T, Mitsui T, et al. Platelet and growth factor concentrations in activated platelet-rich plasma: a comparison of seven commercial separation systems. J Artif Organs. 2014;17(2):186–92.
55. Magalon J, Brandin T, Francois P, Degioanni C, De Maria L, Grimaud F, et al. Technical and biological review of authorized medical devices for platelets-rich plasma preparation in the field of regenerative medicine. Platelets. 2021;32(2):200–8.
56. Haunschild ED, Huddleston HP, Chahla J, Gilat R, Cole BJ, Yanke AB. Platelet-rich plasma augmentation in meniscal repair surgery: a systematic review of comparative studies. Arthrosc J Arthrosc Relat Surg. 2020;36(6):1765–74.
57. Xu J, Gou L, Zhang P, Li H, Qiu S. Platelet-rich plasma and regenerative dentistry. Aust Dent J. 2020;65(2):131–42.
58. Zheng C, Zhu Q, Liu X, Huang X, He C, Jiang L, et al. Effect of platelet-rich plasma (PRP) concentration on proliferation, neurotrophic function and migration of Schwann cells *in vitro*: effect of platelet-rich plasma on Schwann cells. J Tissue Eng Regen Med. 2016;10(5):428–36.
59. Hee HT, Majd ME, Holt RT, Myers L. Do autologous growth factors enhance transforaminal lumbar interbody fusion? Eur Spine J. 2003;12(4):400–7.
60. Giusti I, Rughetti A, D'Ascenzo S, Millimaggi D, Pavan A, Dell'Orso L, et al. Identification of an optimal concentration of platelet gel for promoting angiogenesis in human endothelial cells. Transfusion (Paris). 2009;49(4):771–8.
61. Creeper F, Lichanska AM, Marshall RI, Seymour GJ, Ivanovski S. The effect of platelet-rich plasma on osteoblast and periodontal ligament cell migration, proliferation and differentiation. J Periodontal Res. 2009;44(2):258–65.
62. Melo L, Lana S. Centrifugation conditions in the L-PRP preparation affect soluble factors release and mesenchymal stem cell proliferation in fibrin nanofibers. Molecules. 2019;24(15):2729.
63. Moojen DJF, Schure R-M, Overdevest EP, van Zundert A, Knape JTA, Castelein RM, et al. Antimicrobial activity of platelet-leukocyte gel against Staphylococcus aureus. J Orthop Res. 2008;26(3):404–10.
64. Tang Y-Q, Yeaman MR, Selsted ME. Antimicrobial peptides from human platelets. Infect Immun. 2002;70(12):6524–33.
65. Lana JF, Macedo A, Ingrao ILG, Huber SC, Santos GS, Santana MHA. Leukocyte-rich PRP for knee osteoarthritis: current concepts. J Clin Orthop Trauma. 2019;10:S179–82.
66. Kovtun A, Bergdolt S, Wiegner R, Radermacher P, Huber-Lang M, et al. The crucial role of neutrophil granulocytes in bone fracture healing. Eur Cell Mater. 2016;32:152–62.
67. Rossi LA, Piuzzi N, Giunta D, Tanoira I, Brandariz R, Pasqualini I, et al. Subacromial platelet-rich plasma injections decrease pain and improve functional outcomes in patients with refractory rotator cuff tendinopathy. Arthrosc J Arthrosc Relat Surg. 2021;37(9):2745–53.
68. Collins T, Alexander D, Barkatali B. Platelet-rich plasma: a narrative review. EFORT Open Rev. 2021;6(4):225–35.
69. Phillipson M, Kubes P. The healing power of neutrophils. Trends Immunol. 2019;40(7):635–47.
70. Zhou Y, Wang JH-C. PRP treatment efficacy for tendinopathy: a review of basic science studies. Biomed Res Int. 2016;2016:1–8.
71. Fedorova NV, Ksenofontov AL, Serebryakova MV, Stadnichuk VI, Gaponova TV, Baratova LA, et al. Neutrophils release metalloproteinases during adhesion in the presence of insulin, but cathepsin G in the presence of glucagon. Mediat Inflamm. 2018;2018:1–9.
72. Stevens J, Khetarpal S. Platelet-rich plasma for androgenetic alopecia: a review of the literature and proposed treatment protocol. Int J Womens Dermatol. 2019;5(1):46–51.
73. Ubezio G, Ghio M. Bio-modulators in platelet-rich plasma: a comparison of the amounts in products from healthy donors and patients produced with three different techniques. Blood Transfus. 2014;12:S214. https://doi.org/10.2450/2012.0128-12. Accessed 8 Jul 2020.
74. Italiani P, Boraschi D. From monocytes to M1/M2 macrophages: phenotypical vs. functional differentiation. Front Immunol. 2014;5:514. http://journal.frontiersin.org/article/10.3389/fimmu.2014.00514/abstract. Accessed 8 Jul 2020.
75. Weirather J, Hofmann UDW, Beyersdorf N, Ramos GC, Vogel B, Frey A, et al. Foxp3^{+} CD4^{+} T cells improve healing after myocardial infarction by modulating monocyte/macrophage differentiation. Circ Res. 2014;115(1):55–67.

76. Ogle ME, Segar CE, Sridhar S, Botchwey EA. Monocytes and macrophages in tissue repair: implications for immunoregenerative biomaterial design. Exp Biol Med. 2016;241(10):1084–97.
77. Das A, Sinha M, Datta S, Abas M, Chaffee S, Sen CK, et al. Monocyte and macrophage plasticity in tissue repair and regeneration. Am J Pathol. 2015;185(10):2596–606.
78. Wynn TA, Vannella KM. Macrophages in tissue repair, regeneration, and fibrosis. Immunity. 2016;44(3):450–62.
79. Repsold L, Joubert AM. Eryptosis: an erythrocyte's suicidal type of cell death. Biomed Res Int. 2018;2018:1–10.
80. Mercuri SR, Di Nicola MR, Brianti P, Bianchi VG, Paolino G. Pilot study on the use of the "monocyte-rich" platelet-rich plasma in combination with 1927 nm fractional and 308 nm excimer lasers for the treatment of vitiligo. Medicina. 2021;57(9):904.
81. Helms CC, Gladwin MT, Kim-Shapiro DB. Erythrocytes and vascular function: oxygen and nitric oxide. Front Physiol. 2018;9:125.
82. Schaer DJ, Buehler PW, Alayash AI, Belcher JD, Vercellotti GM. Hemolysis and free hemoglobin revisited: exploring hemoglobin and hemin scavengers as a novel class of therapeutic proteins. Blood. 2013;121(8):1276–84.
83. Woodell-May JE, Sommerfeld SD. Role of inflammation and the immune system in the progression of osteoarthritis. J Orthop Res. 2020;38(2):253–7.
84. Cognasse F, Laradi S, Berthelot P, Bourlet T, Marotte H, Mismetti P, et al. Platelet inflammatory response to stress. Front Immunol. 2019;10:1478.
85. Vasina EM, Cauwenberghs S, Feijge MAH, Heemskerk JWM, Weber C, Koenen RR. Microparticles from apoptotic platelets promote resident macrophage differentiation. Cell Death Dis. 2011;2(9):e211.
86. Gros A, Syvannarath V, Lamrani L, Ollivier V, Loyau S, Goerge T, et al. Single platelets seal neutrophil-induced vascular breaches via GPVI during immune-complex-mediated inflammation in mice. Blood. 2015;126(8):1017–26.
87. Clark SR, Ma AC, Tavener SA, McDonald B, Goodarzi Z, Kelly MM, et al. Platelet TLR4 activates neutrophil extracellular traps to ensnare bacteria in septic blood. Nat Med. 2007;13(4):463–9.
88. Kapur R, Zufferey A, Boilard E, Semple JW. Nouvelle cuisine: platelets served with inflammation. J Immunol. 2015;194(12):5579–87.
89. Dale DC, Boxer L, Liles WC. The phagocytes: neutrophils and monocytes. Blood. 2008;112(4):935–45.
90. Henn V, Slupsky J, Gräfe M, Anagnostopoulos I, Förster R, Müller-Berghaus G, et al. CD40 ligand on activated platelets triggers an inflammatory reaction of endothelial cells. Nature. 1998;391(6667):591–4.
91. Yu Y, Ma X, Gong R, Zhu J, Wei L, Yao J. Recent advances in CD8+ regulatory T-cell research (Review). Oncol Lett. 2018;15:8187. http://www.spandidos-publications.com/10.3892/ol.2018.8378. Accessed 7 Sep 2020.
92. Semple JW, Italiano JE, Freedman J. Platelets and the immune continuum. Nat Rev Immunol. 2011;11(4):264–74.
93. Deppermann C, Kubes P. Start a fire, kill the bug: the role of platelets in inflammation and infection. Innate Immun. 2018;24(6):335–48.
94. Hara GR, Basu T. Platelet-rich plasma in regenerative medicine. 2014;1:25.
95. Brill A. Differential role of platelet granular mediators in angiogenesis. Cardiovasc Res. 2004;63(2):226–35.
96. Lansdown DA, Fortier LA. Platelet-rich plasma: formulations, preparations, constituents, and their effects. Oper Tech Sports Med. 2017;25(1):7–12.
97. Richardson TP, Peters MC, Ennett AB, Mooney DJ. Polymeric system for dual growth factor delivery. Nat Biotechnol. 2001;19(11):1029–34.
98. Crowley JS, Liu A, Dobke M. Regenerative and stem cell-based techniques for facial rejuvenation. Exp Biol Med. 2021;246(16):1829–37.
99. Cervantes J, Perper M, Wong LL, Eber AE, Villasante Fricke AC, Wikramanayake TC, et al. Effectiveness of platelet-rich plasma for androgenetic alopecia: a review of the literature. Skin Appendage Disord. 2018;4(1):1–11.
100. Jiménez Gómez N, Pino Castresana A, Segurado Miravalles G, Truchuelo Díez M, Troya Estavillo M, Anitua Aldecoa E, et al. Autologous platelet-rich gel for facial rejuvenation and wrinkle amelioration: a pilot study. J Cosmet Dermatol. 2019;18(5):1353–60.
101. Vanaman M, Fabi SG, Carruthers J. Complications in the cosmetic dermatology patient: a review and our experience (Part 1). Dermatol Surg. 2016;42(1):1–11.
102. Zein M, Tie-Shue R, Pirakitikulr N, Lee WW. Complications after cosmetic periocular filler: prevention and management. Plast Aesthet Res. 2020;7:44. https://parjournal.net/article/view/3605. Accessed 20 Nov 2021.
103. Gilbert E, Hui A, Meehan S, Waldorf HA. The basic science of dermal fillers: past and present Part II: adverse effects. J Drugs Dermatol. 2012;11(9):1069–77.
104. Safran T, Gorsky K, Viezel-Mathieu A, Kanevsky J, Gilardino MS. The role of ultrasound technology in plastic surgery. J Plast Reconstr Aesthet Surg. 2018;71(3):416–24.
105. Lee S-H, Gil Y-C, Choi Y-J, Tansatit T, Kim H-J, Hu K-S. Topographic anatomy of the superior labial artery for dermal filler injection. Plast Reconstr Surg. 2015;135(2):445–50.
106. Miao Y, Sun Y-B, Sun X-J, Du B-J, Jiang J-D, Hu Z-Q. Promotional effect of platelet-rich plasma on hair follicle reconstitution in vivo. Dermatol Surg. 2013;39(12):1868–76.
107. Andia I, Maffulli N. A contemporary view of platelet-rich plasma therapies: moving toward refined

clinical protocols and precise indications. Regen Med. 2018;13(6):717–28.
108. Vedamurthy M. Beware What you inject: complications of injectables-dermal fillers. J Cutan Aesthet Surg. 2018;11(2):60–6.
109. Wang Y, Massry G, Holds JB. Complications of periocular dermal fillers. Facial Plast Surg Clin N Am. 2021;29(2):349–57.
110. Lee A-L, Chen Y-F, Yao W-T, Liu Y-C, Yu C-M, Yu C-M, et al. Laser Doppler imaging for treating vascular complications from procedures involving dermal fillers: case series and literature review. Diagnostics. 2021;11(9):1640.
111. Beitzel K, Allen D, Apostolakos J, Russell R, McCarthy M, Gallo G, et al. US Definitions, current use, and FDA stance on use of platelet-rich plasma in sports medicine. J Knee Surg. 2014;28(1):29–34.
112. Maisel-Campbell AL, Ismail A, Reynolds KA, Poon E, Serrano L, Grushchak S, et al. A systematic review of the safety and effectiveness of platelet-rich plasma (PRP) for skin aging. Arch Dermatol Res. 2020;312(5):301–15.
113. Roohaninasab M, Goodarzi A, Ghassemi M, Sadeghzadeh-Bazargan A, Behrangi E, Najar NN. Systematic review of platelet-rich plasma in treating alopecia: focusing on efficacy, safety, and therapeutic durability. Dermatol Ther. 2021;34(2):e14768. https://onlinelibrary.wiley.com/doi/10.1111/dth.14768. Accessed 14 Nov 2021.
114. Argentati C, Morena F, Bazzucchi M, Armentano I, Emiliani C, Martino S. Adipose stem cell translational applications: from bench-to-bedside. Int J Mol Sci. 2018;19(11):3475.
115. Andrzejewska A, Lukomska B, Janowski M. Concise review: mesenchymal stem cells: from roots to boost: MSCs: from roots to boost. Stem Cells. 2019;37(7):855–64.
116. Karastergiou K, Mohamed-Ali V. The autocrine and paracrine roles of adipokines. Mol Cell Endocrinol. 2010;318(1–2):69–78.
117. Cinti S. Reversible physiological transdifferentiation in the adipose organ. Proc Nutr Soc. 2009;68(4):340–9.
118. Zuk PA, Zhu M, Ashjian P, Ugarte DAD, Huang JI, Mizuno H, et al. Human adipose tissue is a source of multipotent stem cells D. Mol Biol Cell. 2002;13:17.
119. Zuk PA. The adipose-derived stem cell: looking back and looking ahead. Kellogg D, editor. Mol Biol Cell. 2010;21(11):1783–7.
120. Yang HJ, Kim K-J, Kim MK, Lee SJ, Ryu YH, Seo BF, et al. The stem cell potential and multipotency of human adipose tissue-derived stem cells vary by cell donor and are different from those of other types of stem cells. Cells Tissues Organs. 2014;199(5–6):373–83.
121. Wagner SJ, Leiby DA, Roback JD. Existing and emerging blood-borne pathogens: impact on the safety of blood transfusion for the hematology/oncology patient. Hematol Clin. 2019;33(5):739–48.
122. Baer PC. Adipose-derived mesenchymal stromal/stem cells: an update on their phenotype in vivo and in vitro. World J Stem Cells. 2014;6(3):256.
123. Dmitrieva RI, Minullina IR, Bilibina AA, Tarasova OV, Anisimov SV, Zaritskey AY. Bone marrow- and subcutaneous adipose tissue-derived mesenchymal stem cells: differences and similarities. Cell Cycle. 2012;11(2):377–83.
124. Miranville A, Heeschen C, Sengenès C, Curat CA, Busse R, Bouloumié A. Improvement of postnatal neovascularization by human adipose tissue-derived stem cells. Circulation. 2004;110(3):349–55.
125. Fraser JK, Wulur I, Alfonso Z, Hedrick MH. Fat tissue: an underappreciated source of stem cells for biotechnology. Trends Biotechnol. 2006;24(4):150–4.
126. Yun S, Ku S-K, Kwon Y-S. Adipose-derived mesenchymal stem cells and platelet-rich plasma synergistically ameliorate the surgical-induced osteoarthritis in Beagle dogs. J Orthop Surg. 2016;11(1):9.
127. Gonzalez-Rey E, Gonzalez MA, Varela N, O'Valle F, Hernandez-Cortes P, Rico L, et al. Human adipose-derived mesenchymal stem cells reduce inflammatory and T cell responses and induce regulatory T cells in vitro in rheumatoid arthritis. Ann Rheum Dis. 2010;69(1):241–8.
128. Kim E, Kim W, Oh K-J, Han B, Lee S, Bae K-H. Recent advances in proteomic studies of adipose tissues and adipocytes. Int J Mol Sci. 2015;16(3):4581–99.
129. Zimmerlin L, Park TS, Zambidis ET, Donnenberg VS, Donnenberg AD. Mesenchymal stem cell secretome and regenerative therapy after cancer. Biochimie. 2013;95(12):2235–45.
130. Coelho M, Oliveira T, Fernandes R. State of the art paper Biochemistry of adipose tissue: an endocrine organ. Arch Med Sci. 2013;2:191–200.
131. Brown JC, Shang H, Li Y, Yang N, Patel N, Katz AJ. Isolation of adipose-derived stromal vascular fraction cells using a novel point-of-care device: cell characterization and review of the literature. Tissue Eng Part C Methods. 2017;23(3):125–35.
132. Gimble JM, Katz AJ, Bunnell BA. Adipose-derived stem cells for regenerative medicine. Circ Res. 2007;100(9):1249–60.
133. Gentile P, Calabrese C, De Angelis B, Pizzicannella J, Kothari A, Garcovich S. Impact of the different preparation methods to obtain human adipose-derived stromal vascular fraction cells (AD-SVFs) and human adipose-derived mesenchymal stem cells (AD-MSCs): enzymatic digestion versus mechanical centrifugation. Int J Mol Sci. 2019;20(21):5471.
134. Bora P, Majumdar AS. Adipose tissue-derived stromal vascular fraction in regenerative medicine: a brief review on biology and translation. Stem Cell Res Ther. 2017;8(1):145.
135. Sugii S, Kida Y, Berggren WT, Evans RM. Feeder-dependent and feeder-independent iPS cell derivation from human and mouse adipose stem cells. Nat Protoc. 2011;6(3):346–58.

136. Varma MJO, Breuls RGM, Schouten TE, Jurgens WJFM, Bontkes HJ, Schuurhuis GJ, et al. Phenotypical and functional characterization of freshly isolated adipose tissue-derived stem cells. Stem Cells Dev. 2007;16(1):91–104.
137. Alexander RW. Understanding mechanical emulsification (Nanofat) versus enzymatic isolation of tissue stromal vascular fraction (tSVF) cells from adipose tissue: potential uses in biocellular regenerative medicine. J Prolother. 2018;8:e947.
138. Tonnard P, Verpaele A, Peeters G, Hamdi M, Cornelissen M, Declercq H. Nanofat grafting: basic research and clinical applications. Plast Reconstr Surg. 2013;132(4):1017–26.
139. Bianchi F, Maioli M, Leonardi E, Olivi E, Pasquinelli G, Valente S, et al. A new nonenzymatic method and device to obtain a fat tissue derivative highly enriched in pericyte-like elements by mild mechanical forces from human lipoaspirates. Cell Transplant. 2013;22(11):2063–77.
140. Ong WK, Sugii S. Adipose-derived stem cells: fatty potentials for therapy. Int J Biochem Cell Biol. 2013;45(6):1083–6.
141. Hao T, Chen J, Zhi S, Zhang Q, Chen G, Yu F. Comparison of bone marrow-vs. adipose tissue-derived mesenchymal stem cells for attenuating liver fibrosis. Exp Ther Med. 2017;14:5956. http://www.spandidos-publications.com/10.3892/etm.2017.5333. Accessed 2 Nov 2021.
142. Pendleton C, Li Q, Chesler DA, Yuan K, Guerrero-Cazares H, Quinones-Hinojosa A. Mesenchymal stem cells derived from adipose tissue vs bone marrow: in vitro comparison of their tropism towards gliomas. Najbauer J. PLoS One. 2013;8(3):e58198.
143. Puissant B, Barreau C, Bourin P, Clavel C, Corre J, Bousquet C, et al. Immunomodulatory effect of human adipose tissue-derived adult stem cells: comparison with bone marrow mesenchymal stem cells. Br J Haematol. 2005;129(1):118–29.
144. Fang Y, Zhang Y, Zhou J, Cao K. Adipose-derived mesenchymal stem cell exosomes: a novel pathway for tissues repair. Cell Tissue Bank. 2019;20(2):153–61.
145. Salgado AJBOG, Reis RLG, Sousa NJC, Gimble JM. Adipose tissue derived stem cells secretome: soluble factors and their roles in regenerative medicine. Curr Stem Cell Res Ther. 2010;5(2):103–10.
146. Naik S, Larsen SB, Cowley CJ, Fuchs E. Two to tango: dialog between immunity and stem cells in health and disease. Cell. 2018;175(4):908–20.
147. Mitchell R, Mellows B, Sheard J, Antonioli M, Kretz O, Chambers D, et al. Secretome of adipose-derived mesenchymal stem cells promotes skeletal muscle regeneration through synergistic action of extracellular vesicle cargo and soluble proteins. Stem Cell Res Ther. 2019;10(1):116.
148. Wang K, Yu L-Y, Jiang L-Y, Wang H-B, Wang C-Y, Luo Y. The paracrine effects of adipose-derived stem cells on neovascularization and biocompatibility of a macroencapsulation device. Acta Biomater. 2015;15:65–76.
149. Sorop O, Olver TD, van de Wouw J, Heinonen I, van Duin RW, Duncker DJ, et al. The microcirculation: a key player in obesity-associated cardiovascular disease. Cardiovasc Res. 2017;113(9):1035–45.
150. Tran K-V, Gealekman O, Frontini A, Zingaretti MC, Morroni M, Giordano A, et al. The vascular endothelium of the adipose tissue gives rise to both white and brown fat cells. Cell Metab. 2012;15(2):222–9.
151. Planat-Benard V, Silvestre J-S, Cousin B, André M, Nibbelink M, Tamarat R, et al. Plasticity of human adipose lineage cells toward endothelial cells: physiological and therapeutic perspectives. Circulation. 2004;109(5):656–63.
152. Koh YJ, Koh BI, Kim H, Joo HJ, Jin HK, Jeon J, et al. Stromal vascular fraction from adipose tissue forms profound vascular network through the dynamic reassembly of blood endothelial cells. Arterioscler Thromb Vasc Biol. 2011;31(5):1141–50.
153. Rehman J, Traktuev D, Li J, Merfeld-Clauss S, Temm-Grove CJ, Bovenkerk JE, et al. Secretion of angiogenic and antiapoptotic factors by human adipose stromal cells. Circulation. 2004;109(10):1292–8.
154. Bosman FT, Stamenkovic I. Functional structure and composition of the extracellular matrix: structure and composition of the extracellular matrix. J Pathol. 2003;200(4):423–8.
155. Bauer AL, Jackson TL, Jiang Y. Topography of extracellular matrix mediates vascular morphogenesis and migration speeds in angiogenesis. Czirók A. PLoS Comput Biol. 2009;5(7):e1000445.
156. Docheva D, Müller SA, Majewski M, Evans CH. Biologics for tendon repair. Adv Drug Deliv Rev. 2015;84:222–39.
157. Narayanan AS, Page RC, Swanson J. Collagen synthesis by human fibroblasts. Regulation by transforming growth factor-beta in the presence of other inflammatory mediators. Biochem J. 1989;260:463.
158. Newman AC, Nakatsu MN, Chou W, Gershon PD, Hughes CCW. The requirement for fibroblasts in angiogenesis: fibroblast-derived matrix proteins are essential for endothelial cell lumen formation. Adams JC, editor. Mol Biol Cell. 2011;22(20):3791–800.
159. Bourin P, Bunnell BA, Casteilla L, Dominici M, Katz AJ, March KL, et al. Stromal cells from the adipose tissue-derived stromal vascular fraction and culture expanded adipose tissue-derived stromal/stem cells: a joint statement of the International Federation for Adipose Therapeutics and Science (IFATS) and the International Society for Cellular Therapy (ISCT). Cytotherapy. 2013;15(6):641–8.
160. Marino G, Moraci M, Armenia E, Orabona C, Sergio R, De Sena G, et al. Therapy with autologous adipose-derived regenerative cells for the care of chronic ulcer of lower limbs in patients with peripheral arterial disease. J Surg Res. 2013;185(1):36–44.
161. van Dongen J, Harmsen M, van der Lei B, Stevens H. Augmentation of dermal wound heal-

ing by adipose tissue-derived stromal cells (ASC). Bioengineering. 2018;5(4):91.
162. Nepal S, Venkataram A, Mysore V. The role of adipose tissue in hair regeneration: a potential tool for management? J Cutan Aesthet Surg. 2021;14(3):10.
163. Epstein GK, Epstein J, Nikolic J. Successful short-term hair transplantation results in two patients with primary scarring alopecia of the scalp pre-treated with autologous fat grafting. Dermatol Surg. 2021;47(5):729–31.
164. Simonacci F, Bertozzi N, Grieco MP, Raposio E. From liposuction to adipose-derived stem cells: indications and technique. Acta Bio Medica Atenei Parm. 2019;90(2):197–208.
165. Berry M, Davies D. Liposuction: a review of principles and techniques. J Plast Reconstr Amp Aesthetic Surg. 2011;64(8):985–92.
166. Illouz Y. Body contouring by lipolysis: a 5-year experience with over 3000 cases. Plast Reconstr Surg. 1983;72(5):591–7.
167. Klein JA. The tumescent technique: anesthesia and modified liposuction technique. Dermatol Clin. 1990;8(3):425–37.
168. Coleman SR. Structural fat grafting: more than a permanent filler. Plast Reconstr Surg. 2006;118(Suppl):108S–20S.
169. Kurita M, Matsumoto D, Shigeura T, Sato K, Gonda K, Harii K, et al. Influences of centrifugation on cells and tissues in liposuction aspirates: optimized centrifugation for lipotransfer and cell isolation. Plast Reconstr Surg. 2008;121(3):1033–41.
170. Dimitriou R, Mataliotakis GI, Angoules AG, Kanakaris NK, Giannoudis PV. Complications following autologous bone graft harvesting from the iliac crest and using the RIA: a systematic review. Injury. 2011;42:S3–15.

Body Sculpting

13

Marc J. Salzman

Abstract

HRUS is most useful to plastic surgeons in the surveillance of the integrity of silicone gel breast implants. HRUS is also being used to facilitate the diagnosis and aspiration seromas of the breast and abdomen. Reconstructive plastic surgeons have found HRUS useful in the planning of fasciocutaneous flap surgeries. This chapter explores how HRUS can help esthetically enhance plastic surgery procedures and help the procedures in their accuracy.

Keywords

HRUS · Breast implants · Fat grafting · Brazilian Buttock Lift · Fillers · Nerve block · Cellulite

13.1 Introduction

Plastic surgeons have been one of the last medical specialties to embrace the use of ultrasound in the care of their patients. High-resolution linear probes with frequencies in the 7–13 MHz range are commonly used for both diagnostic and therapeutic plastic surgical applications. The advent of portable ultrasound devices with acquisition costs in the $2000–$ 12,000 range have made the addition of high-resolution ultrasound (HRUS) more available to plastic surgeons. Wireless HRUS devices, which can more easily be used intraoperatively, have made it easier for plastic surgeons to utilize ultrasound to improve the accuracy of procedures such as fat grafting and the "Brazilian Buttock Lift."

13.2 HRUS for Breast Implants

One of the most commonly performed reconstructive or cosmetic plastic surgery procedures involves the placement of silicone gel breast implants. According to the American Society of Plastic Surgeons 2018 Plastic Surgery Statistics report, there were 101,657 breast reconstructions and 313,735 cosmetic breast augmentations performed in 2018 [1]. Breast implants all contain a silicone elastomer shell and can be filled with either saline or silicone gel (Fig. 13.1).

The vast majority of breast implants contain a single lumen or chamber. Other breast implant types that are clinically encountered have a dual lumen construct with either saline on the inside chamber and silicone gel within the outer or the reverse. These dual lumen breast implants allow for intraoperative adjustability of the size of the implant. The silicone elastomer can have either a textured or smooth surface (Fig. 13.2).

M. J. Salzman (✉)
Plastic Surgery, University of Louisville, Louisville, KY, USA
e-mail: mjs@itbecomesyou.com

R. L. Bard (ed.), *Image-Guided Aesthetic Treatments*, https://doi.org/10.1007/978-3-031-36266-8_13

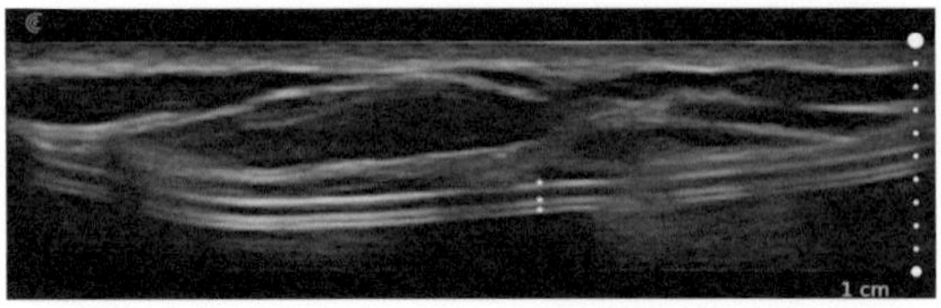

Fig. 13.1 Grayscale ultrasound image of smooth silicone gel breast implant. Top * represents the capsule surrounding the breast implant. The bottom pair of * represent the elastomer shell of the breast implant

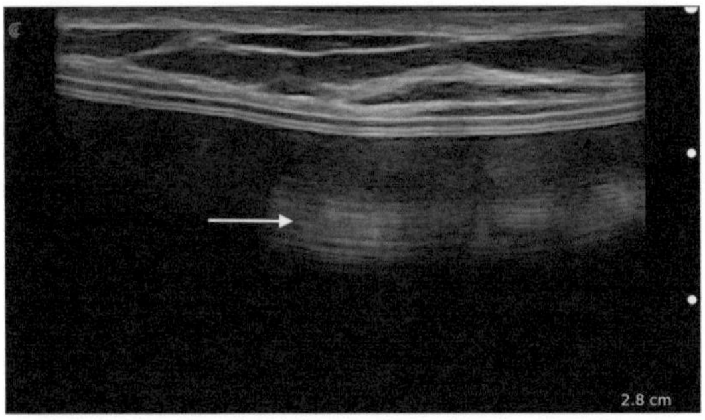

Fig. 13.2 Grayscale ultrasound image of smooth silicone gel breast implant. Arrow shows reverberation artifact of implant elastomer shell

The thickness of the silicone elastomer shell varies from less than a millimeter to just over 2 mm. Almost all silicone gel breast implants are formed over a dome-shaped mandrel and are filled with silicone gel through an opening on the posterior surface of the implant. This posterior opening is covered with a thicker segment of a silicone patch that is glued to the surface of the shell during the last stages of the manufacturing process. A relative newcomer to the choice in breast implant construction is the structured saline implant (Ideal Implant, Dallas, Texas) (Fig. 13.3).

A structured saline implant contains two saline filled chambers and a series of internal implant shells nested together. Breast implants can be round or shaped. Modern breast implants are made with varying height to base width ratios allowing for multiple choices to meet the needs of a myriad of anatomical corrections. Breast implants can be placed below the pectoralis major muscle (submuscular), below the fascia overlying the pectoralis major muscle (subfascial) or above the fascia of the pectoralis major muscle

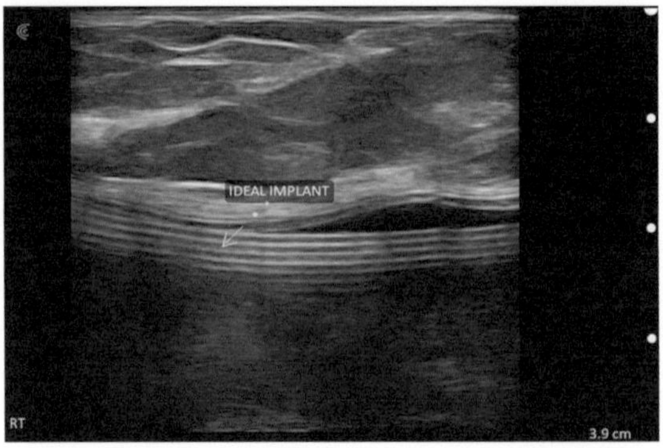

Fig. 13.3 Grayscale ultrasound image of a structured saline implant (Ideal implant, Dallas, Texas) showing a shell within a shell configuration

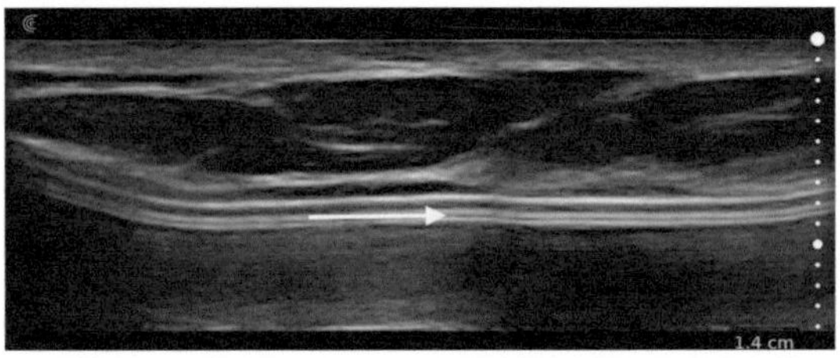

Fig. 13.4 Grayscale ultrasound image of smooth silicone gel breast implant. Arrow depicts the elastomer shell with smooth contour

(subglandular). Common access incisions for placement of breast implants include the inframammary crease, periareolar margin, axilla, and umbilicus. After the placement of breast implants, the body forms a fibrous capsule around the implant. Breast implants have been used since the 1960s [2]. Early generation silicone gel breast implants had very thin elastomeric shells and a honey-like internal gel consistency. The unpolymerized silicone gel could leak through the implant shell and migrate into the surrounding breast capsule (silicone gel bleed). Because of the high rupture rate of this type of implant, later generations of silicone gel implants have an internal barrier to gel diffusion and have a thicker gel consistency due to the higher amount of cross-linked silicone. Breast implant manufacturers have an array of breast implant softness or "feel" that the implant can have based on the ratio of polymerized to unpolymerized gel (Figs. 13.4 and 13.5).

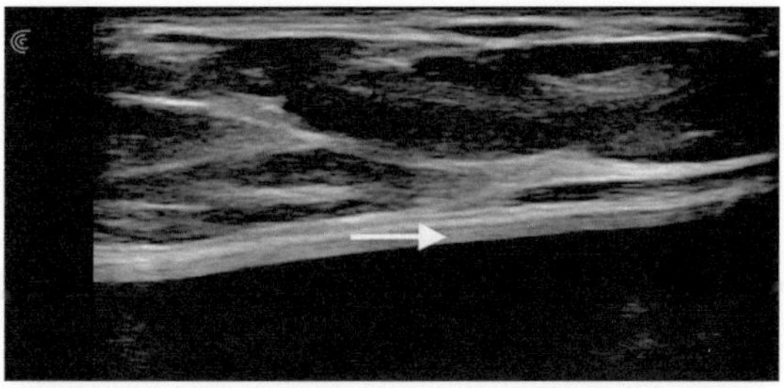

Fig. 13.5 Grayscale ultrasound image of textured silicone gel breast implant. Arrow depicts the elastomer shell with fuzzy contour

Higher cross-linked amounts of silicone cause a firmer feel. Newer, 5th generation silicone gel breast implants are all classified as containing a cohesive gel or "gummy bear" consistency. The failure rate of silicone breast implants has been described [3–5]. Symptoms of silicone breast implant rupture can include capsular contracture, distortion of implant shape, neurogenic pain, a palpable lump, or an axillary mass. Many of the silicone gel breast implant failures are "silent," and the patient has no symptoms and no visible or palpable changes on physical exam. In 1992, because of a suspicion of a relationship between silicone gel breast implants and autoimmune disease, a moratorium was placed by the U.S. Food and Drug Administration (FDA) on the use of silicone gel breast implants for breast augmentation [6]. This decision was reversed in 2006 [7]. One of the concerns of the FDA was the detection of "silent rupture" of silicone gel breast implants. For that reason, the FDA recommended that patients having silicone gel breast implants have an MRI at 3 years post implantation and every 2 years thereafter [8]. MRI is costly and inconvenient for surveillance of the integrity of silicone breast implants. At the FDA General and Plastic Surgery Panel in March 2019, the American College of Radiology reported on the ACR Appropriateness Criteria that MRI for asymptomatic women with silicone gel breast implants is not recommended and that consideration should be made for recommendation of later and less often screening with ultrasound [9]. The ability of ultrasound to diagnose rupture of silicone gel breast implants has been compared in the literature to MRI and mammography [10–14]. Because of the inability of mammography to visualize the internal aspects of the silicone gel breast implant, the sensitivity of mammography in detecting silicone gel breast implant rupture reported at a range of 11–69% is higher for extracapsular rupture [15–19]. The reported sensitivity of ultrasound for the detection of a rupture of a silicone gel breast implant is reported at a range of 30–75% [10, 12–14, 18, 20]. Ultrasound is more likely to correctly predict when a silicone gel breast implant is intact with reported negative predictive values of 50–90% [21].

With lower cost, convenience, and availability within the plastic surgeons' office, ultrasound is a better first screening tool in examining the plastic surgery breast implant patient than an MRI. An economic analysis of screening tests for the detection of ruptured silicone gel breast implants done at the University of Michigan suggested that considering the costs and diagnostic accuracy of ultrasound compared to MRI, it was concluded that initial screening with ultrasound followed by MRI was best in asymptomatic patients, and ultrasound was the preferred screening modality in symptomatic women [22].

13.3 The Breast Implant Exam

It may be useful prior to beginning the ultrasound evaluation of breast implants to inquire what type of breast implant was placed. Occasionally, the patient might retain the breast implant card provided to them at the time of their surgery with the information about the manufacturing company, size, type, shape, and volume of their implants. After multiple prior breast implant surgeries, the patient's recollection of the implant specifics may be unreliable. The patient lays in the supine position with the arm over her head. A high-frequency linear probe, 7–15 MHz, is used to scan all four quadrants of the breast. Slightly lower frequencies in the 5–7.5 MHz range may be used for larger breasts and to better image the posterior portion of the breast implant. Attempt is made to scan with the probe oriented transversely with the angle of ultrasound beam directed perpendicular to the surface of the shell/capsule interface. When examining the surface of the breast implant, depth of the scan is superficial such that the shell/capsule interface lies in the near field to increase visualization of small imperfections in the shell. Depth can then be increased to best visualize the posterior surface of the implant along the chest wall. Breast implants with suggested pathology such as folds or loss of continuity of the elastomer shell should have compression images and videos taken with pressure applied from the opposite side of the imaging quadrant in attempt to unfurl the fold or visualize separation of the shell at the sight of discontinuity. The ability of the sonologist to manipulate the image with pressure application is one of the advantages of ultrasound over the static image achieved by MRI. The lateral border of the pectoralis major muscle and axilla should be scanned for lymph nodes containing silicone.

13.4 The Normal Silicone Breast Implant

In the unbroken, single lumen silicone gel breast implant, the double-line echogenic elastomer shell is seen just below the echogenic fibrous capsule. This creates the normal trilaminar line seen in the unbroken silicone breast implant. The outermost echogenic line corresponds to the breast implant capsule. The middle echogenic line is a fusion of the inner aspect of the breast capsule and the outer aspect of the breast implant elastomer shell. The innermost echogenic line represents the inner aspect of the elastomer shell [23]. A small amount of fluid with some mild echogenicity can usually be seen between the fibrous breast capsule and the elastomer shell of the implant. Textured surface implants will sometimes have more of this normal fluid interface than a smooth walled device. Breast implant placement can be under the gland (subglandular), below the pectoralis major muscle (subpectoral), or less frequently below the fascia of the pectoralis major (subfascial). The inferior aspect of the subpectoral breast implant will extend below the inferior border of the pectoralis muscle and lie above the rectus abdominis and serratus fascias but below the breast gland. The periprosthetic breast implant capsule can be located below or above the pectoralis muscle depending upon the plane of implant placement and position of ultrasound probe relative to the inferior border of the pectoralis muscle. Inside the unbroken, normal implant, just below the elastomer shell, reverberation artifact is represented by echogenic parallel lines seen below the shell. In comparison to the "subcapsular sign" representing collapse of a portion the elastomer shell into the gel of the interior of the implant, the reverberation artifact echogenic lines seen below the elastomer shell of the implant tend to be parallel to the shell, of similar length to each other and fairly evenly spaced apart from each other [24]. Often, these artifactual echogenic lines can be reduced in the image with application of less pressure on the transducer over the implant. The remaining interior of the implant appears mostly anechoic. The anterior and side aspects of the implant shell can usually be visualized. The posterior wall of the implant may be difficult to assess. Ultrasound images of smooth and textured implants can usually be differentiated. The smooth wall device is seen to be more sharply demarcated from the underlying anechoic gel. The textured device appears to be fuzzier in appearance and thicker than its smooth counterpart. Breast implants, despite being placed properly into the surgically created pocket in an upright position, can spontaneously flip upside down such that the posterior patch now lies in the more anterior position and can be visualized easily by HRUS. On ultrasound, the upside-down breast implant image shows an overlap of a double echogenic line representing the elastomer shell overlying a slightly thicker, single echogenic line representing the posterior patch. The consistent distance of the overlap is symmetric with the opposite side of the patch. This symmetry of overlap and single line echogenic structure of the patch separates this otherwise normal implant from the "subcapsular line" of the broken silicone gel breast implant (Fig. 13.6).

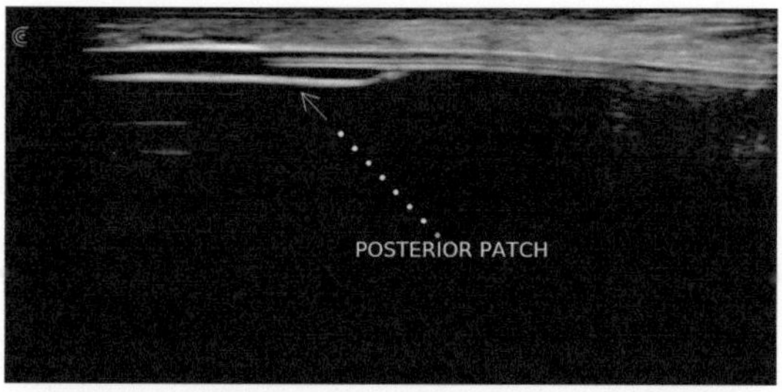

Fig. 13.6 Grayscale ultrasound image of the posterior patch of a silicone gel breast implant

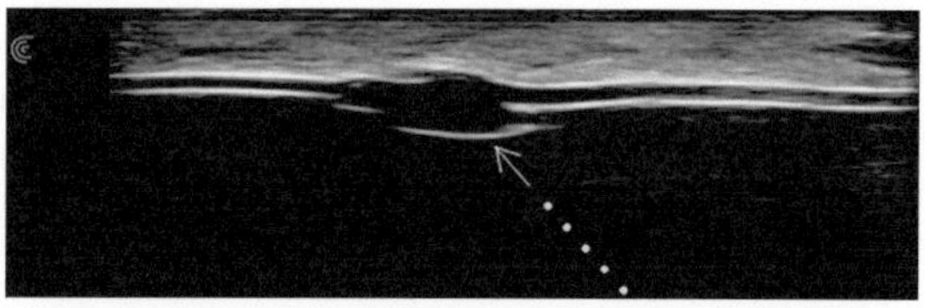

Fig. 13.7 Grayscale ultrasound image of smooth saline filled breast implant. Arrow shows the filling valve on the anterior surface of the implant

13.5 Saline and Structured Saline Breast Implants

Saline breast implants are made from the same elastomer shell as silicone breast implants. Rather than being filled with a silicone gel, these implants are filled with sterile saline. Saline implants contain a filling valve on the anterior surface of the implant, which is readily identifiable by ultrasound. The valve appears as a discontinuous outer shell with a saucer-shaped echogenic line just below the anterior surface of the shell. A new type of saline breast implant is referred to as being a "structured saline implant." These implants contain more than one saline filled chamber and each chamber has its own filling port. One port is on the anterior surface of the shell and the other on the posterior (Fig. 13.7).

The structured saline breast implant has a distinctive ultrasound appearance of an implant within an implant. The peripheral edge of a saline implant will differ in ultrasound appearance from that of a silicone gel filled elastomer. Because of the slowing ultrasound waves as they travel through silicone gel compared to saline, the soft tissues seen posterior to the silicone gel implant seem to appear to be further away creating a "step off phenomena." Broken saline breast implants do not represent the diagnostic challenge of a broken silicone gel breast implant. Most commonly, saline implant failures become self-evident in a matter of day as the saline within the lumen of the implant escapes the confines of the elastomer as the implant collapses from volume loss. On ultrasound, the broken saline breast implant is seen as a series of superimposed echogenic lines with a variable amount of anechoic

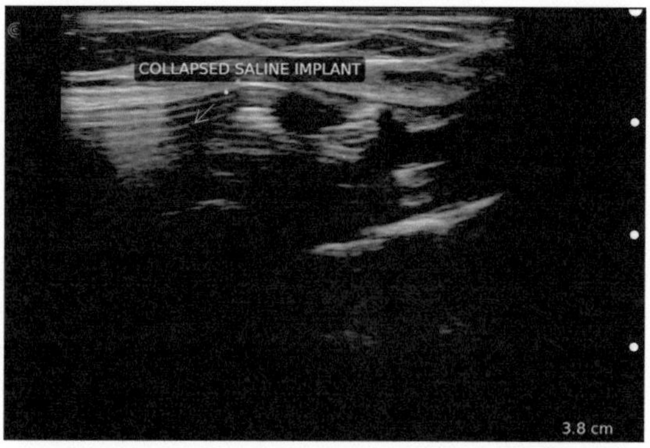

Fig. 13.8 Grayscale ultrasound image showing a saline breast implant that has collapsed with loss of most of its saline volume

space between representing retained saline within the elastomer. HRUS can be helpful in intraoperative localization of the collapsed broken saline implant (Fig. 13.8).

The periprosthetic breast capsule can retract to accommodate the decreased volume of the broken saline breast implant. This can make it difficult for the plastic surgeon to locate the implant through an infra-mammary crease approach as the broken saline implant migrates upward towards the axilla. Using HRUS during the procedure, the plastic surgeon can better adjust the plane of dissection to more easily locate the broken implant.

13.6 Ultrasound Imaging of Broken Silicone Gel Breast Implants

The incidence of silicone breast implant rupture is presently unknown. Older silicone gel breast implants with thin elastomeric shells and honey-like gel viscosity are known to have rupture rates of 50% at 12 years or more since implantation [25]. Rupture rates with newer 5th generation silicone gel breast implants have improved to 10–14% at 8–10 years post implantation [26]. Breast implant rupture can be contained within the fibrous capsule surrounding the implant and is called intracapsular rupture. Should the implant filler silicone gel migrate beyond the confines of the fibrous capsule, this is termed extracapsular rupture. Seventy-seven to eighty nine percentage of silicone gel breast implant ruptures are intracapsular and are usually asymptomatic [15]. In older, thin elastomer shell implants filled with a less cohesive gel, one of the ultrasound signs of implant failure is the "stepladder sign" [13, 24, 27–34]. The stepladder sign on HRUS appears as a series of multiple, discontinuous linear echoes representing the folding of the elastomer shell into the inside of the silicone gel of the implant (Fig. 13.9).

This corresponds to the "linguine sign" seen on MRI. As silicone gel extravasates beyond the confines of the elastomer shell, it may come into contact with fluid surrounding the implant. The ensuing phase aberration of the ultrasound beam causes the silicone gel to take on a "snowstorm" appearance [28, 35] (Fig. 13.10).

This snowstorm appearing gel can be seen in both intracapsular implant failure as well as silicone blebs seen outside of the fibrous capsule and silicone filled lymph nodes seen along the lateral border of the pectoralis major and in the axilla. Another commonly seen sign of intracapsular rupture is the "noose" or "keyhole" [36, 37] (Fig. 13.11).

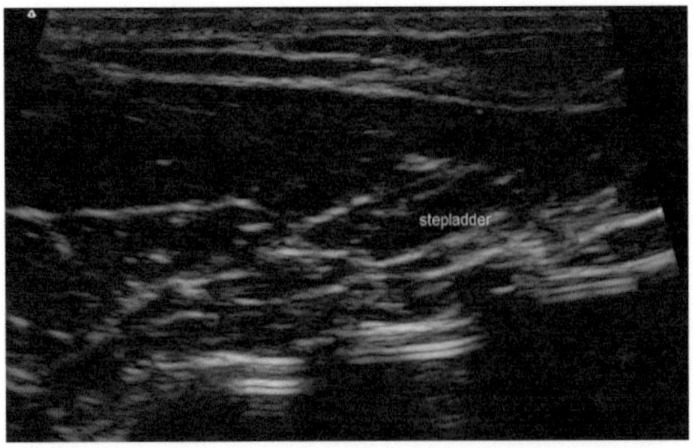

Fig. 13.9 Grayscale ultrasound image of broken silicone gel breast implant exhibiting the stepladder sign

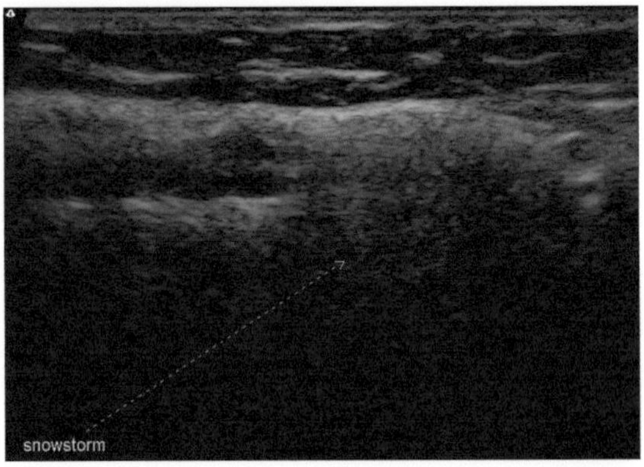

Fig. 13.10 Grayscale ultrasound image of broken silicone gel breast implant exhibiting the snowstorm sign

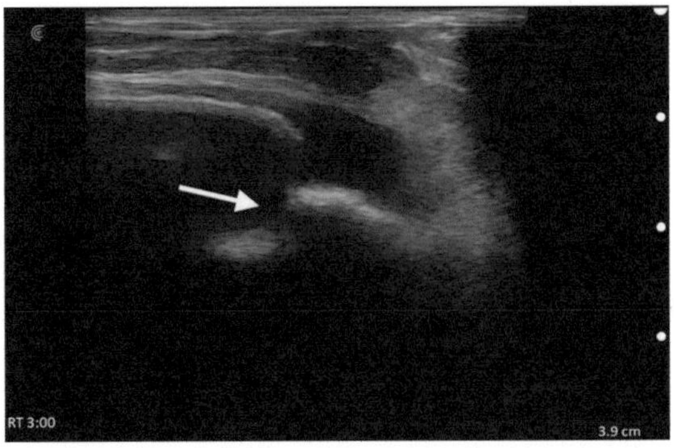

Fig. 13.11 Grayscale ultrasound image of broken silicone gel breast implant exhibiting the keyhole sign. Arrow depicts the midportion of the keyhole

Seen more often in older, less cohesive silicone gel implants, the in-folding of the implant elastomer shell produces a fold which can allow the internal silicone gel to escape through small disruptions of the elastomer shell and occupy the apex of the fold. One of the advantages of using HRUS in the evaluation of possible silicone gel breast implant failure in comparison to MRI is the dynamic nature of the HRUS exam. Using HRUS, the sonographer has the ability to change the configuration of the shell of the implant by the placement of extrinsic pressure on the implant. The finding of a deep fold in an implant may look like a "Noose or Keyhole sign" until extrinsic pressure is applied opposite the fold. As the shell distends and unfolds, the sonographer

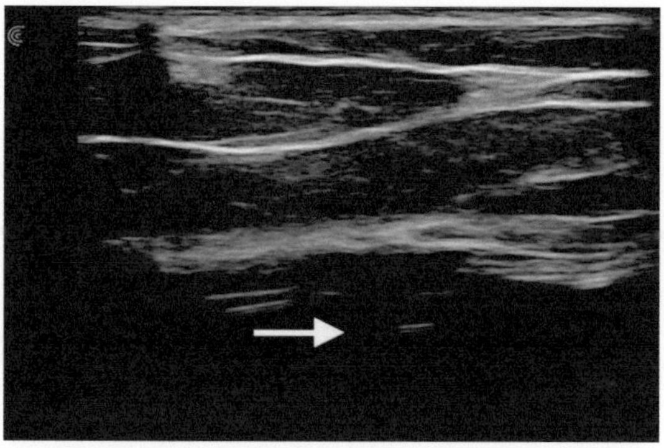

Fig. 13.12 Grayscale ultrasound image of broken silicone gel breast implant exhibiting the subcapsular sign. Arrow depicts the fragment of elastomer

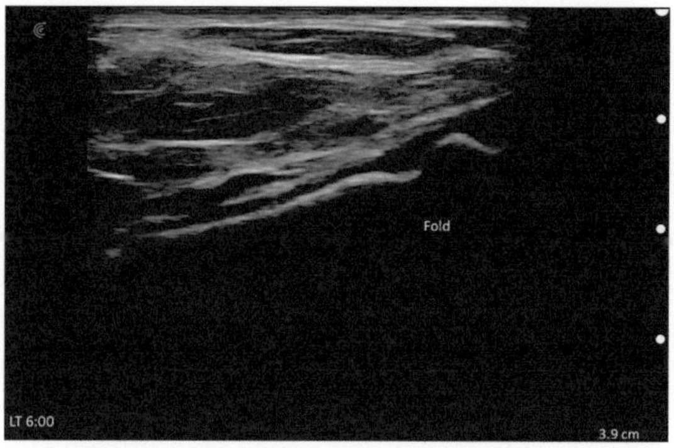

Fig. 13.13 Grayscale ultrasound image of a silicone gel breast implant exhibiting the wavy folds of the elastomer shell

may be able to visualize a filling out of the fold. The actual continuity of the shell would suggest that this is merely a fold and the implant is actually intact. The elastomer shell may fragment with pieces of the shell appearing within the internal silicone gel as a linear echogenic line. This linear echo is referred to as the "subcapsular line" [29, 38–41] (Fig. 13.12).

In the situation where there is complete or near complete collapse of the elastomer shell, the segment of shell embedded into the depths of the remaining silicone gel may be deeper than can be visualized with high-frequency transducers. It may be necessary to image the deeper aspect of the silicone gel breast implant with lower frequencies [42].

13.7 Mimic Signs of Intracapsular Rupture

There are several ultrasound findings that may confound the diagnosis of a ruptured silicone gel breast implant. One of the more common findings seen in an intact silicone gel implant is a fold (Fig. 13.13).

Until the most recent iteration of cohesive silicone gel implants, most implants were not filled to the maximum capacity of the silicone elastomer shell. This would allow for some collapse of the implant shell along the periphery of the implant. Normal folds can have either an anechoic or mildly echoic fluid between the implant shell and the fibrous capsule. In the presence of capsular contracture, where the breast periprosthetic fibrous capsule becomes tight and nondistensible, numerous folds may be visualized. In the situation of a tight capsular contracture, an infolding of the breast implant may be so deep that the ultrasound appearance may appear to be a "keyhole" or "noose" sign giving a false positive ultrasound reading of a broken silicone gel implant. Long standing silicone gel implant capsules may become calcified. This will present as areas of higher echogenicity within the fibrous capsule. Scattered, fine calcifications may not obscure visualization of the breast implant elastomer. More dense, confluent calcifications may cause acoustic shadowing and obscure the normal trilaminar appearance of the shell–capsule interface making diagnosis of rupture difficult (Fig. 13.14).

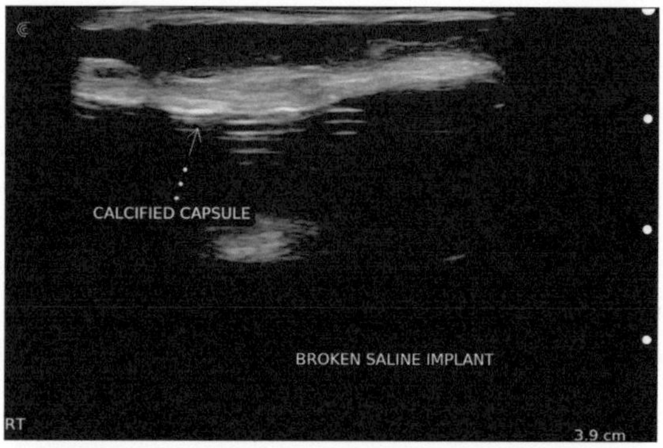

Fig. 13.14 Grayscale ultrasound image of broken saline breast implant with a hyperechoic appearance of the implant capsule suggesting calcification of the capsule

Over time, newer, highly cohesive silicone gel implants may develop changes to the structure of the internal gel while maintaining the integrity of the elastomer shell. Gel fractures or gel bubbles may occur within the internal gel of the implant (Fig. 13.15). The normal anechoic internal gel of the implant may contain echogenic areas within the implant fill material. The ultrasound images of these cohesive gel changes within the internal confines of the implant may mimic the "stepladder" or "subcapsular line" seen with broken silicone gel implants. These internal echoes with an overlying intact shell are poor predictors of the loss of shell integrity. Gel bubbles can also mimic the appearance of a broken silicone gel breast implant. The differentiating clue is the consistent width of a reverberation-type artifact appearance seen just below an intact overlying elastomer shell (Fig. 13.16). Seen in an ex vivo implant, the reverberations take on a cylindrical appearance matching the dimensions of the bubble (Figs. 13.15 and 13.16).

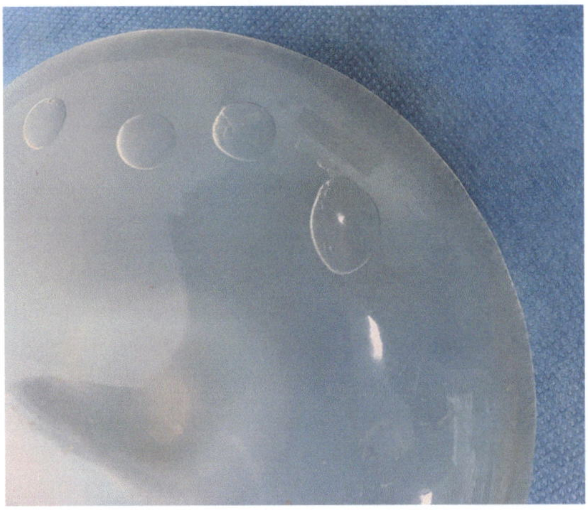

Fig. 13.15 Silicone gel breast implant with bubbles within the internal gel. The elastomer shell is intact

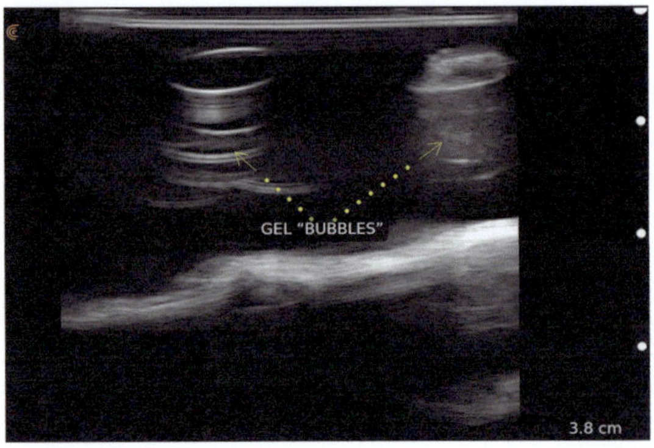

Fig. 13.16 Grayscale ultrasound image of an ex vivo silicone gel breast implant exhibiting echogenic swirling lines indicative of gel bubbles

13.8 Shaped Breast Implant Rotation

Silicone and saline breast implants can be manufactured in both round and anatomically shaped configurations. The Allergan 410 (silicone gel) and 468 (saline) have orientation "knobs" of an additional thicker silicone elastomer strategically placed on the anterior surface of the implant to aid the plastic surgeon in vertical alignment of the implant in the pocket (Fig. 13.17).

These orientation "knobs" can be visualized with HRUS on the anterior surface of the implant. Although the implant may have been orientated vertically during its initial insertion, these implants may rotate causing a distortion of the look of the augmented breast. HRUS may be used to locate the orientation "knobs." By transposing the location of both of the orientation "knobs" found on HRUS to the skin, an assessment of the rotation of the implant from vertically can be determined.

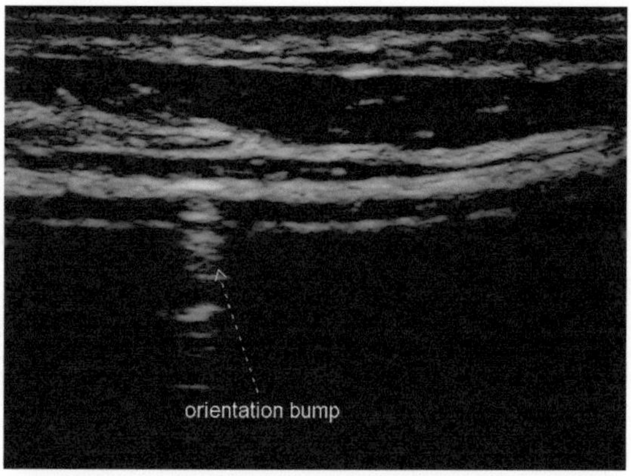

Fig. 13.17 Grayscale ultrasound image of a shaped Allergan 410 silicone gel breast showing the orientation bump on the surface of the elastomer. Posterior acoustic shadowing is seen below the echogenic line indicating the location of the palpable bump

13.9 Capsular Contracture

One of the known common adverse outcomes of the placement of breast implants is the formation of an unyielding fibrous capsule surrounding the breast implant called capsular contracture [42, 43] (Fig. 13.18).

The Baker classification is used to describe fibrous breast implant capsules [44]. Grade 1 capsules allow for a normal feeling and appearing breast. Grade 2 capsules feel more firm than normal. Grade 3 capsules feel firmer and make for a visible distortion of breast shape. A Grade 4 capsule has the characteristics of a Grade 3 capsule and adds the fact that the patient experiences pain as well. The most commonly seen finding on HRUS for a breast implant with capsular contracture is folds. There may be a series of multiple folds or a single deep fold. HRUS is used by plastic surgeons in the evaluation of capsular contracture. Capsular contracture does not usually appear for many months to years after breast implant placement. Patients will sometimes be seen and complain of a breast implant that remained high on the chest wall and never dropped into the more desired position where the middle of the implant corresponded to the overlying nipple. In submuscular implant placement, the post-surgical subsequent tightening of the pectoralis major muscle will disallow gravitational descent of the breast implant. HRUS can be used to evaluate early capsular contracture and distinguish inherent thickening and lack of distensibility of the capsule (true capsular contracture) from incomplete division of the rib origins of the pectoralis major muscle which leave muscle fibers below the mid portion of the implant thereby holding it higher on the chest wall than its more inferior desired position. By scanning the medial aspect of the breast implant capsule at the level of the areola, the point of transition of the submuscular and subglandular position of the breast implant can be visualized and compared to the side with the correct implant position (Fig. 13.19).

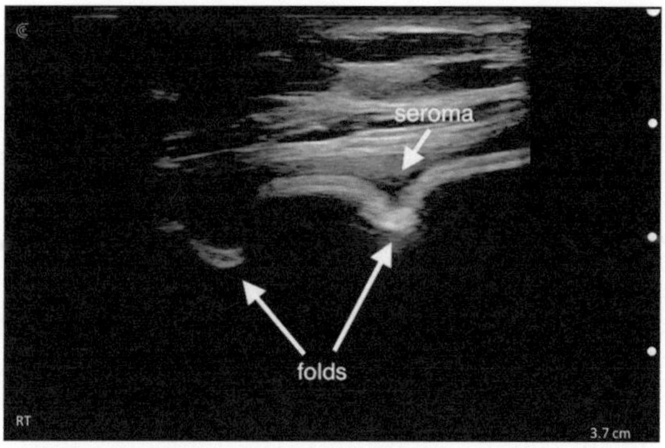

Fig. 13.18 Grayscale ultrasound image of a breast implant exhibiting capsular contracture. Multiple folds and a small amount of seroma are seen

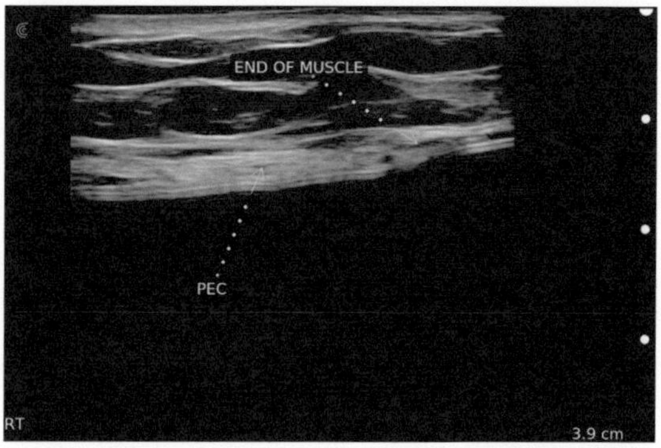

Fig. 13.19 Grayscale ultrasound image of a breast implant imaged at the medial border of the implant at the level of the mid portion of the areola. The transition of the implant from the submuscular to the subglandular position is demonstrated

Based on the visualization of the level of muscle division being different on the affected side, the plastic surgeon may decide to divide some of the muscle origins of the pectoralis muscle as well as the capsule in an attempt to lower the involved implant.

13.10 Seroma and Hematoma

Small fluid collections surrounding breast implants can occur in the absence of any pathology. Anechoic or slightly diffuse hyperechoic fluid collections can be visualized between the capsule surrounding the implant and the elastomer shell. These small seromas may be seen relatively soon after implantation of implants or any surgical manipulation of the breast implant capsule such as a capsulotomy, capsulectomy, or capsulorraphies. Late seroma, 1 year or more after breast implant placement occur in 0.1–0.2% of textured silicone gel breast implants [45] (Fig. 13.20).

Etiology of breast implant seroma can be post traumatic, post-surgical, infectious, idiopathic, or rarely due to breast implant-associated (BIA) anaplastic large cell lymphoma (ALCL). BIA-ALCL is a rare T cell lymphoma that presents a delayed periprosthetic fluid collection (60–90%) or a capsular mass (40%) at an average of 8–10 years after textured breast implant placement [46]. The cases are almost evenly split between post reconstructive and cosmetic placement of textured breast implants. Late breast implant seromas will require evacuation. Ultrasound is useful to allow visualization of the breast implant during breast seroma aspiration. The patient is placed in the supine position on the bed with the head slightly elevated to allow gravitational descent of the fluid. The breast implant is pushed upward and away from the site of needle penetration, usually at the inframammary crease. Various types of needles such as the Veress® needle [47], Sonosite® needle, and blunt cannulas such as the Seromacath® [48] have been described as being useful and safe for periprosthetic fluid aspiration. A linear high-frequency probe (9–14 MHz) is used (Fig. 13.21).

The ultrasound transducer is placed on the skin of the breast overlying the needle and oriented as parallel to the plane of the needle as possible. This is termed the "in-plane technique." Some HRUS devices have a software enhancement of the underlying needle making it easier to visualize. As the plane of the transducer moves away from parallel to the plane of the needle, only portions of the needle may be visualized. Because of the importance of visualization of the tip of the needle in order to best avoid penetration of the implant shell, enhancements of the external geometry of needles such as the Sonosite® allow reflection of the ultrasound waves at sharper angles such that needle visualization is improved at steep beam

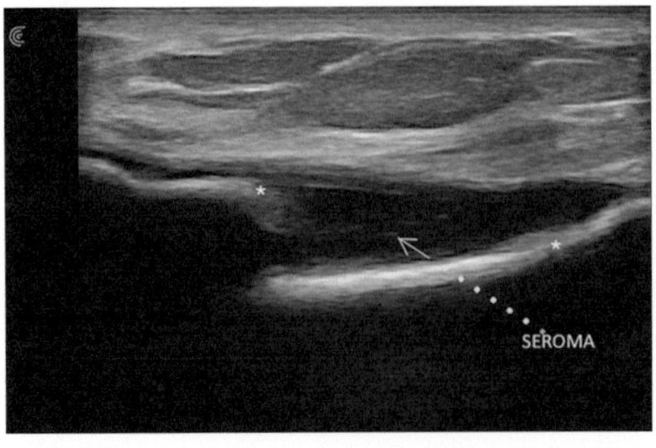

Fig. 13.20 Grayscale ultrasound image of a broken silicone gel breast implant with mostly anechoic fluid between the elastomer shell and the periprosthetic capsule. * denotes the elastomer shell

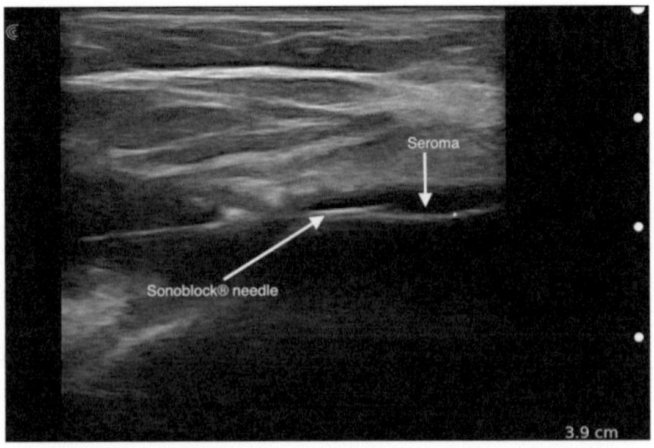

Fig. 13.21 Grayscale ultrasound image of a breast implant seroma being aspirated with a needle. * denotes the elastomer shell of the breast implant

angles. Examination of the fluid aspirate includes culture and sensitivity for infectious etiology and CD30 immunohistochemistry for the diagnosis of BIA-ALCL. At least 50 mL of fluid is necessary for CD30 testing. Ultrasound may be useful in the evaluation of the swollen breast in the immediate postoperative time period. In mastopexy with breast implant placement, there are two potential cavities in which blood or fluid may collect. Early hematoma after mastopexy with implants can appear in the subcutaneous tissue surrounding the areola or within the newly established pocket created for the breast implant. Ultrasound is useful in separating the diffuse echogenic soft tissue appearance of edema from an actual collection of fluid. Seromas will appear anechoic on ultrasound, while a hematoma may have areas of echogenicity within a mostly anechoic space. New hematomas may be difficult to evacuate through a small-bore cannula or needle because of the semi-solid nature of the blood. After clot retraction takes place naturally over a 7–10-day period of time, the ultrasound image becomes less echogenic and takes on the look of an anechoic seroma. At this point in time, the more liquid consistency of the seroma makes HRUS guided aspiration easier.

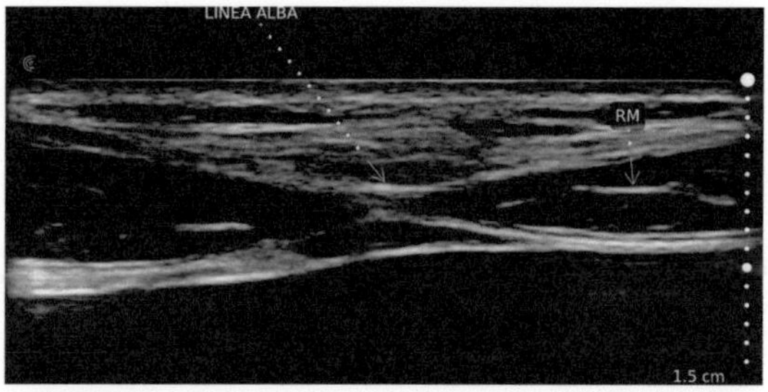

Fig. 13.22 Grayscale ultrasound image of the normal appearance of the abdominal midline with transducer oriented transversely just above the umbilicus. RM is rectus abdominis muscle

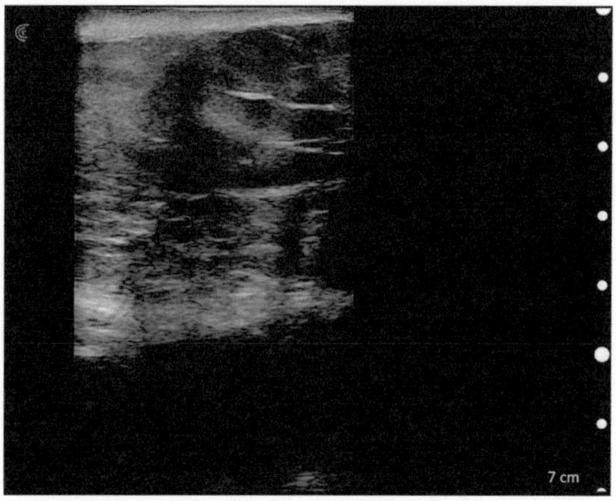

Fig. 13.23 Grayscale ultrasound image of edema of the abdominal wall. Diffuse hyperechoic shadows obscure the normal hypoechoic soft tissue

13.11 Abdomen

The typical ultrasound appearance of the unoperated abdomen, with the transducer in the transverse orientation over the midline replicates the appearance of a “bowtie.” The confluence of the anterior rectus fascia from each side form the linea alba of the rectus abdominis as its center and the sides of the “bowtie” represent the splitting of the anterior and posterior fascias as they separate to include the rectus abdominis muscle within (Fig. 13.22).

HRUS evaluation of anterior abdomen in the plastic surgical patient considering abdominoplasty or suction-assisted lipectomy of anterior abdominal wall may be a useful adjunct to physical exam in detecting unrecognized ventral hernias. Where separation of the midline fascia is seen, a Valsalva maneuver may reveal escape of preperitoneal fat or actual peritoneal contents such as small bowel through the fascial opening. HRUS has demonstrated to be useful in the evaluation of the postoperative body contouring patient. When patients present with a contour deformity after plastic surgery of the trunk, the question that needs to be addressed is whether this represents edema or a collection of blood or serum. The ultrasound image of edema is easily recognized as a diffuse, homogeneous increase in echogenicity throughout the entire image (Fig. 13.23)

In contrast to the image of edema, the HRUS image of a seroma is that of a well-demarcated anechoic area within the surgical area and corresponds to the visual location of the contour deformity (Fig. 13.24).

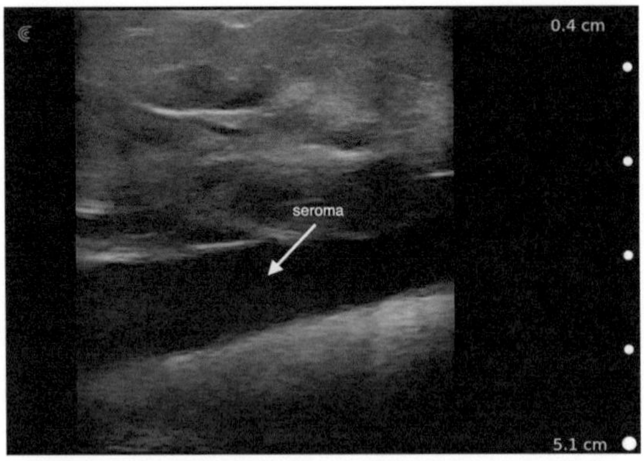

Fig. 13.24 Grayscale ultrasound image of a seroma of the anterior abdominal wall

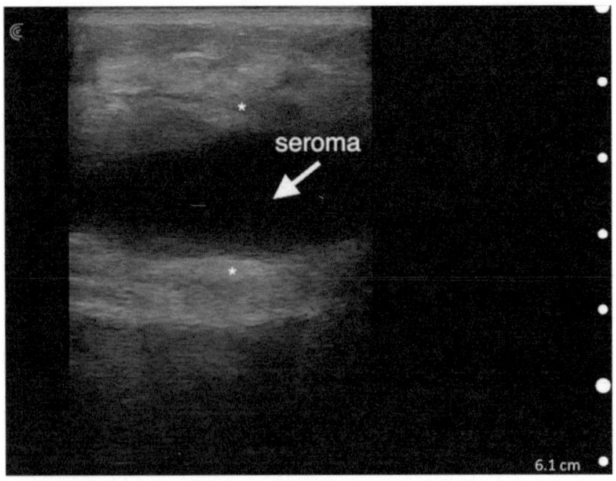

Fig. 13.25 Grayscale ultrasound image of a pseudo-bursae of the anterior abdominal wall. * denotes the hyperechoic hyalinized thickened tissue surrounding the fluid

Abdominal seromas can be easily aspirated under HRUS guidance. Using sterile technique, an ultrasound enhancing needle such as the Sonosite® can be inserted using an "in-plane" technique to aspirate the seroma. Post aspiration ultrasound can confirm the removal of the seroma and follow-up ultrasounds can be done to confirm that the seroma does not reoccur. Recurrent seromas, despite successful serial aspirations, may allow for a thickened scar capsule to surround the seroma cavity. The internal lining becomes hyalinized and continues to produce fluid. These persistent seromas are called pseudo-bursae. HRUS imaging of a mature pseudo-bursae shows an echogenic capsule surrounding an anechoic center (Fig. 13.25).

Minimally invasive techniques such as injections of a sclerosant solution into the pseudo-burse have been described. Should these minimally invasive procedures not be successful in eliminating the pseudo-bursae, a surgical approach may become necessary. Complete excision of the pseudo-bursae with subsequent elimination of the dead space between the abdominal fascia and the overlying fat is usually curative in restoring the normal contours of the trunk.

HRUS has shown to be helpful in marking the patient prior to high-definition liposuction. In high-definition liposuction, the goal is to accentuate the visualization of the underlying musculature of the abdomen, chest, or extremities. The muscle interfaces such as the plica semilunaris, where the external abdominal oblique muscle attaches to the lateral aspect of the rectus abdominis can be visualized with HRUS. The rectus abdominis has transverse thickened areas of fascia that correspond to the location of vascular perforators. These inscriptions can be visualized with HRUS and marked in the overlying skin to indicate an area where more fat will be removed. While transition zones between muscles can then be accentuated with more superficial fat removal, the addition of fat into the muscle can accentuate its visibility through the skin. HRUS can be used during the fat grafting procedure to visualize the direct transfer of the fat graft to the intramuscular position.

13.12 Nerve Blocks

Regional nerve blocks, once only performed by anesthesia providers, can also be administered to plastic surgery patients by the plastic surgeon using HRUS. The 2 most commonly done HRUS-guided nerve blocks done by plastic surgeons are the pectoralis nerve block (PECS block) and the transversus abdominis plane block (TAP block). The placement of breast tissue expanders for post mastectomy breast reconstruction and breast implants for cosmetic enhancement of the breast both can be done with placement of the prosthesis under the pectoralis muscle.

The post procedure spasm of the pectoralis major muscle can lead to a painful experience for the patient and can delay the descent of the breast prosthesis into the more desired, inferior aspect of the submuscular pocket. The pectoralis major and minor muscles are innervated by the medial and lateral pectoral nerves. The lateral pectoral nerve originates from the lateral cord of the brachial plexus (C5, C6, C7). It penetrates the clavipectoral fascia to directly innervate the pectoralis major muscle. The medial pectoral nerve originates from the medial cord of the brachial plexus (C8, T1). It penetrates the deep surface of the pectoralis minor muscle, traverses this muscle, and innervates the pectoralis major muscle from its deep surface. The original PECS block was first described by Blanco [49]. He described a cranial to caudal approach over the clavicle with a linear probe. Using a high-resolution linear probe, the thoraco-acromial artery was located with color Doppler in the fascial plane between the pectoralis major and minor muscles. The lateral pectoral nerve travels in the fascial plane between the pectoralis major and minor muscles along with the thoraco-acromial artery. A 50 mm ultrasound block needle was inserted with an "in-plane" technique through the pectoralis muscle and into the fascial plane between the pectoralis major and minor muscles. Levobupivacaine 0.25% was injected at a volume of 0.4 mL/kg. Perez described an alternative approach at the lateral third of the clavicle with the transducer aligned perpendicular to the axis of the body and passing the needle from medial to lateral after locating the thoraco-acromial artery [50]. The author has described another approach called the lateral approach pectoralis block (LAP). In this method, the ultrasound needle is passed in plane from under the lateral border of the pectoralis major muscle toward the previously located thoraco-acromial artery in a lateral to medial direction. After needle visualization in the fascial plane between the pectoralis major and minor muscles, a test dose of normal saline will confirm the correct location with an anechoic space that separates the two muscles (Fig. 13.26)

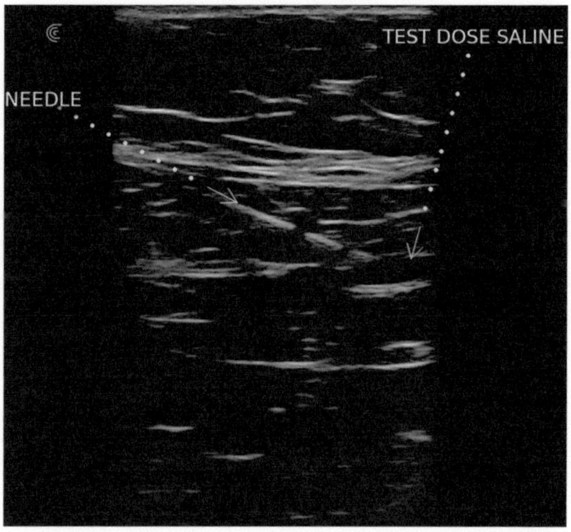

Fig. 13.26 Grayscale ultrasound image of chest wall showing Sonoblock® needle in the space between pectoralis major and minor muscles. A test dose of saline is injected producing an anechoic space between the muscles

The local anesthetic is then deposited in the plane between the pectoralis major and minor muscles along the entire path of the needle from the lateral border of the pectoralis major to the location of the lateral pectoral nerve. This approach has several advantages. It can be done from the side of the bed while the anesthesia provider is attending to tasks at the head. The path of the needle deposits the local anesthetic over the perforating branches of the medial pectoral nerve as they pierce the undersurface of the pectoralis major for an improved block of the inferior aspect of the pectoralis major muscle (Fig. 13.27).

The original PECS block can be augmented with a second injection (PECS 2) placed between the pectoralis minor and serratus anterior muscles. The PECS 2 block adds anesthesia to the lateral chest wall and axilla by blocking intercostal nerves 3–6, intercostobrachial and long thoracic nerves. The PECS blocks have been shown to be effective in lowering visual analog pain scores as well as opiate requirements after breast surgeries [51–53].

HRUS can also be used to provide anesthesia to plastic surgery procedures performed on the anterior abdominal wall. This block can be useful

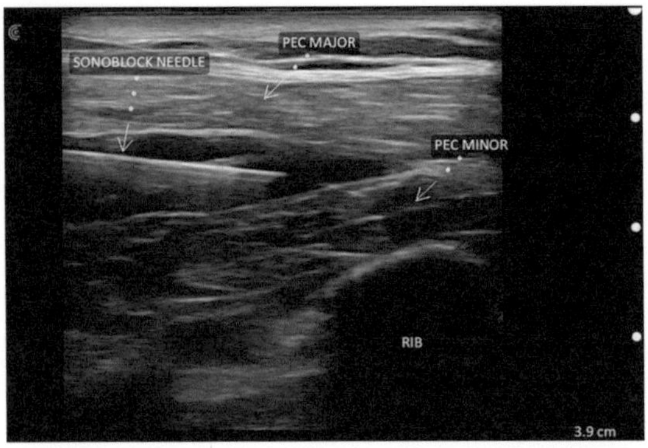

Fig. 13.27 Grayscale ultrasound image of chest wall showing an increased size of the anechoic space separating the pectoralis major and minor muscles

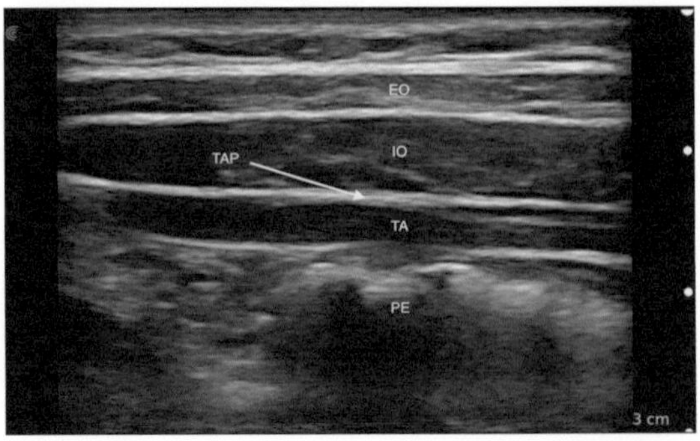

Fig. 13.28 Grayscale ultrasound image of abdominal wall. Transverse view above umbilicus at the anterior axillary line. *EO* external abdominal oblique muscle, *IO* internal abdominal oblique muscle, *TA* transversus abdominis muscle, *TAP* transversus abdominis plane, *PE* peritoneum

for abdominal wall reconstruction, transverse rectus abdominis muscle (TRAM) or deep inferior epigastric flaps (DIEP) and abdominoplasties. Sensory innervation of the anterior abdominal wall is from the anterior branches of the intercostal nerves T 7-12 and the anterior rami of the first lumbar spinal nerve which travel in the plane between the transversus abdominis muscle (TA) and the internal oblique muscle (IO). The transversus abdominal plane (TAP) block was first described by Hebbard [54] (Fig. 13.28).

There are three distinct locations where the (TAP) block can be administered. The Lumbar approach injects at the triangle of Petit. The lateral approach is done in the mid abdomen and the oblique subcostal approach between the posterior rectus sheath and the (TA). The lateral mid abdominal TAP block is typically done with the patient in the supine position after the induction of anesthesia. A high-resolution linear probe (7–14 MHz) is positioned at the anterior to mid axillary line, halfway between the subcostal region and the iliac crest. Depth is adjusted such that the TAP plane is visible in the midfield of the image. External abdominal oblique (EO) muscle can readily be seen below the subcutaneous fat layer. The 3 muscles of the abdominal wall, (EO), (IO), and transversus abdominis (TA) can be visualized from superficial to deep with the (IO) usually being the most prominent in thickness. Below the (TA) is the preperitoneal fat and the contents of the peritoneum. Small bowel peristalsis is often visible. If difficulty in finding all three muscles is encountered, the probe can be moved more medially over the rectus abdominis muscle (RA). Tracing out laterally toward the mid axillary line, the (RA) will be seen to taper and a single echogenic fascia, the plica semilunaris, will become evident. Moving the probe toward the anterior axillary line, the 3 distinct muscle layers will become apparent. A 100 mm, 20-gauge to 22-gauge Touhy tip, sonographic needle (Sonosite® or Braun®) is introduced from medial to lateral. As the TAP is entered, there is usually the feeling of a "pop," and a rebound of the (TAP) in an upward direction is seen on the ultrasound image. In order to confirm the needle tip location within the (TAP), a small 1–2 cc dose of normal saline can be given. A hydro-dissection of the (TAP) is seen as a confluent anechoic separation of the (IO) and the (TA). Should the needle tip not be properly positioned within the (TAP), injection into either the (IO) or the (TA) will produce a diffuse echogenic cloudy appearance within the muscle. Should intramuscular injection proceed proper location of the (TAP), it is prudent to pull the needle back toward the (IO) and try to enter the (TAP) in a new location where the anechoic spread can be more easily identified. The use of local anesthetics in a TAP block, such as liposomal bupivacaine (Exparel®, Pacira

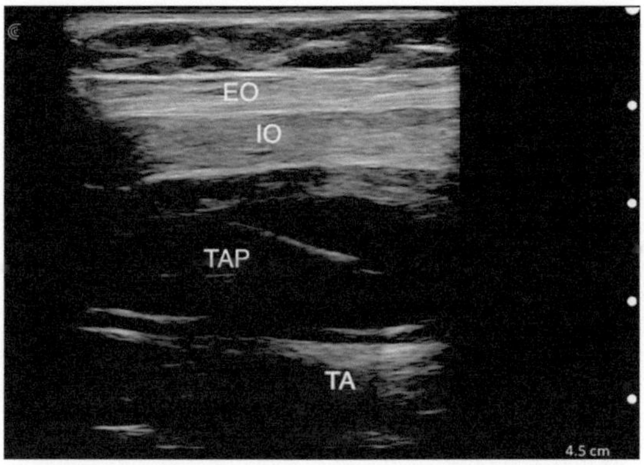

Fig. 13.29 Grayscale ultrasound image of abdominal wall. Transverse view above umbilicus at the anterior axillary line. *EO* external abdominal oblique muscle, *IO* internal abdominal oblique muscle, *TA* transversus abdominis muscle, *TAP* transversus abdominis plane. Anechoic spread of local anesthetic in TAP

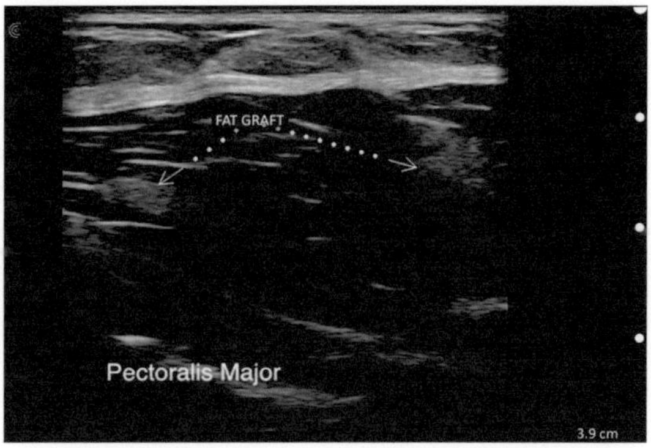

Fig. 13.30 Grayscale ultrasound image of chest wall. Hyperechoic parcels of fat are seen the normal striations of the pectoralis major muscle

Pharmaceuticals, San Diego, Ca) with 72 h durations of effect, has been shown to be effective in pain relief and a decrease in the use of opiates for patients undergoing surgery of the anterior abdominal wall [55–57] (Fig. 13.29).

13.13 Ultrasound Use in Fat Grafting

Autologous fat grafting was first described by Gustav Neuber in 1893 [58]. He grafted fat from the arm to the inferior orbital rim for a depressed scar caused by osteomyelitis. Plastic surgeons today use fat grafting in both reconstructive and cosmetic procedures. Fat is harvested with liposuction cannulas under lower negative pressures to preserve the integrity of the adipocytes. The fat is usually processed by filtration, centrifugation, or gravity-based decantation to remove the cell fragments, blood, and fluid. Fat survival is better with intramuscular injections where vascularity is more robust than the subcutaneous fat layer. Intramuscular fat injections are used by plastic surgeons for cosmetic enhancement of muscles such as the pectoralis, deltoid, and abdomen (Fig. 13.30).

In high-definition liposuction, the deep fat below the superficial fascia is removed and superficial sub dermal fat is removed over natural muscle depressions. Fat grafting can then be used under ultrasound guidance to ensure proper placement of fat within the muscle and avoid penetration of the fat grafting cannula into undesirable locations such as the chest wall, peritoneal cavity, or breast implant. The "in plane" technique is used with a linear high-frequency probe under sterile conditions. Newer wireless ultrasound devices such as the Clarius L7 and L15, (Clarius, Vancouver, BC) have made the intraoperative, sterile, application of ultrasound easier than having an ultrasound transducer covered by a sterile condom to a fixed length cord draped over the sterile field. The wireless devices have the advantage of transmitting the ultrasound image to a wide variety of both Android and IOS devices, which can be more easily moved during the procedure allowing comfortable viewing angles by the operating plastic surgeon. The ultrasound-guided fat grafting procedures are usually begun by first identifying the muscle target. Depth of the ultrasound beam can be adjusted such that the needle penetration is in the mid field of the image. Color Doppler imaging of the surrounding vasculature will help make entry points for the fat grafting cannula in safe locations to avoid vascular injury. The fat grafting procedure can be done in real time by first introducing the cannula into the muscle under ultrasound visualization. The fat can then be injected as the cannula is withdrawn. Post injection visualization of the injected fat will confirm proper location of the fat graft and allow the plastic surgeon to discern what areas of the desired fat graft location still have not been grafted. This will allow for a more even distribution of the fat graft and improve fat graft viability. Fat grafting may also be done in a subcutaneous plane. For breast reconstruction patients, fat may be added to improve symmetry and add volume to the breast. Liposuction soft tissue defects can also be improved by fat grafting into the subcutaneous plane. Ultrasound can be used to measure the size of the defect and monitor the progression of fat taken to the recipient site.

According to the American Society of Plastic Surgeons Procedural Statistics, gluteal fat grafting or the so-called Brazilian buttock lift (BBL) was the fastest growing cosmetic procedure in 2018 with a 19% increase over 2017 and 256% increase since 2000 [1]. However, there has been an alarming number of deaths reported associated with this procedure [59–61]. All of the fatalities have been attributed to fat embolism. It is postulated that the injected fat gains access to the gluteal veins either by direct injection or by injury to the vessel allowing the fat nearby to migrate into the vessel due to the negative pressure of the large gluteal vein [61]. In 2018, the American Society of Plastic Surgeons produced a Gluteal Fat Grafting Advisory stating that gluteal fat grafting should only be done in the subcutaneous space [62]. The use of ultrasound in real time to visualize the location of fat graft deposition into the subcutaneous space of the gluteal region has been described [63]. A linear transducer with a frequency range of 7-12 MHz will allow for good visualization of the buttock in the vast majority of patients. Lower frequency probes will allow for better visualization at deeper locations but will have less resolution. Depth is adjusted such that the gluteal muscle and fascia are visualized. The superficial gluteal fascia is identified as an echogenic line separating the superficial and deep fat compartments of the buttock (Fig. 13.31).

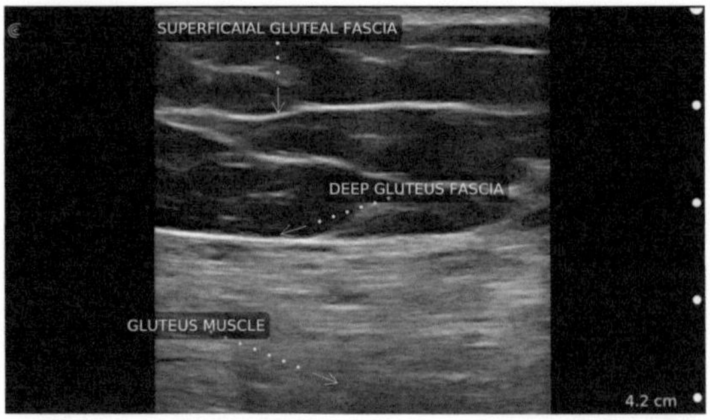

Fig. 13.31 Grayscale ultrasound image of gluteal region. Normal anatomy of buttock showing the subcutaneous space separated by the echogenic superficial gluteal fascia. The deeper echogenic line represents the deep gluteal fascia overlying the gluteal muscle

Vertically oriented fibrous septae can be seen emanating from the superficial gluteal fascia and attaching to the deep surface of the overlying dermis. Doppler ultrasound is used to locate and mark on the skin surface the location of the superior and inferior gluteal arteries. The fat is harvested with a variety of different liposuction techniques and processed with various filtration methods. Using stiff fat grafting cannulas, from access sites that will allow for cannula location to remain superficial to the deep gluteal fascia, the fat is injected under visualization of ultrasound. It is preferable to begin the fat deposition in the plane between the deep and superficial gluteal fascias. Ultrasound image of fat in the subcutaneous space appears as a diffuse echogenic infiltrate that obscures the normal mostly hypoechoic subcutaneous space (Fig. 13.32).

Post fat injection imaging will allow the plastic surgeon to visualize areas that are either incompletely filled or have not had fat injected allowing the surgeon to produce a more homogenous result. Subcutaneous only placement of fat grafts during a BBL is thought to be protective of inadvertent fat injection into the gluteal muscles and will therefore allow for safe placement of fat grafts without the risk of fat embolism [51].

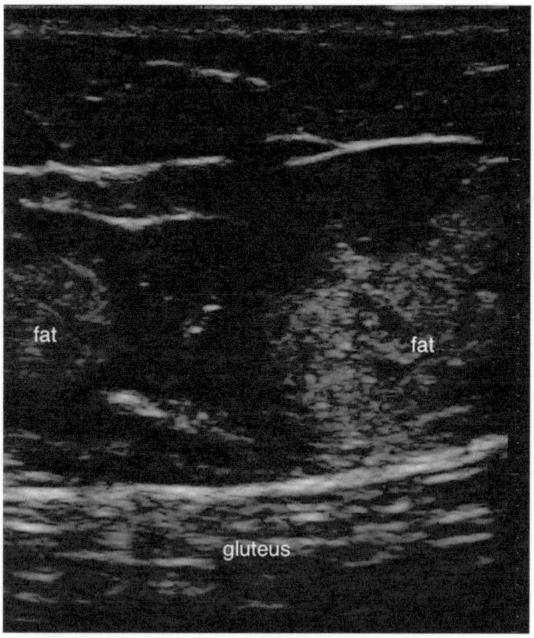

Fig. 13.32 Grayscale ultrasound image of gluteal region. Hyperechoic deposits of fat grafts obscure the normal hypoechoic fat of the buttock region

13.14 Fillers

Dermal fillers are the second most common non-invasive cosmetic procedure (after Botulinum toxins) done by plastic surgeons in the US. According to the American Society of Plastic Surgeons Procedural Statistics for 2018, 2,676,970 soft tissue fillers were done by Board Certified Plastic Surgeons [1]. Soft tissue fillers are used primarily in the face to enhance volume loss, fill in subcutaneous defects, smooth out wrinkles and folds, and improve the appearance of surgical and acne scars. Soft tissue fillers can be separated into two broad categories: biologic fillers and synthetic fillers. Biologic fillers, such as hyaluronic acids (HA), are resorbable sugars and are the most commonly used filler. Permanent fillers such as calcium hydroxyapatite (CaHA) and polymethyl methacrylate (PMMA) are also used to add volume to the dermis and subcutaneous tissues. Hyaluronic acid is a high-molecular-weight polysaccharide which binds water. HA can be either of avian source or made from synthetic fermentation from bacteria. The variables in the formulations of the currently available HAs are particle size, concentration, and the amount of cross-linking. Larger particle size and more cross-linking in the HA formulation will lead to more duration of effect. Higher concentrations of HA will osmotically bind more water and have a more profound effect on increasing the apparent volume correction from the filler. The immediate appearance of HA after injection into the soft tissues using HRUS is that of mostly anechoic spaces of ovoid shape that may contain some internal debris echoes (Fig. 13.33).

As the HA becomes more integrated into the surrounding soft tissues, the HRUS image of the filler becomes more difficult to discern from normal tissue. Calcium hydroxyapatite, Radiesse® (Merz, Raleigh, NC), is a suspension of microspheres of calcium hydroxyapatite crystals in an aqueous gel carrier consisting of sterile water, glycerine, and sodium carboxymethylcellulose. Radiesse® is considered a biostimulator as it causes neocollagenesis in response to the injected calcium hydroxyapatite crystals. On HRUS, Radiesse® appears as multiple hyperechoic deposits with variable degrees of posterior acoustic shadowing (Fig. 13.34).

Polymethylmethacrylate, BellaFill®, is PMMA microspheres in a bovine collagen matrix with 0.3% lidocaine. It is considered a permanent filler with duration of effect lasting 5 years or more. It is mostly used as an intradermal filler for the naso-labial folds, acne scars, and soft tissue defects. Early, less than 3 months after PMMA injection, HRUS images reveal multiple

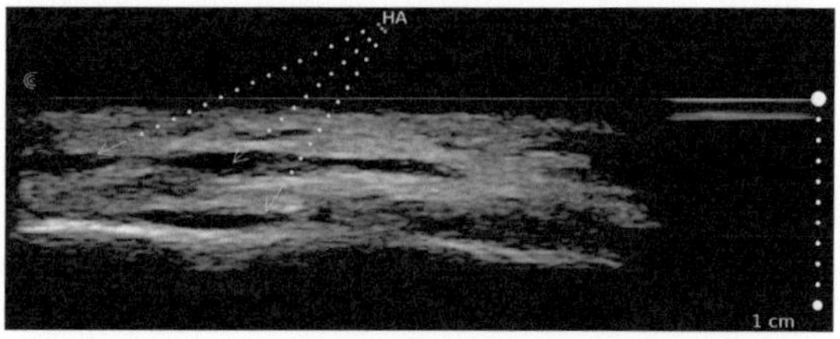

Fig. 13.33 Grayscale ultrasound image of cheek immediately after injection of hyaluronic acid filler. Anechoic deposits of the filler are seen within the fat of the cheek

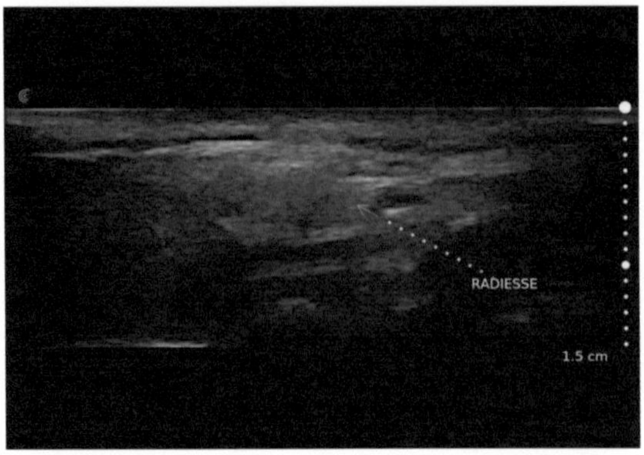

Fig. 13.34 Grayscale ultrasound image of the cheek after calcium hydroxyapatite filler (Radiesse®) injection. The diffuse hyperechoic nature of the filler is seen

hyperechoic dots. Later HRUS imaging of PMMA may show some coalescence of echogenic deposits, some showing posterior acoustic shadowing.Adverse sequelae after soft tissue augmentation with dermal fillers are fortunately rare. Early adverse events, less than 2 weeks after injection, including edema, bruising, and allergic reactions, are usually self-limited and resolve without intervention in 7–10 days. Late adverse events such as infection, nodules, biofilm, or pigmentation changes may be manifested months to years after the injection. HRUS has been used to both diagnose the type, amount, and depth of placement of dermal fillers [64]. Romana et al. described the use of HRUS in evaluating 80 patients with both permanent and temporary fillers. They were able to identify and quantify the presence of filler in the soft tissues in 97% of patients [65]. One of the more challenging adverse long-term sequelae of permanent fillers is the late development of nodules. Inflammatory complications of nonresorbable filler injections are thought to be caused by the formation of granulomas. Histologically, granulomas consist of multinucleated foreign body cells, macrophages, and angiogenesis. HRUS evaluation of late filler nodules may reveal a hypoechoic mass with a hyperechoic pseudocapsule. Various treatments have been suggested for late post filler injection granulomas including intralesional steroids and injections of 5 flouro-uracil. Cassuto et al. described using HRUS to differentiate late nodules into 2 separate categories [66]. Cystic nodules caused by bolus injections were treated with intralesional, 808 nm fiber laser and stab wound evacuation, while an infiltrating pattern caused by retrograde crisscross injection techniques were treated with intralesional fiber laser alone. Seok et al. described treating late nodules caused by injections of L poly lactic acid fillers with HRUS directed curettage [67]. HRUS can also be used to directly target injection of steroids or 5-fluorouracil into the offending mass.

One of the more dreaded complications of soft tissue filler injections of the face is the occlusion of arterial vessels leading to ischemic necrosis of skin and blindness. As there has been a worldwide increase in the use of fillers for cosmetic enhancement of the aging face, the adverse events of ischemic necrosis of soft tissues and blindness have more frequently been reported. HA is the most widely used filler for facial rejuvenation. Unlike the permanent fillers, HA filler effect can be reversed by enzymatic degradation with the injection of hyaluronidase (Hylenex®, Halozyme Therapeutics, San Diego, CA). Hyaluronidase functions as a spreading factor, breaking the glycosidic bonds of the HA inducing depolymerization. In the cases where impending ischemic necrosis of soft tissue is suspected after filler injections, hyaluronidase injection is the treatment of choice. Hyaluronidase is able to penetrate the thin vessel walls and gain access to the HA. One of the leading treatment algorithms for the use of hyaluronidase for impending soft tissue necrosis involves the use of pulsed high-dose injections of hyaluronidase at hourly intervals until the signs of ischemia have been reversed [68]. The empiric nature of this approach and the time involvement of both physician and patient have made this method difficult to employ. Because the amount of injected filler and the precise location of the vessel obstruction are not elucidated in this technique, the final amount of hyaluronidase injected may approach toxic amounts. Schelke et al described the use of Doppler ultrasound to demonstrate a change in the normal laminar flow pattern of unobstructed blood flow to that of a turbulent pattern when some type of obstruction secondary to the filler exists [69]. Under ultrasound guidance, 35–50 units of hyaluronidase were injected directly into the obstructing filler with resolution of the ischemia in 14 of 21 patients after a single dose. Seven patients required a second treatment. In comparison to the hourly, blind injection pulsed therapy regimen, ultrasound-guided hyaluronidase treatment required less time to administer and less volume of hyaluronidase administered.

One of the newer described uses of CaHA is a hyperdilution technique. CaHa, when used undiluted, acts first by volume enhancement due to the carboxymethylcellulose gel component of the filler. The late-volume enhancement is through biostimulation with the production of collagen, elastin, dermal cell proliferation, and angiogenesis leading to duration of effect of 9–18 months. When CaHa is diluted (1.5 mL CaHA with 1.5 mL or more of sterile saline), the immediate volume correction of the hydrogel is minimized, and the product can be injected more superficially to improve skin quality and thickness. One of the off-label uses of dilute CaHA injection is to improve fine wrinkles, skin texture, and skin tightening of the neck and dĕcolletage. When a cannula injection technique is used, HRUS can be used to visualize the correct plane of filler placement as close to the subdermis as possible. Post injection ultrasound imaging can confirm homogeneous dispersion of the filler.

13.15 DVT

One of the more dreaded complications of plastic surgical procedures is deep vein thrombosis (DVT) and the possibility of subsequent pulmonary embolus (PE). One of the accepted methods of risk assessment for thromboembolism is the application of the Caprini score in the decision-making process for chemoprophylaxis [70, 71]. Several studies have disputed the validity of the Caprini scores showing that it was not predictive of which patients would best be served by chemoprophylaxis [72, 73]. Swanson reported on 1000 consecutive cosmetic plastic surgery patients who underwent screening Doppler ultrasound examination of the lower extremities preoperatively, the day after surgery and 1-week post operatively [74].

Compression, longitudinal color flow and waveform analysis were included. Ultrasound image of DVT shows lack of Doppler blood flow in lower extremity veins. Resolution of clot with restoration of Doppler blood flow is visualized weeks later. Nine patients developed DVT and 1 patient had a PE. Eight of the 9 patients were treated successfully with oral anticoagulants. One patient with PE required hospitalization. No patients were anticoagulated prophylactically. Hematoma formation in anticoagulated patients having abdominoplasty is higher than those patients not having anticoagulation. Ultrasound surveillance can obviate the need for chemo prophylactic anticoagulation of plastic surgery patients thought to be at a higher risk for DVT and possible PE.

13.16 Ultrasound of Soft Tissues

Plastic surgeons regularly diagnose and treat soft tissue masses and are involved in evaluating superficial soft tissue irregularities. Common causes of soft tissue masses include seroma, fat necrosis, benign tumors, inclusion cysts, and foreign bodies. Ultrasound evaluation of soft tissue masses by the plastic surgeon has several advantages. Ultrasound can be readily available at the time of consultation, lacks ionizing radiation, is cost effective, and has high spatial resolution. Ultrasound can also be used to assess blood flow without the necessity for contrast administration. Ultrasound is useful for subcutaneous masses that are more superficial and smaller in size. Deep, large, and subfascial masses are best evaluated with MRI. History from the patient as far as the date the mass was first found, change in size, prior trauma or surgery and associated pain is first elicited. Physical examination can assess mobility, tenderness, firmness, and evaluate overlying changes in the skin. A linear, high-frequency probe is used with the highest frequency possible that will allow visualization of the deep aspect of the mass as it relates to the soft tissues. Typically, 2–3 cm of depth will be adequate. Lower frequencies may be needed to assess soft tissue masses in the obese patient or in locations with significant adiposity. Doppler ultrasound can be useful in assessment of soft tissue masses. As many soft tissue masses are hypo vascular, detection of slow blood flow will necessitate higher frequency transducers and the use of presets for detection of slow blood flow. It is helpful to both minimize the size of the doppler box to maximize frame rate and to decrease the color Doppler scale to best visualize blood flow. The transducer is floated over the skin with minimal pressure to decrease movement artifacts. Increasing the Doppler gain is done until slow flow is seen. In the event of no visible flow, some artifact in the periphery of the image may be seen.

Lipomas are the most frequently seen benign soft tissue tumor. In one series, lipomas represented 54% of superficial masses sent for ultrasound evaluation over a 3-year period [75]. Ultrasound images of lipomas will frequently appear isoechoic, hyperechoic, or hypoechoic to the surrounding normal fat (Fig. 13.35)

In the series referred to previously, 59% of the masses were isoechoic, 26% hyperechoic, and 15% hypoechoic to the surrounding normal fat [75]. There may be some wavy echogenic lines within the mass. There is minimal to no Doppler signal and no acoustic shadowing is seen. One variant of the lipoma is the angiolipoma, which can be tender to palpation. The ultrasound image of an angiolipoma is homogeneously hyperechoic and will lack the echogenic lines seen in the lipoma.

Soft tissue infections are often evaluated by plastic surgeons. Whether due to a previous surgery, trauma, or other reasons, plastic surgeons need to differentiate cellulitis from abscess (Fig. 13.36).

Ultrasound has been shown to be an excellent tool to aid in this distinction. The ultrasound appearance of cellulitis is that of an expansion of the subcutaneous space with a diffuse hyperechoic nature of the fat. Noninfectious edema of the soft tissues looks similar on ultrasound to that of cellulitis. Ultrasound images of a soft tissue abscess can be diffuse or well circumscribed. There is a surrounding hyperechoic area and may contain poorly defined pockets of hypoechoic spaces. With compression of the abscess, real-time visualization of mobility of the fluid is diagnostic of an abscess. Anechoic pockets of air within the abscess cavity suggest a diagnosis of necrotizing fasciitis.

Fat necrosis presents as a tender firm mass in the superficial soft tissue space. Plastic surgeons will encounter fat necrosis after procedures where ischemia of tissues can be the causative factor. Free and pedicle flap transfers, breast

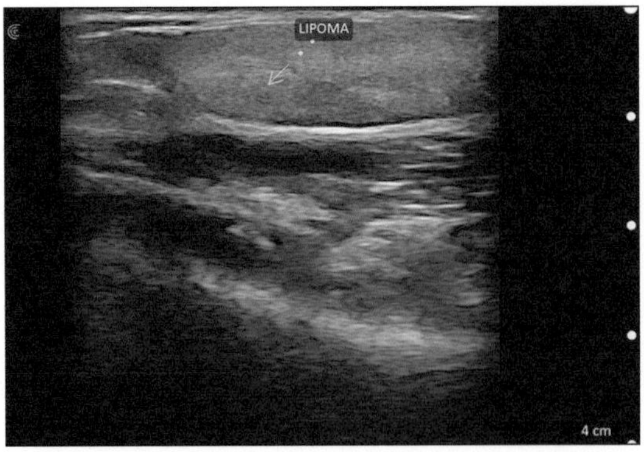

Fig. 13.35 Grayscale ultrasound image of lateral arm. Longitudinal orientation of the transducer over the lateral distal arm shows the well demarcated, homogeneous hyperechoic nature of the lipoma

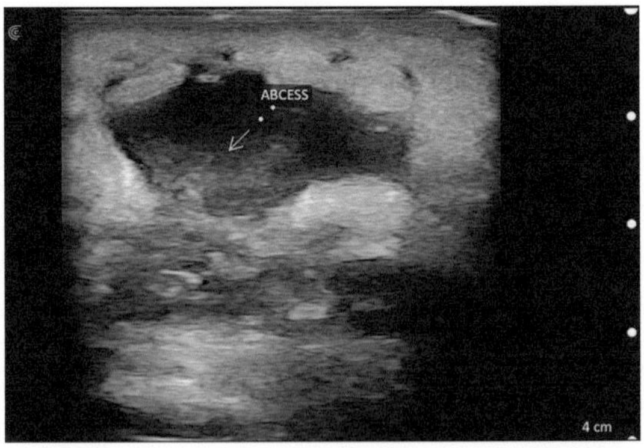

Fig. 13.36 Grayscale ultrasound image of medial knee showing an abscess. The hyperechoic edematous soft tissue surrounds a mostly anechoic chamber with internal debris echoes

reductions, and fat grafting are common causes of fat necrosis. Ultrasound can be used to diagnose and aid in the following clinical course of these benign masses as they tend to resolve without intervention over time. Ultrasound images of fat necrosis can be from isoechoic to hyperechoic to the surrounding normal fat. Anechoic to hypoechoic areas within the mass represent oil cysts (Fig 13.37).

Foreign bodies can present as soft tissue masses. Ultrasound is useful to both diagnose the etiology of and depth of the foreign body and may aid in intraoperatively locating it. Plastic surgeons will on occasion use permanent nonabsorbable sutures made of polypropylene, nylon, polytetrafluorethylene, (PTFE), silk, and polyester. These sutures can develop suture abscesses months to years later and present as soft tissue masses. Ultrasound imaging of suture abscesses reveals the suture material to be hyperechoic with a surrounding area of a hypoechoic halo representing chronic granulation tissue (Fig 13.38).

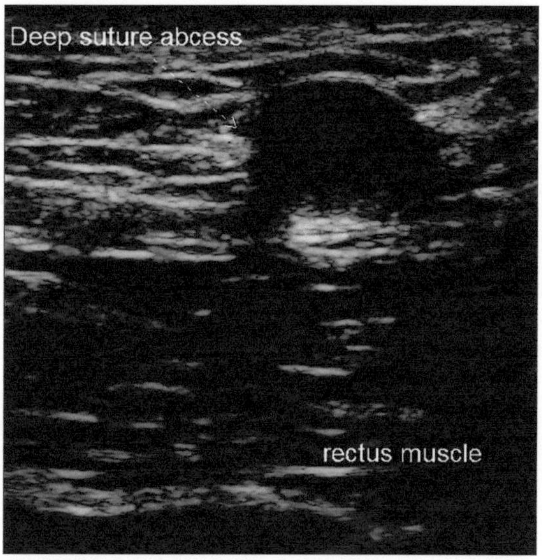

Fig. 13.38 Grayscale ultrasound image of anterior abdominal wall showing a hyperechoic mass representing the suture. The anechoic area surrounding the suture represents the chronic granulation tissue. Acoustic shadowing from the suture is seen deep to the suture

There may be some posterior acoustic shadowing behind the suture material. Using small skin incisions over the offending suture abscess, ultrasound used intraoperatively can aid in removal of the suture with minimal tissue trauma to the surrounding area.

In plastic surgery patients requesting body contour enhancement procedures such as abdominoplasty and trunk liposuction, ultrasound may be useful in the preoperative evaluation of the anterior abdomen. Occult hernias of the abdominal wall may be difficult to palpate in the patient with a high BMI. Ultrasound can be used in the upright position or with the addition of the Valsalva maneuver to assess the integrity of the anterior abdominal wall. Ventral, epigastric, and spigelian hernias are the most common locations. With the linear, high-frequency transducer placed over the midline or lateral rectus abdominis border, the abdominal wall can be evaluated as the patient does a Valsalva maneuver. Preperitoneal fat, small or large bowel contents may be seen to emanate through the fascial opening. This can be differentiated from the postpartum change of the female abdominal wall where there is an attenuation of the linea aspera of the rectus abdominis, but no true hernia opening is present.

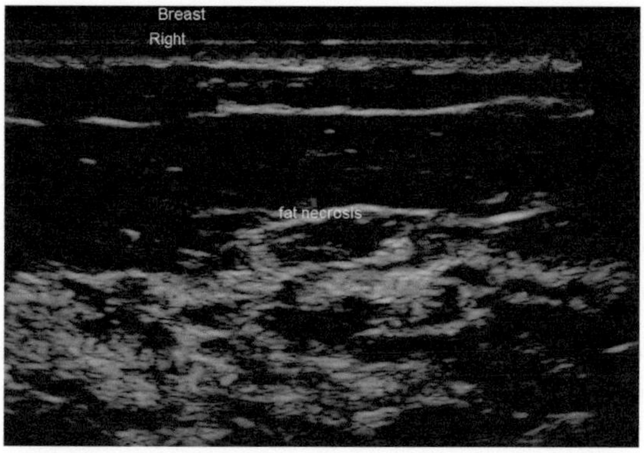

Fig. 13.37 Grayscale ultrasound image of breast showing the diffuse hyperechoic areas with areas of relatively anechoic chambers representing a more liquid oil cyst

Ultrasound can be useful in detecting hematoma in the post-surgical or post traumatic presentation of acute swelling. The differentiation between edema and blood can be important in dictating whether surgical intervention will be necessary. In the acute phase, hematoma can appear hyperechoic on ultrasound. Hematomas, by the time they are evaluated by the plastic surgeon using ultrasound, will usually appear as hypoechoic with some linear hyperechoic lines. As clot retraction liquifies the semi solid blood, the ultrasound appearance will change to an anechoic fluid like appearance.

13.17 Cellulite

Cellulite is one of the most common undesired alterations in the topical appearance of the skin of the posterolateral thigh and buttock. It is much more common in women and affects 85–98% of women at some point in their life [76]. There are a multitude of theoretical causes of cellulite including accumulation of toxins in the hypodermis, obesity, changes in the microcirculation, genetic predisposition, and structural alterations in the relationship of the fibrous septa to the dermis. The dermal and hypodermal architecture of the male and female differ in the orientation and number of septa that attach the fascia to the overlying dermis. In the male, there are numerous septa emanating from the deep fascia in a crisscross fashion. There is only one fat compartment between the muscle and skin. The female architecture is different in that there is a superficial and deep fat compartment separated by a fascial layer. There are fewer septa, and they tend to be more vertically oriented. HRUS can be used by the plastic surgeon to assess the pathology of cellulite, aid in planning its treatment, and provide documented visual ultrasonic evidence of treatment progress. A linear high-frequency probe (10–15 MHz) is used. In the image of the male and female patient, when the probe is oriented along the long axis of the leg, the muscle of the thigh appears slightly echogenic with visible striations. The fascia and septa are more echogenic lines easily visualized between the muscle fascia and dermis. In the absence of cellulite, there is a constant distance between the fascia and the dermis. Where the dimples and orange peel quality of the skin are evident, the superficial fascia undulates upward toward the dermis, and there is usually a visualized septae at the apex of the upward arc. At the skin hypodermis junction, fat can be seen herniating upward into the dermis. Numerous noninvasive as well as invasive treatments for cellulite have been described. Topical application of aminophylline and retinols have been described as having modest success in reduction in the appearance of cellulite [77, 78]. Injected lipolytic agents such as phosphatidylcholine and deoxycholic acid have been used in mesotherapy treatment of cellulite [79, 80]. High-frequency ultrasound has been used to demonstrate the efficacy of mesotherapy, topical creams, and electro-mechanical massage in the reduction of cellulite. Mechanical vacuum-assisted massage with the addition of heat in the form of lasers or radiofrequency devices have also been described as being effective in temporary reduction in the appearance of cellulite [81–83]. Invasive procedures utilizing fiber laser delivery of energy directed at the fibrous septa thought to be causative of the dimpled appearance of cellulite have been described [84]. Using wavelengths of 1440 nm, a side firing, 1000-µm fiber encased within a hollow cannula was used to treat patients with cellulite of the thighs. A high-frequency linear probe was used to measure dermal thickness. Serial ultrasound images demonstrated an increased thickness of the dermis and a more homogeneous appearance of the dermal–epidermal junction.

13.18 Evaluation of Flaps

For the repair of complex soft tissue defects of the torso, extremities, and face, plastic surgeons have relied upon the use of both pedicled and free tissue transfer of muscle flaps with or without the overlying skin as a primary reconstructive option. Lack of availability of donor site muscle, high donor site muscle morbidity, or requirement of less bulky tissue corrections have led to the increased use of fasciocutaneous flaps as a viable alternative to musculocutaneous flaps. Because of the anatomic variability of the perforating vessels of the fasciocutaneous flaps, several presurgical imaging techniques have been suggested as being useful in locating these fasciocutaneous perforators. Color Doppler ultrasound (CDU), computed topographic angiography (CTA), and magnetic resonance angiography have all been suggested as viable options for preoperative planning of fasciocutaneous flaps (Fig 13.39).

The deep inferior epigastric perforator flap (DIEP) is one of the more commonly used methods for free flap post mastectomy breast reconstruction. CTA has been shown to be a fast, accurate method of preoperative assessment of the deep inferior epigastric artery (DIEA) showing its intramuscular course and perforator branching pattern as the vessel exits the rectus fascia and enters the subcutaneous tissue [85]. CTA, however, has small risks of contrast toxicity as well as ionizing radiation exposure. Magnetic resonance angiography (MRA) has been shown to be a viable alternative to CTA with no ionizing radiation [86]. MRA image quality may be affected by motion artifact, and the exam may be contraindicated in patients with claustrophobia or ferrous metallic implants [87]. The use of CDU was described by Hallock in the early 1990s in the planning of 8 fasciocutaneous flaps [88, 89]. A 7.5 MHz, linear transducer was used to locate the dominant perforator or perforators in each case. In a comparison study of CDU and CTA, 98 patients underwent 125 DIEP flaps (91). CDU was found to be statistically superior in accuracy of perforator detection and predictor of vessel size compared to CTA.

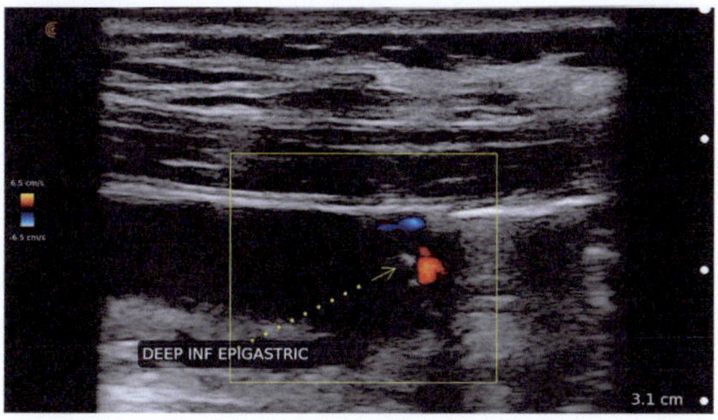

Fig. 13.39 Color Doppler ultrasound image of abdominal wall. Transducer is oriented longitudinally over the rectus muscle below the umbilicus. The deep inferior epigastric artery and vein are seen just below where they enter the rectus abdominis muscle

References

1. American Society of Plastic Surgeons 2018 Cosmetic Plastic Surgery Statistics. American Society of Plastic Surgeons Website.https://www.plasticsurgery.org/documents/News/Statistics/2018/plastic-surgery-statistics report-2018.pdf. Accessed 19 Jan 2020.
2. Cronin T, Gerow F. Augmentation mammoplasty: a new "natural feel" prosthesis. In: Transactions of the third international congress of plastic surgeons. Amsterdam: Excerpta Medica Foundation; 1964. p. 41–9.
3. Ho Lmich LR, Friis S, Fryzek JP, et al. Incidence of silicone breast implant rupture. Arch Surg. 2003;138(7):801e6.
4. Seigle-Murandi F, Lefebvre F, Bruant-Rodier C, Bodin F. Incidence of breast implant rupture in a 12-year retrospective cohort: evidence of quality discrepancy depending on the range. J Plast Reconstr Aesthet Surg. 2017;70(1):42e6.
5. Handel N, Garcia ME, Wixtrom R. Breast implant rupture: causes, incidence, clinical impact, and management. Plast Reconstr Surg. 2013;132(5):1128e37.
6. Kessler DA. Food and Drug Administration. U.S. Department of Health and Human Services. HHS News. No. P92–11. Statement on Silicone Gel Breast Implants. 1992.
7. Food and Drug Administration. Device approvals. 2006. www.fda.gov/MedicalDevices/ProductsandMedicalProcedures/DeviceApprovalsandClearances/Recently-ApprovedDevices/ucm073317.htm.
8. Paetau AA, McLaughlin SA, McNeil RB, et al. Capsular contracture and possible implant rupture: is magnetic resonance imaging useful? Plast Reconstr Surg. 2010;125(3):830e5. FDA General and Plastic Surgery Panel in March, 2019, https://www.fda.gov/media/122960/download.
9. Ikeda DM, Borofsky HB, Herfkens RJ, Sawyer-Glover AM, Birdwell RL, Glover GH. Silicone breast implant rupture: pitfalls of magnetic resonance imaging and relative efficacy of magnetic resonance, mammography, and ultrasound. Plast Reconstr Surg. 1999;104:2054e62.
10. O'Toole M, Caskey CI. Imaging spectrum of breast implants complications: mammography, ultrasound, and magnetic resonance imaging. Semin Ultrasound CT MR. 2000;21:351e61.
11. Di Benedetto G, Cecchini S, Grassetti L, et al. Comparative study of breast implant rupture using mammography, sonography, and magnetic resonance imaging correlation with surgical findings. Breast J. 2008;14(6):532e7.
12. Berg WA, Caskey CI, Hamper UM, et al. Diagnosing breast implant rupture with MR imaging, US, and mammography. Radiographics. 1993;13:1323–36.
13. Scaranelo AM, Marques AF, Smialowski EB, et al. Evaluation of the rupture of silicone breast implants

by mammography, ultrasonography and magnetic resonance imaging in asymptomatic patients: correlation with surgical findings. Sao Paulo Med J. 2004;122(2):41e7.
14. Brown SL, Middleton MS, Berg WA, Soo MS, Pennello G. Prevalence of rupture of silicone gel breast implants revealed on MR imaging in a population of women in Birmingham, Alabama. AJR Am J Roentgenol. 2000;175(4):1057–64.
15. Destouet JM, Monsees BS, Oser RF, Nemecek JR, Young VL, Pilgram TK. Screening mammography in 350 women with breast implants: prevalence and findings of implant complications. AJR Am J Roentgenol. 1992;159(5):973–978; discussion 979–981.
16. Middleton MS. MR evaluation of breast implants. Radiol Clin N Am. 2014;52(3):591–608.
17. Everson LI, Parantainen H, Detlie T, et al. Diagnosis of breast implant rupture: imaging findings and relative efficacies of imaging techniques. AJR Am J Roentgenol. 1994;163(1):57–60.
18. Berg WA, Caskey CI, Hamper UM, et al. Single- and double-lumen silicone breast implant integrity: prospective evaluation of MR and US criteria. Radiology. 1995;197(1):45–52.
19. Rietjens M, Villa G, Toesca A, et al. Appropriate use of magnetic resonance imaging and ultrasound to detect early silicone gel breast implant rupture in postmastectomy recon struction. Plast Reconstr Surg. 2014;134(1):13e–20e.
20. Venta LA, Salomon CG, Flisak ME, Venta ER, Izquierdo R, Angelats J. Sonographic signs of breast implant rupture. AJR Am J Roentgenol. 1996;166(6):1413–9.
21. Chung KC, Malay S, Shauver MJ, Kim HM. Economic analysis of screening strategies for rupture of silicone gel breast implants. Plast Reconstr Surg. 2012;130(1):225–37.
22. Stavros AT. Breast ultrasound. Philadelphia, PA: Lippincott Williams & Wilkins; 2004. p. 199–275.
23. Caskey CI, Berg WA, Anderson ND, Sheth S, Chang BW, Hamper UM. Breast implant rupture: diagnosis with US. Radiology. 1994;190(3):819–23.
24. Robinson OG Jr, Bradley EL, Wilson DS. Analysis of explanted silicone implants: a report of 300 patients. Ann Plast Surg. 1995;34:1e6.
25. US Food and Drug Administration data. http://www.fda.gov/MedicalDevices/ProductsandMedicalProcedures/ImplantsandProsthetics/BreastImplants/ucm063871.html. Accessed 18 Jan 2020.
26. DeBruhl ND, Gorczyca DP, Ahn CY, Shaw WW, Bassett LW. Silicone breast implants: US evaluation. Radiology. 1993;189(1):95–8.
27. Juanpere S, Perez E, Huc O, et al. Imaging of breast implantsda pictorial review. Insights Imaging. 2011;2:653e70.
28. Papadia A, Menada MV, Ragni N, et al. Extended field of view and three dimensional ultrasound imaging of silicone breast implant lesions. Ultrasound Obstet Gynecol. 2007;29:360–1.
29. Sastre G, Rojas R, Roja R, et al. Revisión de implantes mamarios con metodología mamográfica y ultrasonográfica. Rev Argent Radiol. 2005;69:107–12.
30. Gori R. Evaluación ultrasonográfica de la mama con implantes. Rev Argent Ultrason. 2007;6:273–8.
31. Sagi L, Lyakhovitsky A, Barzilai A, et al. Silicone breast implant rupture presenting as bilateral nodules. Clin Exp Dermatol. 2009;34:99–101.
32. Palmon LU, Foshager MC, Parantainen H, et al. Ruptured or intact: what can linear echoes within silicone breast implants tell us? AJR am J Roentgenol. 1997;168:1595–8.
33. Ahn CY, DeBruhl ND, Gorczyca DP, et al. comparative silicone breast implant evaluation using mammography, sonography, and magnetic resonance imaging: experience with 59 implants. Plast Reconstr Surg. 1994;94:620–7.
34. Harris K, Ganott M, Shestak K, et al. Silicone implant rupture: detection with US. Radiology. 1993;187:761–8.
35. Soo MS, Kornguth PJ, Walsh R, et al. Complex radial folds versus subtle signs of intra-capsular rupture of breast implants. MR findings with surgical correlation. AJR Am J Roentgenol. 1996;166:1421e7.
36. Soo MS, Kornguth PJ, Walsh R, et al. Intracapsular implant rupture: MR findings of incomplete shell collapse. J Magn Reson Imaging. 1997;7:724–30.
37. Chung KC, Greenfield ML, Walters M. Decision-analysis methodology in the work-up of women with suspected silicone breast implant rupture. Plast Reconstr Surg. 1998;102:689–95.
38. McNamara M Jr, Middleton M. Ultrasound of breast implants and soft tissue silicone. Ultrasound Clin. 2011;6:345–68.
39. Huch RA, Kunzi W, Debatin JF, et al. MR imaging of the augmented breast. Eur Radiol. 1998;8:371–6.
40. Hold P, Shabana A, Pilbrow W, et al. How should we investigate breast implant rupture. Breast J. 2012;18:253–6.
41. Galdiero M, Larocca F, Iovene MR, et al. Microbial evaluation in capsular contracture of breast implants. Plast Reconstr Surg. 2018;141(1):23–30. https://doi.org/10.1097/PRS.0000000000003915.
42. Wan D, Rohrich RJ. Revisiting the Management of Capsular Contracture in breast augmentation: a systematic review. Plast Reconstr Surg. 2016;137(3):826–41. https://doi.org/10.1097/01.prs.0000480095.23356.ae.
43. Baker JL Jr. Augmentation mammaplasty. In: Owsley Jr JQ, Peterson RA, editors. Symposium on aesthetic surgery of the breast. St Louis: Mosby; 1979.
44. McGuire P, Reisman NR, Murphy DK. Risk factor analysis for capsular contracture, malposition, and late seroma in subjects receiving Natrelle 410 form-stable silicone breast implants. Plast Reconstr Surg. 2017;139:1–9.
45. Adrada BE, Miranda RN, Rauch GM, et al. Breast implant-associated anaplastic large cell lymphoma: sensitivity, specificity, and findings of imaging

studies in 44 patients. Breast Cancer Res Treat. 2014;147:1–14.
46. Mazzocchi M, Dessy LA, Marchetti F, Marchetti F, Carlesimo B. The use of the veress needle to drain mammary periprosthetic fluid. In Vivo. 2010;24(2):219–22.
47. Becker H, Klimczak J. Aspiration of periprosthetic seromas using the blunt SeromaCath. Plast Reconstr Surg. 2016;137(2):473–5. https://doi.org/10.1097/01.prs.0000475795.84725.c4.
48. Blanco R. The 'pecs block': a novel technique for providing analgesia after breast surgery: correspondence. Anaesthesia. 2011;66(9):847–8. https://doi.org/10.1111/j.1365-2044.2011.06838.x.
49. Pérez MF, Duany O, de la Torre PA. Redefining PECS blocks for postmastectomy analgesia. Reg Anesth Pain Med. 2015;40(6):729–30. https://doi.org/10.1097/AAP.0000000000000243.
50. Hebbard P, Fujiwara Y, Shibata Y, Royse C. Ultrasound-guided transversus abdominis plane (TAP) block. Anaesth Intensive Care. 2007;35:616–7.
51. Matsumoto M, Flores EM, Kimachi PP, et al. Benefts in radical mastectomy protocol: a randomized trial evaluating the use of regional anesthesia. Sci Rep. 2018;8:7815.
52. Wang K, Zhang X, Zhang T, et al. The efficacy of ultrasound-guided type ii pectoral nerve blocks in perioperative pain management for immediate reconstruction after modified radical mastectomy: a prospective, randomized study. Clin J Pain. 2018;34:231–6.
53. Bashandy GM, Abbas DN. Pectoral nerves I and II blocks in multimodal analgesia for breast cancer surgery: a randomized clinical trial. Reg Anesth Pain Med. 2015;40:68–74.
54. Neuber F. Fat transplantation report on the negotiations of the Deutscht Gesellsch Chir. Zentralblatt fur Surgery. 1893;22:66.
55. Fiala T. Transversus abdominis plane block during abdominoplasty to improve postoperative patient comfort. Aesthet Surg J. 2015;35:72–80.
56. Sforza M, Andjelkov K, Zaccheddu R, Nagi H, Colic M. Transversus abdominis plane block anesthesia in abdominoplasties. Plast Reconstr Surg. 2011;128:529–35.
57. Cansancao AL, Condé-Green A, Vidigal RA, Rodriguez RL, D'Amico RA. Real-time ultrasound–assisted gluteal fat grafting. Plast Reconst Surg. 2018;142(2):372–6. https://doi.org/10.1097/PRS.0000000000004602.
58. Mofid MM, Teitelbaum S, Suissa D, et al. Report on mortality from gluteal fat grafting: Recommendations from the ASERF task force. Aesthet Surg J. 2017;37:796–806.
59. Cárdenas-Camarena L, Bayter JE, Aguirre-Serrano H, Cuenca-Pardo J. Deaths caused by gluteal lipoinjection: what are we doing wrong? Plast Reconstr Surg. 2015;136:58–66.
60. Cárdenas-Camarena L, Durán H, Robles-Cervantes JA, et al. Critical differences between microscopic (MIFE) and macroscopic (MAFE) fat embolism during liposuction and gluteal lipoinjection. Plast Reconstr Surg. 2018;141:880–90.
61. American Society of Plastic Surgeons. Gluteal fat grafting advisory. https://www.plasticsurgery.org/for-medical-professionals/advocacy/key-issues/gluteal-fatgrafting-advisory. Accessed 31 Jan 2018.
62. Salibian AA, Frey JD, Thanik VD, Karp NS, Choi M. Transversus abdominis plane blocks in microsurgical breast reconstruction: analysis of pain, narcotic consumption, length of stay, and cost. Plast Reconstr Surg. 2018;142(3):252e–63e. https://doi.org/10.1097/PRS.0000000000004632.
63. Cassuto D, Pignatti M, Pacchioni L, Boscaini G, Spaggiari A, De Santis G. Management of complications caused by permanent fillers in the face: a treatment algorithm. Plast Reconstr Surg. 2016;138(2):215e–27e. https://doi.org/10.1097/PRS.0000000000005203.
64. Grippaudo FR, Mattei M. The utility of high-frequency ultrasound in dermal filler evaluation. Ann Plast Surg. 2011;67(5):469–73. https://doi.org/10.1097/SAP.0b013e318203ebf6.
65. Cassuto D, Pignatti M, Pacchioni L, Boscaini G, Spaggiari A, De Santis G. Management of complications caused by permanent fillers in the face: a treatment algorithm. Plast Reconstr Surg. 2016;138(2):215e–27e. https://doi.org/10.1097/PRS.0000000000002350.
66. DeLorenzi C. New high dose pulsed hyaluronidase protocol for hyaluronic acid filler vascular adverse events. Aesthet Surg J. 2017;37:1–12.
67. Wagner JM, Lee KS, Rosas H, et al. Accuracy of sonographic diagnosis of superficial masses. J Ultrasound Med. 2013;32(8):1443–50.
68. Schelke LW, Velthuis P, Kadouch J, Swift A. Early ultrasound for diagnosis and treatment of vascular adverse events with hyaluronic acid fillers. J Am Acad Dermatol. 2019;88:79. https://doi.org/10.1016/j.jaad.2019.07.032.
69. Murphy RX Jr, Alderman A, Gutowski K, et al. Evidence-based practices for thromboembolism prevention: summary of the ASPS venous thromboembolism task force report. Plast Reconstr Surg. 2012;130:168e–75e.
70. Pannucci CJ, Barta RJ, Portschy PR, et al. Assessment of post-operative venous thromboembolism risk in plastic surgery patients using the 2005 and 2010 Caprini risk score. Plast Reconstr Surg. 2012;130:343–53.
71. Swanson E. Caprini scores, risk stratification, and rivaroxaban in plastic surgery: time to reconsider our strategy. Plast Reconstr Surg Glob Open. 2016;4:e733.
72. Keyes GR, Singer R, Iverson RE, Nahai F. Incidence and predictors of venous thromboembolism in abdominoplasty. Aesthet Surg J. 2018;38:162–73.
73. Swanson E. Prospective study of doppler ultrasound surveillance for deep venous thromboses in 1000 plastic surgery outpatients. Plast Reconstr

Surgery. 2020;145(1):85–96. https://doi.org/10.1097/PRS.0000000000006343.
74. Seok J, Kim JM, Kwon TR, Kim JH, Li K, Kim BJ. Ultrasonography-guided curettage of polyDL-lactic acid filler granulomas. J Am Acad Dermatol. 2018;78(1):e5–6. https://doi.org/10.1016/j.jaad.2017.08.026.
75. Khan MH, Victor F, Rao B, Sadick NS. Treatment of cellulite: part I. pathophysiology. J Am Acad Dermatol. 2010;62(3):361–70.
76. Kligman AM, Pagnoni A, Stoudemayer T. Topical retinol improves cellulite. J Dermatol Treat. 1999;10:119–25.
77. Collis N, Elliot LA, Sharpe C, Sharpe DT. Cellulite treatment: a myth or reality: a prospective randomized, controlled trial of two therapies, endermologie and aminophylline cream. Plast Reconstr Surg. 1999;104:1110–4.
78. Palmer M, Curran J, Bowler P. Clinical experience and safety using phosphatidylcholine injections for the localized reduction of subcutaneous fat: a multicentre, retrospective UK study. J Cosmet Dermatol. 2006;5:218–26.
79. Rotunda AM, Suzuki H, Moy RI, et al. Detergent effects of sodium deoxycholate are a major feature of an injectable phosphatidylcholine formulation used for localized fat dissolution. Dermatol Surg. 2004;30:1001–7.
80. Alster TS, Tanzi EL. Cellulite treatment using a novel combination radiofrequency, infrared light, and mechanical tissue manipulation device. J Cosmet Laser Ther. 2005;7:81–5.
81. Sadick N, Magro C. a study evaluating the safety and efficacy of the VelaSmooth system in the treatment of cellulite. J Cosmet Laser Ther. 2007;9:15–20.
82. Kulick M. Evaluation of the combination of radiofrequency, infrared energy, and mechanical rollers with suction to improve skin surface irregularities (cellulite) in a limited treatment area. J Cosmet Laser Ther. 2006;8:185–90.
83. DiBernardo BE. Treatment of cellulite using a 1,440-nm pulsed laser with one-year followup. Aesthet Surg J. 2011;31:328–41.
84. Cina A, Salgarello M, Barone-Adesi L, Rinaldi P, Bonomo L. Planning breast reconstruction with deep inferior epigastric artery perforating vessels: multidetector CT angiography versus color doppler US. Radiology. 2010;255(3):979–87. https://doi.org/10.1148/radiol.10091166.
85. Cina A, Barone-Adesi L, Rinaldi P, et al. Planning deep inferior epigastric perforator flaps for breast reconstruction: a comparison between multidetector computed tomography and magnetic resonance angiography. Eur Radiol. 2013;23(8):2333–43. https://doi.org/10.1007/s00330-013-2834-x.
86. Schaverien MV, Ludman CN, Neil-Dwyer J, McCulley SJ. Contrast-enhanced magnetic resonance angiography for preoperative imaging of deep inferior epigastric artery perforator flaps: advantages and disadvantages compared with computed tomography angiography: a United Kingdom perspective. Ann Plast Surg. 2011;67(6):671–4. https://doi.org/10.1097/SAP.0b013e3181fab9ea.
87. Hallock GG. Evaluation of fasciocutaneous perforators using color duplex imaging. Plast Reconstr Surg. 1994;94(5):644–51. https://doi.org/10.1097/00006534-199410000-00012.
88. Mijuskovic B, Tremp M, Heimer MM, et al. color doppler ultrasound and computed tomographic angiography for perforator mapping in DIEP flap breast reconstruction revisited: a cohort study. J Plast Reconstr Aesthet Surg. 2019;72(10):1632–9. https://doi.org/10.1016/j.bjps.2019.06.008.
89. Wortsman X, Wortsman J, Orlandi C, Cardenas G, Sazunic I, Jemec GBE. Ultrasound detection and identification of cosmetic fillers in the skin: ultrasound of fillers complications. J Eur Acad Dermatol Venereol. 2012;26(3):292–301. https://doi.org/10.1111/j.1468-3083.2011.04047.x.

14 Image-Guided Breast Oncologic Treatment

Robert L. Bard, Noelle Cutter, and Stephen Chagares

Abstract

Three-dimensional vascular imaging has provided a quantifiable measure of treatment success or failure in breast diseases. The ability to presurgically map the vessel distribution allows for targeted surgical planning. The vessel density correlates with activity in both the breast cancer and the locoregional disease. Postoperative pathologic analysis is assisted by focusing on tumor tissue rather than benign disease associated with a primary or recurrent malignancy. The new advances of volumetric analysis make this exam less operator dependent as the probe is fixed in position. The addition of ABUS-automated whole-breast ultrasound has improved screening on dense breasts, while 3D elastography guides biopsy options making this diagnostic menu a sentinel advance in breast conservation. Prevention of breast disease is possible by reducing exposure to environmental factors, better nutrition, and genetic counseling.

Keywords

Dimensional vascular imaging · Breast diseases · Image-guided biopsy · 3D doppler

14.1 Introduction

While the best esthetic outcome of breast disease is to have normal dermal and glandular tissues, the reality is 1 out of 8 women will develop cancer, and women with dense breasts are more likely to develop a benign or malignant tumor according to the American College of Radiology and the AreYouDense Foundation. Our health is related to our genes, nutrition, and environmental exposure. With the advent of plastics and chemicals from petroleum, our environment has been polluted with toxins with short-term and long-term side effects. This is evident as "cancer clusters" have been acknowledged nationwide, especially in Long Island, New York and other areas sporadically in the news headlines.

Women are searching for a diagnosis on any palpable lesion that may be subdermal in location and, thus, invisible to the spatially restricted human eye. Patients are currently concerned about possible side effects from biopsy, radiation, and gadolinium-based MRI contrast agents. Athletic

R. L. Bard (✉)
The Angio Foundation and Bard Diagnostics, New York, NY, USA
e-mail: rbard@cancerscan.com

N. Cutter
Biology, Chemistry, and Environmental Sciences, Molloy University, Rockville Centre, NY, USA
e-mail: ncutter@molloy.edu

S. Chagares
Tinton Falls, NJ, USA

R. L. Bard (ed.), *Image-Guided Aesthetic Treatments*, https://doi.org/10.1007/978-3-031-36266-8_14

women, due to their low fat/body mass ratio, are prone to dense breast tissue and are at 400–700% higher risk of developing cancer than women without dense breasts. Over 40,000 women in the U.S. are expected to die in 2021 from breast cancer. Unfortunately, death rates have been steady in women under 50 since 2007, despite advancements in treatment options. For women in the U.S., breast cancer death rates are higher than those for any other cancer, besides lung cancer.

As of January 2021, there are more than 3.8 million women with a history of breast cancer in the U.S. This includes women currently being treated and women who have finished treatment. Breast cancer is the most commonly diagnosed cancer among American women. In 2021, it is estimated that about 30% of newly diagnosed cancers in women will be breast cancers. Breast cancer became the most common cancer globally as of 2021, accounting for 12% of all new annual cancer cases worldwide, according to the World Health Organization. A woman's risk of breast cancer nearly doubles if she has a first-degree relative (mother, sister, and daughter) who has been diagnosed with breast cancer. About 5–10% of breast cancers can be linked to known gene mutations inherited from one's mother or father. Mutations in the *BRCA1* and *BRCA2*genes are the most common. On average, women with a *BRCA1* mutation have up to a 72% lifetime risk of developing breast cancer. For women with a *BRCA2* mutation, the risk is 69%. Breast cancer that is positive for the *BRCA1* or *BRCA2* mutations tends to develop more often in younger women. About 85% of breast cancers occur in women who have no family history of breast cancer. The most significant risk factors for breast cancer are sex (being a woman) and age. But recent research is beginning to clarify additional risk factors associated with BC.

14.1.1 Physical Activity

Physical activity is considered a significant modifiable factor in breast cancer risk, and since exercise reduces fatty tissue and BMI, it has been thought to increase breast density. However, studies into the relationship between physical activity and breast density have been inconclusive. Other factors, such as alteration in metabolism of endogenous hormones, are suggested to influence mammographic density (MD) as well. Therefore, it is evident that the links between physical activity and breast cancer risk need to be clarified. One of the challenges in promoting the widespread utility of breast cancer risk prediction models has been the assertion that most women with a diagnosis of breast cancer have no established clinical breast cancer risk factors or are not considered to be high risk [1, 2]. Although it is impossible to determine the cause of breast cancer in any individual case [3], easily assessed risk factors that explain a substantial proportion of incident breast cancers can be used to stratify breast cancer risk for targeted screening and primary prevention [4] and improve public health interventions to reduce breast cancer risk.

Recent research has suggested that for women with dense breasts, a screening strategy that also takes into account a woman's risk factors and protective factors may be the best predictor of whether a woman will develop breast cancer after a normal mammogram and before her next scheduled mammogram. A common question that invariably comes up when discussing breast density relates to breast density in *athletes*. As an athlete myself who has dense breasts, I was struck by the number of individuals in my athletic community who also have dense breasts. A shocking trend was seen in the overwhelming amount of young women with dense breasts who subsequently had received false-negative mammogram reports. What we do know is that your breast tissue tends to become less dense as you age, though some women may have dense breast tissue at any age. Women with less body fat are more likely to have more dense breast tissue compared with women who are obese. Athletic women are also more likely to have dense breast tissue.

14.1.2 Purpose of Research

It is not clear why some women have a lot of dense breast tissue and others do not. You may be more likely to have dense breasts if you:

1. **Are younger.** Your breast tissue tends to become less dense as you age, though some women may have dense breast tissue at any age.
2. **Have a lower body mass index.** Women with less body fat are more likely to have more dense breast tissue compared with women who are obese.

14.1.3 Importance

Breast density is associated with breast cancer risk in women aged 40–65 years, but there is limited evidence of its association with risk of breast cancer among women 18+. Furthermore, a high proportion of women with low BMI present with dense breasts, making them likely candidates to receive false-negative readings on a mammogram. We aimed to estimate the proportion of breast cancers attributable to breast cancer risk factors commonly documented in clinical practice and used in breast cancer risk prediction models, including BI-RADS breast density and ultrasounds to confirm mammography readings. Our data will be collected from a cohort of women undergoing ultrasound density scans at the Bard Cancer Center

14.1.4 Methods

Endurance athletes are defined as those who participated in one or more endurance events (long course) in the year or as well as those who are younger (low BMI cohort). Classification of "dense breasts" was heterogeneous and extremely dense as noted by the BI_RADS code (heterogeneously or extremely dense vs scattered fibroglandular densities). The data will be collected as odds ratio (ORs), and 95% confidence intervals included in our outcomes.

14.1.5 JAMA Study

A recent report in *Journal of the American Medical Association* found that first-degree family history of breast cancer dense breasts was associated with an increased population-associated risk proportion of breast cancer. Among premenopausal women, the largest individual population-associated risk proportion was for breast density, with 28.9% (95% CI, 25.3–32.5%) of breast cancers potentially removed by reducing breast density from BI-RADS heterogeneously or extremely dense breasts to scattered fibroglandular densities. The population-associated risk proportion for breast density increased to 65.5% (95% CI, 60.4–70.6%) if all premenopausal women reduced their breast density to the lowest category of almost entirely fat tissue.

14.1.6 Project Goals

Although breast density is a well-established, strong, and prevalent breast cancer risk factor, its biological connection is not clearly understood. More research is needed to support the population-associated risk proportion in athletic premenopausal women. Our data will start with a cohort of women undergoing imaging ultrasounds at the Bard Cancer Diagnostic Center. Our population will include premenopausal women with dense breasts. Anecdotally, 50 years ago, one never saw a 35 year old with breast cancer. Twenty years ago, it was common to see women in their 20s with cancer. Environmental factors and toxic substances may be a by-product of the research outcome.

14.1.7 Summary

Given that greater breast density as categorized by the BI-RADS remains a factor associated with breast cancer for all ages of women, information about breast density together with life expectancy may benefit clinical decision making regarding screening. In March 2019, the US Food and Drug Administration recommended changes to the Mammography Quality Standards Act to make it mandatory to report breast density information to both patients and their physicians. However, how women and their physicians should use this information to inform screening recommendations is unclear. Very dense breasts may increase the risk that cancer will not be detected on a mammogram.

What is clear is that additional research is needed to elucidate the mechanisms underlying the observed associations between breast density and risk of breast cancer. As newer and more advanced breast density assessment techniques are developed, evaluation of the diffusion of such innovations with an aim of developing individualized screening strategies will be important, particularly among athletic women, for whom dense breasts are more likely seen.

Diagnostic ultrasound advances meet these requirements and are performed in the office setting accurately and rapidly due to the high resolution and low cost of today's sonographic equipment. These diagnostic technologies require extensive experience and specialized training in image interpretation. However, advances in the computerization of the imaging, blood flow, and tumor measures of exact volume and vessel density are now less operator dependent. That provides for an accurate and repeatable diagnosis and a means to follow the individual's unique pattern of cancer development, progress, and response to treatment. Recent technological advances also make these procedures available to much broader clinical application, without requiring years of very unique training and clinical experience, for example, with diagnoses of cystic versus solid lesions. Accuracy in assessing breast [1] tumors and metastatic foci has been documented. It must be emphasized that the beginner will find many confusing artifacts and findings should be confirmed with all pertinent imaging modalities.

3D Doppler ultrasound with dynamic contrast-enhanced MRI are the gold standards by which cancers are initially diagnosed or confirmed and serially followed after treatment. The percentage of malignant vessels can be quantified and re-evaluated in the identical tumor volume as serial follow ups to the standard treatments using: radiation, surgery, hormones, chemotherapy, cryotherapy, watchful waiting, and the nonstandard regenerative treatments: ablation using focal laser, focal ultrasound, photodynamic, radiofrequency, and microwave technologies. Since vessel mapping is possible, embolic treatments may be considered.

3D sonography can demonstrate the tumor volume and marginal capsule of locally affected lymph nodes more accurately than the MRI since the resolution is 100 microns at 18 MHz. The exam takes about 10 min, and the probes are automated meaning that this is less operator dependent than other sonographic procedures. Vessel density index (VI) imaging is performed on the data set at an independent workstation and comparison made with prior exams if available.

3D power Doppler indices vary according to the tumor stage, the histologic grade, capsular disruption, and lymph node metastases. Histologic grade has been studied with this technology, and the following approximation has proven useful in prostate tumor staging. This quantitative measure of neovascularity was initially applied to prostate cancer [2]. While it does not exactly correlate with histologic Gleason grading since this is a current functional measure while the microscopy is purely anatomical and may not represent current aggressive potential. It is predictive value of aggression could be studied in the context of breast and other cancers [3, 5].

Medical imaging can map the arteries, veins, and nerves providing preoperative landmarks reducing postoperative bleeding and avoiding nerve damage. Tumors of low aggressive potential may be treated medically and followed by interval scans or locally reduced by radiation or laser ablation. Biopsies of certain abnormalities may be averted or postponed (Fig 14.1)

14.1.8 Breast Cancer

High tumor vessel density correlates with greater aggression. Axillary and mediastinal imaging can document lymphadenopathy. Abdominal scans simultaneously performed may detect ascites and metastases to the liver, periaortic nodes, and pelvic organs. Response to neoadjuvant chemotherapy may be assessed by MRI, CT,

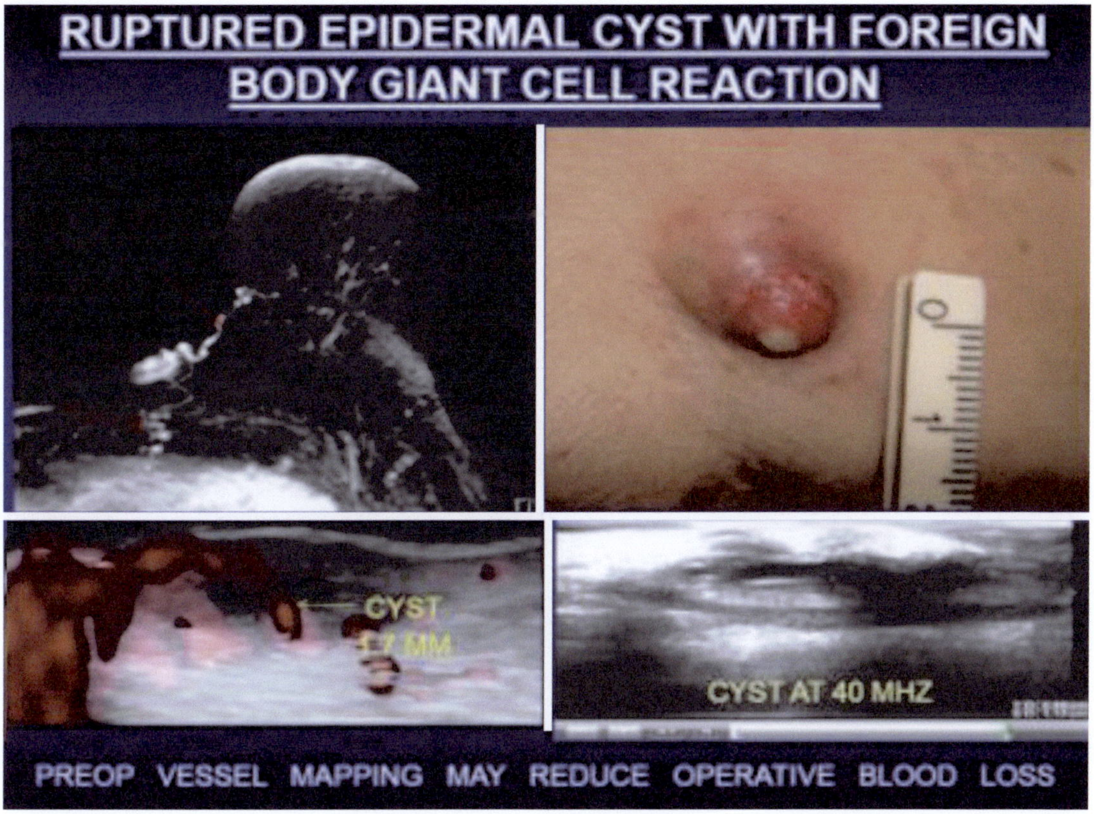

Fig. 14.1 Ruptured intradermal cyst mimicking breast cancer on MRI, Doppler, sonogram, and 3D

mammography, PET/CT, and ultrasound. The new technology of ultrasound elastography, assessing tumor stiffness, predicts response to treatment accurately and may indicate better therapeutic strategies on a timelier basis [4]. Residual cancer burden scoring could provide better treatment options since the treatment response for evaluation of neoadjuvant chemotherapy needs a more comprehensive and authoritative standard than that is currently available.

14.1.9 Lymph Node Disease

Lymph node assessment is possible at the same time. Under sonographic guidance, biopsies may be obtained. Sonographic criteria for malignancy are published elsewhere. Image guidance of enlarged nodes can distinguish between active tumor and necrotic areas, diminishing the necessity of repeated aspirations for indeterminate findings (Fig 14.2). Pathologic assessment of a large postoperative specimen may be facilitated by high-frequency scanning to relocalize the suspect region for targeted study that has been removed from its previous anatomic position [6]. Elastography is useful in targeting subcentimeter foci in large nodal masses.

14.1.10 Image-Guided Biopsy and Treatment

New computer programs use nanotechnology and cybernetic modalities for accurate image-guided biopsy and treatment options. Lesions as small as 3 mm have been successfully imaged at frequencies above 14 MHz. Employing 3D sonography with Doppler, the physician manually targets the area of highest tumor neovascularity. This is critical since only part of a mass may be cancerous and missed on nontargeted

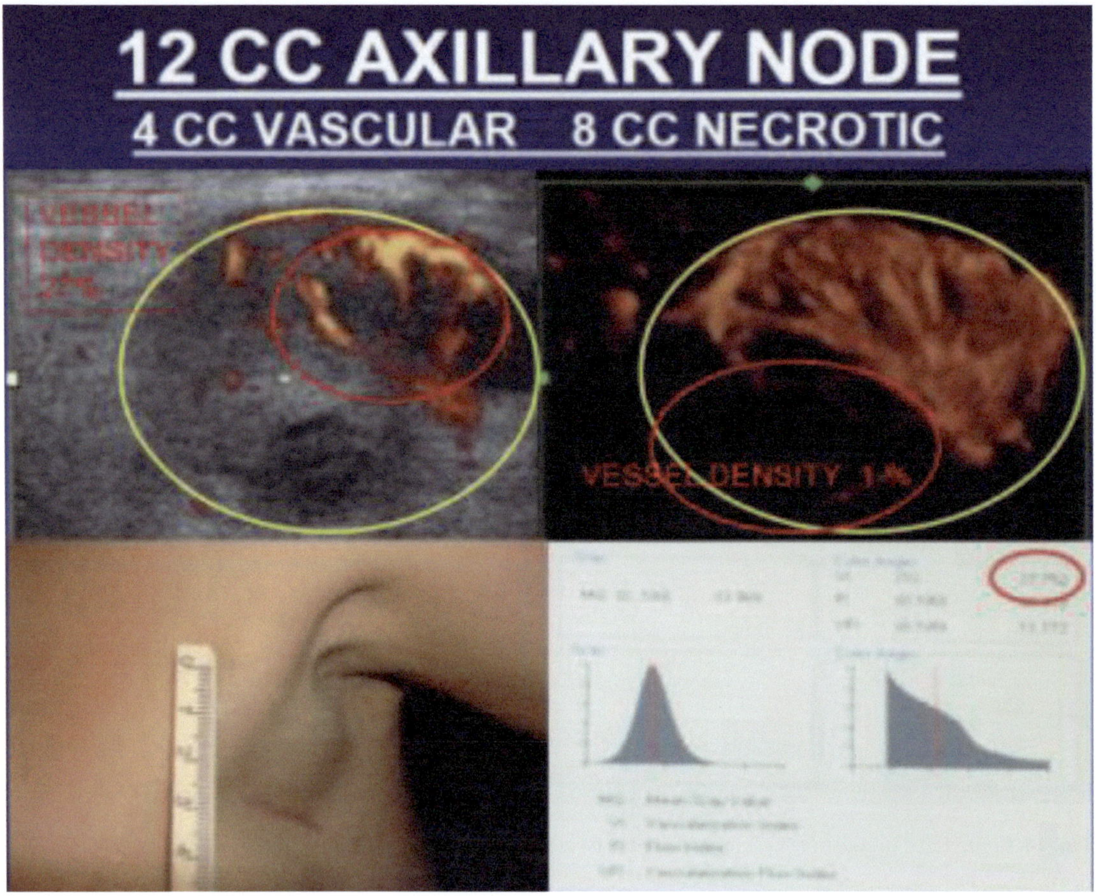

Fig. 14.2 Mixed solid/necrotic axillary lymph node-vessel density allows targeting of active disease

punch biopsies. The marriage with fusion of MRI with ultrasound permits image-guided biopsies that spare the adjacent vascular channels. The same technology allows customized ultrasound or MRI-guided biopsies to be performed under local anesthesia. Immediate cytologic confirmation of tumor cells permits the withdrawal of the biopsy needle and insertion of a LASER fiber or cryogenic probe immediately treating the proven tumor. MRI thermocouple sensors prevent overheating of the adjacent nerves and sensitive tissues. Following ablation, the zone of destruction is confirmed with Doppler, contrast ultrasound or DCE-MRI. Inflammatory lesions that are deeply seated may be approached by robotic image-guided subdermal injections or targeted biopsies if necessary. This outpatient procedure allows the patient to return to work immediately. RF thermoprobes with temperature auto cutoffs prevent thermal skin damage [7]. Similar user-friendly and cost-effective modalities may replace other therapies in the near future. At the 2016 AMERICAN SOCIETY OF LASERS IN MEDICINE meeting in Boston, cutaneous melanoma with intransit metastases was successively treated by laser technologies [8] MRI fusion biopsies with CT and/or ultrasound are routine adding further to the accuracy of image-guided biopsies and focal treatment procedures [9]. Advances in ultrasound elastography progressed from simple strain imaging to shear wave sonography to 3D coronal shear wave elastography where the plane of the image corresponds to the surgical field as the tumor is dissected in the most superficial plane. The tumor desmoplasia in the coronal plane creates a sawtooth irregular border with a central echo pattern simulating a "donut" and is termed the "crater" sign in this increasingly popular imaging paradigm. Elastography is used worldwide primarily in the diagnostic workup of breast, thyroid, and prostate tumors and has reduced the number of biopsies on false-positive findings from mammography, b-mode ultrasound, and MRI [10].

14.1.11 Summary

3D sonography and power Doppler angiography are techniques that contribute new morphologic parameters and noninvasive functional tumoral angiogenic markers for evaluation and treatment follow-up of hyperplastic diseases and cancers. The addition of in vivo real-time volume density measurements of tumor neovascularity may prove to be of value in determining the risk of tumor recurrence noninvasively.

The widespread availability of point-of-care sonography units means a cancer survivor with a new lump can have certainty that it is indeed a benign lipoma or cyst, which can be readily differentiated from a metastatic node or recurrent cancer. The more oncologists, dermatologists, and plastic surgeons use the imaging capacities of sonography, the more they will find its attributes essential to the modern practice of skin disorder therapies.

Axillary mass with 3D histogram targeting region of interest.

14.1.12 Robotic Mastectomy: A Revolutionary Procedure

Stephen Chagares, MD, FACS

- RM introduction in Italy—include statistics from Antonio paper and number of patients performance in Italy we have been watching it for 5 years, finally saw equivalence to current mastectomy procedure, safe to bring to US, time to take action.
- Include countries where RM expanded to after Antonio seminars.
- First-person perspective of Chagares witnessing surgery.
- Brings it to US.

14.1.12.1 Current Spread Worldwide and the United States

- Six (6) Clinical trials active worldwide.
- One (1) Clinical Trial is Texas, Illinois, New York, Pennsylvania, and Minnesota
- One (1) University of Ohio.
- Intuitive is working with locations and the FDA.
- I performed two patients, one risk reducing, one for gynecomastia. first cancer patient in the US and first male worldwide.

Prophylactic risk-reducing mastectomy procedures have existed and seen minimal innovation over the past twenty years. Robotic surgical system technology has offered an alternative to these traditional approaches that has taken mastectomy into the twenty-first century. It follows a similar process to the traditional mastectomy, yet incorporates the robot to provide a more refined method of excising the breast tissue. The use of a robot, most commonly that of the Intuitive *da Vinci*® Surgical System, provides a method of operating through a smaller incision, decreasing the amount of scarring resulting from a procedure.

Robotic-assisted surgical techniques have been performed in various specialties, initially including radical prostatectomy, radical cystectomy, colorectal surgery, and hysterectomy, with the majority of earlier cases dedicated to oncological procedures. Over the ensuing years, robotic-assisted surgery has extended out to general surgery and subspecialties including cardiac surgery, head and neck surgery, and thoracic surgery. The abdomen and thorax have potential spaces making minimally invasive surgery possible. These patients benefit from superior esthetic outcomes and improved postoperative conditions. Despite the lack of a natural cavity in the breast needed for minimally invasive procedures, applications of robotic-assisted surgery have emerged including mastectomy performed both as a risk-reducing treatment for patients at high risk for developing breast cancer and as a therapeutic treatment for those with breast cancer. Specific to mastectomies, a robotic nipple sparing mastectomy (RNSM) is a surgical procedure performed to remove the breast tissue for breast cancer treatment or as a preventative measure for those at risk of developing breast cancer. While I have been performing mastectomies throughout my career, I have incorporated robotic surgery into his skillset since the inception of the technology in 2015.

By performing the same long-held mastectomy procedure with robotic assistance, I am able to operate using a significantly smaller hidden incision created on the side of the chest wall in an RNSM, leaving the nipple and areola intact, compared to the traditional technique which leaves a scar spanning the length of the breast. Currently, insurance bills the procedure at the same cost as a traditional mastectomy, making it all the more accessible to patients interested in receiving the new-age technique.

In October 2015, Dr. Antonio Toesca and his team were the first to describe the surgical technique of using a single small hidden axillary incision to perform RNSM and immediate robotic-assisted implant-based breast reconstruction. The subsequent reports described more than a hundred successful cases around the world, demonstrating the feasibility and safety of this procedure. With this procedure on my radar over the past three years, I knew I had to keep on the cutting-edge and offer my patients a better alternative once these studies were published, reinforcing the safety of the procedure.

I traveled to Milan, Italy, in June 2018 where Dr. Toesca performed the world-renowned RNSM procedure at his operating rooms in the European Institute of Oncology. I, along with surgical teams from South Korea and France, observed Dr. Toesca expertly removed the breast tissue of two middle-aged women with breast cancer, leaving behind the nipple and areola in the process and following the procedure with immediate reconstruction of the breasts.

Following the procedure, I talked to him about expanding the procedure, making it more widely available for patients in the US. Dr. Toesca was familiar with his own initial troubles in kick starting the procedure in Italy, including the regulations and patient trials required to approve the revolutionary process. In adapting his practice to the American health system, I designed a study to assess patient outcome following the procedure to further show its comparable efficacy to traditional mastectomy. I was excited to pursue this route as it allowed me to provide the already proven procedure to patients while building on the collection of positive data supporting its outcomes. By working directly with intuitive surgical, myself, along with a collection of other surgeons, would be able to bring the procedure closer to full FDA approval in the US, making it more available for patients.

The use of robotics in breast surgery is an exciting development, creating new treatment options in the field of breast cancer while setting a precedent for the continued use of the robot in other surgical areas. The precision and increased mobility that the robot provides enables a less-invasive procedure, especially in the case of mastectomy where scarring traditionally spanned the width of the breast, acting as a reminder to the patient of their prior condition. A robotic mastectomy procedure that does not have to sacrifice the accuracy of the procedure to create an improved esthetic outcome becomes an essential tool in providing patients an alternative to the current process, while also paving the way for the future of surgery. This also takes into account the current trend in breast care. Breast cancer affects 1 in 8 women and is the second-leading cause of cancer death, trailing only lung cancer. Some women can be treated with lumpectomies, which conserve the breast. But more women are turning to mastectomies, not only to treat breast cancer but also to prevent it; the rate of mastectomies increased 36% from 2005 to 2013, according to the U.S. Department of Health and Human Services.

Yvonne Z, a patient in her mid-50s, was diagnosed with Stage IIA breast cancer, undergoing a four-month chemotherapy treatment regimen. After receiving information from her referring physician, she opted to undergo RNSM to further decrease her chances of the cancer recurring. Ms. Z became my first RNSM patient, which opened the door to a new era of mastectomy and a new outlook for her, offering a modern approach to an operation that had been so physically, emotionally, and psychologically scarring until now. Following her procedure, Ms. Z recalled, "to be able to wake from surgery, look down, not see any visible scars and have my nipples and areolas intact with implants in, is amazing." Unfortunately, two years later, Ms. Z passed away due to distant metastases. On my last visit with Ms. Z, she was happy to say she never had locally recurrent breast cancer. She passed knowing that she played a role in showing the efficacy of RNSM.

I followed this successful case in using mastectomy to address breast cancer by moving into a more esthetically geared procedure. BT, a 34-year-old patient with gynecomastia, had quickly developed excess breast tissue, growing large painful lumps in both breasts. In assessing Mr. T for the procedure, I applauded his dismissal of the stigma most men have against male breast cancer and pursued the RNSM treatment option. After removing Mr. T's breast tissue, I saw his outstanding postoperative state, having almost complete range of motion in his arms. He advocates for others that, "if there's men out there who have problems, who have breast cancer, lumps, anything, talk to someone about it."

I look forward to providing this comprehensive breast care technique to a greater population of patients while allowing more surgeons to become certified to work with the RNSM technique. In providing further patient outcome information to intuitive, combined with their four additional research institutions, I hope to quickly advance the success and prevalence of RNSM. Seeing robotic mastectomy migrate from Italy into our healthcare system will prove beneficial to both patients and health providers.

14.1.13 Breast Disease in Athletic Women

A special case is younger women who are involved actively in athletic pursuits as well as women under 50 who have low body mass ratios [11]. Inspired by Dr. Cutter's program, the last 50 years of dense breast imaging, first presented at the Breast Ultrasound Congress in 1979 in Philadelphia, was reviewed to date at our institution, revealing a higher incidence of tumors in younger women with many incidences of palpable cancer totally missed by mammography and generally detected by real-time ultrasound which used 7 MHz probes in the 1970s and now uses 18–24 MHz 3D technology. The addition of elastography, automated whole-breast ultrasound, thermography, Doppler histogram, reflectance confocal microscopy, autofluorescence and optical computed tomography with biopsy guidance employing state of the art fusion practices continues to improve our detection rate.

For women under the age of 30 years, the American College of Radiology (ACR) has followed a group of probably benign (Birads 3) with sequential imaging. After 2 years of stability, biopsy determined that most stable lesions had low compliance with cancer. Findings suggested that probably benign tumors were most likely fibroadenomas, which may only warrant a follow-up study of 6 months. Note that the study uses ultrasound with Doppler but not other modalities discussed above for correlation [12]. Most biopsies were requested by the patient implying that the full edition of the advanced imaging may have reduced the biopsy rate by increasing patient confidence in modern diagnostics. Patient education and understanding that biopsies produce scarring and breast distortion that lessens the accuracy of all diagnostics procedures to follow surgical management would be useful as well as full disclosure of the potential complications of surgery. In the last 5 years, patients are opting for nonsurgical tumor treatment of probably benign or low-grade cancers with the newly developed focal treatment technologies, such as cryotherapy, laser, and other thermal treatments such as high-intensity-focused ultrasound (HIFU) and new light therapies. Skin cancers are currently treated with laser without surgical cutting since the depth of the tumor is visible with noninvasive imaging such as ultrasound and confocal microscopy.

14.1.14 Toxins and Environmental Exposure

In 2020, a female computer analyst from San Francisco with breast cancer came into the New York office for evaluation of lymph nodes possibly related to the COVID-19 vaccination. I had recently become aware of the high rate of benign reactive axillary lymphadenopathy from the various vaccines, which are particularly alarming to patients with a previous cancer history. From my military background as a US Air Force radiologist stationed in Vietnam and exposed to Agent Orange, I question patients as to military placement, burn pit duty, and toxic exposure. As I am also trained in Tropical Medicine in Texas, I routinely enquire as to possible parasitic infestation. Furthermore, living 6 miles from Ground Zero at the World Trade Center 2001 holocaust, we query New Yorkers about their presence in the Danger Zone at that site. To my surprise, the lady from Silicone Valley had been a nurse at a hospital and tended to the disaster victims. Since we know from the 911-Occupational Statistics Division at Mt. Sinai Medical Center that skin cancers are the 3 most common comorbidities of toxic exposure. I checked and found a small basal cell skin cancer on the back of her ear. The lesson is clearly for physicians to ask about travel and exposures, while patients must mention potential toxic exposures now commonly found in well water communities.

Evaluation of background toxic environmental exposure including mold and mycotoxins is a modifiable danger if there is personal and public awareness. Toxic exposures have been noted with the COVID-19 virus recently, and it is known that many environmental toxins affect the unborn baby. Early exposure prenatally not only affects both immediate risk but also the lifetime risk of disease, which involves fertility, hormone function, immune system response, and cognitive function. Throughout life, bioaccumulation increases the toxic burden and may exacerbate these biologic functions resulting in chronic health problems. Common environmental exposure includes air pollution, preservatives in food, household products, and most recently body care products, which seem to be contaminated with benzene. The widespread commercial practice of horizontal hydrofracking contaminates freshwater, and a variety of chemicals have been found in fracking wastewater including xylenes, toluene, benzene, styrene, etc. Nationwide groundwater contamination occurs from agricultural development and mass production farming practices. However, in cities, industrial refuse and commercial waste removal including local governmental disposal practices is a common urban contributor to environmental degradation. Municipal water authorities monitor for common contaminants, while in the country private wells are not regulated so administrators do not check for heavy metal, which leaves a significant population vulnerable to well water contamination exposure.

If the toxic load overwhelms the body's detoxification capability, lipophilic chemicals will migrate into adipose tissue, fat cells, or into the cellular mitochondria. The mitochondria are particularly sensitive to chemical exposure and are unable to completely detoxify these compounds leading to cytoplasmic deterioration, and ongoing chemical exposure disrupts biochemical signaling pathways and cellular functions. Toluene, phthalates, and benzene induce inflammation and contribute to atopic dermatitis specifically allergy, asthma, and eczema while possibly increasing the risk of type two diabetes. The health effects of toxic chemicals, industrial plastics, and heavy metal pollutants have been described individually with most of the analysis directed at pregnancy. Additionally, the blood test and urine test for a concentration of toxins such as arsenic and mercury do not correlate very well. Also combinations of exposure to toxins and chemicals have not been studied together. We have learned from the World trade Center testing from 911 that the combined effects of the different by-products of fire and toxins mixed with asbestos have created new and more toxic compounds to the body that are still being a valuated today, such as the discovery that air and surface contamination from 911 debris has produced more skin cancers than lung cancer with prostate cancer being number fifth on the list and lung cancer being number four, while the first three cancers are basal cell, squamous cell and melanomas being second and third on the list of toxic side effects. We have documented from doing high-resolution skin ultrasound with ultrahigh resolution sonography and optical biomicroscopy (reflectance confocal microscopy and optical computed tomography) that the dermal layers are a long-term repository for toxins, which are now imaged and quantified with these new technologies. We may have a better way to measure the long-term risks by looking at the distinctive dermal patterns of skin reflecting cellular aggregates in the intradermal layers, which seem to correlate well with clinical toxic metal, heavy metal, and radioactive contamination.

Detoxification of the body by physical washing and removing the toxin from the skin encourages sweating to increase skin detoxification, improve overall nutrition, and support biochemical pathways or mitochondrial function that reduce the damage to the cellular matrix. Progress is noted that more people are buying liquids in glass rather than plastic containers, and our first responders are washing their fire suits after a fire and no longer parading in their smoke-laden outfits as a show of pride for being a hero at a conflagration.

Regarding mold micro toxins and home detoxification, people are now testing their houses for radon and mold contamination as well as checking their well water level of contamination. Well mold illness is usually related to allergic reactions and can cause respiratory difficulties, and there is a variation of mold disorder called mycotoxin where the mold spore produces toxic chemicals, which then go into the atmosphere or into the food or water. Black mold is the most toxic variety of a mycotoxin and can affect multiple organ systems including the kidney, liver, and brain The constellation of symptoms is variable and different for each person but includes fatigue weakness, poor memory, difficulty concentrating, morning stiffness, joint pain, skin numbness, shortness of breath, increased urinary frequency, red eyes and blurred vision, abdominal pain, diarrhea, and bloating. Extreme cases of vertigo can cause shock [13–18].

References

1. Bard R. Vascular imaging of cancer in the dense breast. 60th Journees Francaises de Radiologie. 2012. Paris.
2. Cruwys C, Pushkin JA. Breast density and impacts on health. Ecancermedicalscience. 2017;11:ed70.
3. Nazari SS, Mukherjee P. An overview of mammographic density and its association with breast cancer. Breast Cancer. 2018;25(3):259–67.
4. Burton A, et al. Mammographic density and ageing: A collaborative pooled analysis of cross-sectional data from 22 countries worldwide. PLoS Med. 2017;14(6):e1002335.
5. Boyd NF, et al. "Mammographic density: a heritable risk factor for breast cancer." cancer epidemiology. Totowa, NJ: Humana Press; 2009. p. 343–60.
6. Azam S, et al. Determinants of mammographic density change. JNCI Cancer Spectr. 2019;3(1):pkz004.
7. Boyd NF, et al. Body size, mammographic density, and breast cancer risk. Cancer Epidemiol Biomarkers Prev. 2006;15(11):2086–92.
8. Bard R. Thermal treatment with 3D Doppler image correlation in image guided cancer treatment. Cham: Springer; 2014.
9. Bard R. Image guided cancer treatment. In: Advances in medical and surgical dermatology, 15th annual Mt Sinai winter symposium. New York: The New York Academy of Medicine; 2015.
10. Merce L, Alcazar J, Lopez C, et al. Clinical usefulness of 3 Dimensional sonography and power Doppler angiography for the diagnosis of endometrial carcinoma. J Ultrasound Med. 2007;26:1279–89.
11. Bard R. Image guided covid-19 lung treatment. Cham: Springer; 2021.
12. Chen Y, Chang C, Zeng W, et al. 3D shearwave elastography of breast lesions. Medicine. 2016;95(39):e4877–91.
13. Mitterberger M. Comparison of contrast enhanced ultrasound targeted biopsy. J Urol. 2007;178:464–72.

14. Jing M, Wen C, Zi L, et al. Early evaluation of relative changes in tumor stiffness by elastography predicts response. J Ultrasound Med. 2016;35:1619–27.
15. Obek C. Core needle biopsy length affects grading and staging. J Urol. 2012;187(6):2051–5.
16. Bard R, Futterer J, Sperling, editors. Image guided prostate cancer treatment. Cham: Springer; 2014.
17. Bard R. Image guided dermatologic treatment. Cham: Springer; 2020.
18. Merchant K, Omar L, Hayes J, et al. ACR Bi-Rads 3 category lesions in women younger than 30. J Ultrasound Med. 2021;40:2699–708.

15 Image-Guided Superficial Radiotherapy and Other Noninvasive Modalities Used in the Treatment of Non-melanoma Skin Cancer and Keloids

Lio Yu, Mairead Moloney, and Robert L. Bard

Abstract

Targeted superficial radiation therapy (SRT) may be used on most skin cancers and certain benign conditions such as keloids. Key to treatment effectiveness is image guidance with ultrasound for depth. SRT is useful in therapy of difficult surgical sites such as the pretibial region, ear, and nose. This chapter is organized with background information on non-melanoma skin cancer (NMSC) and keloids. Followed by a discussion of the various modalities used in the nonsurgical (and surgical) management of NMSC and keloids with an expanded section on the use of image-guided superficial radiotherapy (IGSRT).

Keywords

Radiation therapy · Skin cancer · Basal cell cancer · Image guidance · Squamous cell skin cancer · Keloids

15.1 Introduction

15.1.1 Non-melanoma Skin Cancer (NMSC)

Non-melanoma skin cancer (NMSC) is the most common cancer in the world, including in the United States [1, 2]. NMSC can include various entities including lymphomas, sarcomas, etc., however, the overwhelming proportion consists of basal cell carcinoma (BCC), cutaneous squamous cell carcinoma (cSCC or SCC), and cutaneous squamous cell carcinoma in situ (SCCIS). BCCs are less aggressive than SCCs, with a metastatic rate of 0.0281–0.05%, compared to SCC, which has a slightly higher metastatic rate of 0.5–16% [3, 4]. While NMSC typically have a good prognosis, as they have a low mortality rate and low metastatic potential, the current standard of care is to have these lesions treated surgically with excision, electro-

L. Yu (✉)
Radiation Oncology, Laserderm Dermatology, Smithtown, NY, USA

M. Moloney
New York Institute of Technology, College of Osteopathic Medicine, Old Westbury, NY, USA

R. L. Bard
The Angio Foundation and Bard Diagnostics, New York, NY, USA
e-mail: rbard@cancerscan.com

R. L. Bard (ed.), *Image-Guided Aesthetic Treatments*, https://doi.org/10.1007/978-3-031-36266-8_15

desiccation, and curettage (ED&C), and Mohs micrographic surgery (MMS) to prevent local invasion [4–6].

MMS has been considered the gold standard for NMSC treatment, especially for higher risk lesions, as much research indicates MMS provides the lowest 5-year local recurrence rates for BCC and SCC [7, 8]. Despite surgical excision being the predominant treatment, there are many nonsurgical treatment options available such as topical therapy, photodynamic therapy, cryosurgery, laser therapy, and radiation therapy [7, 8].

Since most (~70%) NMSC lesions occur on the head and neck, tissue conservation is imperative to achieve excellent cosmesis, and thus, surgery may be less desirable or omitted in favor of a nonsurgical approach [5]. With increasing incidence including the younger generation being diagnosed with NMSC, such as BCC and SCC, cosmesis may play an even more important role [9]. The overall goal of treatment is eradication of tumor and preservation of function while achieving optimal esthetics.

Image-guided superficial radiation therapy (IGSRT) may be emerging to be the ideal nonsurgical modality to achieve the 4 "C's" desirable in NMSC treatment: cure, [decreased] complications, cosmesis, and convenience [10] (Figs. 15.1, 15.2, and 15.3).

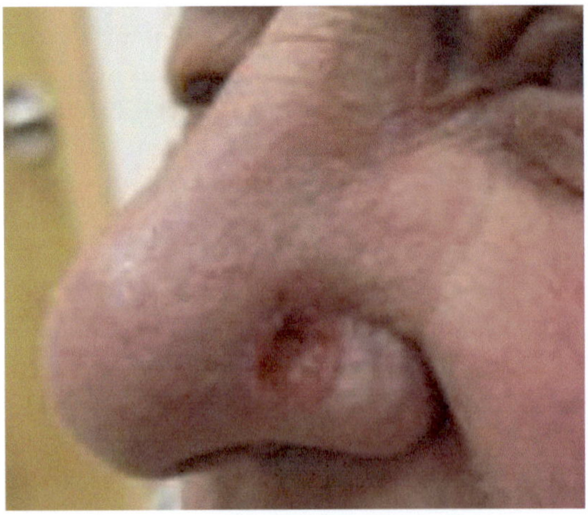

Fig. 15.1 Basal cell carcinoma on the left nostril

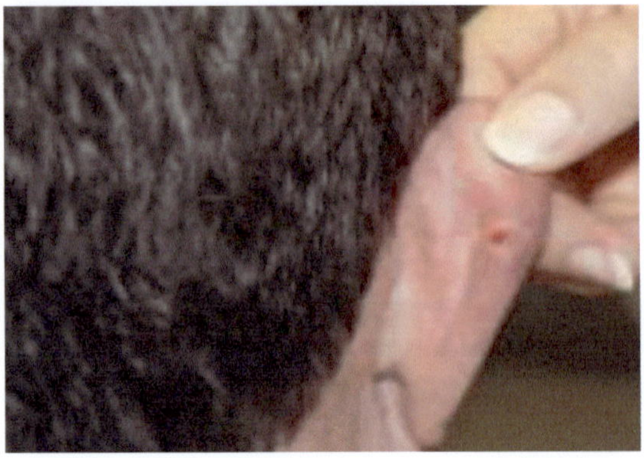

Fig. 15.2 Basal cell carcinoma on the right ear

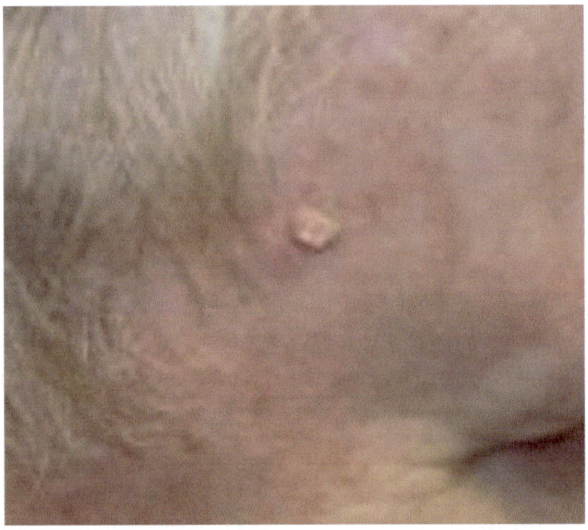

Fig. 15.3 Squamous cell carcinoma on the right forehead

15.2 Keloids

Keloids form as an excessive hyperproliferative scar due to abnormal wound healing [11]. Aside from the cosmetic aspect of keloids, other issues include discomfort, pruritus, pain/hyperesthesia, induration/rigidity of affected tissues, and limitation in the range of motion or mobility of the patient depending on the location of the keloid. They can occur years after a minor injury or spontaneously without any history of injury. When caused by injury, keloids can extend beyond the original borders of the wound. The borders of the keloid are typically irregular, but usually clearly demarcated, firm masses with a shiny surface composed of disorganized type I and III collagen that usually do not regress spontaneously. Patients are plagued with high recurrence rates when keloids are excised. Common locations include ears, cheeks, anterior chest, shoulders, and upper arms where piercing, irritation, or injury often occur.

Keloids occur equally in males and females typically in their 20s to 30s and occur in individuals of all races, but have an incidence of 6–16% in African Americans [11]. Keloid treatment options include 5-fluorouracil (5-FU), Imiquimod, photodynamic therapy (PDT), cryotherapy, radiation therapy, laser therapy, intralesional steroid injection, and surgical treatment [11].

Although many alternative treatments exist for keloids, one of the most effective methods of controlling keloids, particularly refractive keloids having multiple previous attempts at control that have failed, is radiation therapy (Figs. 15.4, 15.5, 15.6, and 15.7).

15.2.1 Nonsurgical Modalities for NMSC and Keloids

15.2.1.1 5-Fluorouracil (5-FU)

5-Fluorouracil (5-FU) is a pyrimidine analog, which is an antimetabolite that interferes with DNA and RNA synthesis leading to decreased cell proliferation and apoptosis [12].

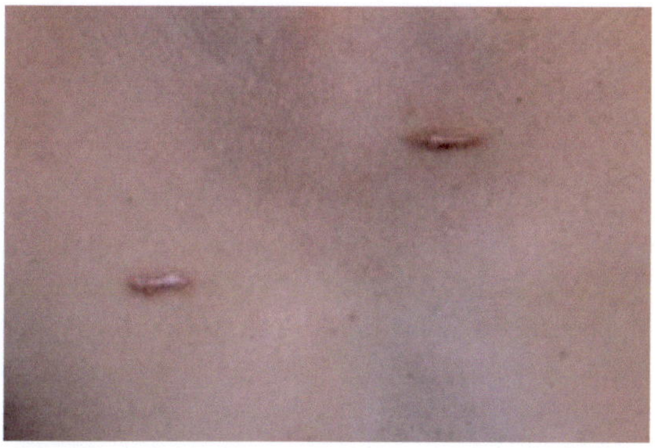

Fig. 15.4 Linear keloids

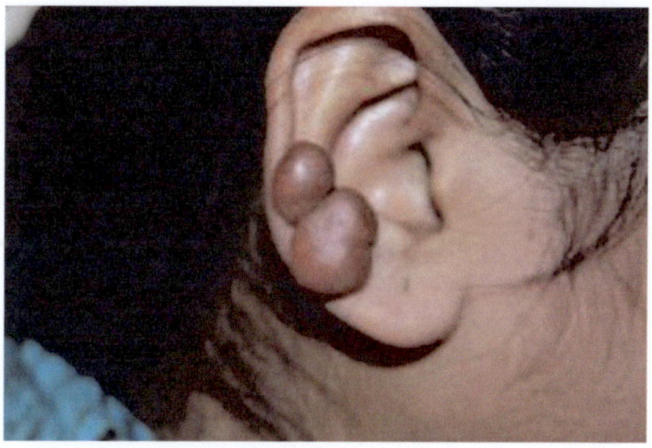

Fig. 15.5 Auricular keloid on right ear

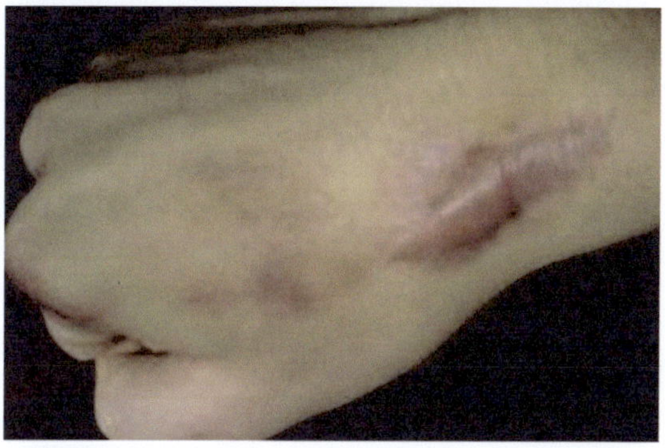

Fig. 15.6 Left wrist keloid

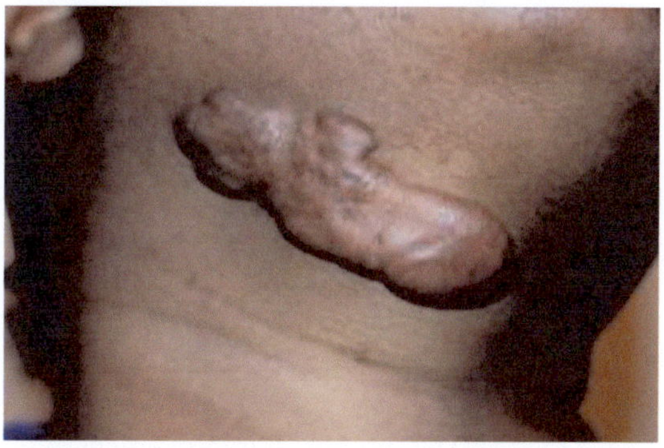

Fig. 15.7 Bulky neck keloid

15.2.1.2 NMSC Treatment with 5-Fluorouracil (5-FU)

Topical 5-fluorouracil (5-FU) is approved by the United States Food and Drug Administration (FDA) for the treatment of superficial basal cell carcinomas (sBCC) and actinic keratoses (AK) [13]. It is also used off-label for select squamous

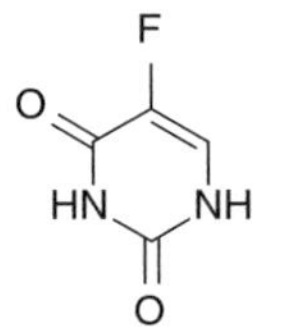

Fig. 15.8 Structure of 5-fluorouracil (5-FU)

cell carcinoma in situ (SCC-IS) [14]. 5-FU is applied topically twice a day for 2 or more weeks [13] (Fig. 15.8).

This topical cream can be used for treatment as opposed to surgery in areas where cosmetic outcome is a concern, such as areas where there are multiple lesions or lesions on the face [13]. Many studies have shown good to excellent cosmesis with 5-FU treatment [14]. One case series reported a 90% histologic cure rate with an average treatment duration of 10.5 weeks [15]. It was reported that good cosmetic results were achieved, and patients were satisfied with their results. Most patients experienced no pain or scarring and only minimal erythema [15]. Another study reported 84.7% (137/153) of sBCC lesions treated with 5-FU had good or excellent cosmesis [9].

Fluorouracil cream can be used over a relatively large area/surface, whereas IGSRT, surgery, ED&C is generally limited to a relatively smaller area. 5-FU can be used to treat BCC's that are too small to be seen by an unaided eye to presumptively treat subclinical tumors in patients with basal cell nevus syndrome [16].

Drawbacks of 5-FU use include that it has small skin penetration, which is why its treatment is limited to superficial BCCs and not thicker or more deeply invading types of BCC or invasive SCC [13, 14]. The superficial improvement of the lesion with 5-FU can deceive dermatologists and the patient. Leaving unseen deeper parts of the lesion to continue to proliferate and grow [13]. Thus, in order to confirm histologic cure, surgical excision is necessary [15].

One of the most concerning drawbacks of 5-FU use is that it has high recurrence rates. One study reported the 5-year tumor-free survival to be 70% after treatment of sBCC with 5-FU [9].

Local skin irritations of 5-FU include erythema, pruritus, dermatitis, crusting, burning sensation, and photosensitivity [12].

Since 5-FU must be applied by the patient twice daily for multiple weeks, making patient selection is a key criterion. Patients must be able to easily reach the lesion for treatment adherence. If the lesion is hard to reach or the patient is elderly, this can lead to noncompliance [12].

15.2.1.3 Keloid Treatment with 5-Fluorouracil (5-FU)

Keloids can be treated with 5-FU (50 mg/mL) via intralesional injection [11]. Particularly for the treatment of keloids, in vitro studies have shown to decrease fibroblast growth, promote fibroblast apoptosis, and decrease collagen growth promoted by TGF-beta. Studies report keloid volume reduction in 58–65% of patients at least 6 months post-treatment of 5-FU monotherapy [17].

One drawback of 5-FU therapy for keloids is that recurrence is common, reported at rates of 21–35% at minimum 3 months after treatment [17].

Side effects after intralesional injection include pain upon injection, ulceration, and hyperpigmentation [17]. Adverse systemic reactions of 5-FU include anemia, leukopenia, and thrombocytopenia, but these systemic side effects have not been observed with intralesional injection [11, 17]. However, 5-FU therapy must be avoided in pregnant women or individuals with bone marrow suppression [11].

15.2.2 Imiquimod

Imiquimod is an immunomodulating agent suggested to stimulate the innate and adaptive immune pathways [18]. It activates the innate immune system by increasing cytokine production and secretion [14]. Imiquimod is approved by the United States Food and Drug Administration (FDA) for the treatment of superficial basal cell carcinomas (sBCC), actinic keratoses (AK), external genital and perianal warts [18]. Imiquimod 5% cream is typically

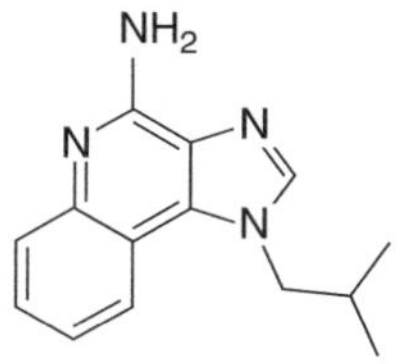

Fig. 15.9 Structure of Imiquimod

applied 2–5 times per week for 6–16 weeks, depending on its use of treatment [12] (Fig. 15.9).

15.2.2.1 NMSC Treatment with Imiquimod

Imiquimod can be used in the treatment of sBCC where surgery is not an option or when patients opt for a nonsurgical treatment option. Imiquimod provides a cosmetic advantage compared to surgery [14]. One study reported 81.8% (121/148) of sBCC lesions treated with Imiquimod had good or excellent cosmesis [9]. Additionally, favorable response rates have been observed, as randomized controlled trials (RCTs) of Imiquimod for the treatment of sBCC with various treatment regimens (i.e., 2×/day, 1×/day, 5×/week, 3×/week) have shown treatment responses up to 100%, and more frequent applications of Imiquimod showed the best responses (i.e. 2×/day or 1×/day) [19].

The most common adverse effects of Imiquimod include local skin reactions, such as erythema, discomfort, erosion, and hypopigmentation/hyperpigmentation [12]. Systemic reactions can include flu-like illness, headache, dizziness, and in rare circumstances urinary retention. Additionally, high recurrence rates may be observed, as one study reported the 5-year tumor free survival to be 80.5% after treatment of sBCC with Imiquimod [9]. As with 5-FU, Imiquimod must be applied by the patient, who must be able to easily reach the lesion for treatment adherence. If the lesion is hard to reach or the patient is elderly, this can lead to noncompliance [12].

15.2.2.2 Keloid Treatment with Imiquimod

Keloids can be treated with adjunctive topical daily Imiquimod 5% cream post-surgical excision [17]. Imiquimod can be useful as it limits collagen production by fibroblasts by increasing interferon-alpha. Adjunctive topical daily Imiquimod 5% cream may help in reducing keloid recurrence post-surgical excision.

However, keloids can still recur despite Imiquimod adjunctive therapy, with reported variable recurrence rates of 0–88.9% with follow-up of 20–24 weeks [17]. Side effects of topical Imiquimod 5% cream include irritation, erythema, and hyperpigmentation, all which resolve upon cessation of Imiquimod.

15.2.3 Photodynamic Therapy (PDT)

15.2.3.1 NMSC and In Situ/Precancerous Lesion Treatment with Photodynamic Therapy (PDT)

Photodynamic therapy (PDT) is used for treating basal cell carcinoma (BCC), Bowen's disease (BD), and actinic keratoses (AK) [20]. An exogenous topical or systemic photosensitizer is taken up by premalignant and malignant cells, which converts the prodrug to protoporphyrin IX (PpIX). Then a light source is introduced, which activates PpIX resulting in the formation of reactive oxygen species (ROS) and selective cytotoxicity of malignant cells. The FDA has approved the use of two topical drugs with PDT [21]. The first drug was a 20% 5-aminolevulinic acid (ALA) solution, known as Levulan Kerastick; ALA-PDT is approved for use of non hyperkeratotic actinic keratoses of the face and scalp. The second drug is Metvixia, which is a methyl ester of ALA (MAL), and MAL-PDT is approved for the effective treatment of NMSC [21]. PDT is generally recommended for actinic keratoses (AKs) and thin NMSC, such as superficial BCC (sBCC) that are less than 1–2 mm thick. sBCC is the most responsive to treatment with PDT (response rates ranging from 75% to 97%) [12] (Fig. 15.10).

An advantage of PDT is that the topical photosensitizers allow for large areas to be treated in a single treatment [14]. The photosensitivity is confined to the area of application of the topical

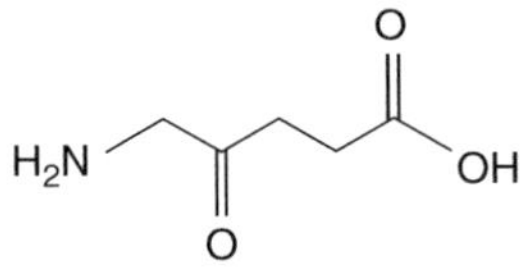

Fig. 15.10 5-Aminolevulinic acid (ALA) structure

photosensitizers, limiting systemic absorption. This is advantageous to patients with larger or multiple lesions; however, treatment does require multiple office visits by the patient [19].

MAL-PDT has been shown to have statistically better cosmetic outcome compared to 5-FU and Imiquimod at 5 year post-treatment with 89.5% (137/153) of sBCC lesions treated with MAL-PDT having good or excellent cosmesis [9]. Additionally, one study of MAL-PDT versus surgical excision for primary nodular BCC found 87% of patients treated with MAL-PDT had good or excellent cosmetic outcome compared to 54% of patients treated with surgical excision who had good or excellent cosmesis [22]. Compared to cryotherapy, cosmesis is found to be superior with PDT [19].

One drawback is potentially high recurrence rates as one study reported the 5-year tumor free survival to be 62.7% after treatment of sBCC with MAL-PDT [9]. Another study reported a 54% primary response for superficial SCC (not SCC-in situ) treated with ALA-PDT, and the projected 36-month disease-free rate was only 8% [23]. Thus, primary treatment of SCC with PDT should be used for early invasive lesions (<1 mm) [14].

Although generally well-tolerated, adverse effects of topical photosensitizers include local skin reactions [12]. During treatment, reactions include stinging, tingling, itching, or burning pain at the treatment site [12, 19]. Oftentimes, this reaction is worse in more sensitive areas, such as the lips and facial lesions can be more painful than scalp lesions [12, 20]. These adverse effects during treatment can be unbearable for some patients. Post-treatment localized skin reactions include oedema, erythema, scaling, and crusting; however, the area usually heals without any scarring [19, 20].

15.2.3.2 Keloid Treatment with Photodynamic Therapy (PDT)

PDT is an emerging therapy for the treatment of keloids either by reducing postoperative recurrence or for keloids refractory to other treatment methods [24]. As an emerging therapy, literature on PDT for the treatment of keloids is minimal and limited to case series and case reports, and there is a need for RCT to determine standard guidelines of treatment.

PDT for keloids acts in a similar manner to PDT therapy for NMSC. A topical photosensitizer ALA and MAL, which are prodrugs, are converted to protoporphyrin IX (PpIX).

Once a light source is added, the PpIX is converted to reactive oxygen species (ROS). For the treatment of keloids, it is proposed that the ROS produced damage the mitochondria and activates cell signaling molecules that induce cell death and thus alter collagen production and ECM organization [24].

Literature review shows that keloid treatment with PDT has the potential to decrease the volume of the keloid scar and recurrence. One case report of a keloid on the chin had reduced keloid volume after five MAL-PDT sessions, and no recurrence was observed 1 year later [24]. Additionally, a case series of ten keloids each treated with three MAL-PDT sessions reported reduced volume with less itching, pain, and pliability of keloids and after 9 months of follow-up, only one of the ten lesions recurred [24]. Another case series of 15 keloids (in 14 patients) that were refractory to 3 or more injections of triamcinolone acetonide were treated with 3 monthly ALA-PDT sessions, and 50% of patients had complete keloid resolution [24].

A drawback of PDT is that it has limited penetration depth, and many keloids are 3 mm or larger [24]. Additionally, PDT is an emerging therapy with no standard guidelines for the treatment of keloids, such as photosensitizer concentration, duration of light, and guidelines on the light source.

15.2.4 Cryotherapy

Cryotherapy uses liquid nitrogen (LN) (−196 °C) to destroy superficial tissue either via direct contact or as a spray [25].

15.2.4.1 NMSC (Early Superficial and In Situ Lesions) Treated with Cryotherapy

Cryotherapy is used to treat small and superficial BCC (sBCC) with freezing times between 10 and 20 s [25]. Cryotherapy treatment has been recommended for use in actinic keratoses (AKs), Bowen disease (BD), superficial BCC (sBCC), small nodular BCC, and small well-differentiated SCC [14]. Treatment of BCC typically requires two freeze–thaw cycles 40–60 s [12] (Fig. 15.11).

Cryotherapy is a simple, quick, and cheap treatment option for NMSC12. Another benefit is that it can be performed with minimal equipment in an outpatient setting [26]. Additionally, 5-year cure rate for NMSC has been reported between 94% and 99% [12, 14].

A drawback to cryotherapy is that this technique is nonselective and will destroy any tissue treated with LN. Thus with cryotherapy, there is no histological margin control [26]. Additionally, several cryotherapy treatments may be necessary as not all malignant cells die during the first freeze–thaw cycle and thus treatment may require multiple office visits [14].

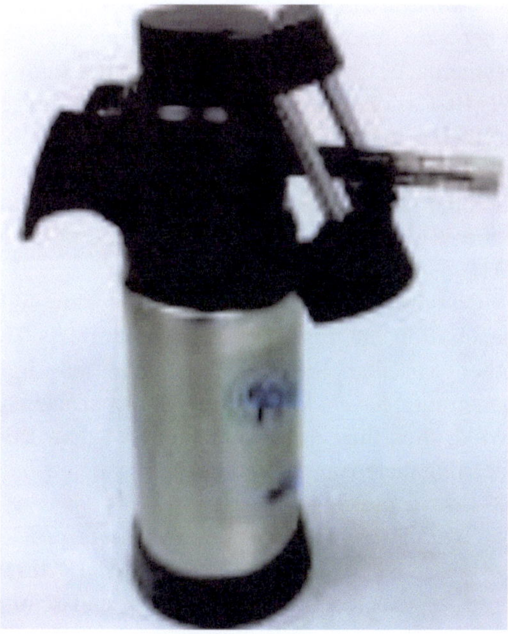

Fig. 15.11 Cryotherapy gun

Adverse local effects of treatment include blisters, crusting, erythema, edema, hypopigmentation, hypertrophic scarring, alopecia, tissue distortion, milia/pyogenic granuloma formation, and pain [12, 25]. Healing can be prolonged taking up to 4–6 weeks [26]. However, there can be excellent cosmetic results as skin tumors heal without significant tissue contraction. Caution should be used when considering treating certain anatomical areas because scaring and retraction can occur. Areas of caution include corners of mouth, vermillion margin of lips, eyebrows, inner canthi, free margin of ala nasi, and auditory canal [14].

Contraindications of cryotherapy include patients with cold urticaria, cold intolerance, cryofibrinogenemia, or cryoglobulinemia [14].

15.2.4.2 Keloid Treatment with Cryotherapy

Keloids can be treated with cryotherapy either via spray, contact, or intralesional [17]. The temperature of the keloid scar is brought below −22 °C, and this treatment aims to reduce keloid size and recurrence. The recommended freeze–thaw cycles for spray and contact LN therapy for keloids are 10–20 s [11]. Additionally, injections of triamcinolone acetonide are recommended in combination with cryotherapy for keloid treatment.

Treatment with LN causes damage to the vasculature and ultimately leads to coagulative necrosis with post-treatment scar biopsies showing more organization of collagen fibers [17]. Studies report keloid volume reduction of 51.4–67.4% after 12 months post-treatment. With intralesional cryotherapy possibly requiring fewer treatment sessions compared to spray or contact.

However, keloids can still recur with reported recurrence rates of 0–24% 6–18 months after treatment [17]. Thus, cryotherapy is typically reserved for smaller scars [11]. Temporary local skin side effects include blistering, pain at treatment site, and hypopigmentation [11, 17].

15.3 Lasers

15.3.1 2 Types of Lasers Are Used for NMSC: Ablative and Vascular

15.3.1.1 Ablative Lasers

Ablative lasers consist of carbon dioxide (CO_2) and erbium yttrium aluminum garnet (Er:YAG). Both lasers have infrared wavelengths of 10,600 nm for CO_2 lasers and 2940 nm for Er:YAG lasers [27]. Depth of tissue ablation is 20 mm per pass for CO_2 lasers and 2 mm for a single pulse for Er:YAG lasers. Most studies involve the use of CO_2 lasers and studies involving the use of Er:YAG for NMSC treatment are far more limited.

Ablative lasers cause lesion destruction via coagulative necrosis, ablation, and hyperthermia [19]. The wavelengths of these lasers are absorbed by the water in the superficial epidermis thus leading to lesion destruction [19, 27].

Treatment with ablative lasers has good cosmesis with minimal skin side effects. One study reported 2 patients of 20 had mild disruption to their eyelash, but otherwise, the CO_2 laser was noted to have produced excellent cosmesis in the treatment of these periorbital BCCs [28]. No ectropion, trichiasis, atrophic/hypertrophic scarring, or damage to eye structure was observed in these patients. Another study of 140 patients with BCC lesions treated with CO_2 laser noted fast recovery time and good cosmetic outcomes [29].

15.3.1.2 Vascular Lasers

Pulse dye laser (PDL) has been efficacious in multiple studies in the treatment of BCC [27]. Typically, a 595 nm laser is used to treat small, superficial BCC as greater efficacy has been observed compared to 585 nm lasers [27]. The 595 nm has a greater maximum coagulation depth than 585 nm with 1.5–2 mm of light penetration, thus the 595 nm laser can treat tumors in the upper 1–1.5 mm of skin. Other vascular lasers with greater depths of light penetration include long-pulsed 1064 nm neodymium-doped yttrium aluminum garnet (Nd:YAG) and the 755 nm Alexandrite. Laser treatment is typically indicated for superficial BCCs and not invasive BCCs or invasive SCCs [14]. Some studies have demonstrated successful treatment of SCC in situ lesions with ablative laser therapy; however, this literature is limited [27].

Treatment with vascular lasers (PDL) can have excellent cosmesis and is well tolerated with only mild skin reactions observed in the initial weeks post-treatment. In one study where 20 BCCs were treated with 4 sessions of 595 nm PDL at 3-to-4-week intervals, 18 of the 20 lesions were noted to have excellent cosmesis via patient's self-evaluations [30]. In one study BCCs were treated with 4 sessions of 595 nm PDL at 2-week intervals. Post-treatment some patients experienced purpura followed by gray discoloration followed by hemorrhagic crusting. However, by 2 weeks all subjects had healed clinically [31]. In another study, BCCs were treated with 4 sessions of 595 nm PDL at 3-to-4-week intervals and post-treatment 15 of the 20 BCCs had hypopigmentation [30]. However, no other skin reaction was observed, no scarring, erythema, or textural changes. In another study of 39 BCCs on the face, patient's experienced erythema, mild edema, and dusky purpura that were clinically healed within 1 week and as with the other studies, no scarring was observed, and patients were happy with the cosmetic outcome [32].

One drawback of PDL is that it has low-light penetration, but this limits its adverse effects. The other vascular lasers with increased light penetration have a lower absorption coefficient in blood, thus they need more fluences than PDL meaning there is increased risk for adverse effects [27].

Overall vascular and ablative lasers provide cosmesis benefits with decreased tissue destruction, bleeding, healing time, and scaring [27]. However, laser treatment can be expensive and inaccessible [14]. Additionally, current studies indicate that tumor recurrence rates are higher than traditional treatment options (i.e., MMS) [27]. Longer follow-up, ideally 5 or more years, is needed to assess if recurrence rates and long-term cure rates are comparable to surgery.

15.3.2 Keloid Treatment with Vascular Lasers

Keloids can be treated with nonablative laser therapy, as there is limited evidence on ablative lasers for the treatment of keloids [17]. The most promising results have been seen with the 585 nm short-pulsed dye laser (PDL) [11]. One recommended dosing schedule is 2–6 treatments every 2–6 weeks at nonoverlapping pulses of 6.0–7.5 or 4.5–5.5 J/cm^2. Other sources suggest a PDL wavelength of 585–595 nm with 12–18 treatments with 4–8 weeks between treatments [17].

Laser therapy can be used for the treatment of keloids by targeting keloid microvasculature by destroying blood vessels and causing ischemia [11, 17]. Specifically, it is proposed that the increased temperature from the 585 nm PDL disrupts disulfide bonds, which allows for collagen fiber rearrangement with decreased fibroblast proliferation [11].

A benefit of PDL therapy is that it can improve scar color, height, volume, texture, and pliability [11, 17]. PDL can also improve keloid symptoms such as pain, itching, and burning [17].

However, laser therapy has high recurrence rates for keloids [11, 17]. Adverse local skin reactions include hyper/hypopigmentation, blistering, crusting, and postoperative purpura that can last up to 10 days [11].

15.4 Radiation (Electrons and Photons) Therapy

15.4.1 NMSC Treatment with Radiation Therapy

Many types of radiotherapy exist for the treatment of NMSC: superficial radiation therapy, electron-beam radiation, and isotype-based brachytherapy [7]. Superficial radiation therapy (SRT) is a type of external radiotherapy that uses low energy, low penetration, kilovoltage (kVp) photons to target the tumor [33]. Electron-beam radiation therapy is another type of external radiotherapy that uses small negatively charged particles/photons to target the tumor [34]. Additionally, there is brachytherapy where the radioactive source is applied directly onto or into the body. For NMSC, brachytherapy typically involves applying the radioactive source to a surface-mold that is fitted to the tumor. Tumor selection for treatment with radiotherapy is imperative and typically recommended for primary, small (<2 cm), and well-defined tumors [26].

A benefit of radiotherapy for NMSC is that it targets the superficial skin, minimizing potential systemic effects of receiving high-energy radiation therapy. Additionally, patients who are not surgical candidates, surgically fatigued, or have large multifocal tumors that would require large resection and reconstruction can be treated with radiation therapy [26]. Since radiotherapy is a nonsurgical modality, it provides excellent cosmetic results, as there is no incision and thus no scarring [35].

However, there are some drawbacks to radiation therapy. Such as tumors that arise in previously irradiated areas or recurrences after previous radiation should not be treated with radiotherapy [26]. Other absolute and relative contraindications of SRT include invasion of underlying bone or muscle, thickness (>6 mm), that cannot be debulked, ataxia telangiectasia, active or uncontrolled lupus or rheumatologic/connective tissue diseases, concomitant administration of radiation sensitizing chemotherapy (i.e., doxorubicin), T4 or node positive status, and others [36]. There is also no histological margin evaluation done with radiotherapy. However, the use of ultrasound in IGSRT may alleviate this latter drawback as ultrasound allows for assessment of tumor depth pre, during, and post-treatment. Additionally, multiple visits are required as radiation treatments are typically fractionated to minimize surrounding normal tissue damage.

As with all treatment methods, post-treatment skin changes can be observed and vary depending on the field size and intensity of the dose [26]. Initial post-treatment skin changes can include erythema, inflammation, blistering, and pain. Long-term sequelae can include telangiectasias, hypopigmentation, poor wound healing, fibrosis, or atrophy [8, 26].

15.4.2 Keloid Treatment with Radiation Therapy

Keloids can be treated with adjunctive radiotherapy post-surgical excision. Adjunctive radiotherapy includes superficial and orthovoltage radiotherapy, electron beam, and brachytherapy [37]. The proposed mechanism of radiotherapy for the treatment of keloids is decreased collagen production by inhibiting neovascularization and fibroblast proliferation [11, 37].

Superficial and orthovoltage radiotherapy deliver X-ray (photon) beams to a depth of 5 mm for superficial radiotherapy and 2 cm for orthovoltage radiotherapy [37]. One retrospective study of keloid excision followed by a 10 Gy dose of 60 or 100 kV superficial radiotherapy within 24 h found a recurrence rate of 9% at 1 year and a recurrence rate of 16% at 5 years.

Advantages of superficial and orthovoltage radiotherapy include treatment targeting the superficial skin and avoiding damage to deeper structures [37]. Treatment is also inexpensive and easy to use.

One disadvantage to superficial and orthovoltage radiotherapy is dose drop off at the periphery leading to uneven treatment [37].

Electron beam radiotherapy delivers electrons via linear accelerator to a depth of 2–6 cm and the dose of radiotherapy depends on the keloid location [37]. Studies recommend that postsurgical radiotherapy with electron beam is most effective within 24 h of keloid excision. One retrospective study of 834 keloids had a local control rate of 88.25% and a recurrence rate of 9.59% with median time to recurrence of 12 months [38].

Advantages include superficial treatment that avoids damage to deeper structures and the ability to treat a broad area of skin without radiation drop off [37]. One disadvantage for electron beam radiotherapy is that it cannot be used on curved surfaces [37]. Additionally, a linear accelerator is also necessary for treatment. High-dose rate (HDR) interstitial brachytherapy and HDR superficial brachytherapy can be used for the treatment of keloids [37]. Both treatments involve a catheter emitting radioactive gamma rays. In HDR interstitial brachytherapy, the catheter is inserted into the target tissue and in HDR superficial brachytherapy the catheter is fixed to the skin.

An advantage of HDR interstitial brachytherapy is that by inserting the catheter into the target tissue, it involves less normal tissue [37]. A drawback of this method is that the total dose must be administered in a short time period. One study found a 3.4% recurrence rate at 7 years for HDR interstitial brachytherapy (12 Gy divided into 4 fractions) given 48 h after keloid excision. Another study found a 3.1% recurrence rate for HDR interstitial brachytherapy (12 Gy divided into 2 fractions) after keloid excision.

An advantage of HDR superficial brachytherapy is that it can be used in the treatment of uneven and long keloids, but as with HDR interstitial brachytherapy, the total dose must be administered in a short time period [37]. One study of keloids treated with HDR superficial brachytherapy (12 Gy divided into 4 fractions or 15 Gy divided into 3 fractions) post keloid excision found a recurrence rate of 9.7% at 12 months.

Overall benefits of radiotherapy for treatment of keloids include that these radiotherapy options treat superficially and target the skin, avoiding damage to deeper tissues [37]. With adjunctive radiotherapy post-excision, there is also a low risk of recurrence and complications. The recurrence rate of excision alone is estimated to be 45–100%.

Overall drawbacks include that radiation therapy is not effective as monotherapy for keloid treatment [11]. Additionally, skin reactions may be observed, and temporary erythema is seen in almost all patients 7–10 days post-radiation and is related to the total dose of radiation received [37]. Other acute post-radiation skin reactions include edema, desquamation, ulceration, and necrosis. Late post-radiation skin reactions seen weeks to months after treatment include pigment changes, atrophy, alopecia, and telangiectasias, which are related to the amount of radiation received per session/fraction. To lower the incidence of these local skin reactions, it is recommended to give an emollient and steroid ointment after radiation, decrease the amount of radiation received per fraction, and lengthen the interval between radiation doses.

One concern with radiotherapy is the risk of carcinogenesis after radiation exposure [11]. A review of keloids treated with radiotherapy from 1901 to 2009 found five cases of carcinogenesis related to the radiotherapy received for keloid treatment [39]. However, the authors determined it was unclear if proper radiation dosing was used and if surrounding tissues were adequately shielded. The authors concluded that keloids can be treated with radiotherapy, and the risk of carcinogenesis is very low when surrounding tissues (i.e., thyroid and mammary glands) are protected. Additionally, in a questionnaire to radiation oncologists around the world, 80% believed that radiation therapy is an acceptable treatment modality for keloids.

15.5 Standard Surgical Modalities for NMSC and Keloids

15.5.1 Electrodesiccation and Curettage (ED&C)

15.5.1.1 NMSC Treatment with Electrodesiccation and Curettage (ED&C)

Curettage is the first step and most vital step in treating NMSC lesions with ED&C. The skin should be held taut, and curettage should be done with a firm hand and pressure circumferentially outward [26]. The end point of curettage is typically a firm resistance, as normal dermis does not curette well compared to tumor tissue. Electrodesiccation should be done after curettage to add superficial destruction, hemostasis, and inflammation to the tumor site. The ED&C cycle should be performed two to three times to maximize cure rates. Estimated cure rates are 92% 5-year cure rate for BCC and 96% 5-year cure rate for SCC.

ED&C can be considered for low-risk, primary BCC and cutaneous SCC in nonterminal hair locations [7, 8]. Lesions in soft tissue areas such as the lip and eyelids should not be treated with ED&C as these areas cannot be curetted properly [26]. Additionally, caution should be used in patients with pacemakers or implantable defibrillators before electrodesiccation is used as these patient's need special monitoring.

Benefits of ED&C include that it is cost effective and can be performed with minimal equipment in an outpatient setting [26].

A drawback of ED&C includes that histological margins are not assessed with ED&C [26]. Additionally, physician experience and training are essential to minimize recurrence of tumors treated with ED&C. Recurrence rates with trainees have been higher (18.8%) compared with experienced physicians (5.7%).

Cosmetic outcome typically includes a firm, white, stellate scar [26]. Uncommon complications include hypertrophic and keloid scars and dysesthesia and pruritus developing within the scar.

15.6 Standard Excision

15.6.1 NMSC Treatment with Standard Excision

Standard excision is recommended for low-risk, primary BCC with 4 mm clinical margins and a histologic margin assessment [7]. Standard excision is also recommended for low-risk, primary cutaneous SCC, and it is recommended that a 4–6 mm margin and depth to mid-subcutaneous adipose tissue is assessed [8]. Overall, 95% of primary, well-defined, BCC and SCC less than 2 cm will be successfully treated with a 4 mm excision margin extending into normal looking skin [26]. However, this margin should be extended to 6 mm for high-risk SCC when treating with standard excision. Standard excision can be considered for both high-risk BCC and SCC, but caution is advised if a complete margin assessment is not done [7, 8].

Benefits of standard excision include high cure rates with an estimated 90% 5-year cure rate for BCC and 92% 5-year cure for SCC [26]. Additionally, vertical frozen sections of tissue are histologically examined to determine tumor margins and confirm tumor removal. However, although histological margins are examined, less than 1% of peripheral margins are examined, which means false-negative margins could be reported.

Drawbacks include that recurrent tumors should not be treated with standard excision as recurrence rates are high and these lesions should be referred to MMS [26]. Additionally, since this is a surgical procedure, patients may be advised to make lifestyle restrictions in the days following surgery to maximize wound healing. Overall complications of skin surgery include infection, excessive bleeding, wound dehiscence, functional defects, and scarring [6, 27].

15.6.2 Mohs Micrographic Surgery (MMS)

Mohs micrographic surgery (MMS) is a tissue-sparing technique to remove skin cancer developed by Fredrick Mohs in 1941 [40]. The procedure includes excising the visible tumor with 0–2-mm margins of normal tissue. The tissue is then fixed and cut into horizontal frozen sections to be examined under the microscope. This fixation process takes about 20–30 min [26]. The Mohs surgeon marks any tumor-positive tissue that was identified under the microscope and samples additional tissue only from the positive tissue plane [26, 40]. This process is continued until clear tissue margins are established, and this process typically requires at least two "cutting" or "stages" [40]. It is important to distinguish Mohs "stages" from tumor staging systems as the former means number of cuts and the latter refers to the overall extent of the cancer.

15.6.2.1 NMSC Treatment with Mohs Micrographic Surgery (MMS)

MMS is recommended for high-risk BCC and cutaneous SCC [8]. This includes BCC and SCC greater than 2 cm, tumors located in high-risk areas (i.e., nose, ear, and lips), recurrent tumors, incompletely excised tumors, aggressive histologic tumors (i.e., basosquamous carcinoma), perineural invasion, tumors without clear clinical margins, tumors arising in chronic ulcers, burns or previously irradiated locations, or in immunocompromised patients [41]. Current evidence suggests MMS offers one of the highest cure rates, with about a 1% 5-year recurrence for BCC and less than 6% 5-year recurrence for SCC [42, 43].

The extremely high cure rates of MMS make it an effective method for treating NMSC lesions. Additionally, despite MMS being a surgical technique, its methods allow for maximizing tissue preservation as wide margins are not excised [40]. As with surgical excision, histological margins are examined to confirm tumor removal, but importantly in MMS, horizontal frozen sections are histologically examined [26]. The horizontal sections allow for complete margin control as 100% of peripheral margins are examined compared to less than 1% in standard excision.

A drawback of MMS being the current standard of treatment for NMSC is with the common anatomical locations that NMSC typically occurs on where conservation of tissue is important, such as the ears, nose, eyes, and neck [6, 8, 44]. MMS removes tissue layer by layer and examines the tissue histologically to determine the margins of the skin cancer, but in a delicate area such as the head and neck, this poses a cosmetic concern due to the initial uncertainty of how much tissue will need to be removed before the margins are cancer free [45].

Similar to standard surgical excision, overall complications of skin surgery include infection, excessive bleeding, wound dehiscence, functional defects, and scarring [6, 27]. MMS can also take several hours and a majority of NMSC occurs in older patients, who might not be able to endure the 2–4 h of MMS required to excise the skin cancer in addition to the sequela that follows after surgery [42, 46] (Fig. 15.12).

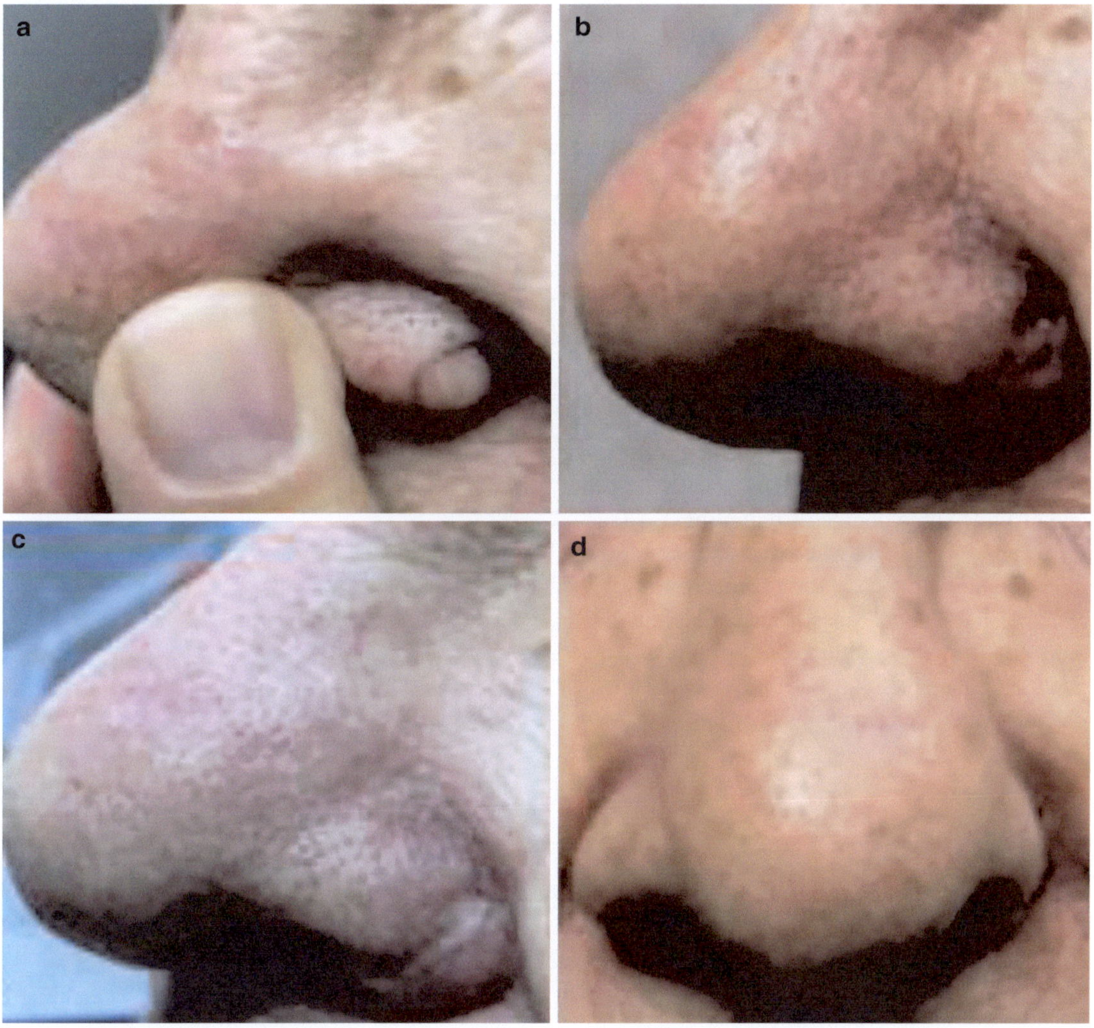

Fig. 15.12 BCC lesion on left nasal ala. (**a**) Biopsy site, pre-Mohs, (**b**) 6-months post-Mohs, (**c**) 19-months post-Mohs, (**d**) head-on photo post-Mohs, can see part of left nostril lost after Mohs. (Courtesy of Dr. Donna Serure, Laserderm Dermatology)

15.7 Intralesional Steroid Injection

15.7.1 Keloid Treatment with Intralesional Steroid Injection

Intralesional injections of triamcinolone (10–40 mg/mL) is the first-line treatment for keloid scars and typically, 2–3 injections are sufficient for treatment [11]. The proposed mechanism of treatment of corticosteroids on keloid treatment is suppression of the inflammatory response. Additionally, corticosteroids decrease the synthesis of collagen and glycosaminoglycans and inhibit fibroblast growth, while increasing the degradation of collagen and fibroblasts (Fig. 15.13).

There are few randomized prospective studies on intralesional injections for keloid treatment [11]. Among the current studies, response rates vary from 50% to 100% and recurrence rates vary from 9% to 50%.

An advantage of intralesional steroid injections is that this treatment option can be com-

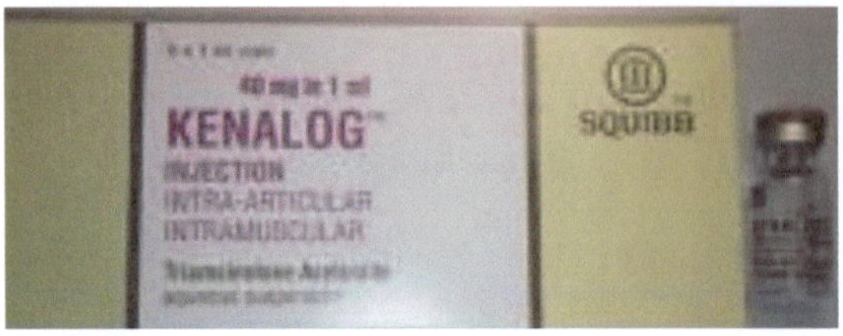

Fig. 15.13 Triamcinolone acetonide (Kenalog)

bined with other keloid treatment modalities, such as surgery or cryotherapy [11]. Intralesional steroid injection monotherapy is most effective in young keloid scars with reports of keloids completely flattening. In older keloids, intralesional steroid injections can provide symptomatic relief and provide some degree of flattening.

Some patients may experience pain at the injection site, which can be avoided with topical anesthesia or local anesthesia injections [11]. Additional adverse skin reactions include skin and subcutaneous fat atrophy, pigmentation changes, and telangiectasias [11, 17].

15.8 Surgical Excision

15.8.1 Keloid Treatment with Surgical Excision

Surgical excision of keloids consists of a linear tension-free closure, split-thickness skin grafting, full-thickness skin grafting, z-plasty, and w-plasty [11].

Disadvantages of surgical excision alone for the treatment of keloids is that the recurrence rate without adjunctive therapy is estimated to be 45–100% [37]. Excision can also result in a larger scar after excision or recurrence of the keloid that is even larger, which is why excisional monotherapy should be used with caution [11].

15.8.1.1 Image-Guided Superficial Radiotherapy (IGSRT)

Image-guided superficial radiotherapy (IGSRT) is a combination of two long standing effective technologies incorporating low penetration ionizing radiation with ultrasound imaging. This reemergent technology of superficial radiation therapy (SRT) has traditionally achieved a high rate of cure for early-stage NMSC while allowing preservation of cosmesis and function without surgery. This spares the patient from having a scar or defect. The SRT component has recently been improved with solid-state technology for reliability and dose/energy consistency. The addition of an ultrasound allows visualization of the lesion with regard to localization and depth in real time prior to, during, and after treatment (Fig. 15.14).

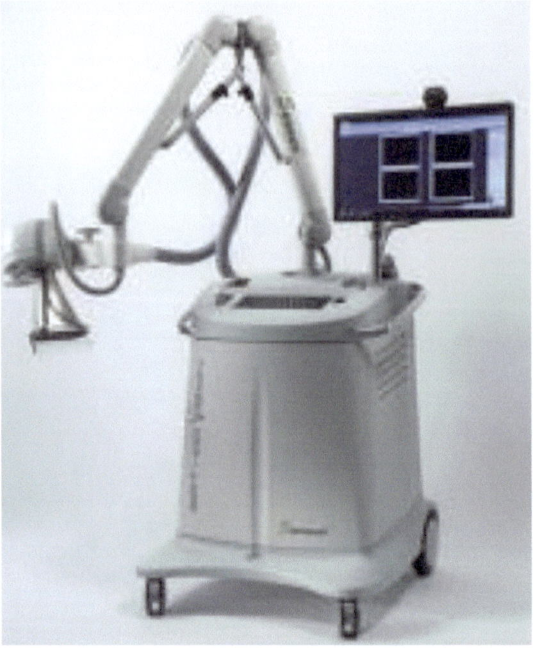

Fig. 15.14 IGSRT machine. (Courtesy of Skin Cure Oncology)

While surgical procedures such as excision, resection, or MOHs typically have very good cosmetic results with high cure rates in general, occasionally a large lesion or one situated in a cosmetically sensitive location may require potentially mutilating and/or function altering surgical management/reconstruction. IGSRT clearly has an advantage cosmetically in these scenarios (Fig. 15.15).

Historically, superficial radiotherapy (SRT) is a long-established modality which included Grenz rays, which were popular and used frequently in the 1950s and 1960s to treat various skin conditions such as acne and skin cancer by

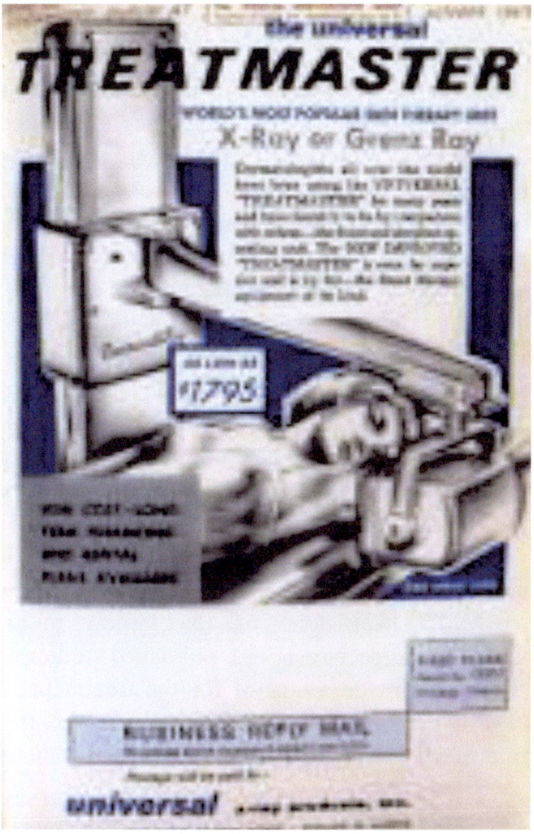

Fig. 15.15 Picture of Grenz ray unit advertisement. (Courtesy of New York Academy of Medicine Library)

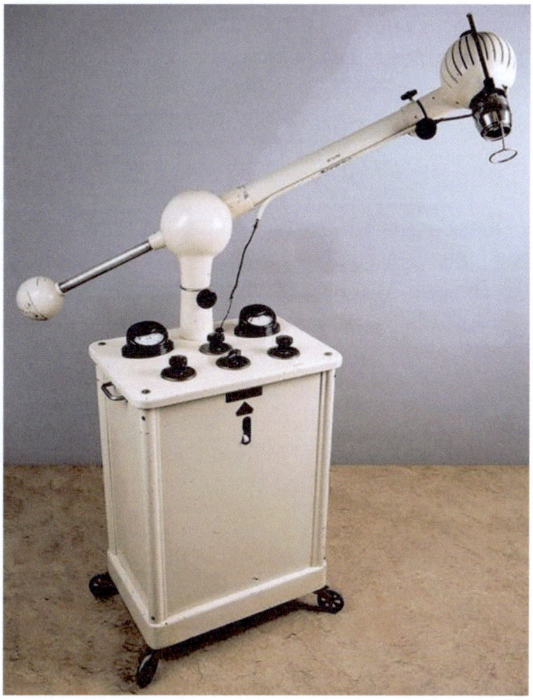

Fig. 15.16 Grenz ray machine. "*File:Grenz ray machine, Germany, 1930-1940 Wellcome L0065506.jpg*" *by Wellcome Images is licensed with CC BY-SA 4.0. To view a copy of this license, visit* https://creativecommons.org/licenses/by-sa/4.0

dermatologists. Dermatologists previously used these Grenz rays because of the low penetrating characteristics of the beam to treat skin conditions. The energy for Grenz rays was usually in the range of 20 peak kilovoltage (kVp). This energy range, however, was unable to adequately treat deeply seated skin cancers. Orthovoltage machines up to 500 kVp could cover deeper tumors, however, were seldom used by most dermatologists in favor of Grenz ray units (Fig. 15.16).

Indeed, radiation for the treatment of NMSC has been used by dermatologists for the past century [43]. Grenz ray treatment by dermatologists has largely fallen out of favor within the last several decades. In the dermatology community, Grenz ray has been replaced in favor of the use of Mohs micrographic surgery (MMS). In 1974, 55% of dermatology clinics in the United States and Canada used superficial and orthovoltage radiation therapy; however, this number dropped to only 12% of dermatology clinics using superficial radiation therapy by 1986 [47]. Despite showing effectiveness for the treatment of NMSC and control rates of 75–100%, the use of radiation therapy decreased and part of this decline was due to the emergence of MMS [44, 45, 48] (see below).

Importantly, SRT has varying energy ranges for varying depths of penetration, and at the upper end of 200 kVp, it still does not penetrate very deeply past the skin dermis unlike higher energy photon radiation. This is particularly well suited to treat superficial tumors with a full 80–100% dose to the skin surface plus up to 5 mm depth, unlike Grenz rays which have much shallower coverage.

Due to the improvement in radiation technology, radiation therapy is experiencing a revival and upgrade for the treatment of NMSC, specifically with superficial radiation therapy [43, 44]. Unlike traditional radiation machines used in oncology, superficial radiation therapy uses low energy, low penetration, kilovoltage photons, typically between 50 and 150 kVp, which targets the skin and spares deeper structures [33, 47]. This makes it ideal for the treatment of early cutaneous malignancies, such as BCC and SCC [43].

The use of image guidance in radiation therapy has been deemed standard of cancer care in recent years. Image guidance in various forms using CT, MRI, and PET fusion has become commonplace in academic and private practice settings. The use of ultrasound guidance has also been established as useful in cancer radiotherapy [49–51] (Fig. 15.17).

In recent years, a resurgence in interest on the use of superficial radiotherapy combined with image guidance has developed and is rapidly gaining acceptance and widespread use. Due to its advantages of avoiding surgical scars, defects, pain, bleeding, infection, and need for reconstruction.

The current commercial IGSRT machine integrates an ultrasound unit with 22 MHz (megahertz) that allows for visualization of skin depths of 0–6 mm [36]. This high-frequency ultrasound is specifically designed for imaging of skin tumors and structures and the tumor and normal dermis can be clearly visualized. This is further enhanced with Doppler technology to help define functional/vascular/tissue parameters to help delineate abnormal cancerous growth/disruption versus normal nontumor areas. The use of ultrasound for image guidance in IGSRT allows clinicians to evaluate the lesion depth before, during, and after treatment. Thus, clinicians can adjust the prescribed energy and daily dose to minimize radiation exposure and adverse reactions.

Nonimage and image-guided superficial radiation therapy is effective, with comparable results to MMS [42]. One of the largest multi-institutional, peer-reviewed, published studies of SRT with image guidance for the treatment of NMSC demonstrated an absolute lesion control rate of 99.3% (2897/2917 lesions) with a mean

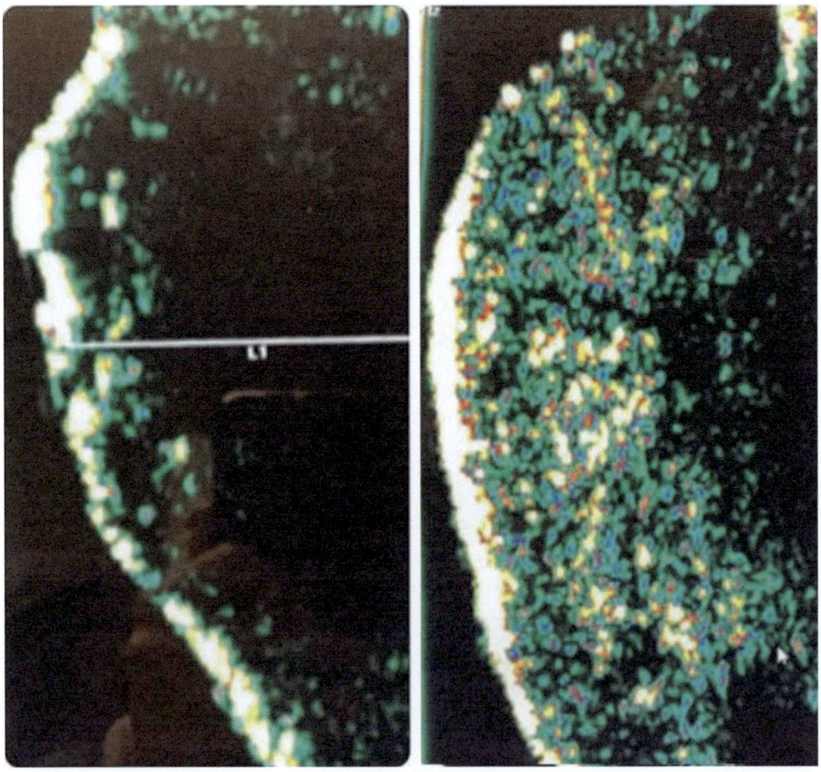

Fig. 15.17 Ultrasound before and 6 weeks after IGSRT treatment of a SCC lesion. (Courtesy of Skin Cure Oncology)

follow-up interval of about 1.3 years and max follow-up of 4.3 years [36]. In subgroup analysis of patients greater than 12 months follow-up (mean follow-up of 2.1 years), the control rate was essentially unchanged at 99.2%. Updated results with additional patients and longer follow-up had an absolute lesion control rate of 99.2% (3027/3050 lesions) with a mean follow-up interval of 2.1 years and max follow-up of 5.5 years [52]. Current research indicates that SRT without image guidance has favorable 2- and 5-year recurrence rates that warrant the use of SRT for treatment of early stage (SCCIS, T1, T2), nonaggressive NMSC [48]. In 2012, Cognetta et al. reported the recurrence rates for 1715 BCC and SCC lesions on the face and scalp treated with SRT from 1149 patients all older than 65.

Overall recurrences for both BCC and SCC were found to be 1.9% at 2 years and 5% at 5 years. Additionally, Rong et al. compared local control rates among studies that used radiation therapy as a modality for treating NMSC [47]. The studies that utilized superficial radiation therapy were from the years 1987 to 2001, and it was found that treatment with superficial radiation therapy without image guidance had a local control rate of 90% or greater in a majority of the studies.

Superficial radiation therapy is safe for treatment of NMSC and has minimal complications [42, 44]. Safety of the patient is ensured during treatment with regard to patient position, patient immobilization, and proper shielding of areas not being treated [44]. Superficial radiation therapy is safe to be used around delicate areas, such as the eye, since the radiation dose specifically targets the skin and not underlying structures [45]. Image-guided SRT on early follow-up and analysis shows at least equivalent or potentially improved results. A recent analysis compared the local control (LC) of IGSRT to nonimage-guided radiotherapy studies for the curative treatment of early-stage NMSC lesions. The results reported that IGSRT LC was statistically superior (p-value ranged from $p < 0.0001$ to $p = 0.046$) to the LC reported in each of the nonimage-guided radiotherapy studies [53].

Absolute and relative contraindications to IGSRT for NMSC include lesion invasive into bone and muscle, lesion thickness >6 mm, previous irradiation at the same location, ataxia telangiectasia, active connective tissue disease, active or uncontrolled rheumatologic disease or lupus, concurrent administration of radiation sensitive chemotherapeutics, and T4 or node positive status [36]. Previous literature stated that certain aggressive forms of BCC, such as morpheaform or micronodular types, should not receive SRT; however, with the advent of image guidance, this may no longer hold true. Higher energy radiotherapy modalities (linear accelerator/electrons) should be selected for deeply invasive BCC/SCC with perineural involvement.

Common reactions expected during treatment include erythema and skin irritation at the treatment site with a healing time of 4 weeks upon completion of treatment [33, 43]. Common late side effects include telangiectasias, hypopigmentation, and atrophy, with systemic reactions being rare. Nestor et al. report that for the lower extremity, below the knee, the post-surgical infection rate for MMS is 2.3% and wide local excisions (WLE) is 8.3% [44]. However, on 151 NMSCs treated on the lower extremity with SRT, there were no post-SRT infections. This is beneficial for individuals, such as the elderly, who are susceptible to poor wound healing in response to surgery.

In addition to the minimal adverse effects of superficial radiation therapy, this treatment modality consists of numerous benefits. SRT is feasible for use in an outpatient office due to the recent advancements in radiation technology making radiation machines smaller, more portable, and less expensive [33, 48]. Additionally, SRT provides excellent cosmetic results, as there are no incisions and thus no scars. Although, in Cognetta et al., cosmesis was not a measured variable, the authors stated that cosmesis in all lesions, which were located on the head and scalp, were rated very good and none were rated as poor [48]. This is particularly beneficial in delicate areas and eradicates the need for removal of tissue or skin grafting, such as the nose, ear, around the eyes and mouth, and lower extremities [42, 44]. The lack of incisions makes SRT beneficial for use in areas of cosmetic concern, individuals unable to tolerate surgery, individuals with comorbidities, individuals on anticoagulants or antiplatelets, and particularly those who are opposed to surgery [6, 44].

In one study of 43 patients with a total of 58 NMSC lesions, all lesions scored a 4 or 5 for cosmesis using a 1–5 Likert scale [54]. Additionally, patients were surveyed about their experience upon completion of IGSRT, and 42 of the 43 patients gave a 4 out of 4 rating of satisfaction. The one patient who did not give a 4/4 rating noted transportation as an obstacle. Overall, all patients said that they would recommend IGSRT and would undergo IGSRT treatment again for treatment of their NMSC lesions.

In view of the efficacy, safety, convenience, and cosmesis of SRT, and in particular image-guided SRT (IGSRT), this nonsurgical modality should be discussed as a standard option with patients in regard to their treatment of early-stage NMSC.

15.8.1.2 Use of IGSRT for Basal Cell Carcinomas (BCC)

Basal cell carcinoma (BCC) represents the most common skin cancer accounting for approximately five million cases per year in the United States [55].

IGSRT has been shown in various studies to be effective in the treatment of BCC with at least equal control rate, generally excellent cosmetic results compared to surgical techniques, and high patient satisfaction.

Typical 5-year control rates using SRT with or without image guidance is expected to achieve at least 95–99% 2- to 5-year control rate [36, 48] (Fig. 15.18).

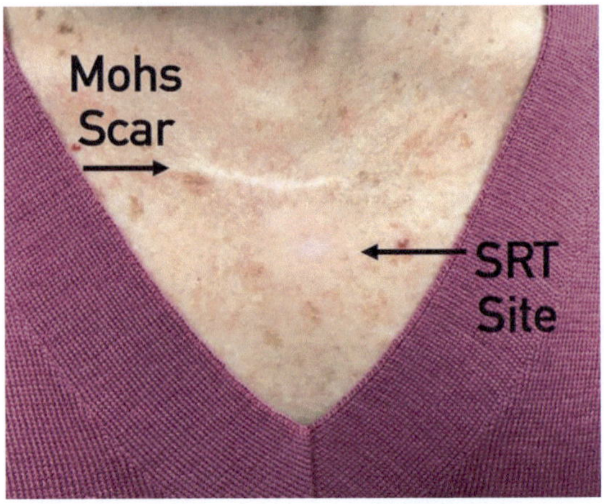

Fig. 15.18 NMSC lesion treated with MMS [top] versus BCC lesion treated with IGSRT [bottom]. (Courtesy of Dr. Donna Serure, Laserderm Dermatology)

One should remember that IGSRT is appropriate only for early-stage BCC in stages 1 and 2 and select superficial stage 3 that is debulked before IGSRT. Advanced stage BCCs are not appropriate for treatment with IGSRT and should be referred for MMS, surgical excision/resection, or high-energy radiotherapy units such as linear accelerators using electrons or combined photons and electrons often requiring surgery beforehand and possibly combined with systemic or immune agents. In certain advanced stages, systemic therapy/immunotherapy such as vascular endothelial growth factor (VEGF) or Hedgehog pathway modulators may be appropriate and can reduce the bulk of the tumor for better local control. Complete response of advanced BCC to Vismodegib is in the order of ~40%. IGSRT has been used in combination or post initiation of Vismodegib to help improve the eradication of localized BCC lesions (unpublished internal data) and is a useful method to palliate symptoms of advanced cases and improve the quality of life of patients where the tumors may cause bleeding, ulceration, pain, infection, or functional limitations.

Nose

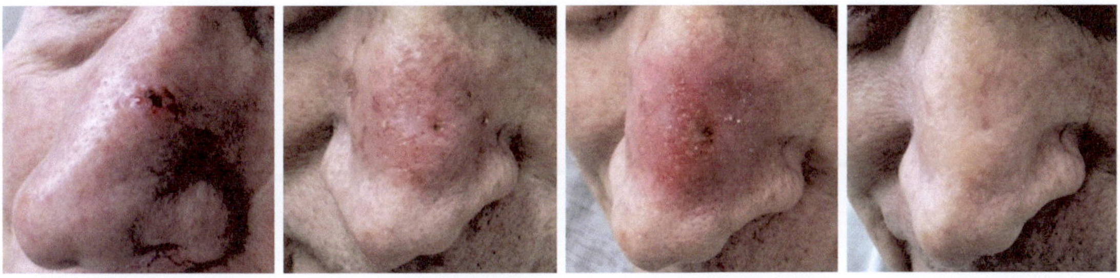

Before Tratment **During Tratment** **Last Tratment** **After Tratment**

Nodular BCC on bridge of nose treated with IGSRT in 78-year-old male. (Courtesy of Skin Cure Oncology)

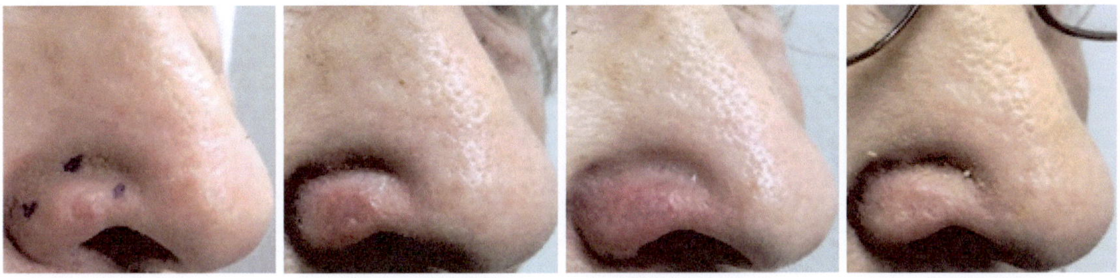

Before Tratment **During Tratment** **Last Tratment** **After Tratment**

Micronodular BCC on bridge of nose treated with IGSRT in a 64-year-old female. (Courtesy of Skin Cure Oncology)

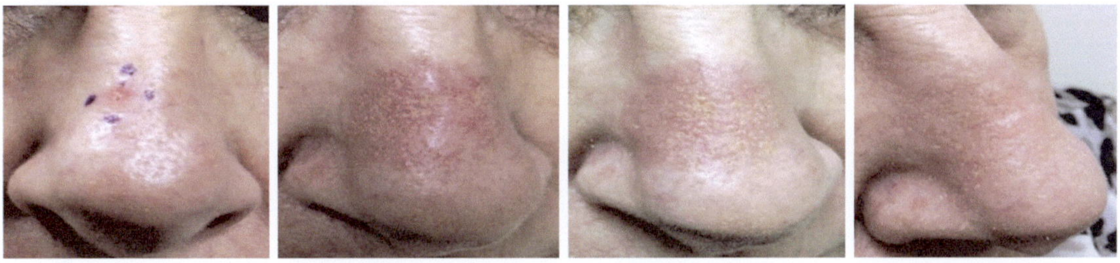

Before Tratment **During Tratment** **Last Tratment** **After Tratment**

BCC on right nasal sidewall treated with IGSRT in a 75-year-old male. (Courtesy of Skin Cure Oncology)

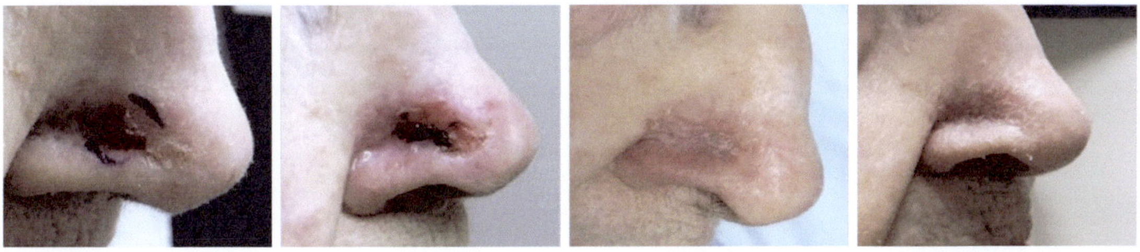

Before Tratment **During Tratment** **Last Tratment** **After Tratment**

Nodular and micronodular BCC on right lateral nose treated with IGSRT in a 74-year-old female. (Courtesy of Skin Cure Oncology)

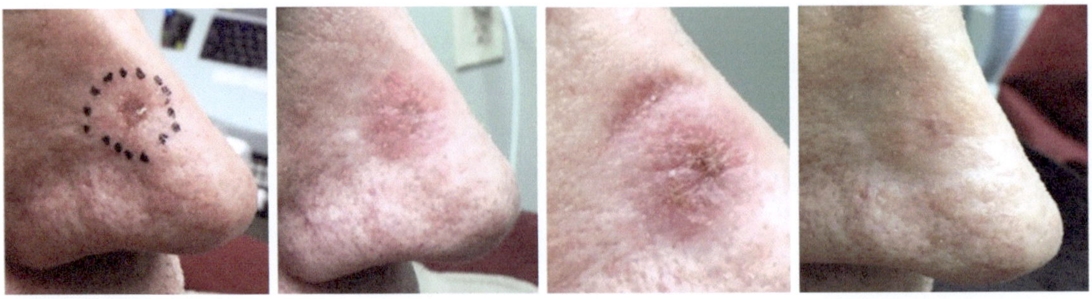

Nodular and ulcerated BCC on right nasal ala treated with IGSRT in a 94-year-old female. (Courtesy of Skin Cure Oncology)

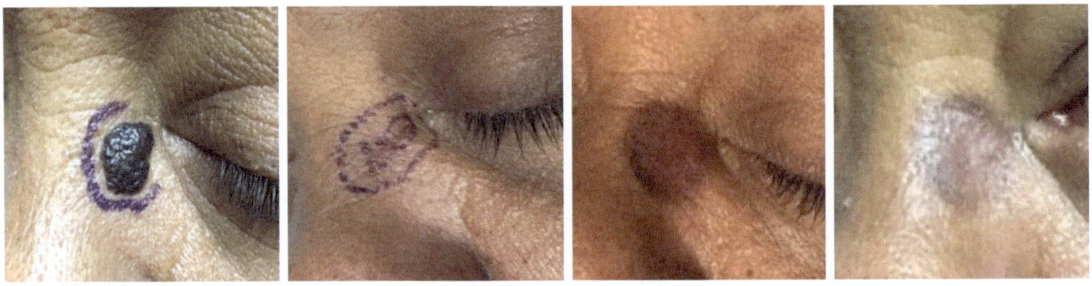

Pigmented BCC on left nasal bridge treated with IGSRT in a 51-year-old female. (Courtesy of Skin Cure Oncology)

Face

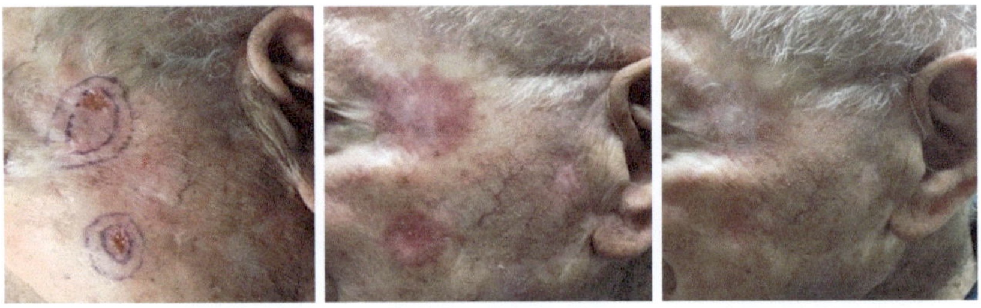

Two BCC lesions on left superior and inferior malar cheek treated simultaneously with IGSRT in a 92-year-old male. (Courtesy of Skin Cure Oncology)

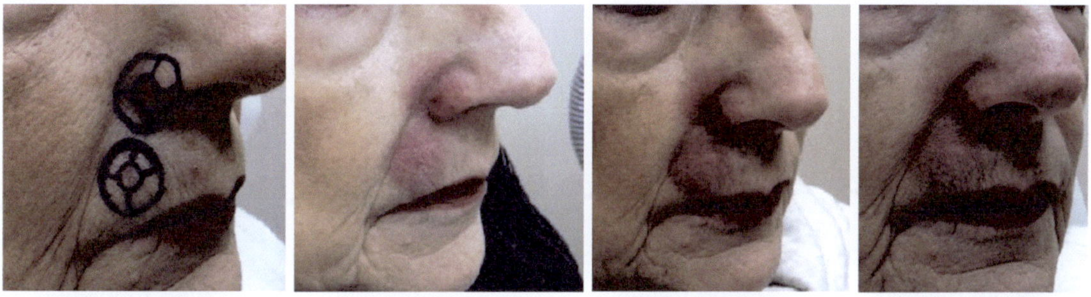

BCC on right upper lip and right nasal ala treated simultaneously with IGSRT in a 70-year-old female. (Courtesy of Skin Cure Oncology)

Neck

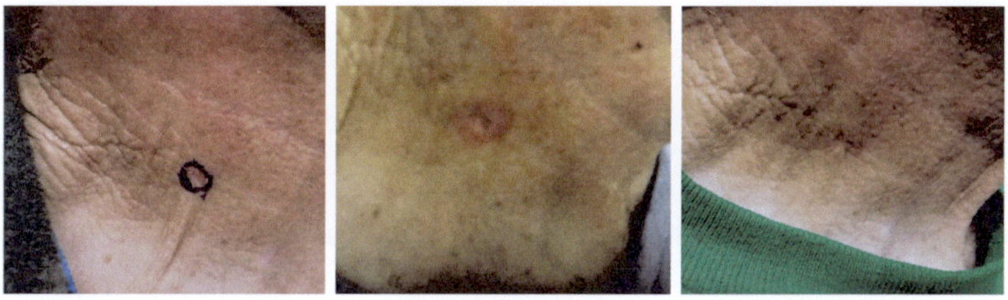

Nodular BCC on right lateral neck treated with IGSRT in a 77-year-old male. (Courtesy of Skin Cure Oncology)

Ear

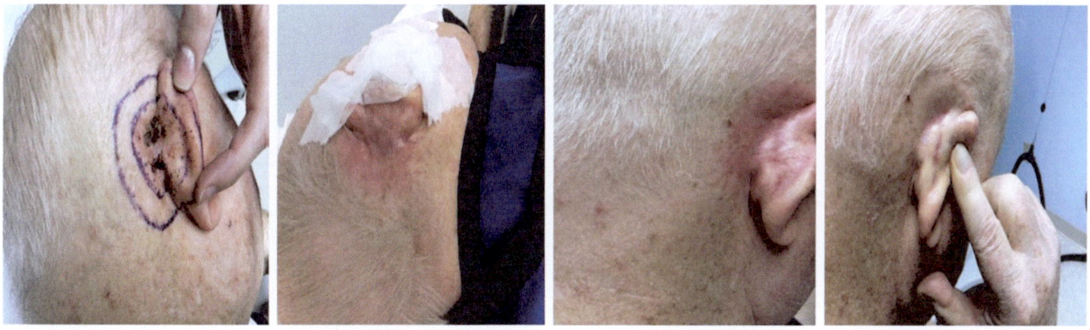

Ulcerative BCC on the right postauricular treated with IGSRT. (Courtesy of Skin Cure Oncology)

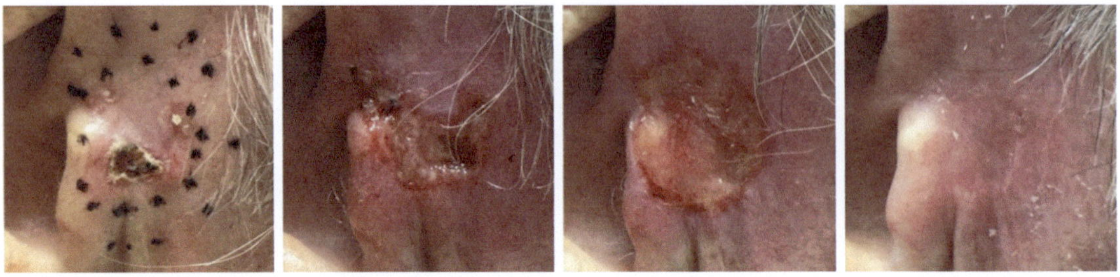

Before Tratment **During Tratment** **Last Tratment** **After Tratment**

Nodular BCC on right preauricular face treated with IGSRT in a 78-year-old male. (Courtesy of Skin Cure Oncology)

Arm

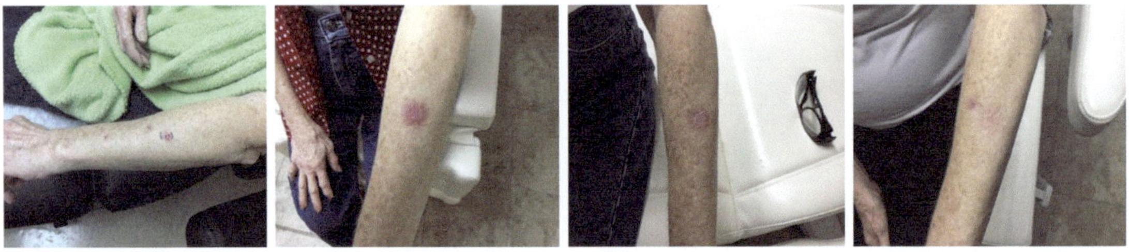

Before Tratment **During Tratment** **Last Tratment** **After Tratment**

Nodular and ulcerated BCC on left mid-forearm treated with IGSRT in a 76-year-old female. (Courtesy of Skin Cure Oncology)

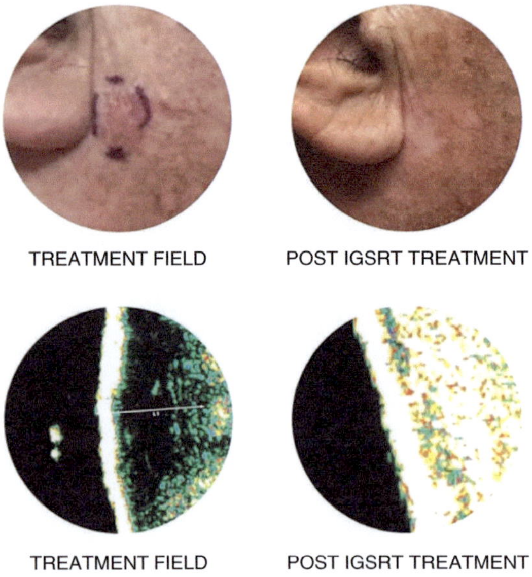

BCC on right preauricular face (lesion and ultrasound) before and after treatment with IGSRT. (Courtesy of Skin Cure Oncology)

15.9 Vismodegib (Erivedge)

The first oral drug for the treatment of BCC, known as Vismodegib (Erivedge), was approved by the FDA in 2012 [52]. This oral drug is approved for adults with metastatic BCC or locally advanced BCC that cannot be treated with surgery or radiation, or for BCC tumors that recurred after surgery [52]. Vismodegib works by targeting the Hedgehog intracellular pathway.

The Hedgehog pathway is activated when Hedgehog protein binds to a cell surface receptor called Patched. The Hedgehog protein and Patched protein then move into the cell where Patched releases an intracellular protein called Smoothened. Smoothened then moves to the cell surface to activate a protein family called glioma-associated oncogene homolog (GLI). Once GLI is activated, cell growth Hedgehog target genes are activated [52].

The Hedgehog pathway is inactive in adults; however, it is reactivated in certain cancers, including BCC. Vismodegib works by binding to the Smoothened protein, inhibiting intracellular signaling and inactivating the Hedgehog pathway [52]. Thus, interfering with BCC tumor growth.

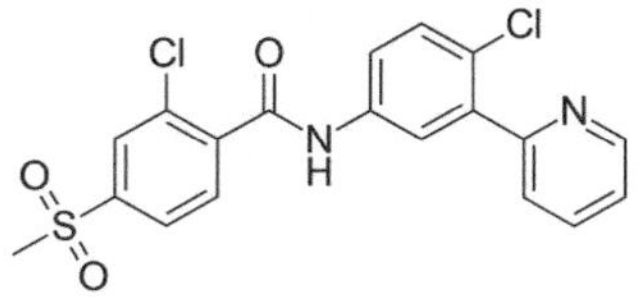

Structure of Vismodegib (Erivedge)

15.10 Use of IGSRT for Squamous Cell Carcinomas (SCC)

Cutaneous squamous cell carcinoma (SCC) accounts for 200,000–400,000 cases per year in the United States [8].

IGSRT is appropriate for the treatment of early-stage 0, 1, and 2 cutaneous SCC. Although the follow-up is still short, there appears to be suggestions of improved local control and cure rates with the use of IGSRT over surgery, particularly Mohs micrographic surgery (MMS). The potential advantage of IGSRT over MMS results from the convention that the tumor is treated with a margin called Umbra, which allows eradication to potential extension of the SCC beyond the visible lesion for up to 5–10 mm or more. Whereas MMS is designed to conserve as much tissue as possible and maintain minimal surgical defect. The margins of MMS could be as small as one cell beyond the visible tumor seen microscopically. With the use of surgery or MMS, the 5-year control rates range from 91% to 96%. Whereas IGSRT early results published by Yu et al. reveal local control as high as 99% at 2 years and 98% at 4 years [48, 51]. For SCC in situ (SCCIS), Yu et al. reported an absolute lesion control of 99.7% and an absolute lesion control of 99.5% for SCCIS lesions that had at least a 12-month follow-up [48].

It should be cautioned that the use of IGSRT in in situ cases of SCC should be limited to lesions that have substantial depth and with at least indications of full-thickness atypia as recommended by NCCN guidelines [53]. It is feasible and advisable to treat very early superficial SCCis, which is predominantly AKs, with simple excision, cryotherapy, or topical chemotherapy, which may be sufficient and does not unnecessarily expose the patient to radiation. Additionally, advantages of saving the use of IGSRT for these situations is that it will be available for treatment of the same area which is prone to develop future occurrences of skin cancer as a result of extensive skin sun damage typical for many patients as they age.

15.11 The Use of IGSRT in Keloids

Keloids represent a form of extreme scarring occurring from incisions or trauma to the skin [11]. Although many alternative treatments exist for keloids, one of the most effective methods of controlling keloids, particularly refractive keloids having multiple previous attempts at control that have failed, is radiation therapy.

Typical regimen used in IGSRT is 3 or 4 fractions of 400–600 centigrade (cGy) given immediately within the first 24–72 h from the time of the excision of the keloid. It is recommended that the first treatment be given on the same day post-surgery if possible and continue on to finish within the first 5–7 days.

In 2019, consensus guidelines on the use of SRT for the treatment of keloid excision lines post-surgery were proposed by Nestor et al. Treatment recommendations for keloid scars on the scalp, forehead, cheeks, nose, neck, arms, and trunk include 100 kV depth of three fractions of 600 cGy for a total of 1800 cGy within the first 3 days postsurgical treatment [43]. Patients should receive 1 dose per day of their first 3 postoperative days to reduce the risk of skin hyperpigmentation [43]. This dosing regimen will reduce the risk of keloid recurrence. [1]

[1] Postoperative external beam radiotherapy regimens are effective in preventing keloid reformation and ranges widely in daily dose and number of fractions (from 200 to 2800 cGy daily fractions from 1 to 20 fractions).

Control of keloids in certain movable areas is a challenge and may also benefit from the substitution of excision with a shaving flat of the keloid scar, which decreases the recurrence of keloid formation in movable areas such as the sternum, elbow joints, or shoulders.

15.12 The Use of IGSRT in Melanoma

Radiotherapy and immunotherapy may be synergistic when it comes to treating metastatic melanoma. As radiotherapy has a potential role in invoking an "abscopal effect," which occurs when the primary tumor site is irradiated, and regression of nonirradiated metastatic sites is observed. This observation has been seen in various malignancies such as hepatocellular carcinoma, lymphoma, and melanoma [54]. This is due to radiotherapy stimulating the immune system and triggering antitumor effects systemically [55]. This effect is rarely seen with radiotherapy alone, but it is observed when combined with immune check point inhibitors (ICI), specifically Ipilimumab [55].

Ipilimumab is an antibody against CTLA-4, which normally functions in turning off cytotoxic T-cells, thus aiding cancer cells in evading immune destruction [55]. Ipilimumab was the first ICI approved for treatment of metastatic melanoma, with a 20% long-term survival [55]. Chicas-Sett et al. conducted a systematic review of 16 studies analyzing the abscopal effect of radiotherapy with Ipilimumab. Overall, the median abscopal effect was 26.5% (10–63%), demonstrating a positive trend in treatment of metastatic melanoma with radiotherapy and Ipilimumab [55]. Additionally, the overall median survival was 19 months (4–39 months), this is a survival benefit of 8 months compared to the overall survival of 11.4 months reported in the phase II and III clinical trials of treatment with Ipilimumab alone [55]. Thus, radiotherapy combined with immunotherapy may potentially increase the cure of even advanced metastatic disease.

Interestingly, there is laboratory evidence that partial treatment of the primary melanoma lesion (using metal, meshes, grids, etc. that partially block out the incident radiation beam) may work better to elicit an abscopal effect.

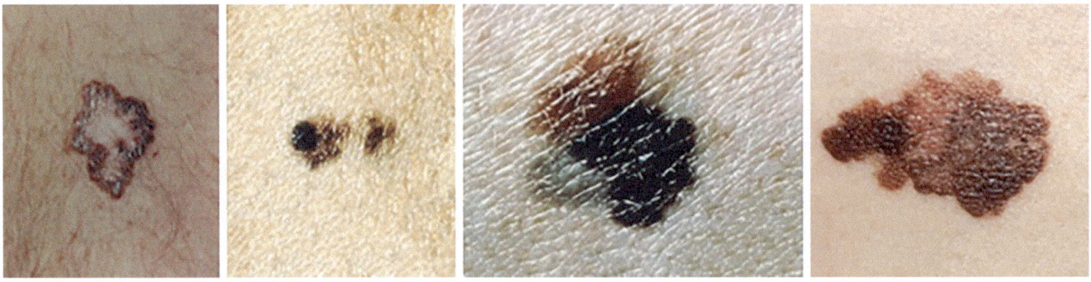

Various photos of Melanoma (National Cancer Institute)

15.13 Conclusion

NMSC is the most common cancer worldwide and exploding in incidence. There are various surgical and nonsurgical modalities to address this problem with cosmesis being a major concern which favors a nonsurgical approach as long as it is effective. Such approaches can also be applied to the management of keloids. While in previous years, the standard management of NMSC has been surgery/MMS, recent years point to an emerging shift in the standard of care to include IGSRT as an equivalent choice with the added benefit of improved cosmesis and function.

References

1. Lomas A, Leonardi-Bee J, Bath-Hextall F. A systematic review of worldwide incidence of nonmelanoma skin cancer. Br J Dermatol. 2012;166(5):1069–80. https://doi.org/10.1111/j.1365-2133.2012.10830.x.
2. Rogers HW, Weinstock MA, Feldman SR, Coldiron BM. Incidence estimate of nonmelanoma skin cancer (keratinocyte carcinomas) in the US population, 2012. JAMA Dermatol. 2015;151(10):1081–6. https://doi.org/10.1001/jamadermatol.2015.1187.
3. Apalla Z, Lallas A, Sotiriou E, Lazaridou E, Ioannides D. Epidemiological trends in skin cancer what does the future hold. Dermatol Pract Concept. 2017;7(2):1–6. https://doi.org/10.5826/dpc.0702a01.
4. Didona D, Paolino G, Bottoni U, Cantisani C. Non melanoma skin cancer pathogenesis overview. Biomedicine. 2018;6(1):1–15. https://doi.org/10.3390/biomedicines6010006.
5. Griffin LL, Ali FR, Lear JT. Non-melanoma skin cancer. Clin Med. 2016;16(1):62–5. https://doi.org/10.7861/clinmedicine.16-1-62.
6. Garcovich S, Colloca G, Sollena P, et al. Skin cancer epidemics in the elderly as an emerging issue in geriatric oncology. Aging Dis. 2017;8(5):643–61. https://doi.org/10.14336/AD.2017.0503.
7. Bichakjian C, Armstrong A, Baum C, et al. Guidelines of care for the management of basal cell carcinoma. J Am Acad Dermatol. 2018;78(3):540–59. https://doi.org/10.1016/j.jaad.2017.10.006.
8. Alam M, Armstrong A, Baum C, et al. Guidelines of care for the management of cutaneous squamous cell carcinoma. J Am Acad Dermatol. 2018;78(3):560–78. https://doi.org/10.1016/j.jaad.2017.10.007.
9. Jansen MHE, Koekelkoren FHJ, Nelemans PJ, et al. Comparison of long-term cosmetic outcomes for different treatments of superficial basal cell carcinoma. J Am Acad Dermatol. 2018;79(5):961–4. https://doi.org/10.1016/j.jaad.2018.04.053.
10. Yu L, Ladd D. Practice changing landmark study-multi-institutional analysis of image guided superficial radiotherapy (IGSRT) for the treatment of non-melanoma skin cancer (NMSC). In: Annual SID meeting.
11. Gauglitz GG, Korting HC, Pavicic T, Ruzicka T, Jeschke MG. Hypertrophic scarring and keloids: pathomechanisms and current and emerging treatment strategies. Mol Med. 2011;17(1–2):113–25. https://doi.org/10.2119/molmed.2009.00153.
12. Bahner JD, Bordeaux JS. Non-melanoma skin cancers: photodynamic therapy, cryotherapy, 5-fluorouracil, imiquimod, diclofenac, or what? Facts and controversies. Clin Dermatol. 2013;31(6):792–8. https://doi.org/10.1016/j.clindermatol.2013.08.020.
13. Naguib YW, Kumar A, Cui Z. The effect of microneedles on the skin permeability and antitumor activity of topical 5-fluorouracil. Acta Pharm Sin B. 2014;4(1):94–9. https://doi.org/10.1016/j.apsb.2013.12.013.
14. Ermertcan AT, Hellings PW, Cingi C. Nonmelanoma skin cancer of the head and neck: nonsurgical treatment. Facial Plast Surg Clin North Am. 2012;20(4):445–54. https://doi.org/10.1016/j.fsc.2012.08.004.
15. Gross K, Kircik L, Kricorian G. 5% 5-Fluorouracil cream for the treatment of small superficial basal cell carcinoma: efficacy, tolerability, cosmetic outcome, and patient satisfaction. Dermatol Surg. 2007;33:433. https://doi.org/10.1111/j.1524-4725.2007.33090.x.
16. Robert S Bader M. Medscape—what is the role of topical 5-fluorouracil 5% cream in the management of basal cell carcinoma (BCC)? https://www.medscape.com/answers/276624-100179/what-is-the-role-of-topical-5-fluorouracil. Published 2020.
17. Blalock TW. Keloids: a review of etiology. Prev Treat. 2020;13(2):33–43.
18. Hanna E, Abadi R, Abbas O. Imiquimod in dermatology: an overview. Int J Dermatol. 2016;55(8):831–44. https://doi.org/10.1111/ijd.13235.
19. Amini S, Viera MH, Valins W, Berman B. Nonsurgical innovations in the treatment of nonmelanoma skin cancer. J Clin Aesthet Dermatol. 2010;3(6):20–34.
20. Griffin LL, Lear JT. Photodynamic therapy and nonmelanoma skin cancer. Cancers (Basel). 2016;8(10):98. https://doi.org/10.3390/cancers8100098.
21. Gold MH. Therapeutic and aesthetic uses of photodynamic therapy part three of a five-part series: chemoprevention utilizing ALA-PDT. J Clin Aesthet Dermatol. 2008;1(4):26–32.
22. Rhodes LE, De Rie M, Enström Y, et al. Photodynamic therapy using topical methyl aminolevulinate vs surgery for nodular basal cell carcinoma: results of a multicenter randomized prospective trial. Arch Dermatol. 2004;140(1):17–23. https://doi.org/10.1001/archderm.140.1.17.
23. Fink-Puches R, Soyer HP, Hofer A, Kerl H, Wolf P. Long-term follow-up and histological changes of superficial nonmelanoma skin cancers treated with topical δ-aminolevulinic acid photodynamic therapy. Arch Dermatol. 1998;134(7):821–6. https://doi.org/10.1001/archderm.134.7.821.
24. Tosa M, Ogawa R. Photodynamic therapy for keloids and hypertrophic scars: a review. Scars Burn Heal. 2020;6:205951312093205. https://doi.org/10.1177/2059513120932059.
25. Berking C, Hauschild A, Kölbl O, Mast G, Gutzmer R. Basalzellkarzinom - therapieoptionen für den häufigsten hautkrebs. Dtsch Arztebl Int. 2014;111(22):389–95. https://doi.org/10.3238/arztebl.2014.0389.
26. Nguyen TH, Ho DQ-D. Nonmelanoma skin cancer. Curr Treat Options Oncol. 2002;3(3):193–203. https://doi.org/10.1007/s11864-002-0009-0.
27. Soleymani T, Abrouk M, Kelly KM. An analysis of laser therapy for the treatment of nonmelanoma skin cancer. Dermatol Surg. 2017;43(5):615–24. https://doi.org/10.1097/DSS.0000000000001048.
28. Ebrahimi A, Rezaei M, Kavoussi R, Eidizadeh M, Madani SH, Kavoussi H. Superpulsed CO2 laser with intraoperative pathologic assessment for treatment of periorbital basal cell carcinoma involving eyelash

line. Dermatol Res Pract. 2014;2014:1. https://doi.org/10.1155/2014/931657.
29. Campolmi P, Brazzini B, Urso C, et al. Superpulsed CO2 laser treatment of basal cell carcinoma with intraoperatory histopathologic and cytologic examination. Dermatol Surg. 2002;28:909. https://doi.org/10.1046/j.1524-4725.2002.02076.x.
30. Konnikov N, Avram M, Jarell A, Tannous Z. Pulsed dye laser as a novel non-surgical treatment for basal cell carcinomas: response and follow up 12-21 months after treatment. Lasers Surg Med. 2011;43:72. https://doi.org/10.1002/lsm.21035.
31. Shah SM, Konnikov N, Duncan LM, Tannous ZS. The effect of 595 nm pulsed dye laser on superficial and nodular basal cell carcinomas. Lasers Surg Med. 2009;41:417. https://doi.org/10.1002/lsm.20787.
32. Minars N, Blyumin-Karasik M. Treatment of basal cell carcinomas with pulsed dye laser: a case series. J Skin Cancer. 2012;2012:1–6. https://doi.org/10.1155/2012/286480.
33. Hamouzadeh P, Darkhor S, Aboie P, Zare M, Gray S. Safety and effectiveness of superficial radiation therapy in the treatment of skin diseases: a systematic review. Heal Technol Assess Action. 2017;1(1). https://doi.org/10.5812/htaa.62068.
34. Alam M, Nanda S, Mittal BB, Kim NA, Yoo S. The use of brachytherapy in the treatment of nonmelanoma skin cancer: a review. J Am Acad Dermatol. 2011;65(2):377–88. https://doi.org/10.1016/j.jaad.2010.03.027.
35. Nestor MS, Berman B, Goldberg D, Cognetta AB Jr, Gold M, Roth W, Cockerell CJ, Glick B. Consensus guidelines on the use of superfi cial radiation therapy for treating nonmelanoma skin cancers and keloids. J Clin Aesthet Dermatol. 2019;12(2):12–8.
36. Cheraghi N, Cognetta AJ, Goldberg D. RADIATION THERAPY for the adjunctive treatment of surgically excised keloids: a review. J Clin Aesthet Dermatol. 2017;10(8):12–5. https://doi.org/10.1007/978-3-662-47181-4_38.
37. Shen J, Lian X, Sun Y, et al. Hypofractionated electron-beam radiation therapy for keloids: retrospective study of 568 cases with 834 lesions. J Radiat Res. 2015;56(5):811–7. https://doi.org/10.1093/jrr/rrv031.
38. Ogawa R, Yoshitatsu S, Yoshida K, Miyashita T. Is radiation therapy for keloids acceptable? The risk of radiation-induced carcinogenesis. Plast Reconstr Surg. 2009;124:1196. https://doi.org/10.1097/PRS.0b013e3181b5a3ae.
39. Bowen GM, White GL, Gerwels JW. Mohs micrographic surgery. Am Fam Physician. 2005;72(5):845–8. https://doi.org/10.5005/jp/books/14212_38.
40. Lane JE, Kent DE. Surgical margins in the treatment of nonmelanoma skin cancer and Mohs micrographic surgery. Curr Surg. 2005;62(5):518–26. https://doi.org/10.1016/j.cursur.2005.01.003.
41. Patel R, Strimling R, Doggett S, et al. Comparison of electronic brachytherapy and Mohs micrographic surgery for the treatment of early-stage non-melanoma skin cancer: a matched pair cohort study. J Contemp Brachytherapy. 2017;9(4):338–44. https://doi.org/10.5114/jcb.2017.68480.
42. McGregor S, Minni J, Herold D. Superficial radiation therapy for the treatment of nonmelanoma skin cancers. J Clin Aesthet Dermatol. 2015;8(12):12–4.
43. Nestor MS, Berman B, Goldberg D, et al. Consensus guidelines on the use of superficial radiation therapy for treating nonmelanoma skin cancers and keloids. J Clin Aesthet Dermatol. 2019;12(2):12–8.
44. Fahradyan A, Howell A, Wolfswinkel E, Tsuha M, Sheth P, Wong A. Updates on the management of non-melanoma skin cancer (NMSC). Healthcare. 2017;5(4):82. https://doi.org/10.3390/healthcare5040082.
45. Linos E, Parvataneni R, Stuart SE, Boscardin WJ, Landefeld CS, Chren MM. Treatment of nonfatal conditions at the end of life: nonmelanoma skin cancer. JAMA Intern Med. 2013;173(11):1006–12. https://doi.org/10.1001/jamainternmed.2013.639.
46. Rong Y, Zuo L, Shang L, Bazan JG. Radiotherapy treatment for nonmelanoma skin cancer. Expert Rev Anticancer Ther. 2015;15(7):765–76. https://doi.org/10.1586/14737140.2015.1042865.
47. Cognetta AB, Howard BM, Heaton HP, Stoddard ER, Hong HG, Green WH. Superficial x-ray in the treatment of basal and squamous cell carcinomas: a viable option in select patients. J Am Acad Dermatol. 2012;67(6):1235–41. https://doi.org/10.1016/j.jaad.2012.06.001.
48. Yu L, Oh C, Shea CR. The treatment of non-melanoma skin cancer with image-guided superficial radiation therapy: an analysis of 2917 invasive and in situ keratinocytic carcinoma lesions. Oncol Ther. 2021;9:153. https://doi.org/10.1007/s40487-021-00138-4.
49. Minka E, Velasquez R, Yu L, Desai A, Lin R. 18845 twelve-month local control and satisfaction results of selected patients with nonmelanoma skin cancer following outpatient superficial radiation therapy. J Am Acad Dermatol. 2020;83:AB222. https://doi.org/10.1016/j.jaad.2020.06.978.
50. Key statistics for basal and squamous cell skin cancers. American Cancer Society. https://www.cancer.org/cancer/basal-and-squamous-cell-skin-cancer/about/key-statistics.html. Published 2021.
51. Yu L, Moloney M, Beers R, Serure D. Enhancing cosmesis while achieving high cure rates for early stage non-melanoma skin cancer in the outpatient dermatology clinic using a novel non-invasive modality. Clin Dermatol Res Ther. 2021;4(1):1–10.
52. Fellner C. Vismodegib (Erivedge) for advanced basal cell carcinoma. P T. 2012;37(12):670–82.
53. NCCN Clinical Practice Guidelines in Oncology (NCCN Guidelines®): squamous cell skin cancer.

National Comprehensive Cancer Network. https://www.nccn.org/professionals/physician_gls/pdf/squamous.pdf. Published 2020.
54. Grimaldi AM, Simeone E, Giannarelli D, et al. Abscopal effects of radiotherapy on advanced melanoma patients who progressed after ipilimumab immunotherapy. Onco Targets Ther. 2014;3(5):e28780. https://doi.org/10.4161/onci.28780.
55. Chicas-Sett R, Morales-Orue I, Rodriguez-Abreu D, Lara-Jimenez P. Combining radiotherapy and ipilimumab induces clinically relevant radiation-induced abscopal effects in metastatic melanoma patients: a systematic review. Clin Transl Radiat Oncol. 2018;9:5–11. https://doi.org/10.1016/j.ctro.2017.12.004.

Aesthetic Podiatric Sonography

16

Robert L. Bard and Richard Kushner

Abstract

High-resolution sonography allows imaging of dermal and subdermal lesions such as ruptured tendons and inflammatory disorders. Foreign body diagnosis is aided by 3D volumetric imaging since the intruding substance may fragment, requiring a search at a distance from the point of entry. Pigmented lesions on the plantar surface may be quickly investigated and biopsy avoided in certain situations. Image guidance accurately targets surgical areas with improved hemostasis. Special attention is given to skin of color and aging effects in our highly diverse society.

Keywords

Podiatry · Dermal ultrasound · Doppler ultrasound · Nail disorders · Claw toe · Onychodystrophy · Melanoma

R. L. Bard (✉) · R. Kushner
The Angio Foundation and Bard Diagnostics, New York, NY, USA
e-mail: rbard@cancerscan.com

16.1 Introduction

A special chapter is devoted to these disorders since the foot is the ultimate and most uniquely human weight-bearing structure where biomechanics play an important role in diagnosis and treatment. The causative factors of aberrant biomechanics create another clinical consideration in lesion formation and therapy of lower extremity disease.

Blood flow evaluation is a measure of inflammatory activity and tumor aggression and is covered elsewhere as is the physics of 3D image reconstruction with Doppler histogram analysis. Benign and malignant cutaneous disorders in previous chapters affect the foot and ankle, including the nail bed.

16.2 Vascular Tumors

Angiomas and similar benign tumors are better treated if the locoregional vasculature is mapped in the preop setting to anticipate potential complications. Vascular disease may be evaluated by blood flow Doppler analysis of the posterior tibial and pedal digital arteries. Intravascular plaque usually producing high-velocity flows may be observed as well as low or absent flow conditions (Fig. 16.1).

A hypovolemic region may be cyanotic casting a blue discoloration of a toe, which may be

R. L. Bard (ed.), *Image-Guided Aesthetic Treatments*, https://doi.org/10.1007/978-3-031-36266-8_16

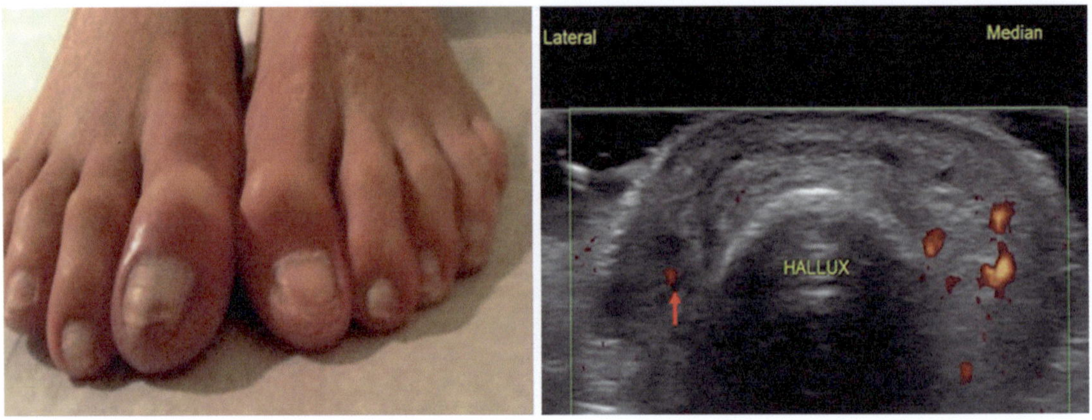

Fig. 16.1 Blood flow differentiates from low flow disorder with incipient necrosis

mistaken for melanoma. The "blue toe" syndrome diffusely and homogeneously discolors the entire nail bed and should not be easily confused with acral melanoma and may also be a cutaneous feature of COVID-19 dermatitis.

Certain verrucae (viral warts) are vascular with a central vessel extending to the surface. A melanoma of the nail has a linear presentation originating from the nail matrix and extending distally as the nail plate grows. The entire nail plate would not be involved thus differentiating blue toe from malignant melanoma.

Differentiating a wart from an amelanotic melanoma is possible due to the vertical Doppler flow commonly found in the benign lesion (simulating a tornado pattern), while the melanoma vascularity tends to be diffuse and horizontal in appearance (hurricane pattern).

16.3 Weight-Bearing Lesions

True bursae and potential or adventitial bursa are initiated and aggravated by chronic repetitive trauma. The subcutaneous lesions may form a subdermal mass and often produce compensatory dermal thickening and occasional discoloration (Fig. 16.2a, b).

Palmar and plantar skin is glabrous meaning hairless with a double-layered epidermis. Epidermal thickening over a joint is termed cornification or clavus, while the common callus is in other areas where intermittent pressure and friction initiate a defense mechanism. The thickness of the epidermis may be demonstrated at high-resolution imaging alerting the podiatrist the safe depth limit for debridement procedures. While there are rare benign hyperkeratotic disorders of the epidermis, thickening of the intraepidermal tissues appears as a black region that is differentiated from fluid by pressure application which shifts liquid content in real-time imaging. The dorsal layer of epidermal thickening often spares the underlying dermis (Fig. 16.3). Acute trauma produces hemorrhagic areas that produce visible pigmentation in the epidermis. This callus is exclusively situated between the dorsal and ventral epidermis (Fig. 16.4a).

The cause of callus formation may also be related to an underlying bone abnormality such as this fragmented tibial sesamoid, thus the presence of thickened epidermal tissues should prompt the search for a causative process (Fig. 16.4b) [1–4]. Callus on the toes is due to friction from poor fitting footwear and repetitive trauma. Contraction of the Achilles tendon and of

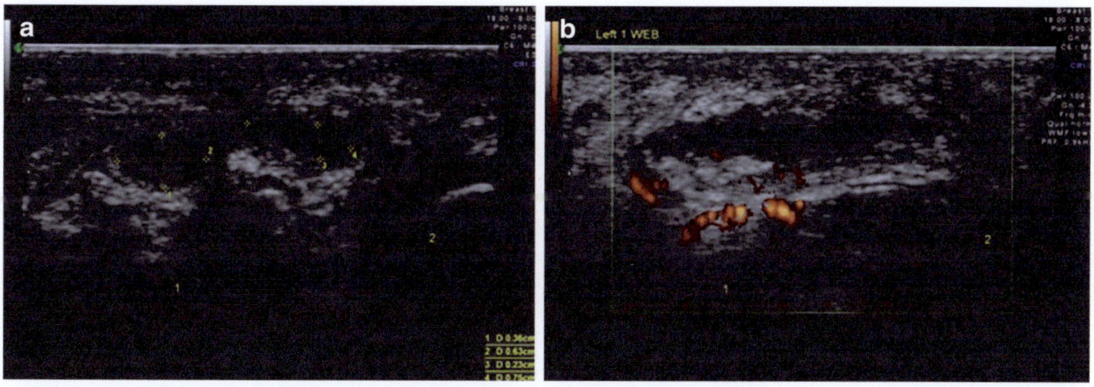

Fig. 16.2 Shearing force induced inflamed bursal sac targeted for image-guided injection. (**a**) Transverse scan shows web space cystic area. (**b**) Doppler longitudinal scan demonstrates thick walled bursal sac and hyperemia in underlying tendon

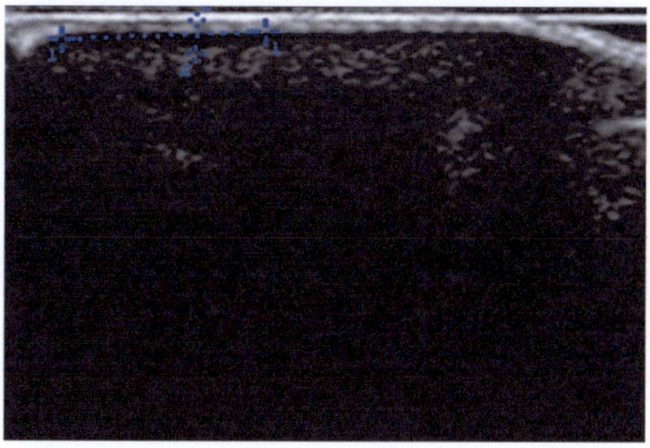

Fig. 16.3 Double-layered epidermis shows depth of callus-sparing dermis

the flexor tendon apparatus causes the tips of the toes to strike the surface with resulting callus formation and nail plate thickening. Abnormal nail plates are misdiagnosed by many patients as a fungus infection due to the increase in anterior–posterior nail plate compensatory hypertrophy. Orthopedic disorders such as clubfoot, hammer toe, or misaligned fracture healing may produce nail impingement on the dermis resulting in asymmetric callus formation or abrasion in the case of penetration of the nail plate.

Doppler imaging ruled out malignant vascularity as would the new optical technologies of OCT (optical coherence tomography) with a imaging depth of 0.2–0.3 mm and RCM (reflectance confocal microscopy) that show surface vessels up to 1.5–2.0 mm in tissue depth. These technologies are discussed in other chapters and will probably have greater application in podiatry in the near future.

Rarely, chronic epidermal thickening will calcify and must be differentiated from subdermal calcinosis or calcinosis cutis (Fig. 16.5a) and crystal forming diseases such as gout and CPDD or pseudogout (chronic pyrophosphate deposition disease) (Fig. 16.5b).

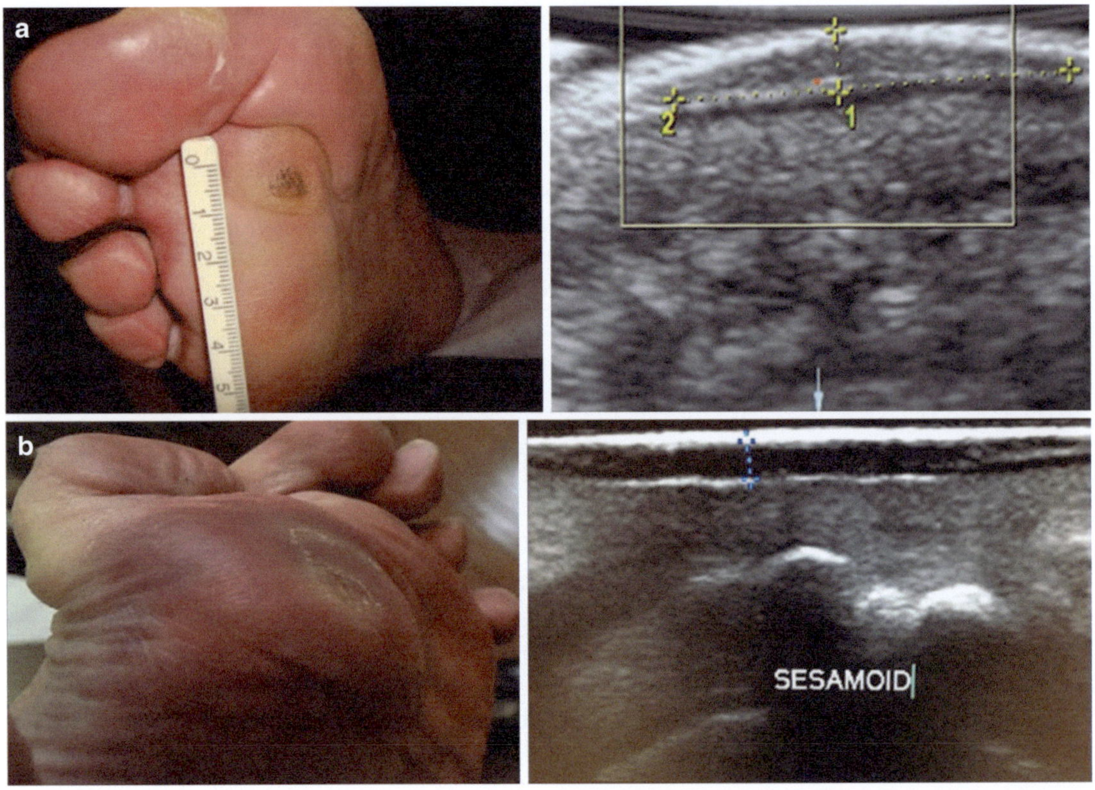

Fig. 16.4 Thickening of epidermal layer causing of blood into callus-simulating pigmented lesion with depth (+...+). (**a**) Vertical dotted yellow line shows echogenic blood within the thickened epidermis. (**b**) Vertical dotted blue line depicts echofree epidermal thickening

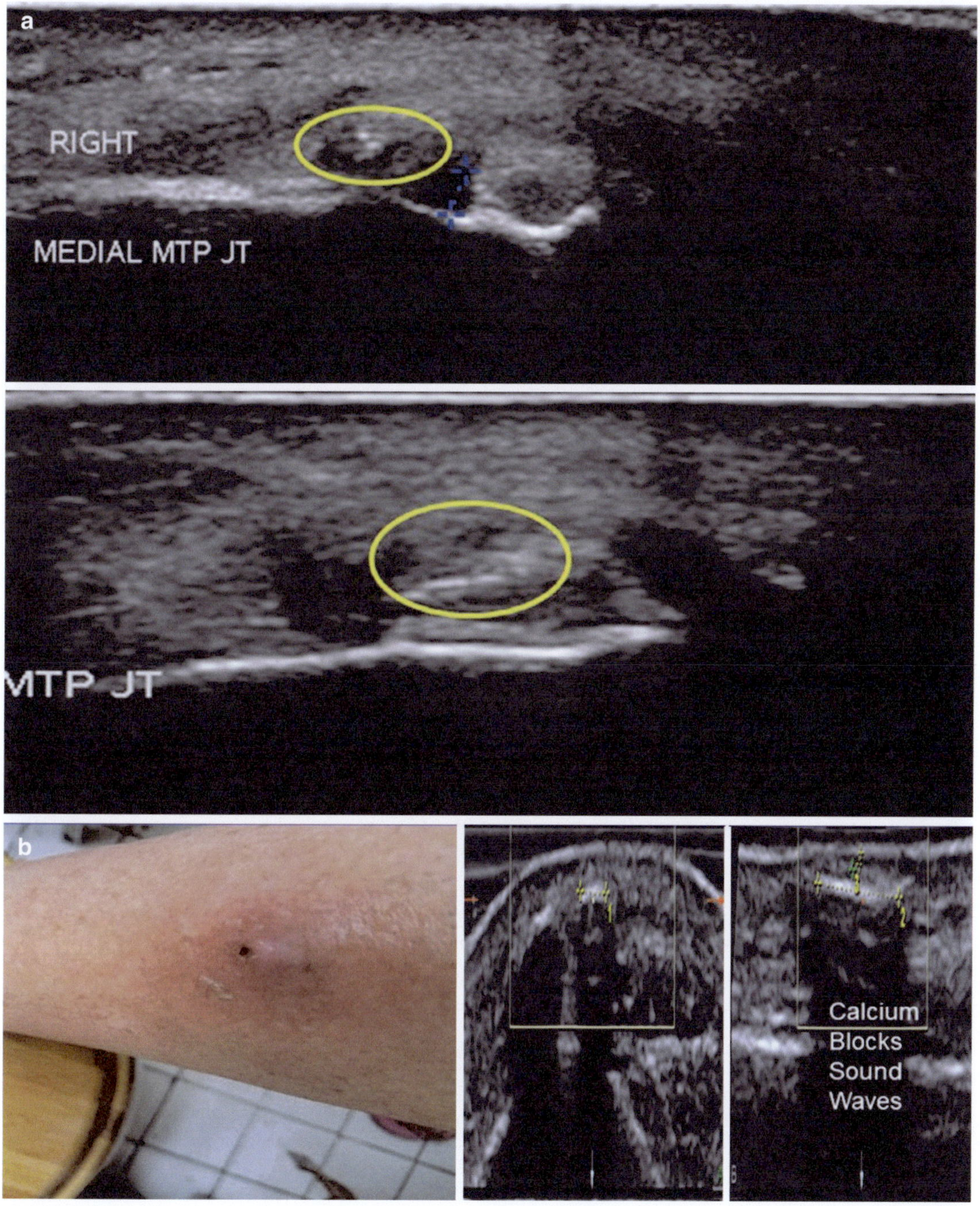

Fig. 16.5 (**a**) Calcinosis cutis-dermal or subdermal calcium may deflect or break needle. (**b**) Crystals from gout or CPDD may be differentiated from calcinosis cutis

16.4 Cysts

The epidermal cyst (formerly called sebaceous cyst) is usually dermally located but extends into the epidermis with a tiny nipple or be wholly located in the subdermal recesses. While new cystic lesions are usually echo free, thin walled and horizontally oriented, older cysts often contain echoes of debris, thick walls, and vertical orientation (Fig. 16.6). Occasionally, longstanding cysts may demonstrate wall calcification and multiple orthogonal image planes to avoid the total sonic shadow may be needed. Since acoustic shadowing is a sign of fibrosis or malignant desmoplasia, the addition of Doppler or MRI sequences may be appropriate. Since a cystic focus appears as a subcutaneous region and may be hard and immobile if chronic, the differential diagnosis must include a bone lesion such as osteoma, or rarely, sarcoma or metastatic focus. Since the bony cortex is easily seen, a protrusion from the bone with intact bone outline and lack of cortical erosion ascertained, a radiographic investigation may be avoided (Fig. 16.7) Certain primary sarcomas and vascular metastases, such as breast, melanoma, and renal cell carcinomas, may show hyperemia on Doppler blood flow imaging.

16.5 Foreign Bodies

Sonography is particularly important in the foot since both weight bearing and movement will affect the distribution in the affected region. The foreign body may fracture with displacement of fragments or be forced into locations unexpected by the initial portal of entry.

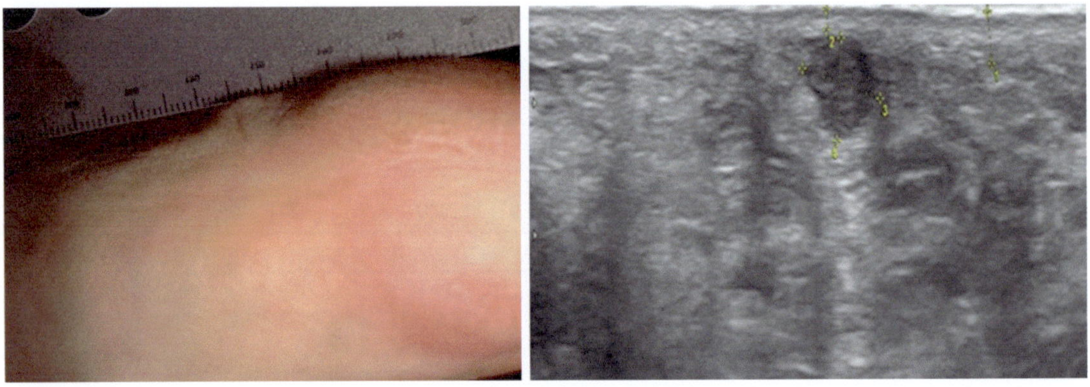

Fig. 16.6 Intradermal location differentiates cyst from scar due to inflammatory or foreign body reaction

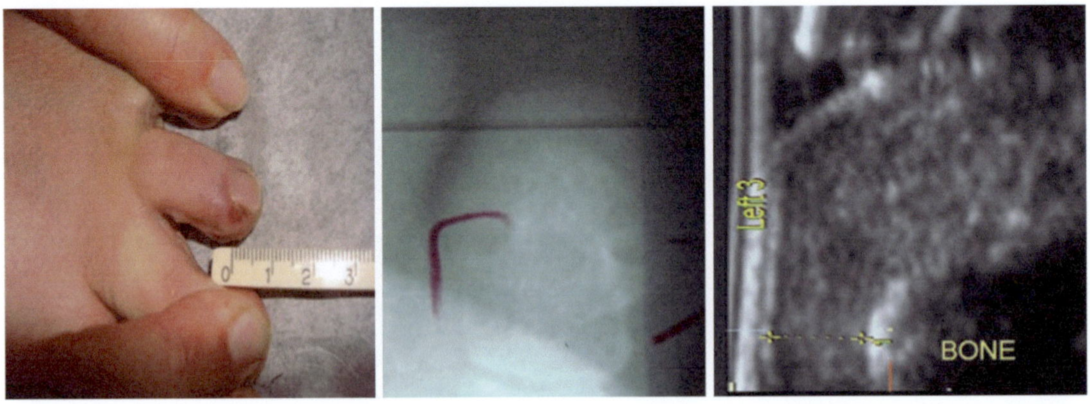

Fig. 16.7 Cortical intact outline differentiates benign osteoma from fracture or osteosarcoma

A completely intratendon location cannot be easily imaged even during visual surgical exploration, whereas sonography pinpoints the site before or during surgery with intraoperative probes. Surgical image-guided foreign body removal has been performed by the US Army field surgeons for over 30 years with highly reduced surgical morbidity and successful resolution of symptoms.

Foreign bodies that lie predominantly in the horizontal plane appear as linear bright echoes with or without the accompanying black shadow on standard 2D imaging. Since the 3D is multiplanar, the greatest dimension will be more easily identified in one of the three planes that occur simultaneously while scanning. A further refinement of 3D imaging is the 4D potential, which is real-time operator adjustment of the probe angle and position while live scanning to optimize the foreign body in its most recognizable silhouette (Fig. 16.8). Note how the fiberglass thread is barely distinguishable from the normal nail bed structures on 2D but appear in stark contrast to the background in the 3D version. Splinter imag-

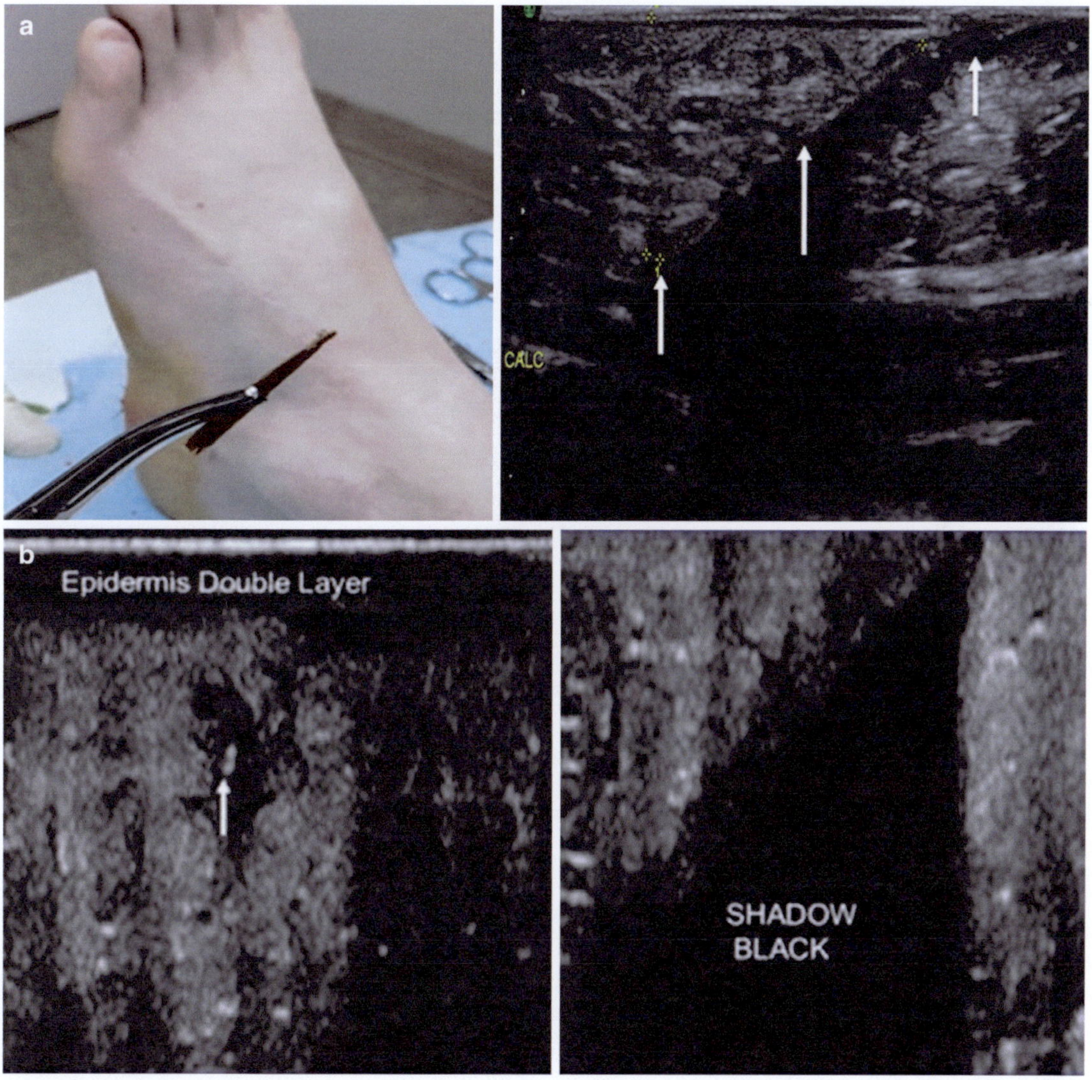

Fig. 16.8 3D volume permits better detection of glass fragment(s) in 4 cm square plane (arrows point to fragment). (**a**) Sonic shadow from foreign body (arrows). (**b**) Echogenic foreign body (arrow). (**c**) Normal dermis (arrow) echogenic 0.1 x 0.8 mm splinter (3 arrows)

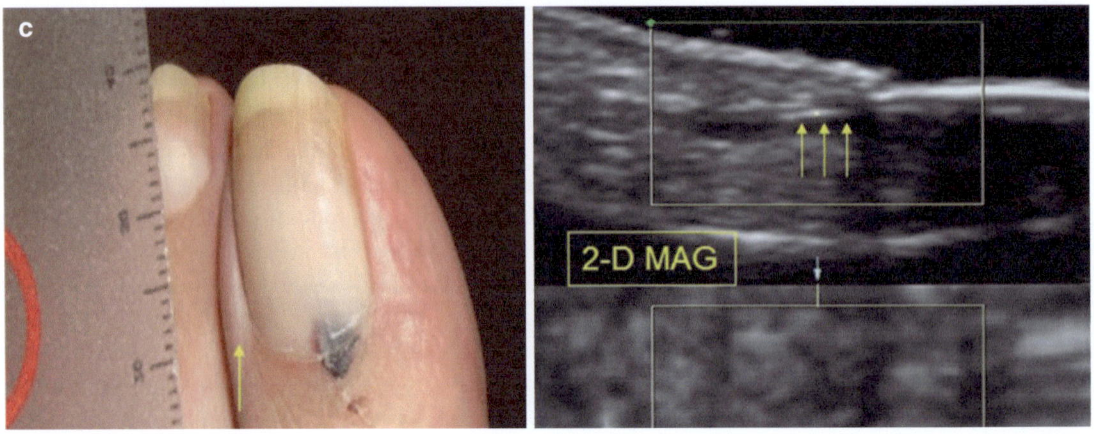

Fig. 16.8 (continued)

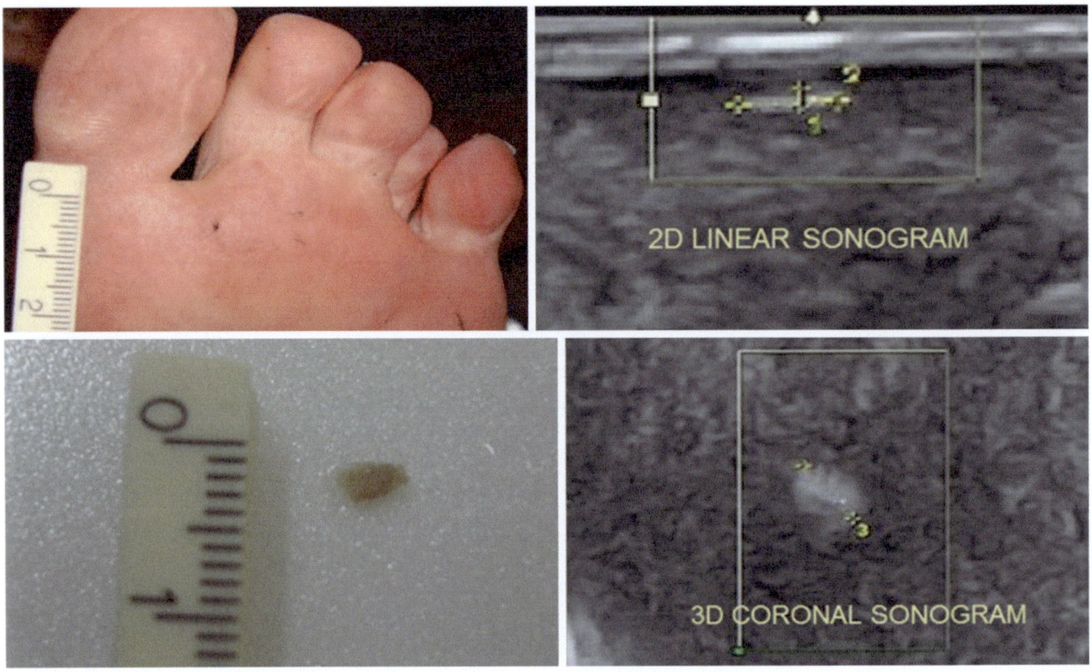

Fig. 16.9 Location above basement membrane allows incisional removal without scar

ing is particularly optimized by the use of very high-frequency probes which can show the fragmented strands (Fig. 16.8a), perilesional fluid and black sonic shadowing which may be missed by lower frequency probes (Fig. 16.8b). Significant perilesional fluid allows easier extraction of splinter and is better mapped at higher frequency potentially permitting minimally invasive removal by forceps.

Similarly, intraepidermal superficial splinters may appear as pigmented lesions to the naked eye but are quickly triangulated in depth by the 2D and 3D technology (Fig. 16.9). The imaging professional must be aware of intradermal echoes related to heavy metal disease or dystrophic calcification that is a common occurrence with the popular use of probes in the 24–70 MHz range. Subdermal lesions are likewise difficult to image

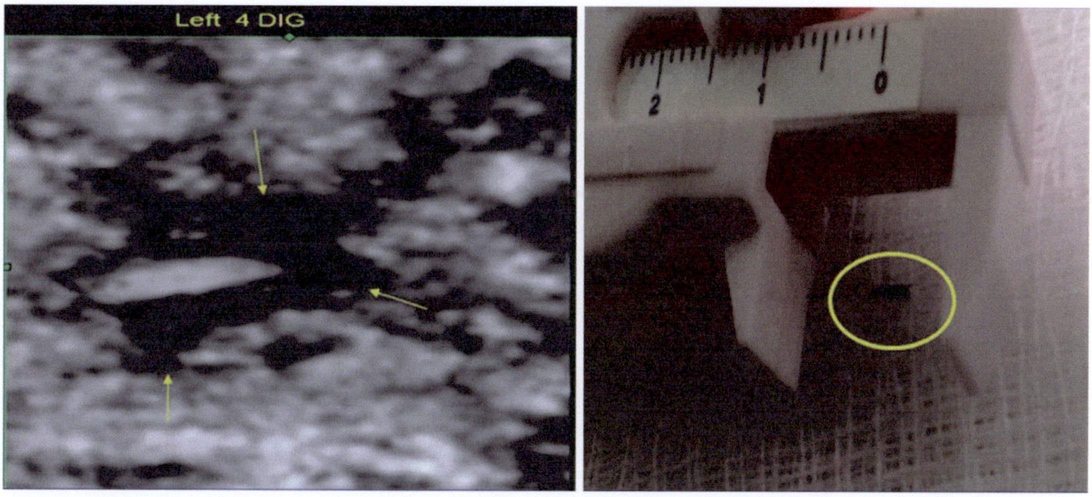

Fig. 16.10 Lack of Doppler flow suggests scarification a possible postop complication

in 2D; however, the frequent occurrence of perilesional fluid due to local inflammatory processes creates a black background for the foreign object to be highlighted. In this case, the sea urchin spine remains uncalcified rendering radiographic imaging useless (Fig. 16.10). The foreign body may remain asymptomatic for prolonged periods or rapidly develop into complications including pain from abscess formation, chronic discharging wound with sinus tracts, necrotizing fasciitis, granulomas leading to bone and joint destruction including tendon infiltration with shredding and tearing, vascular events including thrombophlebitis with or without pulmonary emboli and generalized massive soft tissue injury [5–12].

16.6 Inflammatory Lesions

Subungual granulomas produce dark inflammatory tissue reactions that stand out in the lighter nail bed tissues (Fig. 16.11). Long-standing lesions can erode the adjacent bony cortex and generate pigmented stripes or nail plate irregularities. Very slow growing tumors, including the glomus vascular lesion, often produce scalloping of the underlying bone that may be imaged without radiographs. Angiomatous areas may be associated with other findings such as epidermal thickening due to callus formation (Fig. 16.12) in this biopsy proven hemangioma.

Chronic dermal inflammation in psoriasis, lupus erythematosus, and scleroderma including the growing list of connective tissue disorders with skin manifestations which may use sonography to guide treatment decisions. While epidermal and dermal depth changes are easily performed with standard imaging, the use of 3D Doppler histogram analysis allows a quantifiable marker to demonstrate treatment effectiveness in follow-up scenarios. Since the degree of inflammation is proportional to the number of inflammatory vessels, the 3D volumetric measurement of vessel density in a given volume provides a baseline of the current inflammatory process and serial scans produce a timeline of treatment change by measuring the VESSEL DENSITY INDEX (VDI), which is expressed as a percentage of abnormal vessels in the region under investigation (Fig. 16.13) [13, 14].

Subdermal inflammation is now a common finding in cosmetic procedures and surgical interventions, and panniculitis may appear as dermal discoloration or irregularity. Note the dermal thickening and mottled echo pattern of the subcutaneous fat, which is usually homogeneously dark. Trauma in the metatarsal region also produces this irregularity of the fatty tissues in the region of the hallux (Fig. 16.14).

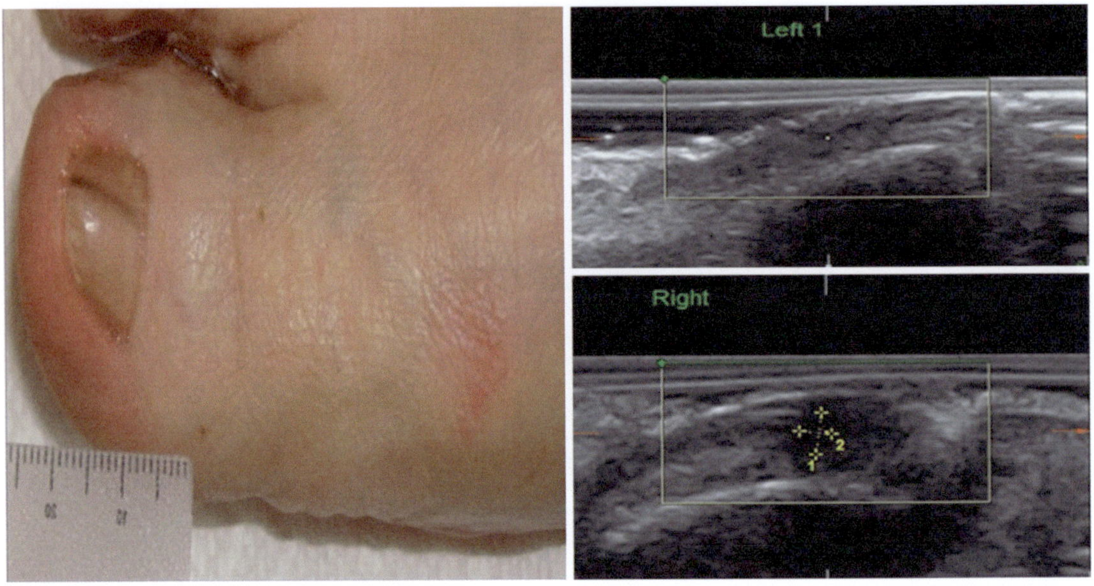

Fig. 16.11 Avascular granuloma differentiated from melanoma-note early cortical erosion

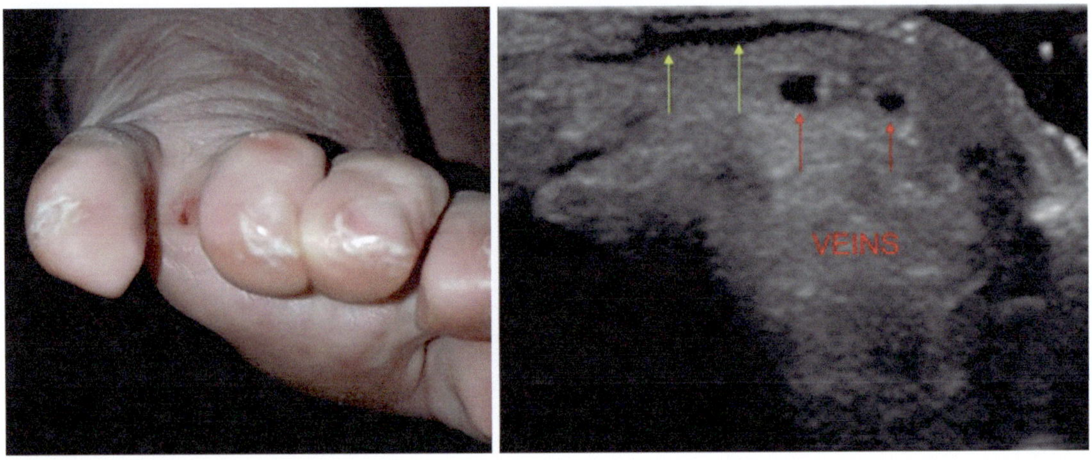

Fig. 16.12 Lesion avascularity rules against melanoma

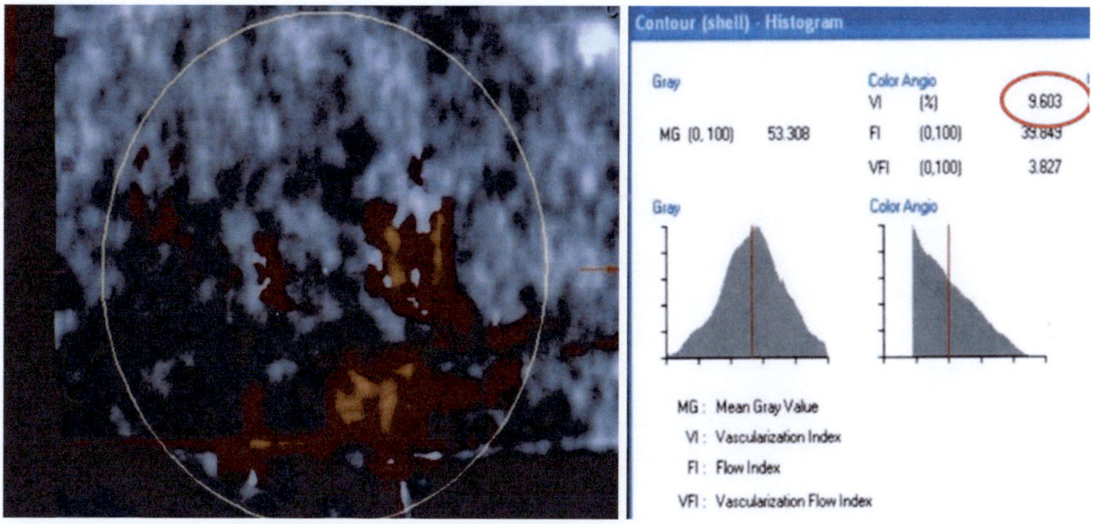

Fig. 16.13 Extravasated epidermal blood differentiated from nevus

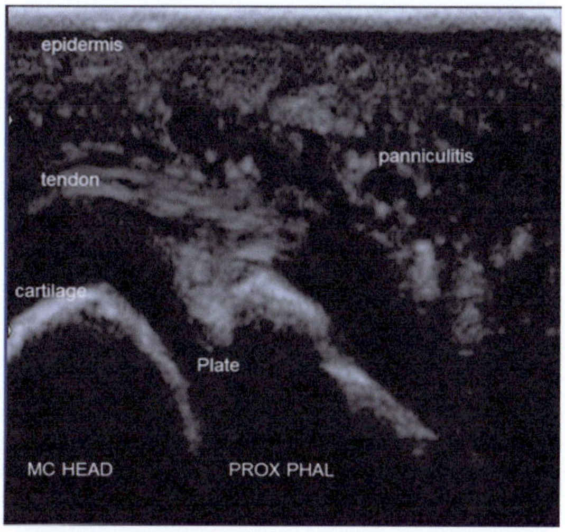

Fig. 16.14 Inflammation from filler injections which have a black box warning for injections on weight-bearing areas

Metatarsalgia associated with plantar plate degeneration or tearing is readily demonstrable by MRI or sonography; however, dynamic ultrasound allows the patient to point out the painful region that may be overshadowed by other findings on MRI such as neuromas or bursitis (Fig. 16.15).

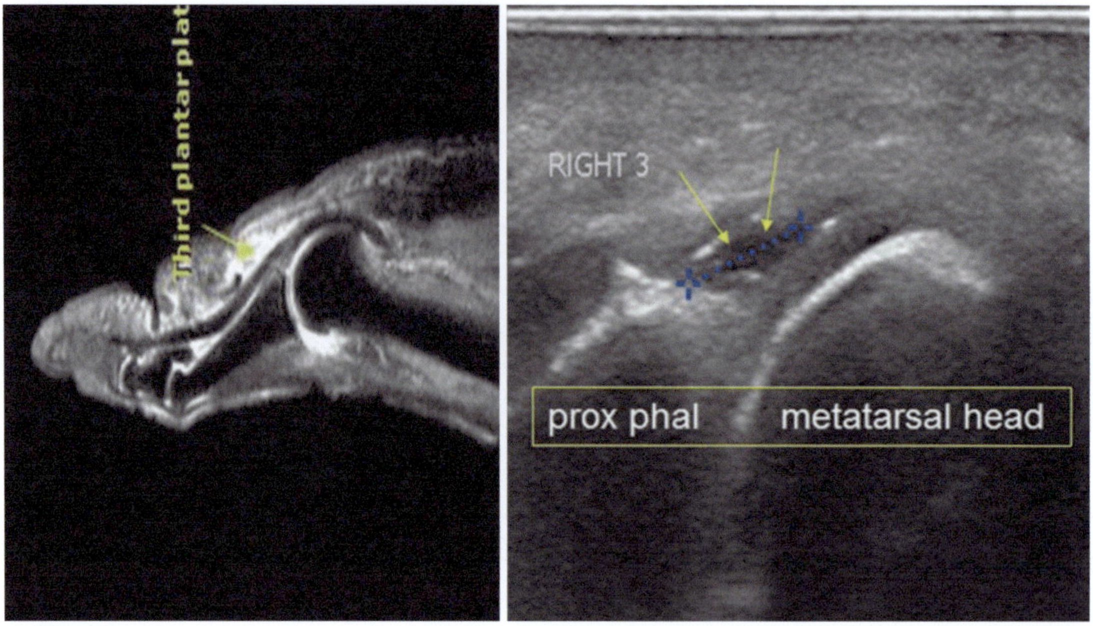

Fig. 16.15 Surgical repair for plantar plate tear is difficult-image-guided prolotherapy with immobilization aids treatment

16.7 Hydrostatic Disorders

Venous reflux increasing capillary and arterial resistance is causative in subdermal fibrosis and dermal inflammation [15]. The depth of the subdermal tissue edema as well as the connective tissue bands connecting the dermis to the deeper fascia is readily ascertainable with the ultrasound and elastographic assets now in use.

Strain elastography using pressure deformation and shear wave elastography with acoustic wave force quantifies the degree of fibrosis within the thickened dermal and subdermal structures. This hydrostatic pressure increase may also lead to the development of "cellulite" appearance in the buttocks and thigh areas. Collagen septal thickening has been studied with high-resolution 7 T MRI that corresponds to the findings depicted by the high-resolution ultrasound probes.

16.8 Melanoma

Given the deadly nature of acral melanoma, especially in the nail and sole of the foot, any pigmented lesion merits serious ultrasound Doppler investigation. While malignant melanoma is classically evaluated by the tumor depth (Breslow) or dermal layer invasion (Clark's level) and signs of surface ulceration, there exist better mechanisms for malignant tumor potential detection. The initial expression in the vertical growth stage of melanoma is usually a dark vertical stripe; however, malignant variations come in every shape and color including flesh tone in the "amelanotic melanoma" variant. Genetic expression testing and optical evaluation are being explored, but the vessel density index mentioned above in the inflammatory processes is a proven criteria that is currently used worldwide. Clearly the lack of dermal invasion and absence of neovascularity are indicative of a nonlethal disorder [16, 17] (Fig. 16.16).

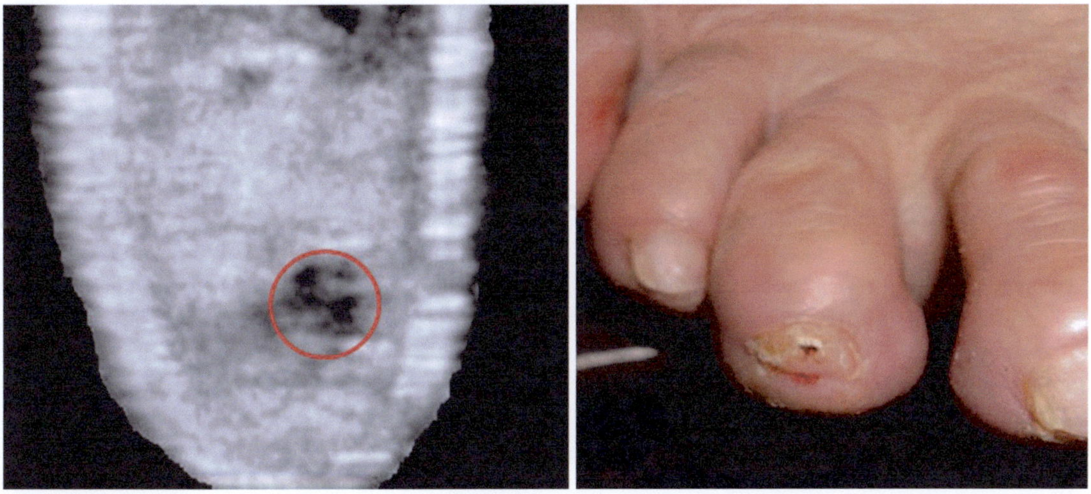

Fig. 16.16 Avascular pigmented lesion favors benign process in skin of color or without recall of injury

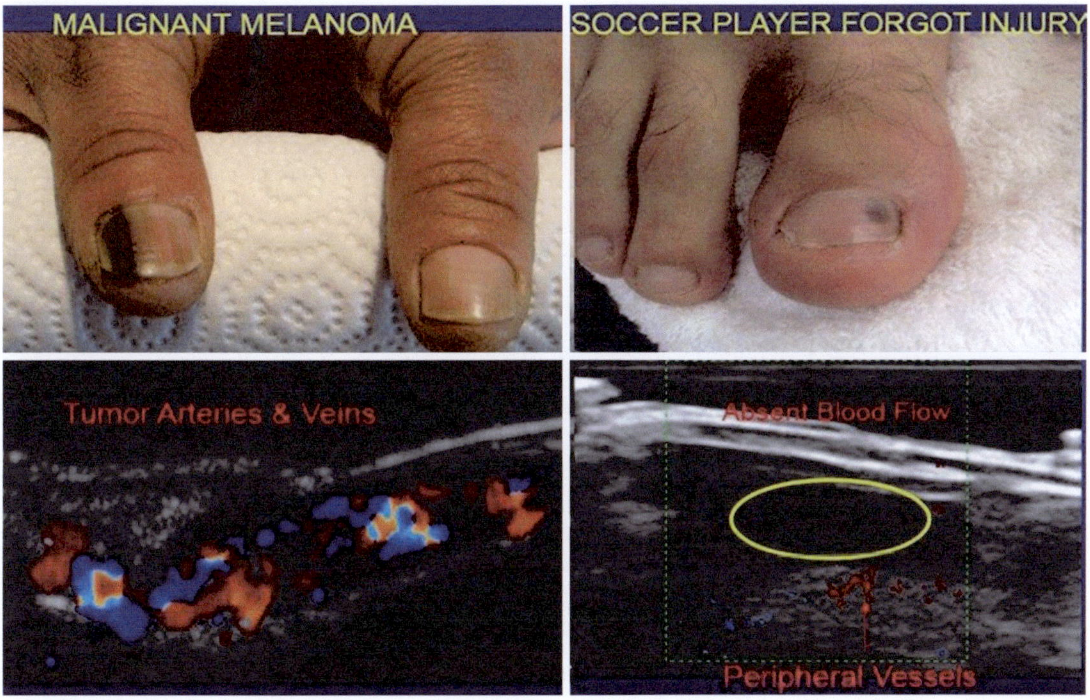

Fig. 16.17 Avascular lesion differentiated from hematoma and melanoma pattern

3D Doppler histogram analysis is the optimal method of determining the malignant potential with a rapid noninvasive study. In the new milieu of oncoimmunology treatments, the progression of therapy will be serially mapped by the 3D Vessel Density Index to predict success or failure [18]. Alterations in vessel density occur earlier than visible or other non-Doppler imaging findings. The possibility of a cancer's biologic nature changing or the tumor response to treatment diminishing can be quickly ascertained and evaluated allowing timely change in therapeutic options (Fig. 16.17). Addition of CEUS improves vascular imaging parameters and produces earlier reliable clinical data on the effect of neovascular changes in regions of interest.

16.9 Special Considerations with Skin of Color Including Aging Effects

Three primary biological substances determine skin coloration in all peoples: melanin in the epidermis, carotene in the dermis, and hemoglobin in the dermal capillaries, which are genetic and/or environmentally determined.

Asian skin is more resistant to aging in part due to more melanin in the basal layer that protects it from premature aging from sun damage. Also many Asian women are conscious of the darkening effect of ultraviolet radiation and purposely limit sun exposure. Although Asian skin has greater trans-epidermal water loss, the larger eccrine glands produce oilier surface characteristics with exaggerated "shine" features and increased risk of post-inflammatory hyperpigmentation. While in some cultures, a mole or pigmented lesion on the sole of the foot is considered good luck, the higher incidence of acral melanoma make this site worthy of increased attention due to the high aggressive potential of this malignancy. When scanning for the depth of the tumor, the adjacent locoregional tissues and the draining nodal basins may be investigated.

Black skin has more sebaceous glands, larger melanosome granules in the basal layer, and a higher percentage of keratinized cells in the stratum corneum, which may account for the increased risk of keloid formation and hypertrophic scarring.

South Asian skin is distinct from Asian or Black skin in that melanosome production is reduced. The tropical climate and higher incidence of parasite infestation make the real-time sonogram of a mass or discolored area important to detect larval motion or the skeleton of a dead parasite.

Latin skin characteristics demonstrate elevated granular mast cell concentrations and melanosome densities that accelerate skin healing but increase the risk of post-inflammatory hyperpigmentation and keloid formation. The higher incidence of diabetes in this group may result in reduced skin healing and lower extremity vascular complications.

Nordic skin from geographically northern climate is pale due to lower melanin values which increases the damage from ultraviolet radiation and possible lack of dietary Vitamin D. Globally, Sweden ranks fourth in highest incidence of skin cancer. Notable are risks of rosacea, sarcoidosis, and ichthyosis almost exclusively found in Norwegians. These inflammatory entities are associated with nail disease, synovitis, and arthritis [19]. Visible changes in skin coloration from trauma, chemotherapy, or collagen diseases are more difficult to assess against the diffusely dark tonal background.

As we learned from allergic skin testing results that measure the wheal response by width and color perhaps a useful addition to this procedure would be to add optical spectral analysis of inconclusive eyeball observation and the wide range of near infrared systems that detect colonies of bacteria on the surface for wound-healing situational analysis. Similarly high-resolution ultrasound measures epidermal and dermal thickness which would support the diagnosis of intradermal and subdermal disorders.

16.10 Optically Assisted Wound Healing

Skin lesions and nail aberrations assessed by optical technologies with image-guided treatment are increasing in medical applications. As the chapter on dental disease notes the presence of bacteria and in some cases malignancies are detectable in the oral cavity and tongue. Nonbiopsy cancer treatment is performed with ultrasound noting the depth of the tumor, while optical coherence tomography or reflectance confocal microscopy verifies the lateral margins before thermal therapies are currently effective in the ablation of basal cell skin cancers.

Improved debridement of wounds is managed in a similar fashion with the optical assistance of violet wavelength at 405 nm to highlight bacterial colonies greater than 10 to the fourth power by their autofluorescence reflective waves calibrated by special filters. The use of quantitative 3D/4D histogram Doppler flow allows the treatment of wounds by mapping the areas of adequate and inadequate tissue oxygenation as well as detecting cancer remnants missed after MOHS micrographic surgery especially in the case of lower extremity squamous cell skin cancers. Large surface dermal wounds are difficult to heal in the vascularly compromised lower extremity so grafts are often applied. The ability to discover unsuspected bacterial foci or malignant cell nests is possible with the early application of image-guided diagnostics [20].

16.11 Minimally Invasive Image-Guided Treatment

Prolotherapy is used to treat musculoskeletal conditions that require an inflammatory process to hasten the healing of fractures, tendon pathology (especially Achilles tendinosis), ligamentous damage, and must be used in conjunction with an understanding of reorienting and reversing the biomechanics that initially created the pathology. This injection therapy assists musculoskeletal reorientation to be achieved with the creation of supporting collagen creation. The inflammatory response to 0.5 g of 50% dextrose mixed with 10 mg of 2% lidocaine and 500 μg of B12 causes an increase of fibroblasts to the area of treatment.

16.12 Nail Treatment Options

Fragile, brittle, or split nails (lamellar splitting) are commonly caused by inflammatory diseases such as psoriasis, rosacea, trauma, onychomycosis, environmental factors, and chemical exposure to detergents, solvents, and cleansers. While removal of external causation and treatment of inflammatory processes is primary, the addition of a hydrosoluble nail lacquer is proving useful and may be applied as an undercoating to nail polish.

16.13 Image-Guided Pedal Microsurgery

Most therapeutic forefoot maneuvers are performed after an Xray, CT scan, or MRI is obtained as a visual road map. The advantage of real-time sonography is that the effect of the treatment is demonstrable during motion including stress, compression, medial/lateral deviation, and distraction of the structures. Applying wearable ultrasound transducer web netting with instantaneous feedback is used in robotic artificial limbs as a guidance tool to modify the voltage output to stimulate the dominant firing muscle group to adjust to the spatially changing environment. The 52 bones of the human foot keep changing with gravity, weight bearing, and structural alignment. For example, when toe is amputated for a nail melanoma or a tendon is cut to straighten a crooked toe, the foot biomechanics are altered as is the alignment of the cephalic fascia and regional joint so that knee pain has been reported in patients with corrective anterior or midfoot procedures (Fig. 16.18).

Injection treatment usually uses small bore needles, but image-guided transdermal surgery often uses 18 gauge needles that could damage the smaller nerves and vessels. While hemostasis is readily controlled and accidentally or deliberately severed tendons may heal the nerves are more delicate and harder to regenerate.

A good example of a crowded field of anatomic entities is the tarsal tunnel in the medial ankle and foot supplying motor and sensory fibers to the toes and is a common site for preoperative anesthetic nerve blocks. The widely used Tinel test is poorly specific, and ultrasound resolution is higher than MRI so it is used for confirmation of the electroneurodiagnostic tests in the often confusing symptomatology of tarsal tunnel syndrome of numbness and burning. From anterior to posterior, the five structures are the posterior tibial tendon, the flexor digitorum longus tendon, the posterior tibial artery with adjacent veins, and the tibial nerve, which later divides into three terminal branches [21]. 4D real-time ultrasound quickly maps the course of the distinctive coarse fibrillar echo pattern of the nerve

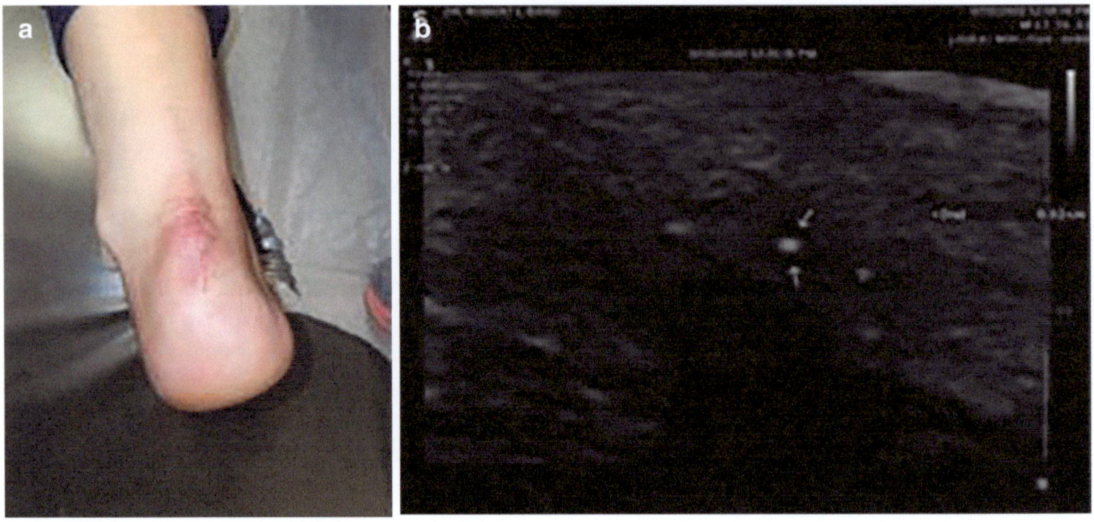

Fig. 16.18 (**a**) FB active postop inflammation following surgery to remove intratendon foreign body. (**b**) 0.5 mm retained foreign body missed at original operation

as contrasted with the adjacent vascular and neighboring tendons (Fig. 16.19).

Common causes of tarsal tunnel syndrome include coalitions and bone spurs, expansile lesions like ganglion cysts, neurogenic and soft tissue tumors, diabetes mellitus neuropathy that increases the nerve volume making it susceptible to compress, gout, xanthoma of hyperlipidemia, and hypothyroidism. Muscle disorders such as exaggerated hypertrophy, accessory flexor digitorum muscle, and the rare accessory muscles like the peroneal calcaneus internus muscle and the tibiocalcaneus internus muscle are to be considered. Overall, tendon disorder and vascular veinous engorgement are the major etiologies for this syndrome. In the examination of the diabetic foot, one must entertain the thought of concomitant inflammation and check carefully for unsuspected nail disease, micro ulcerations, and unrecognized trauma due to loss of nerve sensation. Optical imaging for bacterial colonization invisible to the human eye is sometimes revealed at 405 nm violet light exams. Doppler study for possible arterial and venous conditions is useful. 3D image histogram reconstruction of the diabetically affected nerves for tissue signatures

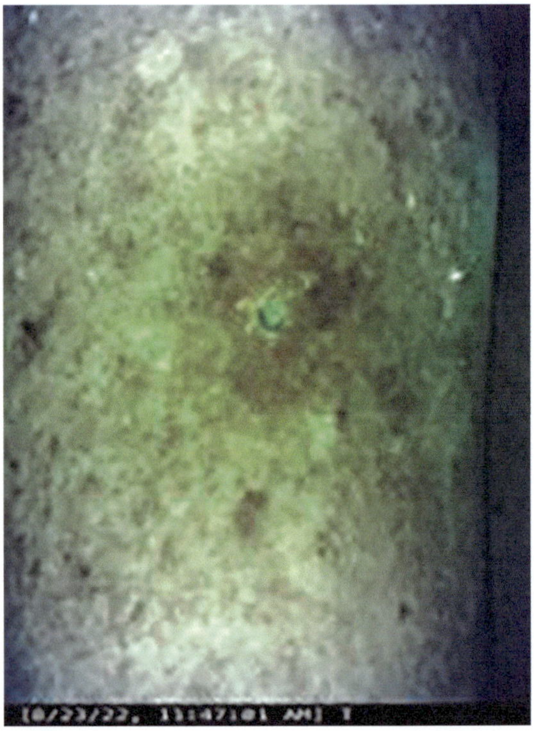

Fig. 16.19 AF diabetic foot ulcer examined at 405 nm violet light reveals eccentric arc of cyan indicating bacterial colonization

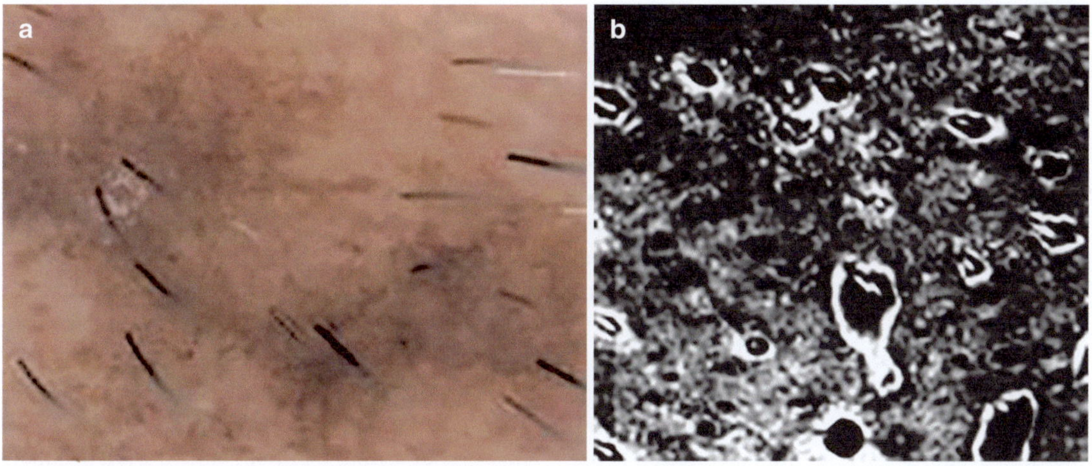

Fig. 16.20 (**a**) Dermoscopic image of pigmented lesion. (Courtesy Dr. Jonathan Ungar). (**b**) Dysplastic nevus imaged by reflectance confocal microscopy showing irregular melanocytes visible in the epidermis. (Courtesy Jonathan Ungar MD)

may become a useful prognosticator of long-term outcomes as we do with breast density and muscle density in multiple sclerosis and amyotrophic lateral sclerosis (Fig. 16.20)

A new tool using MRI-like pulsed electromagnetic waves (PEMF) has been used worldwide and recent German and Israeli advancements now improve blood flow with success in treating diabetic circulatory problems with the feet and delaying amputation for gangrene [22]. Now that 4D imaging accurately depicts sub millimeter nerves and arteries the targeting of focus treatments are more successful. The background for this rejuvenation technology is patient interactive biofeedback control of electromagnetic regenerative waves. Also included in this assortment of new modalities is shock wave therapy commonly used to break up kidney stones and currently useful in treating plantar fasciitis and other musculoskeletal disorders.

16.14 Integrative Energy-Guided Therapies

While surgery, chemo and radiation are the standard treatment for many tumors, patients from other cultures are being diagnosed and treated successfully with alternative minimally invasive or noninvasive options. My investigation into this phenomenon was kindled by my USAF tour of duty in Thailand where suntans were avoided and Buddhism was practiced. American military personnel emulating the local country customs would squat on their knees mingling with the Thai soldiers and soon develop tendinitis because their ligaments were genetically different than this Asian society. The discovery of the efficacy of holistic medicine crystallized while I was studying bone cancer at the Armed Forces Institute of Pathology in Washington DC during the day and attending a Buddhist prayer group nearby. The verbal chanting by the monks is musical but also tonal as is the case with Chinese and many Southeast Asia national languages. Western language is generally monotonal so the subtlety of the speech is not appreciated and often inappropriate when we imitate another dialogue. Practices like acupuncture for pain and light therapies for skin disease are codified in our CPT lexicon. Mind-body medicine is becoming more accessible as we realize that accessing the brain and autonomic nervous system is complementary to western textbook treatments and accepted therapeutic algorithms. An analogy is the piano where a child deliberately plays a tune with one finger while a virtuoso caresses the ivory keys with passion guiding the hands allowing the same musical instrument to make audiences jump up and cheer a great performance. The disciples of the prayer culture in DC included cancer survivors who listened to their bodies internal messaging and thrived on "unacceptable" treatment.

Back to bone cancer and out of the box thinking. US oncologists use radiographs, MRI and PET/CT to adjust treatment of bone sarcomas while the Sarcoma Center in Ulm, Germany uses 4D Doppler histogram analysis of tumor neovascularity to decide if a painful area is a healing fracture or a malignant osteosarcoma. As summertime is shortly arriving this distinction is useful to separate a toddler's healing rib fracture from a deadly Ewing's sarcoma.

16.15 4D Doppler Imaging

3D imaging technologies offer one-step image-guided treatment since the size, depth, margins, and tumor aggression parameters are quantifiably displayed. Real-time 3D Doppler (also called 4D) treatment verification is critical since aggressive cancer types have a high recurrence rate suggesting that earlier imaging missed deep tumor nests or subcutaneous locoregional metastases. 4D systems permit real-time biopsy of the malignant focus while avoiding the areas that are necrotic, fibrotic, immunologically reactive or simply adjacent, inseparable benign disorders (Fig. 16.21)

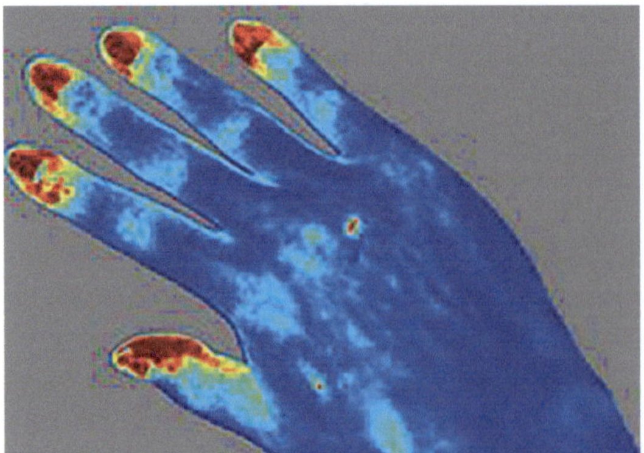

Fig. 16.21 Optoacoustic image laser speckle image of normal extremity with nail capillary flow identified. (Courtesy of RWD Life Sciences)

16.16 Identifying Cancers

Basal cell cancers (BCCs) are the most common malignancy worldwide. BCCs are rarely fatal; however, certain aggressive squamous cell cancer (SCC) types have devastating health consequences via locoregional growth and circulatory dissemination [23]. Metastatic potential of BCC is determined by functional analysis of specific intratumor sonographic findings. Malignant melanoma is the leading cause of death of women in the 25–45 age range and has a 98% diagnostic accuracy using ultrasound 15–22 MHz systems and higher with 24, 30, 48, and 70 MHz frequencies now available. More importantly, there are specific tumor vessel density criteria identifying which melanoma cancer is most aggressive using quantitative Doppler 3D Histogram analysis technologies [24].

16.17 Quantifiable Digital Scanning Versus Biopsy

The optical dermatologic modalities of RCM (reflectance confocal microscopy) and OCT (optical coherence tomography) are highly accurate in ruling out malignant disorders and often flag a biopsy on a visually innocent appearing lesion such as amelanotic melanoma or pigmented basal cell cancer. 4D ultrasound imaging is real-time evaluation of a 3D volume so we know immediately the depth and quickly assess the probability of recurrence. Specific echoes generated by nests of keratin are strong indicators of aggression and analyzed volumetrically. Highly suspect areas are then checked for locoregional spread, and search is performed for draining sentinel node lymphadenopathy so we show our patient that the disease is completely sonographically imaged in real time as the exam proceeds in systematic diagnostic stages. 4D permits image-guided biopsy of the most virulent area of the dermal tumor and allows the pathologist to focus on the most suspicious region of the postoperative lymph node specimen mass excised from the axilla, neck, or groin.

16.18 Digital Imaging Reduces Complications

Fear of complications deters patients from seeking medical advice and possible disfiguring surgical intervention so many opt for noninvasive options. One out of 33,000 moles is malignant meaning high-resolution imaging reduces unnecessary biopsies. Cancer treatment depends on accurate determination of tumor depth and penetration possibly involving facial nerves, periocular muscles, nasal bone, or ear cartilage. Verified superficial tumors may be treated topically or by low-dose non-scarring radiation therapies. Many cancers provoke a benign local immune response or concomitant inflammatory reaction that simulates a larger tumor burden. There is often cicatrix formation accompanying the body's healing response and benign disorders may coexist and appear clinically inseparable from the malignant lesion. Precision 4D imaging highlights the true surgical borders of the cancerous tissue resulting in smaller excisional margins, healthy tissue sparing, and reduced scar formation.

16.19 Margin Delineation

Advances in laser/optical devices allow near microscopic tissue analysis of the cells by rapid, noninvasive testing. Real-time microscopy is performed during surgery to assure that the tumor border is clear in cases of skin cancer and future use in breast and prostate cancer treatment is under clinical study.

Topical treatments are 5-fluorouracil cream and imiquimod for low risk, superficial lesions. Immunotherapies have proven highly effective in the case of malignant melanoma although accompanied by significant side effects such as confusion and cutaneous disorders. Lasers have become popular with very superficial tumors with pretreatment depth determined by high-resolution ultrasound.

Superficial radiation therapy (SRT) for non-melanoma skin cancer has been increasing in use with the aging population and portable units suitable for the office-based setting while in use since the 1900s, it declined in use with the advances in MMS. The precision image-guided radiation technologies are now achieving higher clinical application due to the cosmetic benefit and minimal side effects. While SRT uses low-energy photons with limited penetration the new focused "proton" beams are targeted precisely and limit surrounding tissue damage in spite of very high energy and may be used more frequently more the more aggressive subtypes. Of note, 3D Doppler ultrasound establishes tumor depth and response to therapy and assesses the malignant aggression potential using the specific echo pattern and neovascular findings characteristic of dangerous lesions. It has been used as a template for the image guidance coordinates for radiation therapy planning. High-intensity focused ultrasound (HIFU) and LASER treatments are used sporadically in cases where other options are not feasible and anecdotally have had good results.

16.20 Autonomic Nerve System Autoregulation

Combining western medicine with eastern ideology involves feedback from the autonomic nervous system whereby the real-time reaction to the treatment is monitored both by the patient and the treater. Simple measures using the pulse and breathing changes are common in many techniques and the ability to target the areas showing immediate interactions with the therapeutic modality may be focally energized or radiated as needed.

An Overview of Biofield devices: Buddhist Perspective states:

> *Of particular relevance to biofield science, a large and rapidly growing body of data has demonstrated the existence of nonthermal EMF bioeffects, for which the molecular interaction energies are less than the average thermal energy of the target. The existence of these extremely weak EMF effects suggests the possibility of bioinformation flow at extremely low energies and could foreshadow a paradigm shift away from the biochemical paradigm and towards an information-oriented model, wherein weak signaling (via EMF, light, or vibration) plays an essential role in biological regulation.* [25]

16.21 Treatment Verification

The overall recurrence rate analysis by Cognetta of 1715 NMSCs (BCC and SCC) was 1.9% [15]. Another study by Shulte on 1276 NMSCs showed a combined rate of 5.1% [16]. A paper by Zagrodnik using BCC histopathology for superficial, nodular, and sclerosing (morpheaform) cell types revealed a 5-year recurrence rate of 11.8%, 2.8%, and 27.7%, respectively.

More aggressive histopathologic types recurred up to 27% and this in part may be explained by tumor not treated since it was outside the treatment field as in satellite, in transit, or more distant or deeper subcutaneous metastases not detected by the available imaging technology at the time. The vascular measurement parameters in OCT and RCM add another measure of treatment success by verifying absent blood flow in previously nontreated neovascular tumor tissue. Future tumor neovascularity assessment will use the (off-label FDA approved) contrast-enhanced ultrasound (CEUS) for advanced quantification. Another common heel problem is the pressure ulcer or decubitus ulcer for bedridden patients. Initial erythema that signifies stage one disease is difficult to evaluate in dark skin so a sonogram on a painful area could show dermal thickening and hyperemia and initiate timely treatment to prevent disease progression [26]. The use of optical imaging for bacterial contamination would also be applicable to prevent greater ulceration. Another use of optical microscopy in tumors near bony structures is to differentiate skin cancer from bone sarcoma where a case of acral lentiginous melanoma was erroneously diagnosed as a primary soft tissue sarcoma [27].

Optical scanning using laser speckle interferometry is sensitive to capillary vessels and has been used in burn diagnostics for skin viability and evaluation of the energy medicine treatments to evoke a vascular response in the autonomic nervous system.

16.22 Elastography

Density and elastic physical properties of tumors are different than normal tissue and are trackable with treatment changes widely used in breast, brain, pancreas, thyroid, and prostate cancer imaging [9]. Recently applied to tendinopathy and scarring with strain and shear wave modalities, it has been studied extensively with liver fibrosis with 25% of the world population as non-alcoholic fatty liver disease (NAFLD) [28]. Ultrasound attenuation-based fat quantification relies on energy loss as acoustic waves travel through tissue with fat having a high attenuation factor related to the sound frequency applied and results are similar in most hospital grade units and is FDA approved for measuring liver fibrosis. Most important is the placement of the measuring box and the size and number of the sample [29].

16.23 Autofluorescence

Used for cell cytology, new versions allow for detection of bacteria in concentrations greater than 10(4) power assisting wound-healing processes. Portable point of care (POCUS) ultrasound has created a pathway for possible cancer detection without biopsy [30]. Inflammatory skin diseases may be assessed and sequential treatment progress followed by the optical changes where autofluorescence is lower in atopic dermatitis than psoriasis [31]. This technology may be used to avoid biopsy in the same way that confocal microscopy is currently in clinical practice. Biologically active material illuminated at 405 nm will fluoresce with violet light and special filters.

References

1. Blechschmidt E. Die architecture de fersenpolsters. Morphologisches Jahrbuch. 1934;73:20–68.
2. Tietze A. Concerning the architectural structure of the connective tissue in the human sole. Foot Ankle. 1982;2:252–9.
3. Steiness IB. Vibratory perception in diabetes. Acta Med Scand. 1957;158:327–35.
4. Kim W, Voloshin AS. Role of the plantar fascia in the load bearing capacity of the human foot. J Biomech. 1995;28:1025–33.
5. Tantray MD, Rather A, Gull Y, et al. Role of ultrasound in detection of radiolucent foreign bodies in extremities. Strategies Trauma Limb Reconstr. 2018;13(2):81–5.
6. Fakoor M. Prolonged retention of an intramedullary wooden foreign body. Pak J Med Sci. 2006;22:78–9.
7. Freund EI, Weigl K. Foreign body granuloma: a cause of trigger thumb. J Hand Surg Br. 1984;9:210.
8. Choudhari KA, Muthu T, Tan MH. Progressive ulnar neuropathy caused by delayed migration of a foreign body. Br J Neurosurg. 2001;15:263–5.
9. Meurer WJ. Radial artery pseudoaneurysm caused by retained glass from hand laceration. Pediatr Emerg Care. 2009;25:255–7.
10. Flom LL, Ellis GL. Radiologic evaluation of foreign bodies. Emerg Med Clin North Am. 1992;10:163–76.
11. Little CM, Parker MG, Callowich MC, et al. The ultrasonic detection of soft tissue foreign bodies. Invest Radiol. 1986;21:275–7.
12. Harcke TH. Sonographic localization and management of metallic fragments. Mil Med. 2012;177:988–92.
13. Mehta T, Raza S. Power Doppler sonography of breast cancer: does vascularity correlate with node status or lymphatic vascular invasion? Am J Roentgenol. 1999;173(2):303–7.
14. Merce LT, Alcazar J. Clinical usefulness of 3-dimensional sonography and power Doppler angiography for diagnosis of endometrial carcinoma. J Ultrasound Med. 2007;26:1279–87.
15. Bard R, van der Bent S, Kushner R, et al. 4th inflammatory skin disease summit. New York: Academy of Medicine; 2021. p. 48.
16. Lassau N, Spatz A, Avril MF, et al. Value of high frequency ultrasound for preoperative assessment of skin tumor. Radiographics. 1997;17:1559–65.
17. Wortsman X. Sonography of facial cutaneous basal cell carcinoma. J Ultrasound Med. 2013;32:567–72.
18. Lassau N, Chami L, Chebil M, et al. Dynamic contrast enhanced ultrasonography and anti-angiogenic treatments. Discov Med. 2011;11:18–24.
19. Nielsen M. Fearless beauties. Portland: Skintelligent; 2020.
20. Bard R, Kushner R, Stoff J, et al. Image guided 3D ultrasound of inflammatory disease including Covid-19 presented 4th international skin disease symposium. New York Academy of Medicine; 2021.
21. Soares O, Duarte M, Brasseur JL. Tarsal tunnel syndrome. J Ultrasound Med. 2022;41:1247–72.
22. Graak V, Chaudhary S, Bal B, et al. Evaluation of the PEMF in the management of diabetic polyneuropathy. Int J Diabetes Dev Ctries. 2009;29(2):56–61.
23. Ewing J. Neoplastic diseases. London: WB Saunders; 1940.
24. Lassau N, Koscielny S, Avril M, Margulis A, Duvillard P, Baere T, Roche A, Leclere J. Prognostic value of angiogenesis evaluated with high frequency and color Doppler sonography for preoperative assessment of melanomas. AJR. 2002;178:1547–51.
25. https://www.ncbi.nlm.nih.gov/pmc/articles/PMC4654784/. Accessed 9 May 2022.
26. Sullivan R. A 5 year study of stage one pressure ulcers in darkly pigmented skin. Wounds. 2014;26(12):351–9.
27. Escandor SE. Acral lentiginous melanoma misdiagnosed as soft tissue sarcoma. In: Presented at 2022 Nidiskin symposium, New York.
28. Barr RG. Algorithm for attenuation coefficient of liver fat quantification. J Ultrasound Med. 2022;41:1939–48.
29. Ferraioli GKV. Ultrasound attenuation for liver fat quantification. Radiology. 2021;302:495–506.
30. Choi JH. Autofluorescence analysis of dermatitis and squamous cell carcinoma. Clin Exp Dermatol. 2015;40(2):123–8.
31. Kim JH. Comparative study of skin autofluorescence in atopic dermatitis and psoriasis. Skin Res Technol. 2017;23:1

17 Holistic Integrative Dentistry: Looking Good Versus Functioning Well

Robert L. Bard and Randall L. Weisel

Abstract

Oral health affects the microbiome altering the immune system response to pathogens. Optical evaluation with ultraviolet and violet light systems of oral bacteria is useful in disease detection and optimal prevention with targeted treatment. This chapter focuses on the importance of facilitating oral and dental hygiene as part of typical medical evaluation, as a means of increasing the self-esteem aspect in patients and also as a usage of prevention regarding wide spread bacterial or viral infections.

Keywords

Esthetics · Spectral imaging · Inflammation · Oral health · Microbiome · Ultrasound

Randall L. Weisel has died before the publication of this book.

R. L. Bard (✉)
The Angio Foundation and Bard Diagnostics, New York, NY, USA
e-mail: rbard@cancerscan.com

R. L. Weisel (Deceased)
Clearwater, FL, USA

17.1 Introduction

Our external appearance, the esthetics of our bodies are intimately associated with the health of our physiological parameters of our cardiovascular system, internal tissues, and organ systems. Inflammation plays a primary role in these aging and genetic expressions of disease. Billions of dollars are spent each year on cosmetic procedures to slow the cellular breakdown of external aging or camouflage its effects. Research has proven inflammation and infection have a causal relationship to aging, disease, and our ultimate demise. Healthcare disciplines, such as dermatology, plastic surgery, ophthalmology, dentistry, and others, developed treatment modalities to slow or reverse the external signs of aging. Much of the science within these disciplines are directed to influence inflammation and infection. Many of the clinical signs of external aging and the treatment to slow or reverse these aging processes have been determined by clinical signs and symptoms. Medicine has developed blood tests that objectify the physiologic expression of systemic inflammation. Although most diag-

R. L. Bard (ed.), *Image-Guided Aesthetic Treatments*, https://doi.org/10.1007/978-3-031-36266-8_17

nosis and treatment are done from clinical evaluations and subjective information, such as medical histories, it is apparent, as we accept validation and importance of the information that we can get from blood chemistry and genetic analysis, the overall field of esthetics will evolve to a more informatics guided area within health care.

17.2 General Esthetic Principles

Dentistry has long been conceptualized to be tooth focused. Within the field of health, dentistry is viewed by many to be primarily esthetic procedures and are optional luxuries. For most individuals, tooth removal without consideration of acceptable replacement strategies is a "first-order" treatment choice when dental disease, caries, and periodontal disease exist. Paradigm shifts indicate that dentistry is a vital component of overall systemic growth and development. Teeth and the oral component interact for functions such as mastication, digestion, proprioception of masticatory muscle function, speech, swallowing, respiration, maintaining structural integrity of the stomatognathic system, and self-image. Specifically, in dentistry, dental esthetics has been identified primarily with self-esteem, the psychophysiological component of self-worthiness. Through research, dental esthetics (straight teeth, white teeth, and a nice smile) has been proven to have a profound effect on self-esteem. It has been said, "a good face is a letter of recommendation." One's self-esteem may be affected by the perception of how nice their teeth look. Self-confidence has been demonstrated to be affected by a person's perception of how nice their smile is. Some believe that good dental esthetics is essential for getting the better job. On the other extreme, depression may be linked to low self-esteem. Dentistry is defined by the American Dental Association as the evaluation, diagnosis, prevention and/or of diseases, disorders, and conditions of the oral cavity, maxillofacial area and/or the adjacent and associated structures and their impact on the human body (1997 House of delegates).

17.3 Advanced Dental Esthetics

Within the last century, a heightened awareness has developed within the medical and dental communities that teeth, gums, and the oral environment play important roles as part of the overall systemic health. The concept of oral systemic health has slowly gained acceptance with evidence-based research. Many medical and dental professionals are directing their focus on research to better understand the mouth body interrelationships. Research is clearly exposing that the functionality of structures of the head and neck is intimately connected to the body. The oral systemic links have important roles to the overall physiologic aspects of health and wellness. Recent research has been published pertaining to structural malformations and microbial pathogens within the oral cavity and their impact on overall health. These findings and pathogens may have "probable unfavorable effects" and may have plausible causality for overall systemic diseases. A significant amount of research has been done in both medicine and dentistry to prove that a relationship exists between these disciplines of healthcare. Although it is evident more research must be done to conclusively validate that there is a probable causal relationship and that these two areas are not mutually exclusive, the complete acceptance of these ideas has been slow. The reason for the separation between dentistry (tooth focused) and medicine (systemic disease focused) is unclear. The debate on reasons can be long, in depth and, at best, speculative. It maybe that within both disciplines of health care and lay persons understanding that there is not universal acceptance of the physiologic role of teeth and structures composing the stomatognathic system. Research, discussion of the information gathered, agreement by the experts, and presentation of their findings will be important for a better understanding and acceptance that the health of the oral environment is important for overall esthetics.

17.4 Biometric Dentistry

Dentistry must encompass esthetics. Esthetics is an essential consideration of life. Albeit it may be the key reason for the separation of medicine and dentistry. Physiologic maladaptation is arguably a more important issue than looks. An unwritten false conception is, "if it looks good, it is physiologically functioning well." There is no better example than dental esthetics and the interaction with human systemic function. Just because your teeth look good does not always indicate efficient and healthy function. Addressing dental looks, without the supporting structures being considered, may influence success of the dental procedures delivered and the patient's overall health. The oral systemic interaction is very complex. Our knowledge and understanding of teeth, oral ecosystems, oral pathophysiologic manifestations, and the overall systemic diseases are becoming clearer. It appears as our technological advancements evolve from the laboratory to the clinical settings, we are realizing the importance of oral systemic interdependence. The statement "*complexity is the mother of simplicity*" is demonstrated by a crossword puzzle. Most crossword puzzles are made up of many separate pieces. If you look at the many pieces laying on a table, it can look very complex. When the puzzle is completely put together, it usually has an attractive picture. What was once complex turns out, with mental cognitive energy expenditure and a little physical effort, to be a picture of simplistic beauty. This type of metaphor can be used to describe the evolution of discovery and understanding within both medicine and dentistry. The compartmentalization of both disciplines is a necessity. Our present state of affairs in healthcare diagnosis and recommendation of treatment is solidly founded on this approach. Symptoms of aging, diseases, and our end-of-life processes are approached as pieces of a complex puzzle (organ systems) and with the picture being the overall health and wellness (of the body).

There has been a lack of appreciation of the probable simplicity of the fundamental molecular biologic principles of oral-systemic interaction. We have available advanced informatics, genomics, proteomics, and technology for early detection and treatment of disease and aging. Our compartmental focused healthcare approach, within medicine and dentistry, has blinded us to the realization (simplicity) that understanding the fundamental interactions of the pieces (organ systems) has the potential to afford us with a more healthy and longer existence. There is no argument that our technological advancements have had an impact on our quality of life and longevity. Research that has allowed many technological advancements is very expensive. As in any field, healthcare has become a big business. Big Pharma, third-party payor involvement, big private healthcare alliances, and big government have become the way many of our health and wellness initiatives are funded. Privatization for capitalization for these advances in health care has created great wealth. What has been our main source of funding for these technological advancements may just be the reason that acceptance of plausibility to acceptance of causality of diseases of oral systemic interactions has been slow to come to fruition. If we can detect diseases early and/or are able to reverse disease processes, healthcare dollars could be saved. That means many areas of entrepreneurial businesses that capitalize on diagnosis and treatment without addressing "why" diseases occur may theoretically lose money. Many financial activists within health care resist change. Their mantra is "it is not broken don't fix it." There is no debate that healthcare concerns are major social and political issues. Strong evidence of reason and logic support unlocking the oral systemic connections. This may be important to addressing the key for slowing, if not reversing aging, disease, and death.

17.5 Paradigm Shifts Revisited

The idea that diseases of the oral microbiome effects on diseases of the body is not new. In the early 1900s, the Focal Infection Theory was introduced. Many believed that diseases within the oral cavity had direct implications on systemic diseases. Due to lack of supportive research evidence, the theory died out within 30 years. The oral cavity ecosystem has become one of the most well studied parts of the body. The complex microbial inhabitants of the mouth led to the development of periodontal dental medicine or periodontology. Periodontology, a specialty within dentistry, studies the teeth, gums, and bone within the oral cavity. This specialty of dentistry focuses on the diagnosis and treatment of diseases of these structures. Microbes, mainly bacteria and viruses, have been intensely studied pertaining to their impact on this microbiome. Inflammation, a systemic host response to entities that is perceived to be potentially harmful, has been the primary interest of much research within this specialty. Compartmentalization embraced this field of dentistry. In the mid-1980s, the earlier paradigms of oral systemic pathogenic interrelationships began to regain favor. With the advent of technological diagnostic advancements, the plausibility of causality from oral pathogens and the host responses has become objectively evidenced. At this present time, the medical community has fully embraced that pathogenic bacteria, and host immune responses may cause adverse treatment outcomes. Especially, in the specialties of cardiology, obstetrics, orthopedics, and oncology, the direct causal implications within the body to unhealthy oral conditions are being studied fervently and universally are gaining acceptance.

17.6 The Oral Microbiome

The oral cavity is home to over 700 species of microbes. This ecosystem includes bacteria, virus, fungus, and parasites. It is the second largest environment of microbes in the body. The gut microbiome is the largest microbial colonization. Microorganisms play various and important roles for metabolic functions of the host. Most live in commensal and symbiotic relationships. Their existence assists in digestion, immune function, and waste disposal for the host. In a healthy individual, there exists a homeostasis of these various functions. For these microbes to thrive within the host, they require different nutrients and conditions to live in. Some microbes require oxygen (aerobic) others require no oxygen (anaerobic), and facultative microbes can live in either environment. Like the host, these microbes' food source is glucose. Within the gut microbiome, these microbiotas are mainly anaerobic in nature. Their functional processes are very important in digestion and metabolic function of the host. When a disequilibrium exists within the host and the gut, the microbial inhabitants can escape (leaky gut syndrome) and travel via the blood throughout the body. They usually take nutrients that are needed by the host. When this occurs, they become pathogens and can be harmful.

A similar inhabitants lives within the oral cavity. Anaerobic, aerobic, and facultative microbes coexist within this ecosystem. They cohabitate various hard and soft niches. Microbial habitats that have been researched include the teeth, gums (gingiva and periodontal pockets), the tongue, the tonsils, the oropharynx, and nasopharynx. Genetic testing has been very beneficial for genetic mapping of the oral ecosystem. Since the completion of the human genome project in 2003, our ability to 3 dimensionally visualize the microflora topography has opened understanding of their complex relationships of symbiosis. Also, we have been able to develop theories of pathogenesis. Ease of access for genomic examination has made the various niches of the oral cavity one of the most researched microbiomes of the body. Accepted concepts of pathogenesis within the oral cavity are focused on the teeth and the periodontal pockets. Advances in genetic vetting of pathogens that cause tooth decay and periodontal disease have solidified our understanding how these diseases occur.

17.7 Anatomy

Tooth decay, periodontal disease, and oral cancer rank among the top diseases in the world according to the World Health Organization. Gum disease is high on the list of noncommunicable diseases. Both diseases are caused by pathogenic microflora. Gum disease has a combination of microbial causality and the effects of host response (i.e., inflammation). Oral and oropharyngeal cancer, the 15th most prevalent cancers in the world, has been proven to be caused mainly by the variants of the human Papillomavirus (HPV). A brief overview of tooth decay or cavities in layman's terms reveal two main pathogenic bacteria to be the cause of the destruction of teeth. These anaerobic bacteria are *Streptococcus mutans* and *Lactobacillus*. For us to understand the pathogenesis of tooth decay, we must know about the composition of a tooth.

Teeth are the hardest organs in the body. They are one of the most unique examples of bioengineering within the body. They are functionally involved in multifactorial processes. These processes include mastication, digestion, proprioception of the masticatory muscles, speech, swallowing, respiration, structurally maintaining the integrity of the stomatognathic system, and self-image. Teeth are composed of enamel which is the hardest structure of a tooth and the body. It has an amorphous composition encompassing the coronal portion of a tooth. Dentin lies directly beneath enamel, composing most of a tooth and is the second hardest matter of the body. Dentin is porous. It has a complex lattice structure of interwoven channels called odonto-tubules. Bone is the third hardest structure. Enamel, dentin, and bone are primarily composed of hydroxyapatite. Their composition differs mainly in the amount of water that is present in their structure. The root portion of teeth is covered by a substance called cementum. Teeth are intimately connected to the bone of the jaws with ligaments. These ligaments are called periodontal ligaments (PDL). Periodontal ligaments are attached to the roots of the teeth, primarily in the cementum. Within the area of PDL–cementum connection of the body to teeth are many blood vessels and nerves. The periodontal ligament serves as a suspension structure not unlike shock absorbers. Interposed in this area of suspension are nerve endings called mechanoreceptors. Mechanoreceptors function as a "sensor system" for the central nervous system. There are many other types of nerves that are present that serve various roles. Although the mechanoreceptors are the most important nerve endings surrounding teeth, they relay neural messages that allow the central nervous system to monitor the proprioception of the components of the stomatognathic system.

The innermost portion of the tooth is the pulp. The pulp is in the center of the teeth. It is composed of blood vessels, nerves, and dentin producing cells called odontoblasts. The odontoblasts are specialized cells that transverse through the odonto-tubules. These cells function to propagate the neurovascular biological roles within the dentition to facilitate oral-systemic interactions. The pulp is connected to the cardiovascular system and is the main nutrient source for approximately 2/3 of a tooth. The other portion of nutrient supply is within the vascular supply of the PDL. Having a clear picture of the blueprint of teeth and their connection to the body is imperative to understanding oral systemic interaction. Figure 17.1 is a diagram of the healthy anatomical structure of a tooth and alveolar bone.

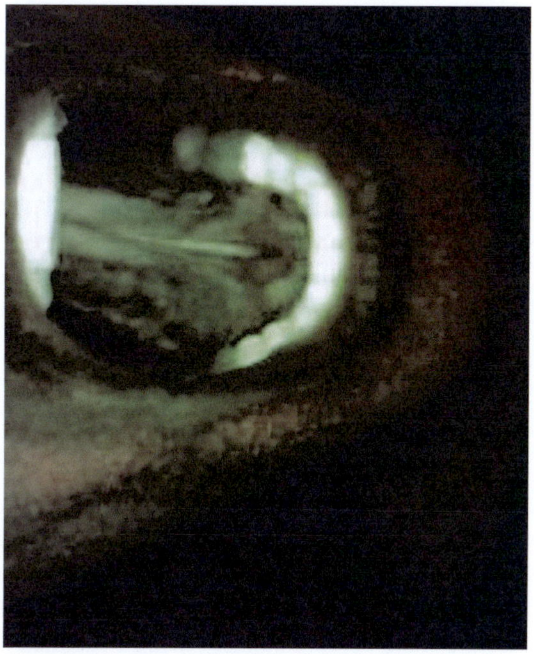

Fig. 17.1 AF examination of the oral cavity with normal tissue green

17.8 Overview of Diseases of Teeth and Gums

When we discuss diseases of the oral cavity, dental decay and periodontal disease are our primary focus. There are many expressions of disease and disorder within the oral cavity. These are evidence of mainly systemic pathogenicity of the host's cardiovascular system. Disease processes such as herpetic ulcers, dry mouth syndrome, enlargements of tissue, and ulcers related to oral cancer are evidenced within the oral cavity.

Dental decay is an acid degradation of tooth structure. This acid is produced by anaerobic microflora that attaches to the hard surface of teeth. The main bacteria involved in this disease are *Streptococcus mutans* and *Lactobacillus*. These bacteria will initially metabolize the food particles that are left within the oral cavity after eating. They utilize the food particles with a complex metabolic process that ends up in lactic acid production. This lactic acid production can cause the hard structures of the tooth to disintegrate. This is called dental caries or a cavity. When these bacteria get into the dentin, they can metabolize the nutrients within the odontoblasts. The main way dentistry attacks these bacteria that have started to demineralized teeth is by attempting to remove these pathogenic bacteria.

In dentistry, the most popular tools to remove this disease are usually pneumatic or electric drills and hand instruments. Lasers have been used to remove these microbes also. Dental professionals restore the defect of the hard structure with a filling that is a resin (glass) or a silver amalgam material. When tooth decay is quite extensive, dentists will use a porcelain or metal crown. The type of restoration used is determined by the amount of destruction of the teeth by the bacterial activity and repetitive mechanical trauma. When there is tooth loss due to the destruction of teeth and supporting periodontal structures, the masticatory system is restored with removable prosthetics and implants. Removable prosthodontics, partials and complete dentures are commonplace within dentistry. Implantology has become a routine way to replace missing teeth. Although these two disciplines within dentistry have improved greatly, there is no argument that natural dentition is the best choice. Early detection and intervention of dental disease have afforded our patients the ability to ward off the oral systemic ramifications of overall health.

Periodontal disease is a pathogenic process of the tissues of the gums and the underlying bone. The causal factors are many anaerobic and facultative microbial pathogens. The host's own immune system plays a role in the process. By virtue of the host trying to protect itself with inflammation, the chemicals within the immune protective cells, manufactured as part of the protective process, will cause harm to the host tissues. In simple terms, periodontal disease is due to infection and inflammation. It is beyond the scope of this chapter to become in depth in these processes, although we will address some of the bacteria that are present in and responsible for periodontal disease. Some of the major destructive microflora are *Porphyromonus gingivalis* (Pg), *Aggregatibacter actinmycetemcomitans* (Aa), *Fusobacterium nucleatum* (Fn), the red complex, and many others. These microbes have the innate enzymatic ability to easily enter the host through mucosal tissues. Research has demonstrated that these microbes can produce and release enzymes that allow entry in the cardiovascular system. The hemidesmosomes that hold epithelial cells together are affected to allow virtually undetected systemic entry. The pathogens use nutrients within the blood and tissues for their metabolism and reproductive processes. The main nutrients that are taken from the host are glucose, iron, and hemoglobin. Consistent efficiency of oxygen transportation and carbon dioxide removal with the body is adversely affected. These metabolic by-products are measurable with analysis of blood chemistry and other advanced medical technologies.

There are numerous hormonal chemicals (proteins) that are released during active periodontal disease. These neuro proteins are called cytokines. A few that are elevated by active periodontal disease are interleukin 1, interleukin 6, tissue necrosis factor, etc. As previously mentioned, these cytokines and the white blood cell responses to assist the host in protecting itself can ultimately cause destruction of the surrounding tissues. These protective mechanisms may be directly or indirectly related to systemic pathogenic disease processes. Research of the oral systemic link has revealed associations to cardiovascular disease (heart attacks and strokes, atherosclerosis, sleep-related breathing disorders (SRBD), diurnal-related breathing disorder (oxygen desaturation syndrome), high blood pressure, atrial fibrillation (A fib), diabetes, adverse pregnancy events and outcomes, respiratory disease, chronic kidney disease, rheumatoid arthritis, cognitive impairment diseases such as dementia and Alzheimer's, obesity, metabolic syndrome, erectile dysfunction, and numerous cancers.

Oral cancer and oropharyngeal cancer is the 15th most prevalent cancer in the world. Human Papillomavirus or HPV is one of the leading causes of these deadly diseases. This virus is a sexually transmitted pathogen. Research has demonstrated that variations of HPV are causally related to oral cancer. The morbidity and mortality related to oral cancer have stimulated medical and dental research to find ways to combat and prevent oral cancer. Pharmaceutical companies have developed vaccines for HPV. A concerted effort to educate the public about oral cancer and preventive pharmacologic treatments have been initiated. In early 2020, marketing media strategies, i.e., TV commercials, and social media campaigns have been very prevalent.

17.9 Oral Systemic Health and the Wellness Connection

Dentistry has been the gateway of novel technological advancements to recognize pathologic conditions that cause diseases and accelerated aging processes. These technologies can be described as "solutions waiting for problems." Healthcare practitioners can utilize the benefits of light technology to induce autofluorescence of pathology. Ultrasound imaging may be used to image pathology within the carotid arteries and thyroid. Genomic testing for human and microbial DNA variants that indicate pathological conditions ia readily available to assist in wellness and health initiatives. Digital radiology and cone beam computed tomography radiology or CBCT of the teeth and gums has become an important part of our screening, diagnostic, and treatment tools.

The understanding of autofluorescence and the potential importance within health care has been recognized for over a century. Approximately 30 years ago, autofluorescence began to be used in the dental field. With the understanding of the light and tissue interaction on a cellular level, technology that utilizes this natural phenomenon was recognized by the FDA (marketing purpose only) for vetting of oral cancer. Several companies have formed to introduce this technology to the marketplace. Early adopters quickly used autofluorescence within their clinical settings. Like other products in various markets that are initially introduced, autofluorescence appeared to be too sensitive. Many dentists sent their patients to the appropriate referral personnel with the suspicion of a deadly disease, oral cancer. Frustration quickly arose from what was called false positives. What appeared to be a great technological advancement that would champion "early detection" of a deadly disease, lost favor within the dental healthcare setting. As with many discoveries in science and commerce, collateral uses of autofluorescence within dentistry were not recognized.

17.10 Autofluorescence

Recently, a review research study has been released demonstrating that autofluorescence technology used within the oral mucosa can objectively demonstrate inflammation, dysplasia, oral cancer, and microbial infection. Numerous other research papers have been published that substantiates the power and importance of autofluorescence to noninvasively recognize these pathologic conditions. Though more research must be done to continue to validate exactly what the visual presentations excited with

AF technology mean. At this point, it is accepted that inflammation and infection can be visualized. This technology is being used within medicine to delineate anaerobic pathogen colonization within nonhealing diabetic wounds. It is also being used to visualize microbes present within dental plaque on teeth and dental caries destroying the dentition. To fully appreciate the importance of this point of care technology, we must understand what we are seeing. By knowing what we are seeing and realizing "why" it should be used, it can be conceived that autofluorescence may be the next big advancement in health care. Until more in depth clinical research studies have been completed and results published, autofluorescence can only be used as a screening technology.

There is no question that the science is valid. Autofluorescence within specified ranges of electromagnetic light spectrums will demonstrate pathology visually. Within the oral cavity, microbial pathogens that have robbed the host of vital nutrients can be objectified. Using AF in the 400 to 460 nm range, we can demonstrate inflammation by complete absorption of this electromagnetic spectrum. Within the same LED spectrum, microflora that has ingested iron from the host's blood will fluoresce an orange-red color. Science principles prove what can be observed. AF reveals mitochondrial activity within the tissues of the host that indicate pathogenic expressions of inflammation, dysplasia, or oral cancer. The importance of the ability to visualize pathology within our patients is monumental. AF used for point of care, noninvasively detect pathologic processes that can lead to catastrophic events, will undeniably make positive impacts on health care.

17.11 Systems

There are several manufacturers that produce LED light in these 400 to 460 nm spectra. Velscope VX, oral ID and reveal from designs for visions are three such technologies within dentistry. Moleculight is a device marketed to the medical community that uses this technology for examination of nonhealing diabetic wounds. Using light to enhance absorption and fluorescence requires filters of ambient light. Expression of the pathologic conditions with LED spectral enhancement require the screening to be done in a dark environment. The closer the light source is to the mucosal tissue, the better the visual representation (Fig. 17.1), an expression of inflammation (Fig. 17.2), and autofluorescence of pathogenic microbial bio load. Figures 17.3, 17.4 and 17.5.

Using this technology within the oral environment will delineate different states of health. If one sees a green presentation, then the oral environment and most likely their systemic environment are within healthy conditions. If orange-red or black presentations are observed the healthcare professional should consider the existence of conditions that support an unhealthy systemic environment. It has been proven the brighter the orange-red expression for microbial colonization, the heavier the bio load and mitochondrial metabolic activity. The same direct

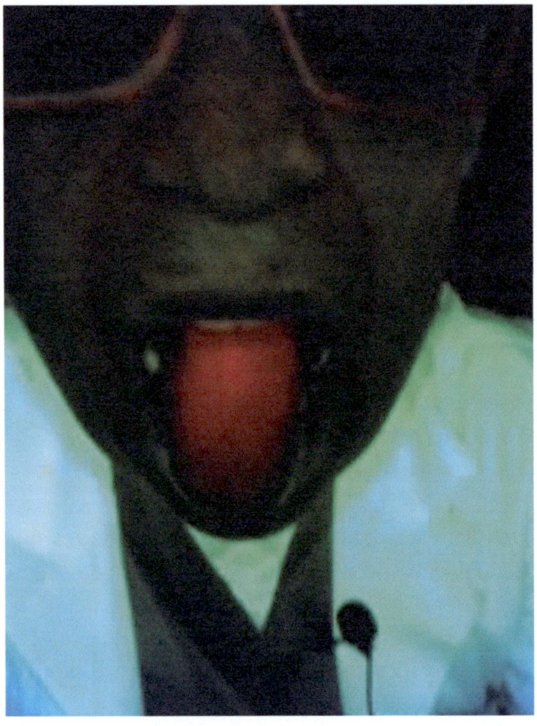

Fig. 17.2 AF examination revealing diffuse bacterial inflammation as orange/red region due to porphyrin fluorescence

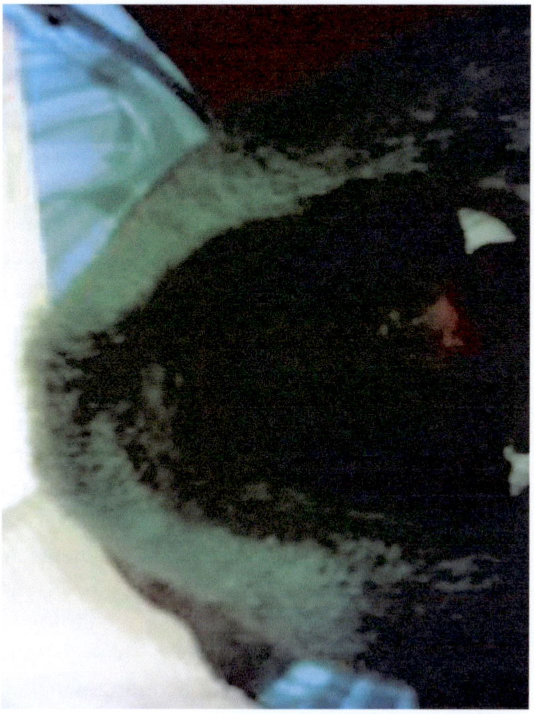

Fig. 17.3 Focal bacterial colonization

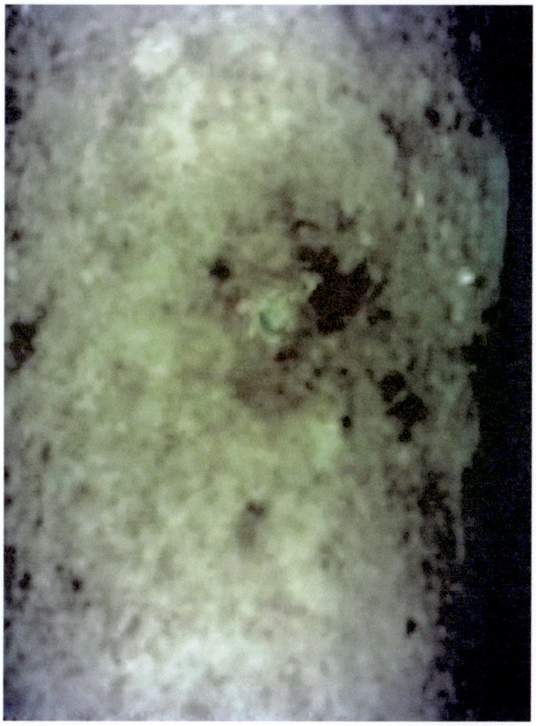

Fig. 17.4 AF exam showing cyan color of inflammation due to mixed fungal/bacteria colonies

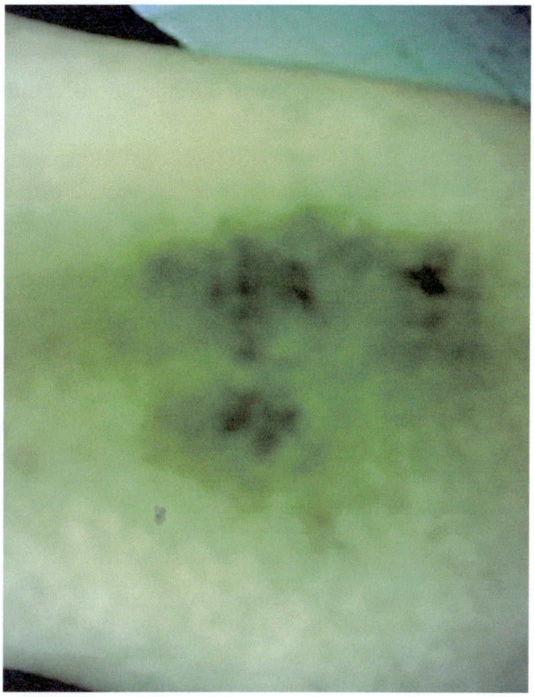

Fig. 17.5 AF shows intradermal hemorrhage as iron molecules reflect 804 nm light

relationship of mitochondrial metabolic inflammatory activity can be inferred for AF visualization of inflammation to oral cancer processes. The darker the appearance of black from the tissue, the more active the inflammation, dysplasia, or cancer. It is known what the expressions of black and orange-red are. It is well accepted that the brighter the orange-red, the heavier the bio load. Also, it can be inferred that the darker the black expression, the higher the mitochondrial cellular activity is occurring. More research must be done to thoroughly substantiate this scientific hypothesis.

17.12 Ultrasound-Guided Optical Imaging

Point of care ultrasonography (POCUS) is defined as the acquisition, interpretation, and immediate clinical integration of ultrasonographic imaging performed by a treating clinician other than a radiologist or a cardiologist.

These clinicians may be medical practitioners or dental physicians. Point of care ultrasonography devices (POCUS) are small, durable, mobile, and have reasonable price points. Studies have demonstrated that non-radiologists and non-cardiologist can become competent in the utilization and performance of pocus. POCUS technology can be utilized for screening and diagnostic imaging. This usually depends on the healthcare practitioner that implements POCUS. As part of the overall health care team, a physician of the head neck (a dentist) can effectively offer ultrasonography as part of the procedures he offers to help his patients. In the hands of a dentist, POCUS is used for screening purposes.

Ultrasound use within dentistry is a novel concept. Less than 1% of the dentists in the world utilize ultrasonography within their clinical settings. The literature supports use of ultrasonography for procedures such as guided biopsies, determination of infections in the fascial planes, and repercussions of internal bleeds from macro and microtrauma. Newer areas of investigation are screening for pathology, such as carotid intima media thickness (CIMT) swelling of lymph nodes of the head neck and thyroid disease and disorders. As a physician of the head neck the American Dental Association, aligning with the definition of the ADA, mandates that a dentist should utilize any technology that he or she understands and is clinically trained to gather information about potential pathologies of the oral systemic condition. Appropriate referral to the discipline of health care is warranted if pathology is suspected.

Figure 17.3 demonstrates the anatomical relationship of the vasculature within the neck (carotid arteries) and the thyroid organ. Trained ultrasonographers can utilize pocus technology to obtain noninvasive images of the carotid arteries and thyroid organ. Empirical research of over 10,000 subjects has demonstrated that pathogenic conditions may exist within the thyroid with patients who suffer diurnal-related breathing disorders (DRBD) and sleep-related breathing disorders (SRBD). A thorough clinical exam of the neck region is warranted on every patient. If hypertrophic conditions exist within the region of the thyroid, recommendations for screening or diagnostic ultrasound are warranted.

Cardiovascular disease is the number one cause of death for men and women in the world. Although there are differing points of view on the cause of heart attack stroke and vascular disease, it is universally accepted that lipo protein buildup within the muscle layer of arteries indicates arterial and cardiovascular disease. Point of care ultrasound is a powerful tool to recognize these pathological conditions. Using the carotid artery as a representation of all arteries in the body and due to ease of access, POCUS examination of the carotid arteries is a very helpful screening for early signs of heart and vascular disease.

As with any technological advancements in health care, ultrasonography has been no different. POCUS is one of those technologies that are "a solution waiting for a problem." Point of care ultrasonography is becoming smaller, easily portable, able to supply more descript noninvasive imaging and affordable. The understanding and need for better images of structures within the body has given this technology more credibility. Disciplines within medicine such as obstetrics and gynecology, cardiology, gastroenterology, orthopedics, and physical medicine have embraced ultrasonography. Many important healthcare decisions are made daily by noninvasive ultrasonographic imaging technology. POCUS has allowed health care the ability to affordably assist within this process.

Within dentistry the use of point of care ultrasonography can have much benefit for our patients. Dentists see more patients per year than primary care physicians. With technologies such as autofluorescence and pocus, objective screening for inflammation, infection, cancer, CIMT, and thyroid maladies will become more commonplace. Early detection of diseases can lead to early interventions of debilitating and fatal health issues. Dental personnel can use these technologies to screen for potential pathologic conditions. The appropriate referral can be made. The objective health information can be provided. Patient healthcare should benefit from information obtained with this emerging imaging technology.

17.13 Genomics

In 2003, the culmination of one of the greatest universal undertakings in history was revealed to the world. The human genome project was a 13-year project of many leading scientists of the world. It cost billions of dollars. The worldwide initiative took countless number of man hours. The human genome project's main goal was to map the genes and location of this information on chromosomes of humans, plants, and various other living species. It truly was a monumental undertaking. Leading research scientists and scientific authors published their findings. Within human beings they documented and archived over 23,000 genes and their alleles, i.e., where they reside on each chromosome. This established a new frontier in health care.

Genomic medicine and dentistry are rapidly becoming a viable way to develop a better understanding of disease processes. We are now able to gene sequence an individual's entire DNA profile within days, if not hours, of obtaining a blood, saliva, or tissue sample. The same mapping strategies are used for microbes and their genetic makeup. A whole frontier of medicine, pharmacological intervention, has opened with bio genomic research. Monoclonal antibody therapy is an example of this. Bioengineering researchers can clone antibodies from humans by slicing them to rodent DNA. Monoclonal antibody strategies have developed medicine for almost any disease process known to man. Drugs focused on treating cancers, diabetes, cardiovascular disease, migraine headaches, depression, neurological disorders, i.e., Parkinson's disease, and Alzheimer's, gastroenterological disorders, and viruses such as SARS-2 and COVID-19 have risen from monoclonal antibody research. More than half the research being done in 2021 involves this type of genetically guided development.

Within the past 20 years, several companies have marketed genetic analysis of suspected microbial pathogens of oral diseases. Health care has available chairside DNA tests for Human Papilloma Virus strains (HPV) that cause oral cancer, Herpes Simplex (HSV) and microorganisms that are recognized to be responsible for periodontal disease. Perio Path and Oravital are two companies that market these genetic tests. Knowing thy enemy is the reasoning behind genomic testing. If we understand the pathogens that are causing the disease, we can develop treatment protocols to combat these specific microorganisms. In the case of discovering the presence of the HPV virus, we can educate the patient, offer vaccinations to enhance adaptive immunity toward HPV, and if the need presents itself, treat with directed pharmacologic and surgical intervention.

17.14 Covid

Viral genetic research has been instrumental for the development of vaccines directed for the human papilloma virus strains that cause cancer. Gardasil and Gardasil 9 are the commercial names for such vaccines [1]. It has been highly recommended by the CDC for adolescents aged persons to participate in vaccination for HPV. Immunization with these vaccines is recommended to activate the adaptive immune system of individuals to develop antibodies against the human papilloma virus. In 2020, our world, as we know it, changed forever. Due to exposure to a deadly, rapidly mutating aerosol transmitted virus, SARS-2 and COVID-19 viruses and their mutations. These viruses that appear to have originated in China, enter the body the nasopharyngeal and oropharyngeal regions. Their center of influence appears to be the respiratory system. These viruses evoke potentially catastrophic immunologic reactions. Genetic analysis is the way researchers can study SARS-2 COVID-19 viruses. Strategies to determine the presence of these viruses have passed FDA approval. Vaccinations to hopefully protect us against the viruses are now available. Numerous companies have manufactured a multitude of different treatments to fight them have been developed.

Usually, it takes many years to analyze a pathogen and develop strategies to recognize and treat them. This is due to the virulence of this virus and its ability to mutate. Worldwide initiatives have rapidly been implemented to find effective, safe ways to build our body's defenses against SARS-2 and COVID-19 viruses. Vaccines have been fast tracked through long-term efficacy and safety research studies by the FDA to hopefully combat the morbidity and mortality of SARS COVID viruses. These initiatives have not been without major social and political confusion and rebellion. The world has become divided by the rapid deployment of ideas and ideals for addressing this global health crisis. It is apparent that we are making headway by disarming the catastrophic effects of SARS-2 and COVID-19 viruses. Through genetic analysis and understanding of the DNA code and their apparent mutations, we will hopefully be able to make the world a safer place.

17.15 Imaging in Dentistry: Digital X-Rays and CBCT

Wilhelm Roentgen discovered X-rays in 1895. This was a turning point for dentistry. The ability to noninvasively see structures and pathology within the head and neck allowed major advances for medicine and dentistry. It allowed for better and more thorough screening, diagnostics, and treatment planning.

In the late 1980s, digital radiology was developed. Advances within computer technology and software allow healthcare practitioners to utilize solid-state semiconductor sensors to be exposed to radiation and an image visualized on a computer screen. The main advantages of this technology are that less radiation is needed to produce an image, and the image can be manipulated to better view the hard and soft structures.

Computer software that analyzes the digital image has high-pass and low-pass spatial filtering. This feature allows manipulation for enhancement of the image. These computer images can be archived within digital imaging and communications in medicine files or DICOM files. DICOM information is a standardization of digital imaging that is universally recognized. This format has allowed for medical and dental radiology files to be transmitted and recognized by another user such as an insurance company or another healthcare provider.

Digital imaging in dentistry has evolved into two platforms. Small digital image producing sensors that can be used within the oral cavity are now commonplace. Cone beam computed tomography or CBCT has revolutionized health care. The small digital imaging sensors produce two-dimensional images without the use of phosphorus screen films and the chemistry needed to develop the image. Evolution of digital technology led to the development of CBCT to produce three-dimensional images.

Besides the obvious cost-effective advantages of this technology, digital imaging offers many more opportunities to enhance healthcare. Less radiation is needed to produce an image. The images are stored within computer DICOM files. This requires less physical space for archiving the information. The images can be viewed almost immediately. The images can be manipulated for better quality unlike screen-film radiology. By the standardization of the DICOM platform, the images can be transmitted electronically with HIPAA compliance. Most of all, the quality of the images can be enhanced to afford healthcare practitioners more precision clarity of the biological structures. This may allow for better diagnostic abilities for more favorable treatment outcomes.

17.16 Protocol for POCAF and POCUS in Clinical Settings

It is this author's opinion that utilization of point of care autofluorescence (POCAF) and point of care ultrasonography (POCUS) will become standard of care technology within medical and dental guidelines as dentistry is a subset of medicine. Trained medical and dental personnel can utilize AF technology and ultrasonography to screen for systemic diseases. The goal of early detection will allow for early intervention of many systemic diseases. If the information gathered warrants a referral, the patient can be guided to the appropriate medical practitioner.

In a dental office or primary care physician (PCP) setting, a point of care autofluorescence test can be performed within the oral cavity. The examination should consist of vetting the dorsum of the tongue, the ventral and lateral aspects of the tongue. The teeth and mucosa should be examined. AF with POCAF technology can reveal local and systemic inflammation, dysplasia, oral cancer, and microbial infection. AF representation of an orange red color indicates infection. Normal and abnormal visual expressions can be objectively recorded from screening with this technology. An abnormal finding of an orange red color will alert the healthcare practitioner that the patient may have a systemic infection. The patient may have a systemic environment that is conducive to anaerobic microbial infestation and colonization.

Recent research with AF has exposed an ecosystem, the oral environment, that reveals pathogenic microbial inhabitance. Utilizing AF techniques and genetic vetting allows objective visualization of these pathogens. The dorsum of the tongue appears to be the primary area of microbial colonization. The teeth and the periodontal pockets are our secondary areas of colonization. Pathogens, such as *Porphyromonoas gingivalis* (Pg), *Aggregatibacter actinomycetans* (Aa), *Fusobacterium nucleatum* (Fn), *Streptococcus mutans* (Sm), and Lactobacillus are anaerobic or facultative anaerobic bacteria that inhabit these niches. Further research uncovered their metabolic mechanisms that allow them to slip, virtually undetected, through the protective mucosal epithelial cells into the bloodstream. It is hypothesized that systemic conditions within the host exist to allow colonization within the body. These microbes become pathogenic when they metabolize the host's blood by-products.

Glucose, iron, and oxygen are nutrients vital for metabolic energy production within the mitochondria of every cell. These nutrients are bound to hemoglobin within red blood cells. Pathogenic microorganisms use these nutrients for their metabolic needs and to reproduce. Their waste metabolites contain iron "stolen" from the host's tissues and blood. AF technology, in the 400-460 nm range, excites porphyrin bound to iron. An orange or red color presentation will be visualized. It appears that the oral cavity is the entry point for these pathogens. Most likely because the mucosa is an area of least resistance for systemic entry. These microbes have genetically evolved. They produce enzymes that can open hemidesmosomes that hold cells together. Nonstratified epithelium is the easiest tissue for these microorganisms to separate and invade the host's systemic ecosystem.

There are several things that can be inferred from a positive finding for anaerobic microbial activity within the oral cavity. (1) Conditions exist systemically and within the oral cavity that allow anaerobic microbial colonization. (2) These microorganisms are stealing nutrients from the host. They are pathogens. (3) The host's defenses are responding to fight these pathogens. There is a high probability that blood markers will be elevated.

The knowledge of the probable existence of systemic anaerobic conditions. That pathogens are entering the cardiovascular system and challenging the immune system. We may be able to develop an understanding and remediation of probable causal conditions for accelerated aging, diseases and ultimate death of the human organism. If there is a positive finding for inflammation, the patient should have specific blood chemistry work performed. There are several inflammatory blood chemistry tests commercially available. One test, hsCRP, enlightens physicians to the immune system's condition of reactiveness to something the body senses will be harmful. The liver is the organ that produces most of this inflammatory protein. It is an indicator of nondescript systemic inflammation. This health data can be very beneficial. A knowledgeable health care provider will be able to suggest the appropriate interventional strategies for patients with elevated hsCRP values.

17.17 Stroke Prevention and COVID-19

Early detection and prevention of arterial and venous disease is key to minimizing the effects of brain aneurysms, strokes from venous thrombosis or arterial hemorrhage, and obstruction. The association of trauma to PTSD is now followed by advanced Doppler ultrasound and functional MRI. This abnormal physiology may also manifest as arterial dissection, collagen disease, inflammatory arthritis, dermatitis, ocular disorders, GI disturbances, limb pain, and aneurysms of the brain and aorta. Devastating strokes in the COVID-19 era occur in the younger age group and the Latin population is at higher risk.

Interest in arteritis was elevated with the study of Tayakasu's disease in the 1970s with advances in contrast arteriography diagnosed diffuse vascular involvement causing strokes and aneurysms in multiple sites. While this arterial inflammation is more common in Asiatics, in the US blacks are nearly three times more likely to have a stroke at age 45 than whites. The pediatric population seems to be at higher risk for this arteritis as evidenced by their unusual rate of COVID-19 affliction affecting the vasculature and called "MULTIPLE ACUTE INFLAMMATORY SYNDROME." Birth control pills are a cause of disease in younger women, and cancer, alcoholism, and obesity raise the incidence at all ages.

We have learned over the last century that the blockage of coronary arteries to the heart and carotid arteries to the brain is precipitated by inflammation of the inner walls of the vessel called the "intima."

While thickening of the interior wall of vessels gradually occurs over time and aggravated by diet, stress, and hypertension (high blood pressure), the event that is acutely disabling is the abrupt tearing of the plaque debris which blocks the flow and often embolized to the brain. Similarly, abnormal heart rhythms, commonly atrial fibrillation, pools blood in the chamber which clots and sends clotted formation (thrombi) to the head. Similar to COVID-19 affecting multiple organs, individually or simultaneously, the vascular tree is distributed to every organ system in the human body. An article in September NEUROLOGY reported by Medscape documented the incidence of COVID-19 first presentation as large artery occlusion was highest in men under the age of 50 years. The mortality rate for over 50 was higher than the under 50 patients.

17.18 History

My group at Metropolitan Hospital in New York first noticed unusual neurologic symptoms in young and middle-aged patients in the late 1960s. As a division of the NY Medical College system, we were fortunate to have an active interventional radiology department specializing in neuroimaging and arteriography. The observation of distortion and occlusion of arteries supplying the brain, kidneys, GI tract, and lower limbs to various degrees from single to multiple locations was closely linked to the Japanese disorder known as Tayakasu's arteritis at the time and recently renamed "arteritis." A clinical finding of this arterial inflammation in the abdominal aorta was pain in the upper abdomen by the great vessels by palpation. Astute physicians were successfully treating this with common "aspirin."

However, the chronic and diffuse nature of arteritis often weakened the vessel wall producing aneurysmal dilation and rupture. Today, we find sophisticate noninvasive or minimally invasive modalities to be the first line of interrogation of vasculitis.

17.18.1 Covid and Stroke

Large vessel occlusion stroke highest in the 2.4x greater in COVID-19 patients and in Hispanic and minority groups. Am Roentgen Ray Society Podcast 9/18/20 Dr Ben Kipper Study on COVID-19 in NYC pandemic. Larger groups and more diverse population needed to corroborate this study on minorities. A recent study of Covid cases found 45.5% with neurologic symptoms.

17.18.2 Diagnosis

Blood flow abnormalities in the arterial system are best studied by Doppler imaging like the weather Doppler showing tornadoes. Multiple options exist for blood flow analysis including:

17.18.3 Carotid Sonogram

While cerebrovascular disease is often diagnosed ex post facto after a catastrophic episode with MRI and CT, the noninvasive Doppler analysis of the vascularity is generally checked with ultrasound for plaque and obstruction. A useful measure of the risk of coronary and cerebrovascular disorder is the carotid intimal thickness (CIMT). Standard depth of the inner wall thickness is a measure best obtained by high-resolution sonograms since a reading over 0.9 mm indicates increased risk. The newer sonogram units have depth resolution of 0.02 mm making this a preferred noninvasive option.

17.18.4 Carotid Doppler

Flow abnormalities of turbulence and absence are commonly evaluated with this modality. Plaque forms more readily in aberrant flow patterns and high-velocity regions accompanying narrowing.

17.18.5 Eye Sonography

Sonofluoroscopy of the orbital soft tissues and eyes is performed in multiple scan planes with varying transducer configurations and frequencies. Power and color Doppler use angle 0 and PRF at 0.9 at optic nerve head. 3D imaging of optic nerve and carotid, central retinal arteries, and superficial posterior ciliary arteries performed in erect position before and after verbal communication. Retinal arterial flow is measured. Optic nerve head bulging is checked as increased intracranial pressure may be demonstrable.

17.18.6 Transorbital Doppler

R/L ciliary arteries have normal Doppler flows of 10 cm/s which is symmetric.

17.18.7 Contrast-Enhanced Ultrasound

Widely used European nonionic contrast injection allows imaging capillary size vessels and perfusion characteristics.

17.18.8 Transcranial Doppler

This measures the flow in the anterior, middle and posterior cerebral arteries as well as Circle of Willis.

17.18.9 3D/4D Vessel Density Histogram

Multiple image restoration and reconstruction show retinal vessel density of 25% at the optic nerve head and adjacent region with quantitative accuracy.

17.18.10 Endoarterial 3D Doppler

Microcatheters inserted into the arterial or venous system provide measurement of wall thickness and presence of inflammatory vessels inside the intima.

17.18.11 Retinal OCT

Subtraction techniques done with OCT optical coherence tomography may show changes in the caliber of the retinal vessels with verbal ideation.

17.18.12 Soft Tissue OCT

The depth of penetration may be extended to 2–3 mm allowing for analysis of vascular changes in erythematous or erythropoor dermal areas. Thrombosis may be observed.

17.18.13 Reflectance Confocal Microscopy

This microscopic analysis of the cells also quantifies microvascular pathology and is a potential modality for studying vasculitis.

17.18.14 Small Coil MRI

High-resolution systems used for animal study and superficial organs can image the intra-arterial anatomy including dynamic contrast imaging on standard 1.5T and 3T units.

17.18.15 7 Tesla MRI

High-field systems analyze signal abnormalities rapidly with high resolutions.

17.18.16 Hybrid Imaging

Hybrid imaging refers to combining diagnostic modalities to assess disease and monitor therapy.

17.18.17 Treatment Options

CEUS and nanoparticle delivery of dexamethasone may be used to reduce plaque inflammation and stroke occurrence. Intraarterial unstable plaque, most commonly found in the carotid artery, readily ruptures (acutely blocking flow) or dislodges causing distal embolism and arterial occlusion often in the brain, extremities, and GI tract. While the composure of this plaque is mostly fibrin and lipid, it is the ulceration, bleeding, and active inflammation that produces catastrophic outcomes. Neovascularization plays a central role in plaque initiation, progression, and rupture. Quantifying these inflammatory microvessels is a surrogate marker of plaque instability and stroke risk. Histopathologic evidence shows plaque with high vessel density is more likely to rupture.

As we learn more about COVID-19, the virus is being associated with several medical conditions and complications in patients that have been infected. A *recent study* found gum disease can be associated with severe COVID-19 outcomes and other medical conditions. To understand how gum disease is associated to COVID-19, it is important to know what gum disease is and how it can be linked to other complications in the body.

Gum disease is a common type of dental disease that affects the supporting structures of the teeth such as the gum tissue and the bones surrounding the teeth. Gum disease is different than tooth decay in that it causes holes in the bones that support the roots of the teeth. Tooth decay causes holes in cavities. Gum disease is so common that 90% of the population has the disease. It is primarily caused by neglect of not brushing and flossing on a daily basis, and not regularly going to the dentist.

A body responds to a bacterial infection in the gums through inflammation. This process may contribute to the term "cytokine storm" in which proteins are released and may be associated with an over-exuberant inflammatory response that destroys tissues elsewhere in the body. "Those same inflammatory products can enter the bloodstream through infected gum pockets around the teeth," says *David Okano, DDS, MS,* section head of periodontics at the University of Utah *School of Dentistry.* "When inflammatory products from gum disease enter the bloodstream, those products can go to other body organs and potentially cause tissue damage."

A study to be published in the *October 2020* issue of the *Journal of the California Dental Association* (JCDA) suggests that hospitalized coronavirus patients with prior underlying gum disease may be at higher risk for respiratory failure. The study indicates that symptoms of chronic periodontitis, such as bone loss, may lead to more severe COVID-19 complications. "They have higher levels of inflammatory products circulating, and, therefore, have more potential to cause damage in the lungs," Okano says. Damage in the lungs can lead to respiratory failure and require hospitalized COVID-19 patients to be put on a ventilator. While this research is in its early stages, what is known is that periodontal health is connected to your overall systemic health.

There is a growing body of scientific evidence that supports gum disease may be associated with other *health complications*. Years of research has found diabetic patients are more susceptible to gum disease. "We know patients who are diabetic and not well controlled can be more prone to infection," Okano says. The effect of gum disease and diabetes is referred to as "bidirectional," which means there's influence both ways. Gum disease is not only more likely to occur in a patient that has uncontrolled diabetes, but inflammation in gum disease makes it harder to control diabetes. *Diabetes* has also been listed as an *underlying health condition* that might increase risk of severe illness from COVID-19. Other evolving research has associated gum disease to other systemic diseases including:

1. *Cardiovascular disease* (heart attacks and stoke).
   (a) Pulmonary disease.
   (b) *Pregnancy* with preterm delivery of babies with low birth weight babies.
2. *Certain* cancers (kidney and pancreatic).
   (a) Alzheimer's disease.
   (b) Everyone is susceptible to gum disease, but some may be a greater risk. According to several NHANES studies, individuals over the age of 65 have a greater severity of gum disease. Hispanic populations and African Americans may also have higher incidences of periodontitis.

Prevention is the key to gum disease, stresses Okano. It is important to brush and floss your teeth daily. An individual should also see their dentist regularly, at least every 6 months. Those with more severe forms of gum disease should see a periodontist.

Periodontal disease, commonly known as gum disease, can cause bleeding gums, bad breath, and if left untreated lead to tooth loss. Research from the AAP and the Centers for Disease Control and Prevention suggests up to half of US adults age 30 and older have some form of periodontal disease. Periodontal disease has been linked to several other serious conditions in addition to COVID-19, including diabetes, heart disease, and Alzheimer's.

Conducted using the national electronic health records of the State of Qatar between February and July 2020, the study analyzed patient cases with severe COVID-19 complications (death, ICU admissions, or assisted ventilation). The control group comprises COVID-19 patients discharged without major complications. Periodontal conditions in the two groups were analyzed using dental radiographs from the same database.

17.19 Summary

COVID-19 affliction of the arterial and venous systems with clot formation and vessel inflammation affects every organ system in the body. Arteritis of the small vessels involves the lungs, heart, brain, kidneys, and liver predominantly, which increases stroke risk in the absence of other contributing factors. Advanced ultrasound imaging offers early detection alerts and image-guided therapeutics are now available. Anti-inflammatory treatments, such as the MATH+ protocol used to treat COVID-19 pulmonary disease, might be useful in reducing intra-arterial inflammation and preventing plaque rupture.

A positive AF exam for infection is an indication for a POCUS examination of the carotid arteries and thyroid organ. Research shows a strong correlation of oral pathogens and cardiovascular disease. Further studies indicate a correlation of sleep-related breathing disorders (SRBD) and most probable diurnal-related breathing disorders (DRBD) for expressions of thyroid disease and cardiovascular disease. A positive finding for infection within the oral cavity is an indication for a point of care ultrasonogram of the neck. A thorough examination of the carotid arteries bilateral and the thyroid organ should be done. Within a dental setting, this would be a screening examination. Within a primary care physician's office, this would be a diagnostic ultrasound. There may be pushback within third-party payer systems due to the resistance of novel use of technology for discovery of early disease processes. Figures 17.6, 17.7 and 17.8 are images taken in a dental setting of carotid artery disease and thyroid disease. The images were sent to the appropriate medical practitioners. Interventional treatment was initiated due to the information from these images. Until a screening ultrasound examination was performed in a dental setting, these patients did not know they had systemic disease. Early intervention of cardiovascular disease and thyroid disease has resulted in favorable life expectancies.

Esthetics in medicine and dentistry is big business. Billions of dollars are spent within these disciplines of this industry each year. There are a countless number and types of procedures and treatments to slow aging, reverse aging, and keep people looking younger longer. Within medicine, there are many technologies that allow the healthcare practitioner, through sound and light image guidance, to plan and complete esthetic procedures.

Dentistry has evolved with uses of light technologies, such as lasers, digital scanning, and digital radiography, to treatment plan and complete procedures for enhancing a patient's looks and function. Sound producing technology has

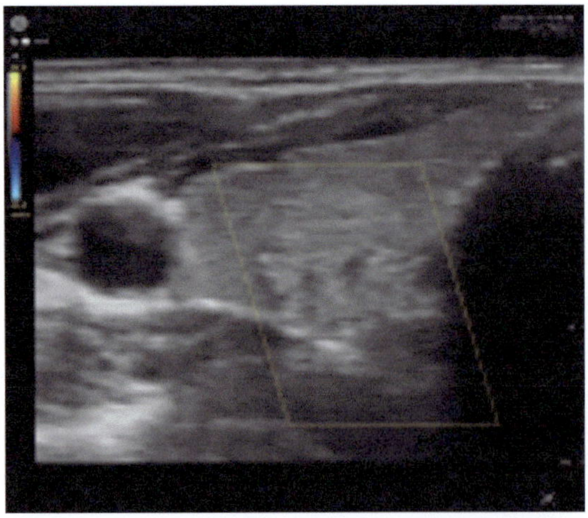

Fig. 17.6 This is an ultrasound image of a normal carotid artery (black) and thyroid gland (gray) in the box

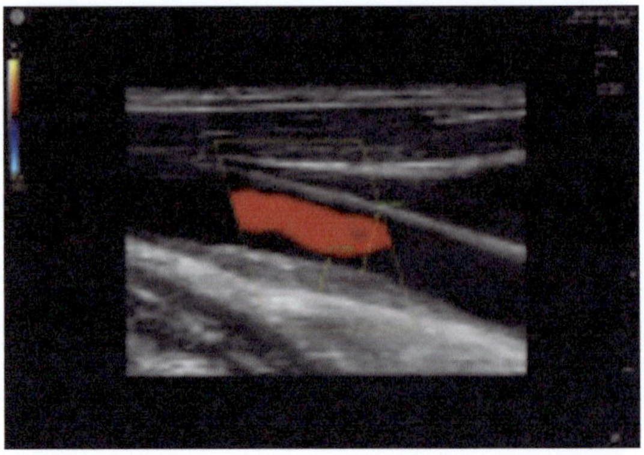

Fig. 17.7 This is a CIMT ultrasound image of cardiovascular disease showing intimal thickening of 13 mm maximal depth indicating increased cardiovascular health risk. The color Doppler flow (red) is noted

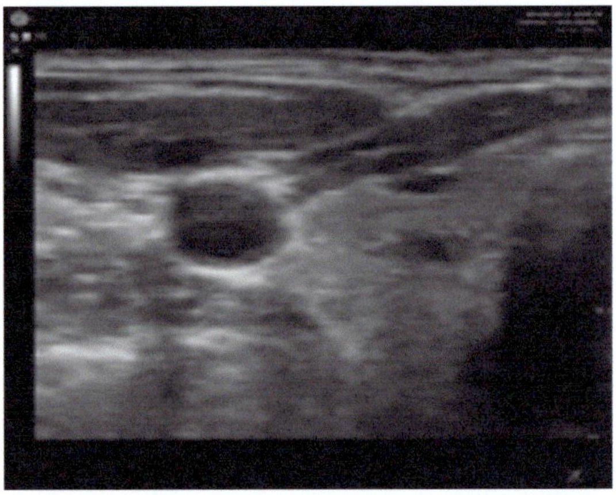

Fig. 17.8 This is an ultrasound image of a thyroid nodule and a midgland lesion that does not have well-defined encapsulation (possible cancer) so follow-up is recommended

been utilized mainly for treatment of periodontal disease, endodontic therapy (root canals), and oral surgery. Novel uses of light and sound technology are establishing themselves within dentistry. Point of care autofluorescence and point of care ultrasonography are two such technologies that may help healthcare practitioners help their patients.

Medicine and dentistry are intimately connected by oral systemic bio physiologic processes. For our patients to look good and remain looking good requires optimum internal health. We must use the knowledge we can obtain with advanced technology. Technologies like autofluorescence devices, ultrasonography, genomics, and digital imaging will give us information about our patient's physiologic health. Artificial Intelligence (AI) can assist in assimilation of the information. Then we can share the findings with all involved in health and wellness.

Above all, the public must be educated. We continue to build on our present understanding of aging, health, and wellness. Biological science continues to develop novel concepts and technology. These advances will allow patients, providers, and insurance providers to make more predictable health-related and esthetic-related decisions on care.

We must decompartmentalize our disciplines within medicine and dentistry and communicate. Advances will occur in esthetics within healthcare. From informatics driven by imaging, DNA analytics, and artificial intelligence, we will obtain vital knowledge. Medicine and dentistry should come together for the benefit of our patients. With open unbiased communication between healthcare providers, researchers, third-party payors and patients, novel promising technologies will be developed and accepted to allow for better treatments and outcomes.

Reference

1. Bard R. Image guided covid-19 management. NewYork, NY: Springer; 2021.

Full-Arch Implant Rehabilitation (FAIR): A Single-Visit Protocol for Restoring Function and Esthetics in Partially and Fully Edentulous Patients

18

Arun K. Garg

Abstract

The introduction of digital imaging and planning tools in dentistry has dramatically changed the traditional workflow and greatly expanded the range of treatment options available for patients with total or near-total edentulism. Although the placement of dental implants is the standard of care for restoring lost dentition, many edentulous patients were not candidates for this treatment in the past because alveolar resorption following tooth loss left them with inadequate bone to support them. Studies have shown that wearing removable dentures can reduce patients' quality of life, causing pain and areas of discomfort, chewing and speaking difficulties, slippage, reduced occlusal force, and poor oral sensation. In contrast to conventional removable dentures, full-arch implant rehabilitation utilizing a digital workflow is a predictable treatment with less morbidity, less laboratory and clinical chair-time, and a substantial increase in patient satisfaction.

Keywords

Edentulous · Dental implant · Arch restoration

18.1 Introduction

According to the Centers for Disease Control and Prevention, the life expectancy of the average American in 2020 was more than 77 years [1]. As a result, a growing number of patients are seeking a solution to the problem of missing teeth that is (1) highly functional, (2) esthetically pleasing, and (3) cost effective. Edentulism negatively impacts overall oral health as well as longevity [2]. Moreover, patients who have complete or partial dentures are often embarrassed because of perceived esthetic shortcomings, and they may suffer from functional discomfort and compromised denture retention accompanied by difficulty speaking and chewing [3]. Although there are denture adhesive applications to combat these esthetic and functional problems, many denture patients consider their use a personal and social burden [4–8].

Fortunately, there is a relatively simple treatment solution for edentulous patients that is far superior to traditional dentures and overdentures and nearly equivalent to natural teeth [9, 10].

A. K. Garg (✉)
University of Miami School of Medicine,
Miami, FL, USA

R. L. Bard (ed.), *Image-Guided Aesthetic Treatments*, https://doi.org/10.1007/978-3-031-36266-8_18

18.1.1 The FAIR Protocol

The full-arch implant rehabilitation (FAIR) protocol provides a step-by-step procedure for restoring the edentulous (and nearly edentulous) maxilla and mandible to nearly natural function and esthetics. Through the application of digital technology, including cone beam computed tomography (CBCT), computer-aided design/computer-aided manufacturing (CAD/CAM), and computer-guided surgery, 4 or 5 implants are spaced throughout the edentulous arch and immediately loaded with a provisional fixed prosthesis. The protocol represents 30 years of clinical evolution, enabling highly skilled clinicians to provide edentulous or near-edentulous patients with the dental appearance and function they increasingly demand. Through this approach, fixed rehabilitation of the total arch is achieved without the complex surgeries, high morbidity rates, high costs, and lengthy perioperative treatments traditionally associated with bone regeneration and grafting procedures.

The FAIR dental prosthesis offers many advantages for the dental patient with a fully or partially edentulous arch (Table 18.1). The prosthesis is immediate, fixed, esthetically pleasing, highly functional, inexpensive, and maintainable. Importantly, the FAIR procedure and similar techniques can frequently be performed without bone grafting, with exceptional success rates [11–24].

Table 18.1 Advantages and disadvantages of removable dentures, overdentures, and the FAIR approach

	Advantages	Disadvantages
Removable dentures	• Relatively inexpensive tooth and gingival replacement • Provide lip support • Easy to remove and clean outside of the mouth	• Uncomfortable • May cause sore spots on gingival tissue • Make it difficult to eat certain foods • Cause accelerated bone loss • Often require relining to improve comfort as bone deteriorates • May make speech difficult • May require creams or adhesives to reduce mobility • Approximately 10% functionality compared with natural teeth
Removable overdenture supported by 2 or 4 implants	• Improves stability and functionality to 60% compared with natural teeth • Relatively inexpensive tooth and gingival replacement • Provides lip support • Easy to clean outside the mouth	• Uncomfortable • May cause sore spots on gingival tissue • Denture must be removed and cleaned outside of the mouth • May still move when chewing or speaking • May require relining to improve fit and comfort as bone deteriorates
FAIR approach	• Improves functionality to 80% compared with natural teeth • Eliminates the need for bone grafting • Can be provided a provisional partial denture on the day of surgery, allowing a soft food diet during healing • Replaces roots and teeth • Preserves bone and soft tissue • No decay; 95% success rate over 30 years • Natural looking esthetics • Allows patients to eat any kinds of foods • Can be cleaned like natural teeth	• Requires healing and restorative time • Involves surgical procedure and anesthesia

18.1.2 The FAIR Difference

The FAIR treatment protocol has two parts: (1) a surgical procedure that concludes with placement of a provisional restoration, accomplished within a single visit; and (2) following a short healing period, delivery of the definitive fixed prosthesis. The provisional prosthesis that is delivered on the day of surgery allows patients to consume soft foods during healing. The definitive prosthesis, which has a 95% success rate over 30 years, gives patients a natural esthetic appearance while imposing virtually no food restrictions.

The ideal candidate for the FAIR protocol has ≤8 teeth per arch, moderate to advanced periodontal disease, financial limitations (e.g., no wish for a crown, partial denture, or graft), and the desire for a same-day fixed provisional restoration (Figs. 18.1 and 18.2). For patients who are good candidates, FAIR prostheses are an excellent functional and esthetic treatment solution that can greatly increase their sense of well-being and self-esteem and enhance their overall quality of life.

18.1.3 Identifying Candidates

FAIR cases fall into four broad categories (Fig. 18.3):

1. The fully edentulous maxilla.
2. The fully edentulous mandible.
3. The partially edentulous maxilla.
4. The partially edentulous mandible.

Each of these categories requires consideration of a specific set of parameters and a unique perioperative approach. Maxillary cases, for example, require surgical avoidance of the sinus and engagement of the sinus wall, whereas mandibular cases require avoidance of the mental foramen. In partially edentulous cases, measurements are based on adjacent teeth; in fully edentulous cases, they are based on the patient's denture. Fully edentulous cases may or may not require bone removal or a blood draw for applying platelet-rich plasma therapies, but partially edentulous cases will involve both bone removal and a blood draw as well as bone grafting and the use of special socket-debriding burs.

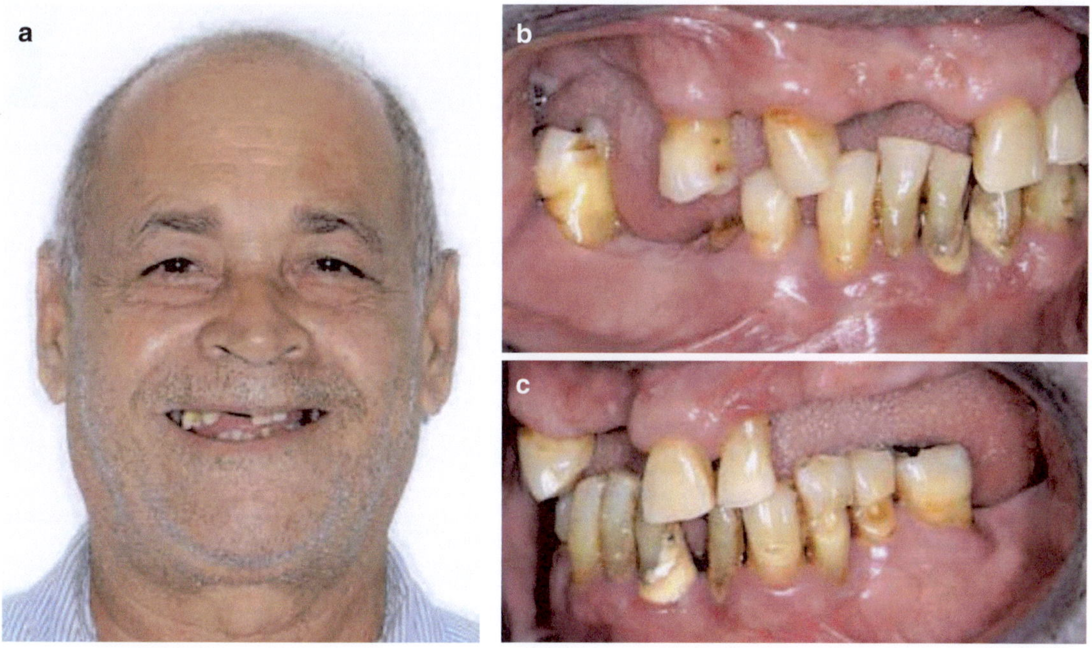

Fig. 18.1 (a–c) A partially edentulous patient with 0 to 8 teeth in an arch and moderate to advanced periodontal bone loss is the ideal candidate for maxillary FAIR treatment

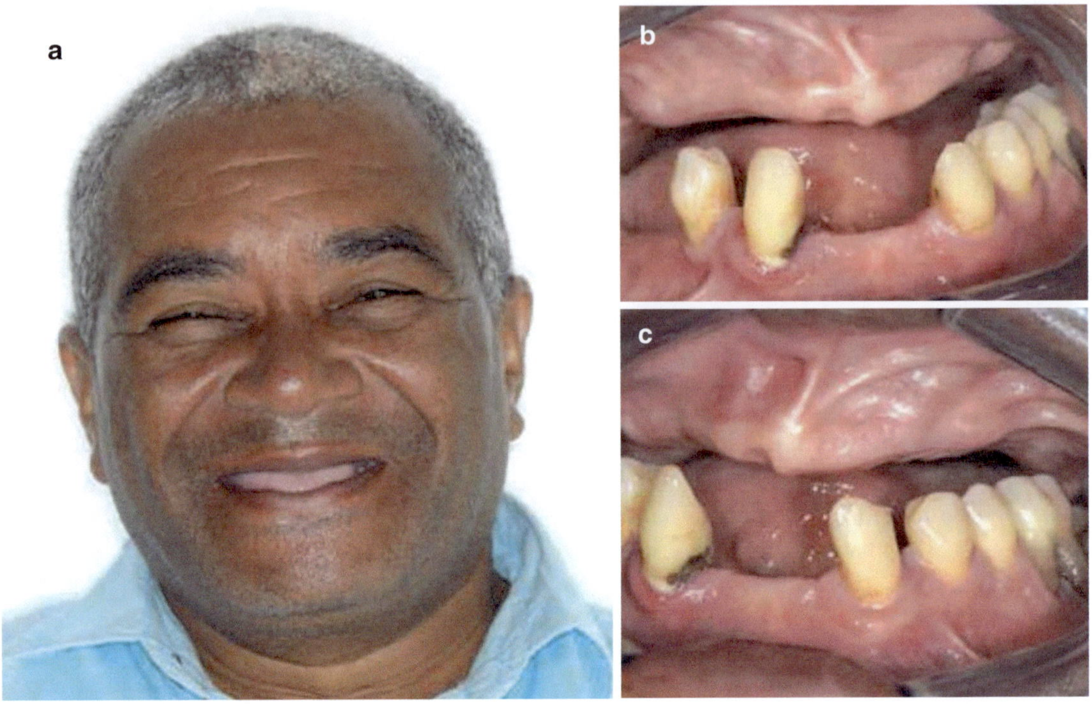

Fig. 18.2 (**a**–**c**) This patient is fully edentulous in the maxilla and is also an ideal candidate for FAIR treatment

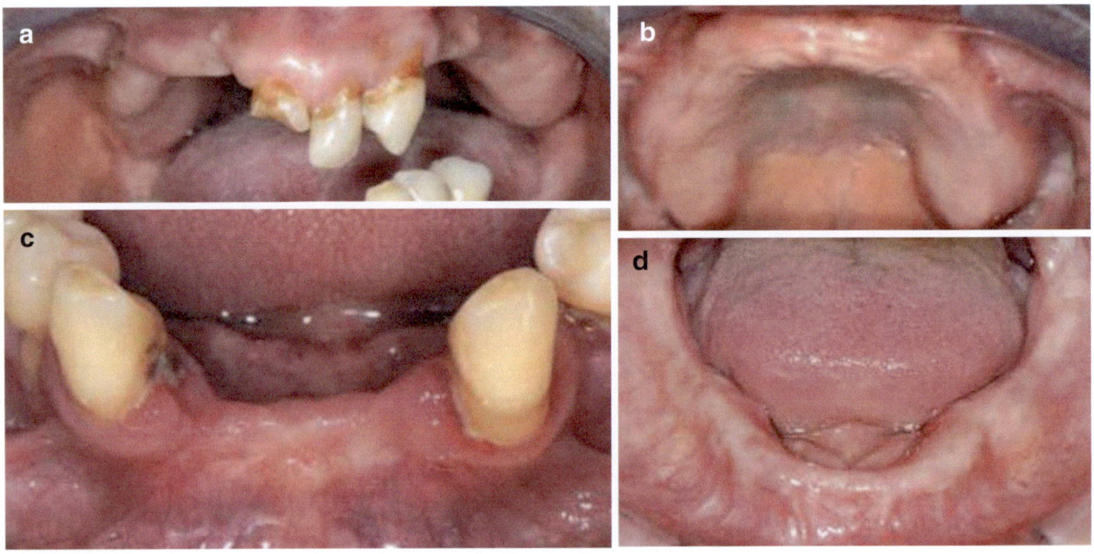

Fig. 18.3 Four broad categories of ideal FAIR candidates. (**a**) Partially edentulous maxilla. (**b**) Fully edentulous maxilla. (**c**) Partially edentulous mandible. (**d**) Fully edentulous mandible

Medical history, chief complaint, and patient expectations
Note any conditions that might affect the patient's treatment outcome or their suitability for a surgical procedure. The patient's expectations should also be discussed and recorded.

Dental history
Understand the patient's expectations and history with dental failure (eg, periodontal disease) as well as habits including clenching and bruxing.

Intraoral and extraoral examination
For patients with remaining teeth, the oral examination is always based on periodontal findings and the disease status of the remaining teeth and soft tissue.

Radiographic analysis
Initial radiographic evaluation can be done with the help of a panoramic radiograph. The practitioner can then decide if other methods are needed, such as a full-mouth periapical series, a cone beam computed tomography (CBCT) scan, or medical CT scan.

Fig. 18.4 A thorough evaluation is necessary to choose the right treatment and to establish a predictable treatment outcome

Before considering any treatment options, of course, the clinician should thoroughly evaluate each patient (Fig. 18.4) [6–9]. Assessment of candidates for the FAIR protocol should include a comprehensive medical history to determine how the patient's overall condition might affect expected outcomes from the surgical treatment. In addition, the patient's dental history must be reviewed carefully to identify any treatment failures potentially caused by a periodontal disease process or other conditions such as clenching or bruxing. A panoramic radiograph should be included in the initial records to help determine if a full-mouth periapical series, a CT scan, or a CBCT analysis will be required.

The esthetics of the smile, as well as all aspects of the patient's oral function (e.g., vertical occlusal space), are crucial determinants for treatment [25]. Preoperative interventions may be required to address poor-fitting dentures, limited interocclusal space, incorrect bite, and insufficient space for a prosthesis. Patients should be asked whether they have noticed any recent changes in their facial appearance and whether they are happy with their appearance and confident when smiling. They should also be encouraged to describe any concerns they have about signs of aging resulting from wearing their denture.

18.1.4 Treatment Planning

18.1.4.1 Patient Examination

The initial evaluation should begin with a thorough intraoral and extraoral examination. The condition of any remaining teeth, the existence of caries, the occlusal status (and discrepancies in the occlusion), and any evidence of tooth migration should be carefully evaluated and documented [26]. For patients with existing dentition, the periodontal status of both their teeth and their soft tissues should be assessed. Patients with partial or complete edentulism should be examined for general and specific soft tissue conditions [27].

A photographic evaluation must be carried out and should include the following views:

- Full face and reposed lips with and without denture or partial denture.
- Full face smiling with and without denture or partial denture.
- Lips retracted and teeth apart with and without denture or partial denture.
- Lips retracted and teeth together: frontal, right, and left.
- Lateral full face.
- Lateral smile.
- Intraoral alveolar ridge without denture.
- Occlusal and intaglio aspects without denture.

All of the collected records and data are used to evaluate critical esthetic and phonetic components of the case, including the nasolabial angle, facial midline, occlusal plane, lips (support, size, and dynamics), tooth display at rest and when speaking, smile line, and transition zone [28]. For edentulous or partially edentulous patients, a base plate and bite rim can be used to capture the vertical dimension of occlusion (i.e., the relationship of the mandible and maxilla with the teeth at maximal intercuspation).

18.1.4.2 Radiographic Analysis

The radiographic evaluation is critical to the success of the treatment, as the type of definitive prosthesis that can be placed is based on the availability of both the hard tissue and the soft tissue. Patients should be evaluated for the quantity and quality of bone that is present in order to maximize the possibility of immediate function of the prosthesis [22]. CT scans are used to plan the treatment and to design the case, including the use of a three-dimensional stereolithographic model (3D STL) based on the patient's CBCT scan (Fig. 18.5).

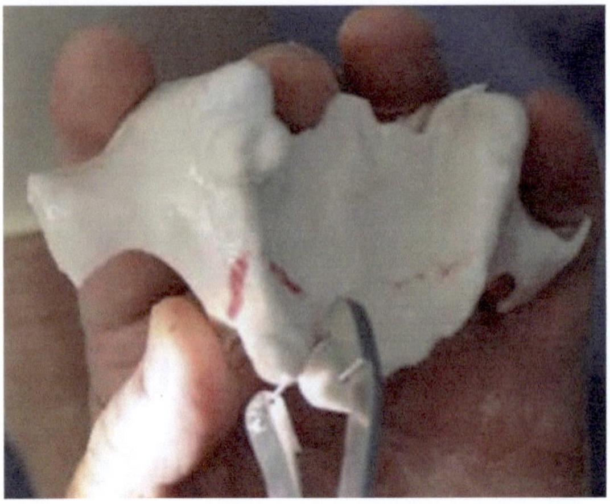

Fig. 18.5 A three-dimensional STL model from the CT scan is extremely helpful in treatment planning for the surgery

18.1.4.3 Smile and Lip Line Evaluation

Evaluating the smile line and the transition line of the prosthesis can help in establishing potential esthetic considerations. The clinician should measure the length of the central incisor and add 6 mm; the transition line must be apical to the smile line for an esthetic outcome (Fig. 18.6a). If the transition line is coronal to the smile line, the outcome will not be esthetically pleasing (Fig. 18.6b). For patients with a high smile line, a measurement of 17–18 mm is preferred to conceal the transitional line from acrylic to gingiva. Conversely, patients with a low smile line may require a measurement of only 14 mm. Less distance than that, however, can compromise the strength of the prosthesis. The 14- to 17-mm protocol combines optimal esthetics with technically sound function based on the length of the implants and the type of bone in which they are placed.

18.1.4.4 Bone Volume and Bone Density Assessments

Bone volume is evaluated with a CT scan and radiographs to help determine the implant and restorative options. Bone resorption is designated as *mild*, *moderate*, or *severe* (Figs. 18.7 and 18.8) [29, 30]. Additionally, accurate records must be made to assess the condition of the oral mucosa and alveolar ridges as well as the quality of facial, cheek, and lip support (including contours). The clinician should take good-quality impressions of both arches along with an occlusal registration that includes the palate and vestibules in the maxilla and the retromolar pads in the mandible.

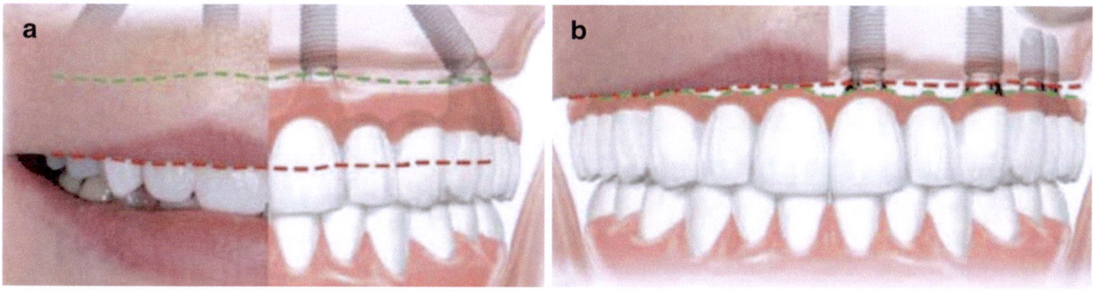

Fig. 18.6 (**a**) This case is successful because the transition line (green dotted line) is apical to the smile line (red dotted line). (**b**) If the transition line is coronal to the smile line, it is a prosthetic failure

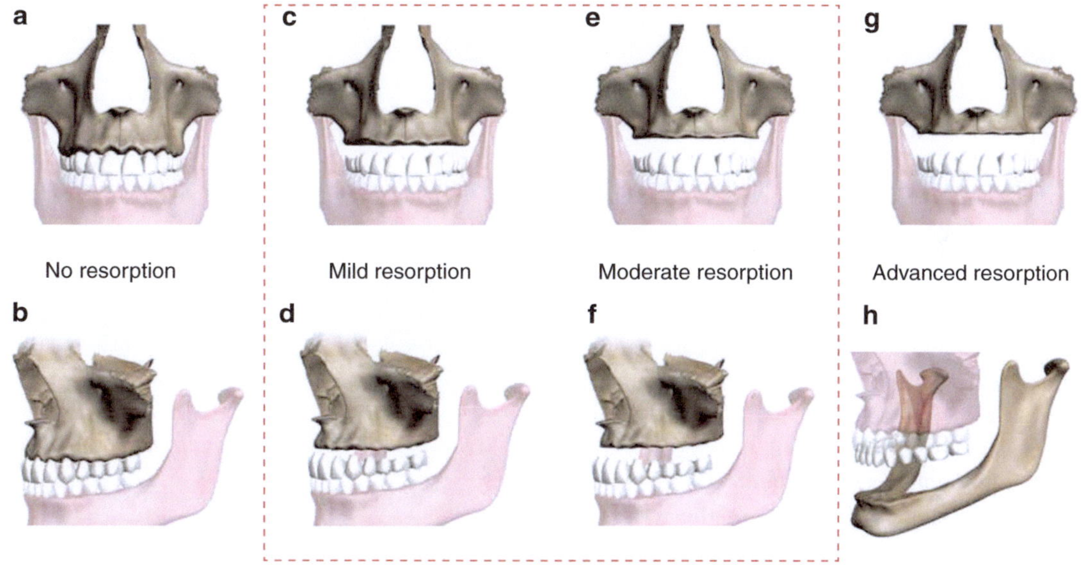

Fig. 18.7 Bone resorption severity in the maxilla. (**a**, **b**) No resorption. (**c**, **d**) Mild resorption. (**e**, **f**) Moderate resorption. (**g**, **h**) Advanced resorption

18.1.4.5 Model Evaluation

Depending on the case type, the clinician can use several different methods to determine how much bone to remove to complete the FAIR procedure. For partially edentulous patients, incisal/bone measurements to determine bone removal can be made based on existing teeth. To obtain proper seating measurements, palatal references should be used in the maxilla and the retromolar pad in the mandible. Another method is to obtain an occlusal registration using the immediate prosthesis from the laboratory in conjunction with occlusal registration materials once all remaining teeth have been extracted. This type of immediate occlusal guide can be used to verify the measurements obtained by more traditional methods. A midline deviation of up to 4 mm is not a concern esthetically, but in cases where the deviation is greater, the occlusal guide can help the clinician avoid complications. The guide can also be used to confirm the proper vertical dimension.

18.1.5 Category 1: The Fully Edentulous Maxilla

Restoring the fully edentulous maxilla using the FAIR protocol requires expert skills [20, 22, 31–37]. The carpentry maxim, "measure twice; cut

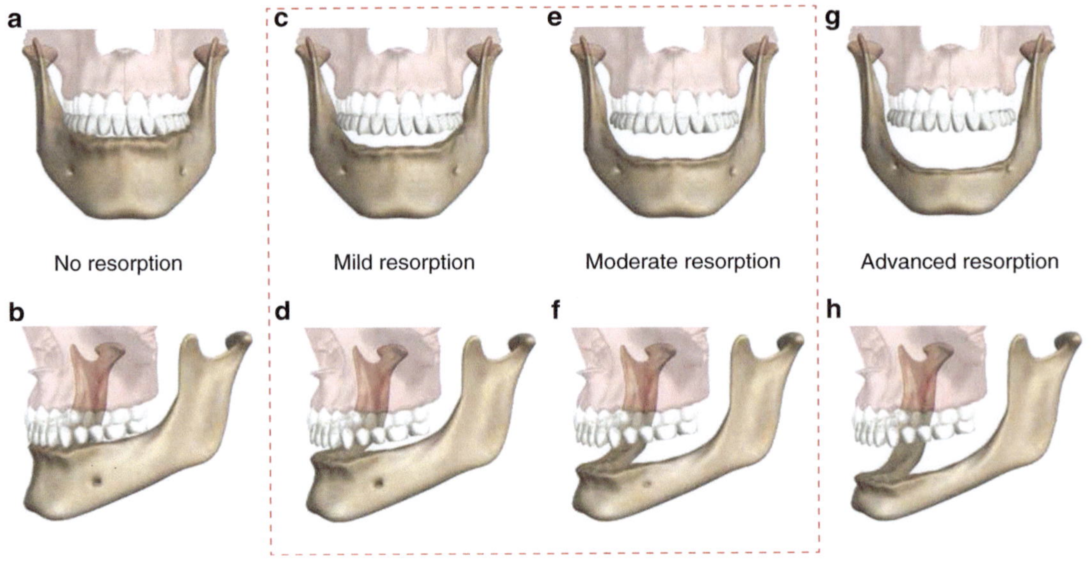

Fig. 18.8 Bone resorption severity in the mandible. (**a**, **b**) No resorption. (**c**, **d**) Mild resorption. (**e**, **f**) Moderate resorption. (**g**, **h**) Advanced resorption

once," is equally apt for the implant surgeon when translated as "visualize the case multiple times; perform surgery once" [38–40]. This process is facilitated by the use of a virtual three-dimensional (3D) computed tomography (CT) stereolithographic (STL) model based on the patient's examination records or the models of similar cases, including, in some cases, physical measurements taken inside the patient's oral cavity. It can also include using and performing a practice surgery on a bone consistency STL model prior to the actual patient surgery. Such planning is particularly important in cases where the alveolar bone is minimal, making the selection of the implants and their angulation and positioning more critical [41–43]. The FAIR procedure usually involves only four implants, but it is deceptively complex, requiring extensive preoperative planning and surgical vision.

18.1.5.1 Preoperative Procedure

A clear denture duplicate template for the procedure is cut (either in the laboratory or by the clinician) so that the buccal flange is only 15 mm from the incisal edge from premolar to premolar (Fig. 18.9). The flanges on the back of the denture are not cut; otherwise, the denture can be overseated. This will provide a measure for the amount of bone recontouring that will be required.

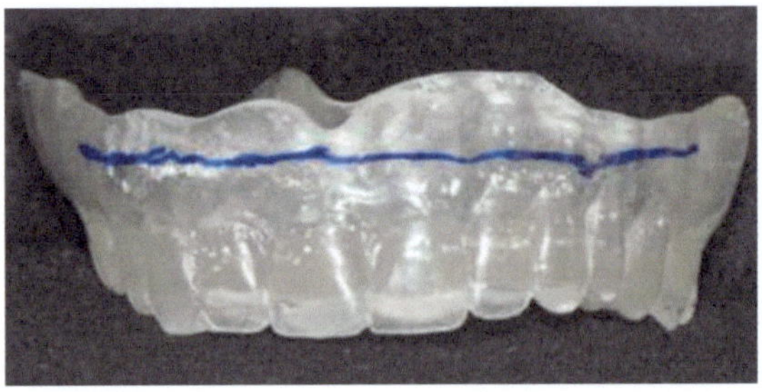

Fig. 18.9 The clear acrylic template should have the buccal flange from premolar to premolar trimmed to 15 mm from the incisal edges of the teeth

The FAIR surgical procedure can be quite lengthy, lasting as long as 4 h, and it therefore requires a unique approach to anesthesia for patient comfort [44–46]. While IV sedation allows the patient to bite and to follow commands, it is not recommended because the clinical cost can be prohibitive due to the extended length of the procedure [47]. General anesthesia is also not a good option because it makes obtaining proper occlusion nearly impossible, even if the patient is nasally intubated, and thus requires the clinician to manipulate the patient's jaws [48].

Bupivacaine (e.g., Marcaine, Pfizer), which lasts 7–12 h but can take up to 30 min to take effect, can be used simultaneously with lidocaine, which typically takes only 5 min for onset but lasts 2½ to 3 h. In this way, if the surgery is lengthy, the bupivacaine will provide the patient with the necessary comfort once the lidocaine has dissipated. Dosage is important, and less bupivacaine is often required if used in conjunction with lidocaine. Triazolam (e.g., Halcion, Pfizer) may be a good supplement to help relax the patient [49].

18.1.5.2 Surgical Procedure

Under local anesthesia, the surgery begins with an incision from the first molar to the contralateral first molar. The incision can be made mid crestal or slightly palatal, depending on the experience of the clinician (Fig. 18.10). The nasopalatine nerve is generally located behind the midline

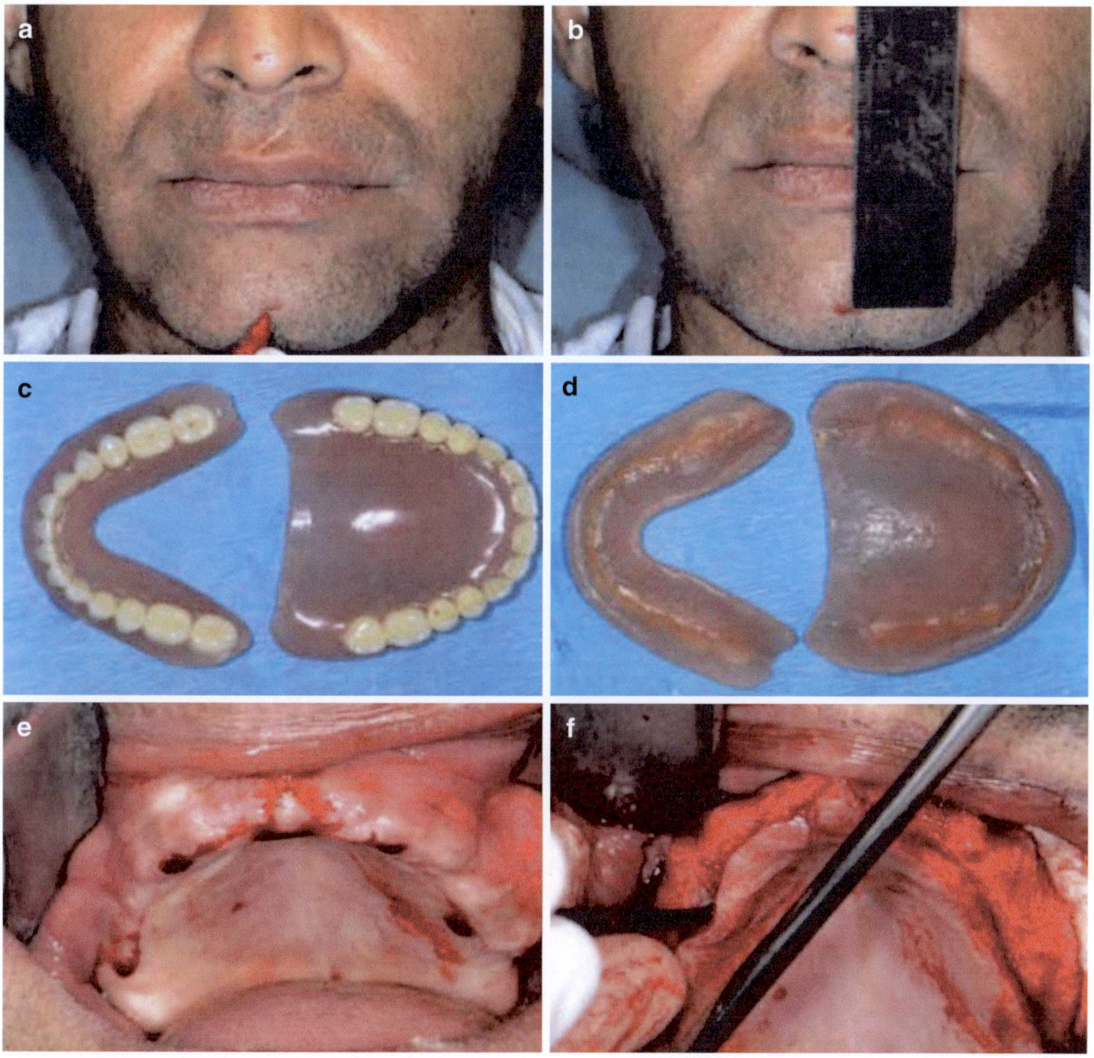

Fig. 18.10 (**a**, **b**) Determine (either clinically or radiographically) if there is 22 mm of interbone space if both arches are being treated. (**c**, **d**) Place the denture in the mouth to get an accurate bite registration to aid in seating the maxillary denture accurately after the maxilla is flapped open. (**e**) In the midline area, create a small outgoing notch of tissue to avoid the nasopalatine nerve in a moderate-to-severely resorbed ridge to allow for accurate repositioning of the flap to its original position. (**f**) Reflecting palatally provides the necessary access for multiple implant placement

palatally, but in cases of bone resorption, it may be located more forward, slightly palatal, or on the ridge because the nerve remains at the point where the ridge resorbed. Consequently, the clinician should cut toward the buccal mid crestal rather than palatally. A notch is cut buccally to avoid the nasopalatine nerve, which not only helps the surgeon avoid the nerve but also facilitates repositioning of the tissues when a flap is reflected, with uniform suturing from the midline back. A 6- to 9-mm vertical incision is made on the buccal side in the molar areas bilaterally.

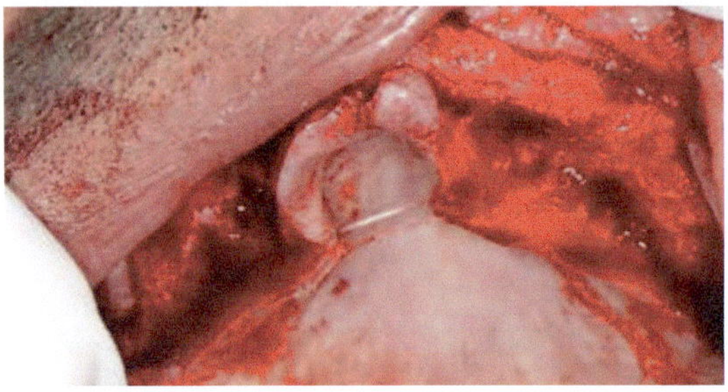

Fig. 18.11 In lieu of surgical assistance, temporary suturing can help the clinician in reflecting a flap

The buccal and palatal sides of the ridge are reflected for different reasons. If a mid crestal incision is made, then the palatal must be reflected properly to enable drilling. If the incision is slightly palatal, less palatal reflection is necessary. Nevertheless, reflecting palatally provides needed access for multiple implant placement. In the absence of sufficient surgical assistance, temporary suturing can aid the clinician in reflecting a flap (Fig. 18.11). By tying off the palatal, the clinician can then focus on the buccal reflection. With the aid of a retractor and the reflected tissue, the clinician can begin reducing the height of the alveolar bone in accordance with a clear guide to ensure a 15-mm clearance from the incisal edge of the denture to the bone. However, if the reduction is only 2 or 3 mm, then a periodontal probe can be used instead to measure the distance for grinding based on radiograph or CT imaging (Fig. 18.12a, b). The clinician should make sure that the bone shelf remains sufficiently wide.

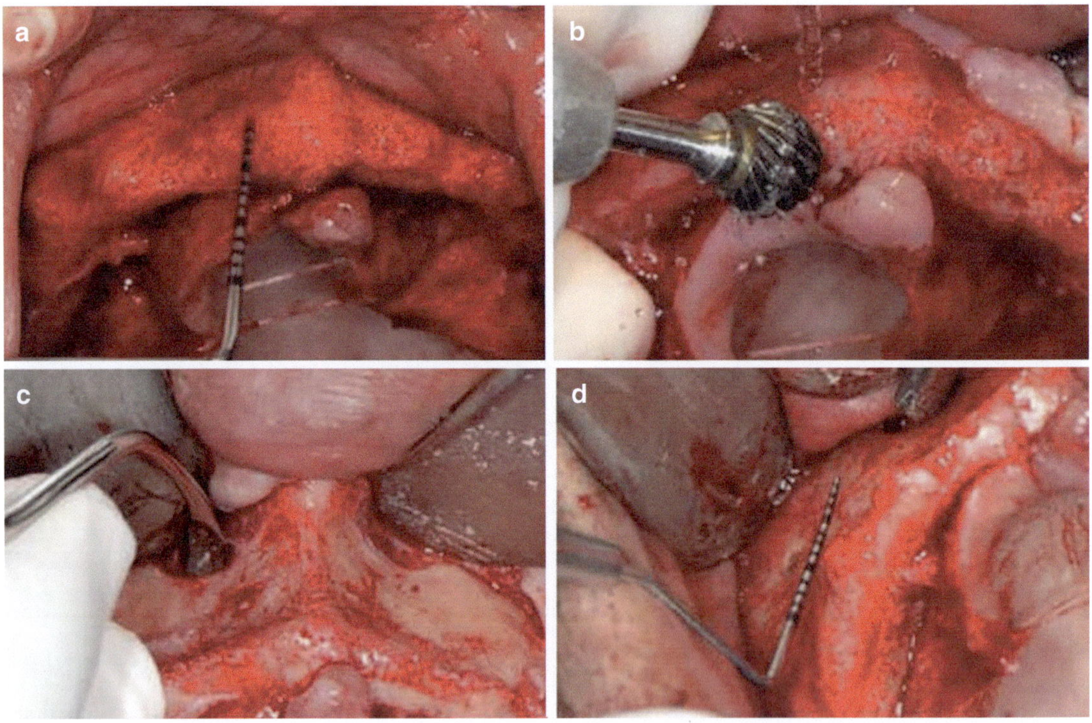

Fig. 18.12 (**a**) A periodontal probe can be used to measure the distance for grinding. (**b**) Reduce as necessary and create the bone shelf. (**c**) Identify the nasal floor and the lateral piriform plate. (**d**) The tilted implants will be aimed from the first/second premolar area to the inferolateral piriform rim

Eliminating cortical bone may result in a lack of unicortical stability. To restore this stability, the apex of the implant must be placed in the nasal floor cortical bone. This can be visually determined via reflection of approximately 2 to 3 mm on the lateral piriform rim or the lateral aspect of the nose (the mesial aspect of the sinus and the distal aspect of the nasal floor) (Fig. 18.12c). The entrance point of the implant is halfway between the first and the second premolar (Fig. 18.12d). However, unlike the sinus membrane, the nasal floor cannot be patched if it is perforated. Instead, the procedure must be aborted due to the risk of infection, and the area must be repaired [50].

P-I Brånemark recommended an alternative approach. To determine the location of the anterior portion of the sinus for placing the apex of the implant, only the sinus floor (and not the nasal floor) should be elevated using a no. 8 round bur to make an opening through which a probe may be placed. The probe must be a periodontal probe, not a straight or a bendable duck probe, which can damage the sinus membrane because of its angle. Brånemark recommended neither grafting nor plugging the hole but simply putting the implant in place [51]. The wall that separates the nasal cavity from the maxillary sinus is the bone-substantive canine area, as reflected in the length of canine teeth. Teeth anterior to the canines have shorter roots. The FAIR method uses canine-length implants as the distal implants.

18.1.6 Category 2: The Fully Edentulous Mandible

The structure and bone composition of the mandible, as opposed to the maxilla, make it the more attractive and successful location for full-arch rehabilitation [17, 52–59]. As with the maxilla, mandibular rehabilitation planning is accomplished via a clear acrylic denture duplicate template (Fig. 18.13) and three-dimensional (STL) modeling based on the patient's bone anatomy cone beam CT. Alveolar bone availability is a crucial factor for the fabrication of models and the selection of implants, positioning, angulation, and complementary abutment attachments [39–42]. The FAIR procedure involves 4–6 implants and requires extensive preoperative planning and creative surgical vision.

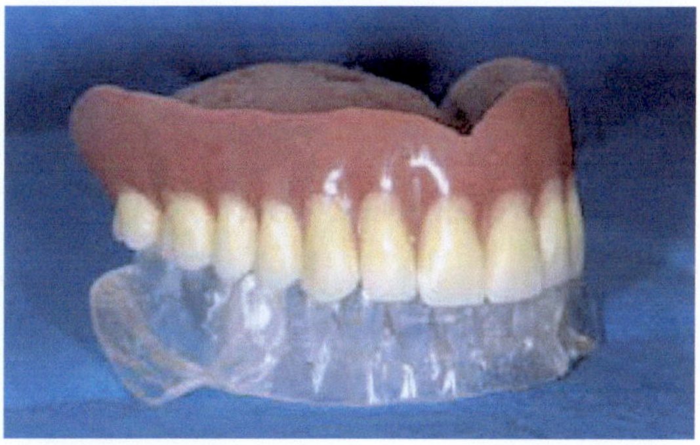

Fig. 18.13 A clear acrylic denture duplicate template for the mandibular FAIR procedure is fabricated and measured

18.1.6.1 Preoperative Procedure

The clear denture duplicate template for the procedure is fabricated in the laboratory or by the clinician. To ensure that the prosthesis will be properly seated, marks are made to determine the proper vertical distance or dimension with dentures in place. The nose and chin points are marked and measured (Fig. 18.14a, b), and the retromolar pad should be used to ensure the accuracy of the denture and/or clear duplicate seating. For the clinician to obtain a bite registration, the maxillary denture is seated first (Fig. 18.14c, d). The mandibular denture is then placed in the patient's mouth for the bite registration, and the patient closes the mouth with dentures in place.

As noted above, because the FAIR surgery and denture conversion can often last up to 4 h, anesthesia and patient comfort are crucial [44–46]. The effects of lidocaine can last up to 3 h after a 5-min onset, but Marcaine (Pfizer) can provide patient comfort for 7–12 h after its 30-min onset. Therefore, the two anesthetics can be given simultaneously for lengthy surgeries, with careful attention to limiting Marcaine dosage in conjunction with lidocaine. While Halcion (Pfizer) may be a viable oral sedation option for anesthetizing the FAIR patient, IV

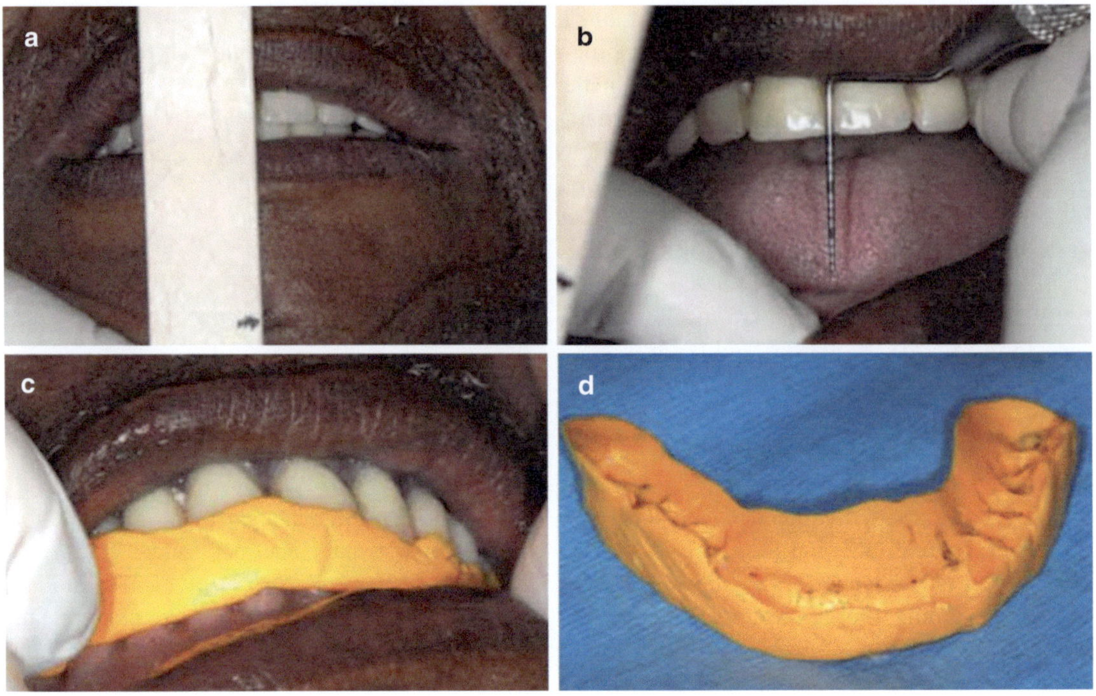

Fig. 18.14 (**a**, **b**) Mark and measure the preoperative vertical dimensions to ensure its replication postsurgery and prosthesis placement. (**c**, **d**) Bite registration material is used to record the occlusion

sedation can be cost prohibitive, and general anesthesia prevents the clinician from obtaining accurate measurements of occlusion [47–49].

18.1.6.2 Surgical Procedure

The incision design is similar to that of the maxilla, but instead of the vertical incisions proceeding posteriorly, there is a single midline vertical releasing incision of approximately 7 mm (Fig. 18.15). As the implants are placed at the sites of the first to second premolars, a mid crestal incision from first molar to contralateral first molar is adequate. Whereas in the maxilla the palate can be used to seat the clear template, in the mandible the retromolar pad area is used for this purpose. A mid crestal incision in the mandible that is too short will prevent placement of the implants, whereas a mid crestal incision that is too long will prevent proper seating of the denture using retromolar pads. The ridge can be recontoured if socket preservation was not completely successful or if 15 mm of intraocclusal space is not available.

To avoid soft tissue sloughing at the crestal area and possible damage from limited blood supply, the clinician should carefully adhere to precautions associated with atrophic mandibular bone, nerve, and vascular structures [60–62]. Careful incision design facilitates the avoidance of nerve damage and the repositioning of the soft tissues after flap reflection and implant/abutment placement to avoid suturing gaps. Lingual and even buccal flap retraction can be accomplished with temporary suturing if desired.

Once flap reflection is completed, alveolar bone height reduction can commence, based on the clear guide, to guarantee a minimum height of 15 mm of clearance from the incisal edge of the clear denture duplicate template teeth to the bone. Using specialized acrylic burs helps to ensure sufficient width and shape of the remaining bone shelf if adjustment is necessary.

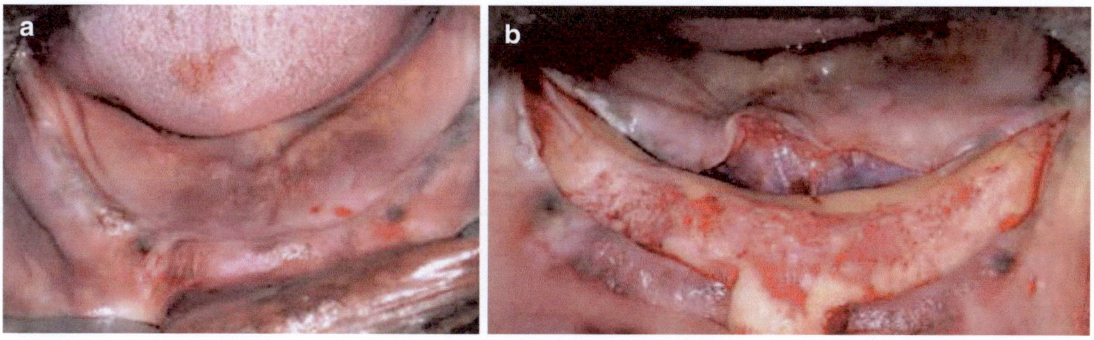

Fig. 18.15 (**a**, **b**) A vertical releasing incision of approximately 7 mm is made with exposure from first molar to first molar

18.1.7 Category 3: The Partially Edentulous Maxilla

18.1.7.1 Preoperative Procedure

The clear denture duplicate template for the procedure is cut (either in the laboratory or by the clinician) so that the buccal flange is only 15 mm from the incisal edge from premolar to premolar (Fig. 18.16). (The flanges on the back of the denture are not cut to prevent it from being overseated in the vestibule.) This will provide a measure for the amount of bone recontouring that will be required.

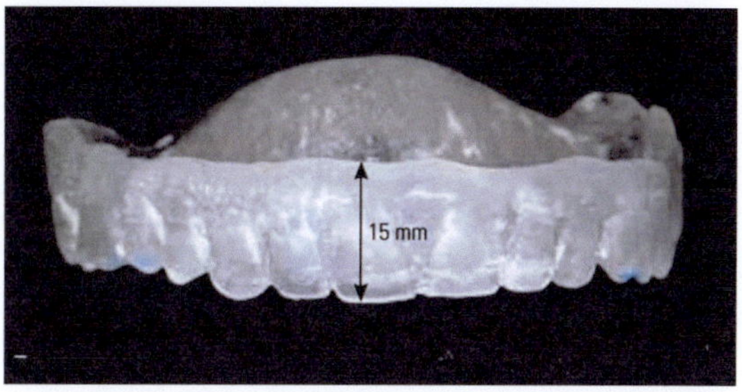

Fig. 18.16 A clear denture duplicate template with the buccal flange cut to 15 mm from premolar to premolar is used as a guide for bone reduction

18.1.7.2 Surgical Procedure

Once anesthesia is employed, the surgery can begin with an incision design made from first molar to contralateral first molar around the existing teeth. Vertical releases are created at the distal extent of the incision bilaterally, and a flap is reflected buccally and palatally (Fig. 18.17a–c) [57]. With the aid of a retractor and the reflected tissue, the clinician can begin reducing the height of the alveolar bone in accordance with a clear guide to ensure a clearance of 15 mm from the incisal edge of the denture to the bone. A clear denture duplicate template with the buccal flange cut to 15 mm is used as a guide (Fig. 18.17d) for bone reduction. The ridge can be reduced with a variety of instruments, such as a sagittal saw, a hall drill with round bur, a piezoelectric surgery unit with a small saw blade, an implant motor handpiece with a large round bur, and more. The author's recommendation is to use the implant motor and handpiece with a specialized bur with the smooth tip to prevent tearing of the palatal soft tissue (Fig. 18.17e) to create the ideal shape for the ridge (Fig. 18.17f, g).

It is important to landmark the positions of the sinus membrane and nasal floor before the anterior implants are placed, usually straight up and down or slightly tilted to reach accessible bone beyond an area of less-than-ideal bone. The distal implants are placed so that the apex of the implant engages the lateral piriform rim (Fig. 18.17h). The anterior implants are placed so that the apex engages the bone of the nasal floor. The entrance point of the distal implants is halfway between the first and the second premolar, but it essentially follows the path of the

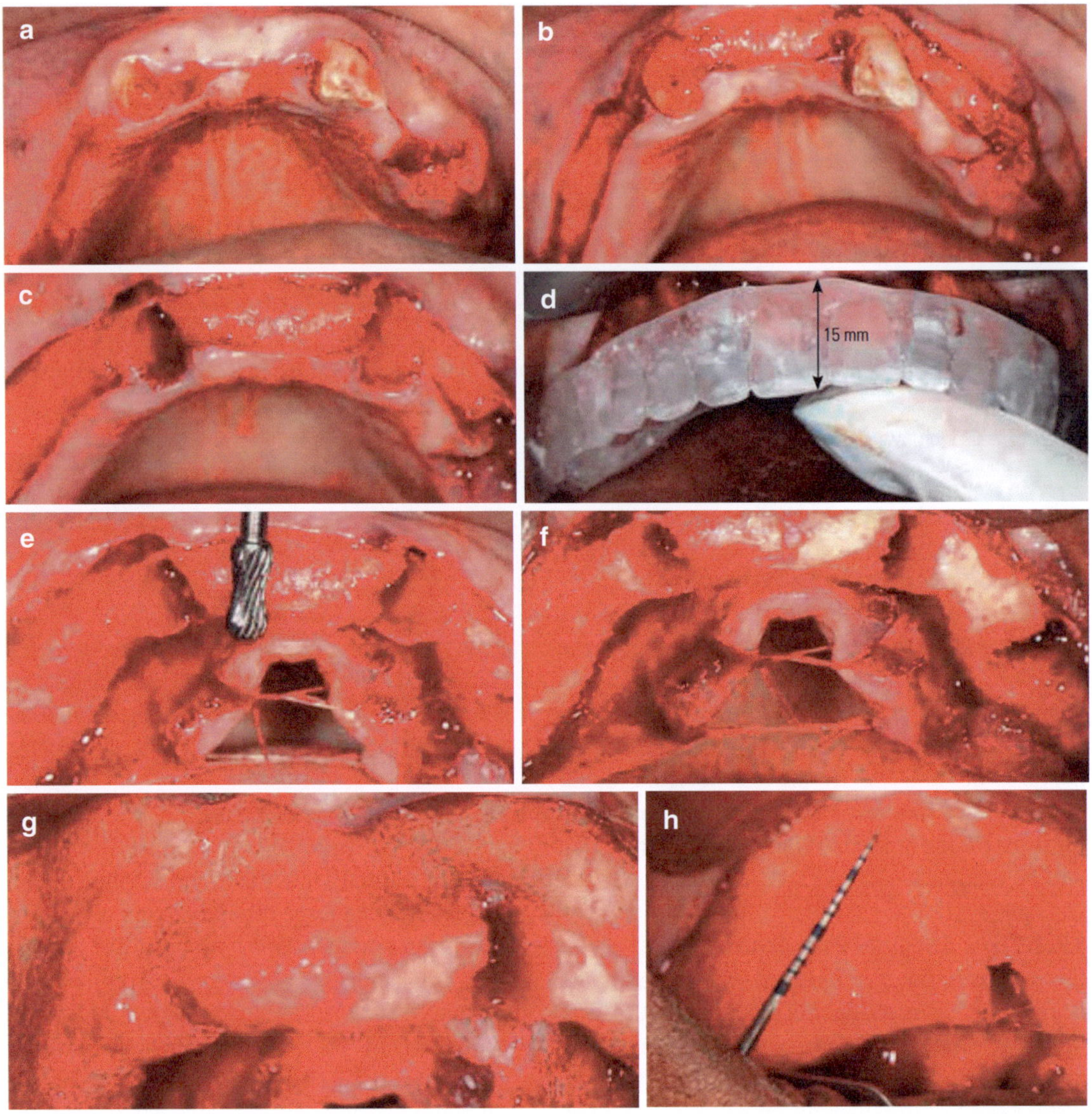

Fig. 18.17 (**a–c**) Vertical releases are created at the distal extent of the incision bilaterally, and a flap is reflected buccally and palatally. (**d**) A clear denture duplicate template with the buccal flange cut to 15 mm from premolar to premolar is used as a guide for bone reduction. (**e, f**) The ridge can be reduced using the implant motor and handpiece with a specialized bur. (**g, h**) Reflecting the flap to expose the bone

anterior maxillary sinus wall. If the soft tissues of the sinus floor are perforated, the procedure should be aborted or the implant repositioned due to the risk of inadequate implant stability or sinus infection [58]. For this reason, it may be beneficial to perform a sinus floor elevation and grafting to avoid the possibility of perforation while attempting to engage the bone of the nasal floor.

18.1.8 Category 4: The Partially Edentulous Mandible

18.1.8.1 Preoperative Procedure

While the structure and bone composition of the mandible make it conducive to full-arch rehabilitation, in partially edentulous cases the clinician will have the additional task of treating one or more fresh extraction sockets [17, 52–59]. To complete the FAIR procedure, these sockets may be grafted to serve as possible implant sites. Therefore, the clinician should draw blood from the patient for platelet-rich plasma (PRP) and use it to hydrate particulated freeze-dried bone allograft [63–65]. In addition to bone grafting, PRP membranes and/or gummy bone (a mixture of autogenous fibrin glue and bone graft) may also be part of the healing therapy for the extraction sites [66].

Bilateral blocks rather than infiltrations (as when simply placing implants) are used when extracting the remaining teeth in the mandible. Once teeth are extracted, a round bur (no. 8 carbide) or piezoelectric unit with a round diamond tip can be used to clean the extraction sockets [67]. If it is necessary to recontour the mandible, handpieces may be used, preferably a 1:1 surgical handpiece (instead of the usual 20:1 gear-reducing implant handpiece). The attachment is usually 1:1 so the speed of the bur will be 40,000 rpm to contour the ridge. For the implant osteotomy, the usual 20:1 gear-reducing handpiece is used, and the osteotomy is created at 1200 rpm in conjunction with a tilted approach. The vertical dimension is determined, and the clinician marks points on the nose and chin and uses a palate or retromolar pad to ensure accurate occlusion estimates for both arches. A bite registration is made by seating the maxillary denture followed by the mandibular denture. The remaining teeth are extracted. Alveolar bone availability enables implant selection, position, angle, and abutment attachments [39–42]. A dental laboratory or the dental office can fabricate the clear denture duplicate template for assistance in proper implant positioning. If the laboratory does not provide a clear duplicate template (Fig. 18.18), one can be fabricated simply with the mandibular denture and a Denture Duplicator Kit (Lang Dental), which uses alginate and a separating medium.

18.1.8.2 Surgical Procedure

The mandibular incision begins at the midline and proceeds posteriorly, from first molar to first molar, or further if more posterior teeth are being extracted. The clinician makes a 7-mm vertical releasing incision in the midline area, exposing the ridge from first molar to first molar on the two terminal ends, which is idea for placing the distal tilted implants in the first to second premolar sites. Because the palate cannot be used to seat the denture in the mandible, an incision that is too short prevents proper implant placement while an incision that is too long prevents proper seating of the denture on the retromolar pads (Fig. 18.19). Recontouring the ridge to remove 2 to 3 mm of bone may be necessary if 15 mm of space is unavailable.

The clinician must adhere to precautions required for the structures of atrophic mandibular bone, nerves, and blood vessels to avoid soft tissue sloughing at the crestal area [60–62]. Careful incision design prevents nerve damage and suturing gaps during implant/abutment

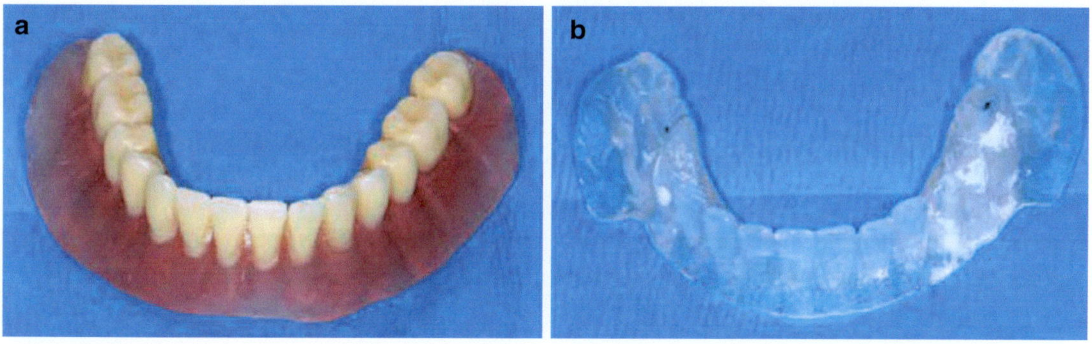

Fig. 18.18 (**a**) The patient's denture. (**b**) A clear denture duplicate template

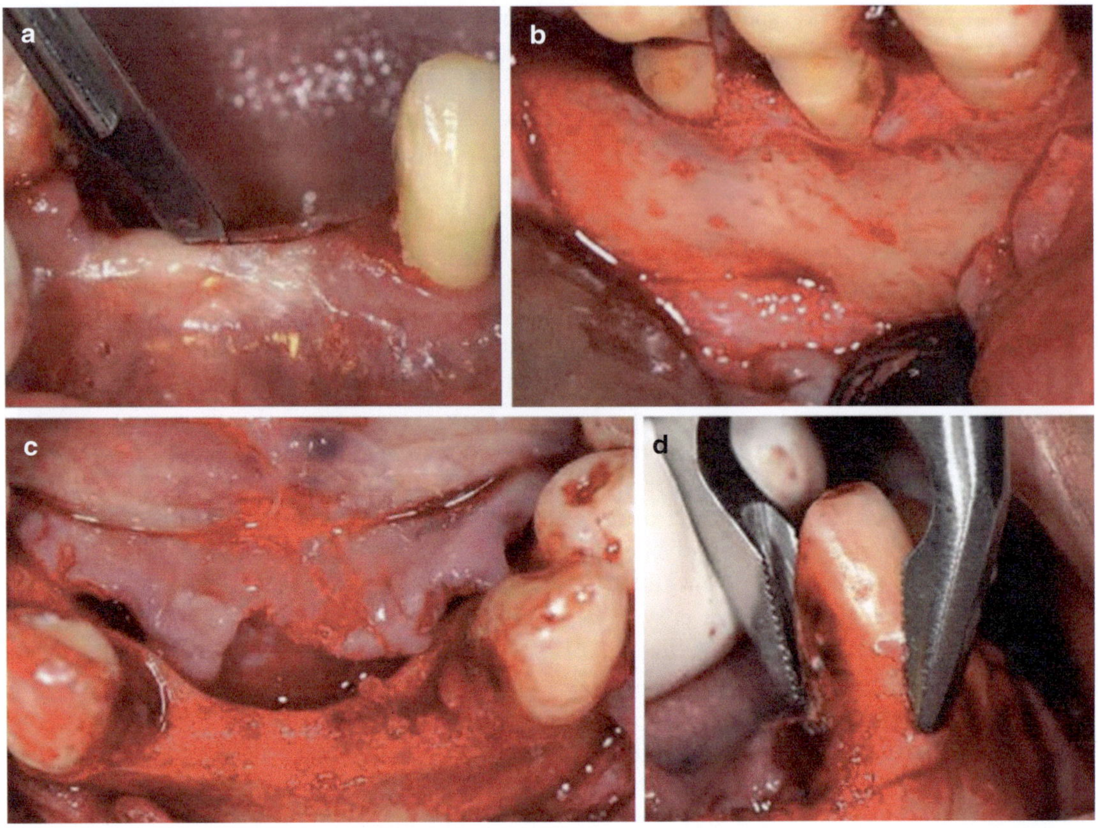

Fig. 18.19 (**a**, **b**) Making the incision and reflecting the flap to identify the mental foramen and nerve and expose the bone. (**c**, **d**) The teeth are extracted atraumatically

placement. After flap reflection, the clear guide is used to reduce alveolar bone height while preserving a minimum clearance of 15 mm from the incisal edge of the denture to the bone. Radiographs or CT scans can help guide the reduction. Sufficient bone width of the remaining bone shelf is preserved and the ridge is ideally recontoured with the use of specialized burs.

18.2 Conclusion

The FAIR protocol is an innovative approach to treatment of the edentulous or nearly edentulous patient. In lieu of single implants replacing individual missing teeth, four or five implants are spaced throughout the arch and immediately loaded with a provisional fixed prosthesis. Studies have shown that wearing dentures can reduce patients' quality of life, causing pain and areas of discomfort, chewing and speaking difficulties, slippage, reduced occlusal force, and poor oral sensation. The FAIR dental prosthesis offers many advantages for the dental patient with a fully or partially edentulous arch. The prosthesis is immediate, fixed, esthetically pleasing, highly functional, inexpensive, and maintainable. Importantly, the FAIR procedure and similar techniques can frequently be performed without bone grafting.

References

1. Centers for Disease Control and Prevention; https://www.cdc.gov/nchs/data/vsrr/vsrr015-508.pdf. Accessed 19 Nov 2021.
2. Kaushik K, Dhawan P, Tandan P, Jain M. Oral health-related quality of life among patients after complete denture rehabilitation: a 12-month follow-up study. Int J Appl Basic Med Res. 2018;8(3):169–73.
3. Allen PF, McMillan AS. A review of the functional and psychosocial outcomes of edentulousness treated with complete replacement dentures. J Can Dent Assoc. 2003;69(10):662.
4. Leles CR, Ferreira NP, Vieira AH, Campos AC, Silva ET. Factors influencing edentulous patients' preferences for prosthodontic treatment. J Oral Rehabil. 2011;38(5):333–9. https://doi.org/10.1111/j.1365-2842.2010.02158.x.
5. Heath MR. The effect of maximum biting force and bone loss upon masticatory function and dietary selection of the elderly. Int Dent J. 1982;32(4):345–56.
6. Wolff A, Gadre A, Begleiter A, Moskona D, Cardash H. Correlation between patient satisfaction with complete dentures and denture quality, oral condition, and flow rate of submandibular/sublingual salivary glands. Int J Prosthodont. 2003;16(1):45–8.
7. Chierici G, Lawson L. Clinical speech considerations in prosthodontics: perspectives of the prosthodontist and speech pathologist. J Prosthet Dent. 1973;29(1):29–39. https://doi.org/10.1016/0022-3913(73)90136-4.
8. Reissmann DR, Dard M, Lamprecht R, Struppek J, Heydecke G. Oral health-related quality of life in subjects with implant-supported prostheses: a systematic review. J Dent. 2017;65:22–40. https://doi.org/10.1016/j.jdent.2017.08.003.
9. Dellavia C, Rosati R, Del Fabbro M, Pellegrini G. Functional jaw muscle assessment in patients with a full fixed prosthesis on a limited number of implants: a review of the literature. Eur J Oral Implantol. 2014;7(Suppl 2):S155–69.
10. Rosenbaum N. Full-arch implant-retained prosthetics in general dental practice. Dent Update. 2012;39(2):108–16. https://doi.org/10.12968/denu.2012.39.2.108.
11. Misch CE, Degidi M. Five-year prospective study of immediate/early loading of fixed prostheses in completely edentulous jaws with a bone quality-based implant system. Clin Implant Dent Relat Res. 2003;5(1):17–28. https://doi.org/10.1111/j.1708-8208.2003.tb00178.x.
12. Motta M, Monsano R, Velloso GR, de Oliveira Silva JC, Luvizuto ER, Margonar R, Queiroz TP. Guided surgery in esthetic region. J Craniofac Surg. 2016;27(3):e262–5. https://doi.org/10.1097/SCS.0000000000002493.
13. Uhlendorf Y, Sartori IA, Melo AC, Uhlendorf J. Changes in lip profile of edentulous patients after placement of maxillary implant-supported fixed prosthesis: is a wax try-in a reliable diagnostic tool? Int J Oral Maxillofac Implants. 2017;32(3):593–7. https://doi.org/10.11607/jomi.4967.
14. Barbosa GA, Bernardes SR, de França DG, das Neves FD, de Mattos M, Ribeiro RF. Stress over implants of one-piece cast frameworks made with different materials. J Craniofac Surg. 2016;27(1):238–41. https://doi.org/10.1097/SCS.0000000000002175.
15. Zoidis P. The all-on-4 modified polyetheretherketone treatment approach: a clinical report. J Prosthet Dent. 2018;119(4):516–21. https://doi.org/10.1016/j.prosdent.2017.04.020.
16. Maló P, Rangert B, Dvärsäter L. Immediate function of Brånemark implants in the esthetic zone: a retrospective clinical study with 6 months to 4 years of follow-up. Clin Implant Dent Relat Res. 2000;2(3):138–46. https://doi.org/10.1111/j.1708-8208.2000.tb00004.x.
17. Maló P, Rangert B, Nobre M. "All-on-Four" immediate-function concept with Brånemark system implants for completely edentulous mandibles: a retrospective clinical study. Clin Implant Dent Relat Res. 2003;5(Suppl 1):2–9. https://doi.org/10.1111/j.1708-8208.2003.tb00010.x.
18. Maló P, Friberg B, Polizzi G, Gualini F, Vighagen T, Rangert B. Immediate and early function of Brånemark system implants placed in the esthetic zone: a 1-year prospective clinical multicenter study. Clin Implant Dent Relat Res. 2003;5(Suppl 1):37–46. https://doi.org/10.1111/j.1708-8208.2003.tb00014.x.
19. Malo P, de Araújo Nobre M, Lopes A, Moss SM, Molina GJ. A longitudinal study of the survival of all-on-4 implants in the mandible with up to 10 years of follow-up. J Am Dent Assoc. 2011;142(3):310–20. https://doi.org/10.14219/jada.archive.2011.0170.
20. Maló P, de Araújo Nobre M, Lopes A, Francischone C, Rigolizzo M. "All-on-4" immediate-function concept for completely edentulous maxillae: a clinical report on the medium (3 years) and long-term (5 years) outcomes. Clin Implant Dent Relat Res. 2012;14(Suppl 1):e139–50. https://doi.org/10.1111/j.1708-8208.2011.00395.x.
21. Lopes A, Maló P, de Araújo Nobre M, Sanchez-Fernández E. The NobelGuide® all-on-4® treatment concept for rehabilitation of edentulous jaws: a prospective report on medium- and long-term outcomes. Clin Implant Dent Relat Res. 2015;17(Suppl 2):e406–16. https://doi.org/10.1111/cid.12260.
22. Maló P, de Araújo Nobre MA, Lopes AV, Rodrigues R. Immediate loading short implants inserted on low bone quantity for the rehabilitation of the edentulous maxilla using an all-on-4 design. J Oral

Rehabil. 2015;42(8):615–23. https://doi.org/10.1111/joor.12291.
23. Maló P, Araújo Nobre MD, Lopes A, Rodrigues R. Double full-arch versus single full-arch, four implant-supported rehabilitations: a retrospective, 5-year cohort study. J Prosthodont. 2015;24(4):263–70. https://doi.org/10.1111/jopr.12228.
24. Maló P, de Araújo Nobre M, Lopes A, Ferro A, Gravito I. All-on-4® treatment concept for the rehabilitation of the completely edentulous mandible: a 7-year clinical and 5-year radiographic retrospective case series with risk assessment for implant failure and marginal bone level. Clin Implant Dent Relat Res. 2015;17(Suppl 2):e531–41. https://doi.org/10.1111/cid.12282.
25. Sheridan RA, Decker AM, Plonka AB, Wang HL. The role of occlusion in implant therapy: a comprehensive updated review. Implant Dent. 2016;25(6):829–38. https://doi.org/10.1097/ID.0000000000000488.
26. Palla S. Occlusal considerations in complete dentures. In: McNeil C, editor. Science & practice of occlusion. Chicago, IL: Quintessence; 1997. p. 457–67.
27. McGarry TJ, Nimmo A, Skiba JF, Ahlstrom RH, Smith CR, Koumjian JH. Classification system for complete edentulism. The American College of Prosthodontics. J Prosthodont. 1999;8(1):27–39. https://doi.org/10.1111/j.1532-849x.1999.tb00005.x.
28. Rosenlicht JL, Ward JA, Krauser JT. Immediate loading of dental implants. In: Babbush CA, Hahn JA, Krauser JT, Rosenlicht JL, editors. Dental implants: the art and science. 2nd ed. St. Louis, MI: Saunders; 2010. p. 340–54.
29. Chugh T, Jain AK, Jaiswal RK, Mehrotra P, Mehrotra R. Bone density and its importance in orthodontics. J Oral Biol Craniofac Res. 2013;3(2):92–7. https://doi.org/10.1016/j.jobcr.2013.01.001.
30. Parel SM, Phillips WR. A risk assessment treatment planning protocol for the four implant immediately loaded maxilla: preliminary findings. J Prosthet Dent. 2011;106(6):359–66. https://doi.org/10.1016/S0022-3913(11)60147-9.
31. Rosén A, Gynther G. Implant treatment without bone grafting in edentulous severely resorbed maxillas: a long-term follow-up study. J Oral Maxillofac Surg. 2007;65(5):1010–6. https://doi.org/10.1016/j.joms.2006.11.023.
32. Agliardi EL, Francetti L, Romeo D, Del Fabbro M. Immediate rehabilitation of the edentulous maxilla: preliminary results of a single-cohort prospective study. Int J Oral Maxillofac Implants. 2009;24(5):887–95.
33. Avrampou M, Mericske-Stern R, Blatz MB, Katsoulis J. Virtual implant planning in the edentulous maxilla: criteria for decision making of prosthesis design. Clin Oral Implants Res. 2013;24(Suppl A100):152–9. https://doi.org/10.1111/j.1600-0501.2011.02407.x.
34. Agliardi EL, Pozzi A, Stappert CF, Benzi R, Romeo D, Gherlone E. Immediate fixed rehabilitation of the edentulous maxilla: a prospective clinical and radiological study after 3 years of loading. Clin Implant Dent Relat Res. 2014;16(2):292–302. https://doi.org/10.1111/j.1708-8208.2012.00482.x.
35. Cavalli N, Barbaro B, Spasari D, Azzola F, Ciatti A, Francetti L. Tilted implants for full-arch rehabilitations in completely edentulous maxilla: a retrospective study. Int J Dent. 2012;2012:180379. https://doi.org/10.1155/2012/180379.
36. Jensen OT, Cottam JR, Ringeman JL, Graves S, Beatty L, Adams MW. Angled dental implant placement into the vomer/nasal crest of atrophic maxillae for all-on-four immediate function: a 2-year clinical study of 100 consecutive patients. Int J Oral Maxillofac Implants. 2014;29(1):e30–5. https://doi.org/10.11607/jomi.te39.
37. Tallarico M, Meloni SM, Canullo L, Caneva M, Polizzi G. Five-year results of a randomized controlled trial comparing patients rehabilitated with immediately loaded maxillary cross-arch fixed dental prosthesis supported by four or six implants placed using guided surgery. Clin Implant Dent Relat Res. 2016;18(5):965–72. https://doi.org/10.1111/cid.12380.
38. Warreth A, McAleese E, McDonnell P, Slami R, Guray SM. Dental implants and single implant-supported restorations. J Ir Dent Assoc. 2013;59(1):32–43.
39. Bryington M, De Kok IJ, Thalji G, Cooper LF. Patient selection and treatment planning for implant restorations. Dent Clin N Am. 2014;58(1):193–206. https://doi.org/10.1016/j.cden.2013.09.009.
40. De Kok IJ, Thalji G, Bryington M, Cooper LF. Radiographic stents: integrating treatment planning and implant placement. Dent Clin N Am. 2014;58(1):181–92. https://doi.org/10.1016/j.cden.2013.09.008.
41. Menini M, Pesce P, Bevilacqua M, Pera F, Tealdo T, Barberis F, Pera P. Effect of framework in an implant-supported full-arch fixed prosthesis: 3D finite element analysis. Int J Prosthodont. 2015;28(6):627–30. https://doi.org/10.11607/ijp.4345.
42. Siadat H, Alikhasi M, Beyabanaki E, Rahimian S. Comparison of different impression techniques when using the all-on-four implant treatment protocol. Int J Prosthodont. 2016;29(3):265–70. https://doi.org/10.11607/ijp.4341.
43. Michelinakis G. The use of cone beam computed tomography and three dimensional printing technology in the restoration of a maxillectomy patient using a dental implant retained obturator. J Indian Prosthodont Soc. 2017;17(4):406–11. https://doi.org/10.4103/jips.jips_106_17.
44. Faraco FN, Kawakami PY, Mestnik MJ, Ferrari DS, Shibli JA. Effect of anesthetics containing lido-

caine and epinephrine on cardiovascular changes during dental implant surgery. J Oral Implantol. 2007;33(2):84–8. https://doi.org/10.1563/0.845.1.

45. Sánchez-Siles M, Torres-Diez LC, Camacho-Alonso F, Salazar-Sánchez N, Ballester Ferrandis JF. High volume local anesthesia as a postoperative factor of pain and swelling in dental implants. Clin Implant Dent Relat Res. 2014;16(3):429–34. https://doi.org/10.1111/cid.12005.
46. Valieri MM, de Freitas KM, Valarelli FP, Cançado RH. Comparison of topical and infiltration anesthesia for orthodontic mini-implant placement. Dental Press J Orthod. 2014;19(2):76–83. https://doi.org/10.1590/2176-9451.19.2.076-083.oar.
47. Schwamburger NT, Hancock RH, Chong CH, Hartup GR, Vandewalle KS. The rate of adverse events during IV conscious sedation. Gen Dent. 2012;60(5):e341–4.
48. Stronczek MJ. Determining the appropriate oral surgery anesthesia modality, setting, and team. Oral Maxillofac Surg Clin North Am. 2013;25(3):357. https://doi.org/10.1016/j.coms.2013.03.008.
49. Dionne RA, Yagiela JA, Coté CJ, Donaldson M, Edwards M, Greenblatt DJ, Haas D, Malviya S, Milgrom P, Moore PA, Shampaine G, Silverman M, Williams RL, Wilson S. Balancing efficacy and safety in the use of oral sedation in dental outpatients. J Am Dent Assoc. 2006;137(4):502–13. https://doi.org/10.14219/jada.archive.2006.0223.
50. de Almeida Ferreira CE, Martinelli CB, Novaes AB Jr, Pignaton TB, Guignone CC, Gonçalves de Almeida AL, Saba-Chujfi E. Effect of maxillary sinus membrane perforation on implant survival rate: a retrospective study. Int J Oral Maxillofac Implants. 2017;32(2):401–7. https://doi.org/10.11607/jomi.4419.
51. Perelli M, Abundo R, Corrente G, Saccone C, Arduino PG. Sinus floor elevation with modified crestal approach and single loaded short implants: a case report with 4 years of follow-up. Case Rep Dent. 2017;2017:7829179. https://doi.org/10.1155/2017/7829179.
52. Ganeles J, Rosenberg MM, Holt RL, Reichman LH. Immediate loading of implants with fixed restorations in the completely edentulous mandible: report of 27 patients from a private practice. Int J Oral Maxillofac Implants. 2001;16(3):418–26.
53. Chiapasco M. Early and immediate restoration and loading of implants in completely edentulous patients. Int J Oral Maxillofac Implants. 2004;19(Suppl):76–91.
54. Morton D, Jaffin R, Weber HP. Immediate restoration and loading of dental implants: clinical considerations and protocols. Int J Oral Maxillofac Implants. 2004;19(Suppl):103–8.
55. Gallucci GO, Bernard JP, Bertosa M, Belser UC. Immediate loading with fixed screw-retained provisional restorations in edentulous jaws: the pickup technique. Int J Oral Maxillofac Implants. 2004;19(4):524–33.
56. Castellon P, Blatz MB, Block MS, Finger IM, Rogers B. Immediate loading of dental implants in the edentulous mandible. J Am Dent Assoc. 2004;135(11):1543–622. https://doi.org/10.14219/jada.archive.2004.0080.
57. Capelli M, Zuffetti F, Del Fabbro M, Testori T. Immediate rehabilitation of the completely edentulous jaw with fixed prostheses supported by either upright or tilted implants: a multicenter clinical study. Int J Oral Maxillofac Implants. 2007;22(4):639–44.
58. Khatami AH, Smith CR. "All-on-Four" immediate function concept and clinical report of treatment of an edentulous mandible with a fixed complete denture and milled titanium framework. J Prosthodont. 2008;17(1):47–51. https://doi.org/10.1111/j.1532-849X.2007.00246.x.
59. Francetti L, Agliardi E, Testori T, Romeo D, Taschieri S, Del Fabbro M. Immediate rehabilitation of the mandible with fixed full prosthesis supported by axial and tilted implants: interim results of a single cohort prospective study. Clin Implant Dent Relat Res. 2008;10(4):255–63. https://doi.org/10.1111/j.1708-8208.2008.00090.x.
60. Greenstein G, Tarnow D. The mental foramen and nerve: clinical and anatomical factors related to dental implant placement: a literature review. J Periodontol. 2006;77(12):1933–43. https://doi.org/10.1902/jop.2006.060197.
61. Tolstunov L. Implant zones of the jaws: implant location and related success rate. J Oral Implantol. 2007;33(4):211–20. https://doi.org/10.1563/1548-1336(2007)33[211:IZOTJI]2.0.CO;2.
62. Greenstein G, Cavallaro J, Tarnow D. Practical application of anatomy for the dental implant surgeon. J Periodontol. 2008;79(10):1833–46. https://doi.org/10.1902/jop.2008.080086.
63. Rutkowski JL, Fennell JW, Kern JC, Madison DE, Johnson DA. Inhibition of alveolar osteitis in mandibular tooth extraction sites using platelet-rich plasma. J Oral Implantol. 2007;33(3):116–21. https://doi.org/10.1563/1548-1336(2007)33[116:IOAOIM]2.0.CO;2.
64. Del Fabbro M, Corbella S, Taschieri S, Francetti L, Weinstein R. Autologous platelet concentrate for post-extraction socket healing: a systematic review. Eur J Oral Implantol. 2014;7(4):333–44.
65. Del Fabbro M, Bucchi C, Lolato A, Corbella S, Testori T, Taschieri S. Healing of postextraction sockets preserved with autologous platelet concentrates. A systematic review and meta-analysis. J Oral Maxillofac

Surg. 2017;75(8):1601–15. https://doi.org/10.1016/j.joms.2017.02.009.
66. Sohn DS, Huang B, Kim J, Park WE, Park CC. Utilization of autologous concentrated growth factors (CGF) enriched bone graft matrix (sticky bone) and CGF-enriched fibrin membrane in implant dentistry. J Implant Advanced Clin Dent. 2015;7:11–29.
67. Arakji H, Shokry M, Aboelsaad N. Comparison of piezosurgery and conventional rotary instruments for removal of impacted mandibular third molars: a randomized controlled clinical and radiographic trial. Int J Dent. 2016;2016:8169356. https://doi.org/10.1155/2016/8169356.

Cardiac Ablation: Energy Sources and Delivery Platforms

19

Kevin Liu and John Catanzaro

Abstract

Cardiac arrhythmia is described as an abnormal cardiac rhythm that can result in various physical symptoms, such as fluttering in the chest, skipped beats, overt heart failure with pulmonary and lower extremity edema, or may even lead to cardiac arrest. Due to the high incidence of myocardial complications from COVID-19 and the side effects of vaccines, the subject of wellness by minimally invasive technologies is discussed. This chapter discusses the different energy forms of cardiac ablation and their delivery platforms.

Keywords

Energy sources · Aesthetics · Ablation · Arrhythmia · COVID-19

K. Liu · J. Catanzaro (✉)
Division of Cardiology, Section of Electrophysiology, University of Florida—Jacksonville, Jacksonville, FL, USA
e-mail: Kevin.Liu@jax.ufl.edu; John.Catanzaro@jax.ufl.edu

19.1 Introduction

While there are options for pharmacologic control, cardiac ablation provides the opportunity for arrhythmia cure in many cases. The concept behind all forms of ablations involves inducing cardiac tissue necrosis to eliminate an arrhythmogenic focus or pathway. Cardiac arrhythmia is defined by three various mechanisms of action, including reentry, automaticity, or triggered activity. Ablation of putative regions of the myocardium allows for restoration to a normal rhythm after the mechanism and location of the arrhythmogenic heart cells are understood.

Arrhythmias such as atrial fibrillation require the delivery of ablation targeted at the pulmonary veins. In contrast, the circuit of typical atrial flutter involves ablation at the cavotricuspid isthmus due to the macro reentrant circuit turning around the tricuspid valve. In other cases, ablating a more localized focus may terminate the recurrence of arrhythmias such as atrial tachycardia or ventricular tachycardia. Diagnostic tests are often performed before ablation therapy, including but not limited to EKGs, Holter monitors, electrophysiology studies, etc.

R. L. Bard (ed.), *Image-Guided Aesthetic Treatments*, https://doi.org/10.1007/978-3-031-36266-8_19

19.2 Radiofrequency Ablation

Due to the high incidence of myocardial complications from COVID-19 and the side effects of vaccines, the subject of wellness by minimally invasive technologies is discussed.

Radiofrequency ablation is originated from initial attempts to treat arrhythmia through surgical procedures. An electrophysiology study is the ability to record electrical stimulation while recording from multiple intracardiac electrodes, which was first started in 1971. In 1981, AV block was accidentally induced through defibrillation shock through a His catheter and spurred the idea of catheter ablation via direct current cardioversion for arrhythmia treatment [1, 2]. Radiofrequency ablation was then further developed in the 1990s stemming from electrocautery, leading to the current era [3]. Since its development, further research, and understanding have created developments to increase efficiency and decrease complication rates with radiofrequency ablation.

Radiofrequency ablation (RFA) is currently the most commonly studied and used form of ablation. It is currently the gold standard for cardiac ablation. Current guidelines for atrial fibrillation recommend ablation as a possible first- or second-line treatment for paroxysmal or persistent atrial fibrillation after antiarrhythmic drugs failure [4–6]. Current RFA success rates stand at an 80% success rate after 5 years, and 60% success rate at 10 years for paroxysmal atrial fibrillation, and 25% first time successes, and 68% after multiple attempts for ablation of persistent atrial fibrillation, although this depends on each patient [3].

Radiofrequency ablation works by creating a current channel between the catheter and a receiving electrode. The electric current is set to oscillate between the radiofrequency range (450–500 kHz) (which was used by other electrosurgical devices, making regulatory approval easier) [7, 8]. Frequencies higher than this result in further tissue heating and less frequency results in cardiac muscle/nerve stimulation (arrhythmia/pain sensation) [9]. The electric current results in ion movement and generation of heat due to friction (electrically resistive heating).

$$\mathrm{SAR} = \frac{\sigma \times \mathrm{E}^2}{\mathrm{m_d}}$$

SAR (specific absorption rate) represents the rate at which a material with conductivity σ and mass density m_d will conduct energy through radiofrequency energy's electric field E. Therefore, as electrical current increases, so does the conducted thermal energy [7]. However, this is primarily for the immediate contact zone (due to the highest current density occurring at the tip), and thus further distance heat is transferred through heat conductance through the formula:

$$\rho c \frac{\Delta \mathrm{T}}{\Delta \mathrm{t}} = \mathrm{k}\nabla^2 \mathrm{T} + \frac{\mathrm{E}^2}{\sigma} - \mathrm{Q_{perf}}$$

where ρ,k, c, and T are constants regarding the tissue's density, thermal conductivity, specific heat, and temperature, respectively. Simplified, this equation represents the change in temperature over time as a component of 3 variables: thermal conduction ($k\nabla^2 T$), the current density (E^2/σ), and the cooling caused by blood perfusion (Q_{perf}).

The rate at which cell death occurs depends on temperature and time: A few minutes at 50 °C, a few seconds >60 °C, which is the ideal temperature aimed for during ablation. However, too low temperature will result in persistent arrhythmic tissue, and too high temperature will result in tissue damage potentially beyond the arrhythmogenic area of interest. Vaporization occurs at >110 °C (electrically insulating vapor), charring occurs at high RF densities preventing RF energy delivery via the ablation catheter. A "steam pop" can occur when water or medium around the tip of the ablation catheter boils and gas is released, resulting in a myocardial perforation. Thus, controlling the power output through voltage, temperature (thermal sensor), and impedance measurements is essential.

There has been a further improvement to the RFA catheter design to allow better current/heat penetration depth. More recent technologies include active cooling of the immediate contact zone allowing for increased depth and penetration

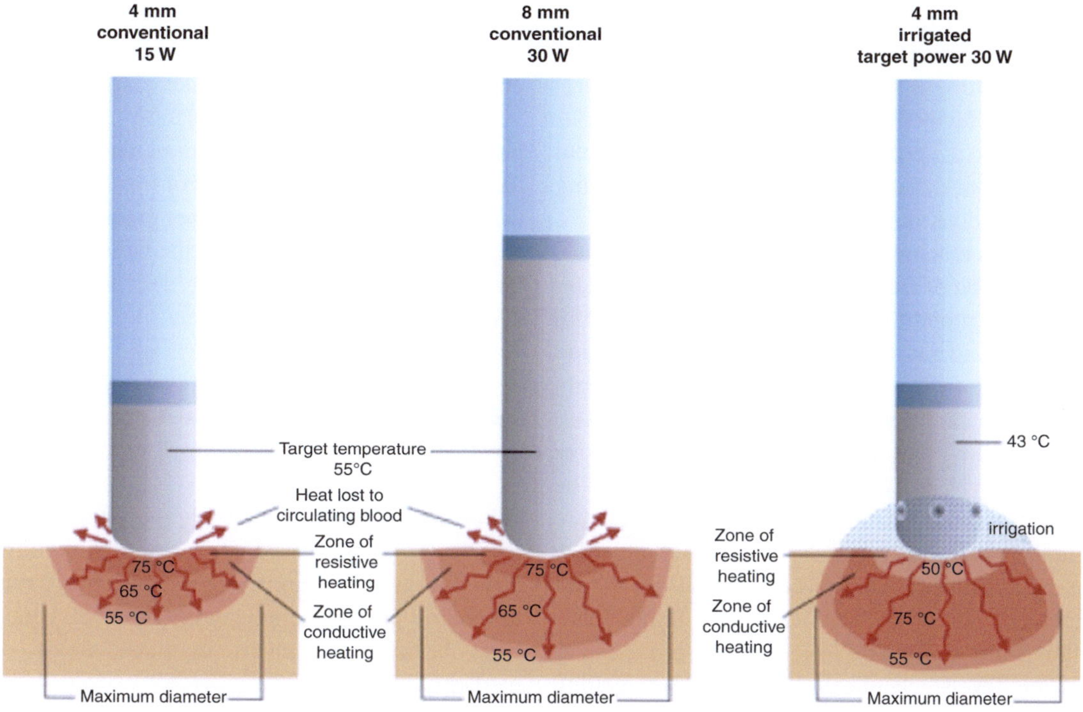

Fig. 19.1 Demonstration of a radiofrequency ablation catheter in relation to zones of resistive and conductive heating and the benefit of irrigation to allow for deeper conductive heating with decreased superficial heating [10]

of current without charring/vaporizing tissue in direct contact and measurement of the contact force at the tip of the catheter [7, 10]. This way, control of surface-level heat can improve penetration depth of heat conductance. Convective cooling is one of the more efficient ways in reducing superficial heat (through surrounding blood/water, or heat sinks from the electrode tip). Heat can be reduced at the surface, allowing for an increased time of radiofrequency application and heat conductance through tissue and increasing lesion size (see Fig. 19.1 below.)

19.3 Cryoablation

Cryoablation developed relatively quickly alongside heat-related ablation. Its use in ablation stemmed initially from cryosurgery as the application of cooling gases and vacuum containers improved in design and use [11] with the eventual patent and application of cryoablation made in 1988. Continued advances eventually led to cryoballoon ablations, with the first-generation arctic front cryoballoon system (Medtronic) in 2010.

Cryoablation is another form of inducing tissue necrosis through freezing instead of heat. It carries the benefit of reversible localized damage, as long as the tissue is not frozen. Once the tissue is frozen, intracellular and extracellular ice crystal formation leads to osmotic cellular damage, microvascular injury resulting in hemorrhage and inflammation, ischemia, fibrosis, and apoptosis of surrounding tissue. The cell membrane becomes disrupted, leading to coagulation injury and irreversible damage [12, 13]. After this initial phase, thawing occurs, which results in the coalescence of intra/extracellular ice crystals. This increases osmotic damage and further shear forces, as well as restoring microcirculatory function allowing for hemorrhage and inflammation leading to coagulative necrosis [14].

Freezing temperature is achieved through the use of high-pressure nitrous oxide or nitrogen storage tanks. Once this highly pressurized gas is pumped into the probe, it has room to expand, resulting in a rapid temperature decrease at the tip to as low as -60 °C (Joule-Thomson effect) [15], and temperatures can stay in this range as gas flow to the probe tip is controlled [12]. Due to solute concentration levels in cells, freezing typically does not occur until they reach -5 °C, and when reaching -20 °C, most cells die. Thus, the duration of freeze time necessary for cellular death is proportional to freezing temperature (lower temperatures need shorter duration), and temperature <-50 °C is always lethal. Interestingly slow and fast freezing rates result in low cell survivability, but intermediate rates allow for better survivability; thus, freezing rates should be <1.67 or >6.67 °C/min [16]. Slow temperature rates lead to extracellular ice crystals, which expel salt, increase ion concentration in the extracellular space, and draw out intracellular fluid osmotically. This leads to rising intracellular solute levels, chemical denaturing/deactivating enzymes, proteins, and intracellular organelles. On the other hand, fast freezing temperatures result in ice crystal formation, which fractures and re-form into larger crystals over time. This results in shearing forces, distension, and disruption of cellular organelles, membranes, and small blood vessels (intracellular ice will result in death in most cases). In most cases, faster freezing rates are used for better insurance of lethality and decrease variability in tissue response to cooling.

Cryoablation lesions are characterized by preserving tissue architecture (fibrocytes and collagen) and reducing the risk of destroying the healthy structure, decreasing the risk of cardiac perforation or thrombogenicity. While penetration of tissue necrosis is relatively similar to RFA, the histologic comparison reveals relatively more defined margins of injury in cryoablation in comparison to the ragged edges of a heat ablation. In addition, compared to the free-floating catheter for RFA ablations, the ice that forms at the tissue contact site during cryoablation allows for the catheter's adherence and stabilization to its ablation target. Finally, because of the reversibility of freezing during cryoablation, it is possible to perform cryo mapping (reaching tissue temperatures of 0 to -5 °C) to demonstrate the electrophysiologic effect and thus create an efficient and safe map before cell necrosis.

There are two cryoablation platforms: traditional tips for focal ablations and balloons for pulmonary vein isolation. For focal ablations, the tip has an expansion chamber to allow for gas expansion. On the other hand, the balloon acts as the expansion chamber and delivers cooling across the surface of the balloon.

19.4 Alternative Modalities of Ablation

While radiofrequency ablation and cryoablation are the two most used forms of ablation for arrhythmias, other modalities are currently being tested for possible application, some of which have been implemented in other fields of medicine.

19.5 Laser Ablation

Laser ablation for cardiac arrhythmias has been introduced relatively recently, with a recent study, leading to FDA approval in 2016 [17]. Currently, this technology is available as the HeartLight (CardioFocus, Massachusetts), the most recent being HeartLight X3. A 980 nm diode laser (with the specific wavelength to not be absorbed by deuterium gas) and endoscope are positioned in a deuterium oxide-inflated balloon, which is inflated in the pulmonary vein, allowing for stabilization and direct visualization of the pulmonary vein. The laser is then administered to the targeted tissue, inducing similar effects to RFA ablation by heating and coagulation necrosis by energy absorbed by water molecules within the cell and conductive heating at more depth. Power can be controlled through the energy applied to the laser (5.5–12W). With higher wavelengths, the laser energy can penetrate past the endothelium, causing less char and endocardial damage [18].

As a new technology, laser ablation has not been adopted into everyday practice to treat paroxysmal atrial fibrillation. However, emerging data suggest comparable efficacy with other ablation modalities, possibly decreasing radiation exposure times and complication rates. The most common complication is diaphragmatic paralysis in 3.5% of cases [17, 19].

19.6 Pulse Field Ablation/ Electroporation

Pulse field ablation is an innovative concept for arrhythmia ablation, with current ongoing studies (ADVENT, PULSED AF, and INSPIRE) [20]. This form of ablation uses short, high-amplitude electrical pulses to induce transient permeability of cell membranes (in this case, specifically the sarcolemmal membrane), allowing for calcium entry and ATP loss, resulting in cell necrosis, which was demonstrated for cancer cells by Frandson et al. [21]. The most attractive features of this ablation modality are that with a controlled time of power output, there should be minimal heating associated and relative tissue specificity for myocardium compared to surrounding tissue like esophageal tissue or the phrenic nerve [22].

Nonthermal ablation permanently creates nanoscale defects in the cell membrane by exposing cells to short and intense electric fields, leading to cell death [7]. This ablation energy could become prominent in the next few years with recent rapid development.

19.7 High-Frequency Ultrasound (HIFU)

Ultrasound uses vibrational energy to mechanically move particles that converts into thermal energy, eventually leading to protein denaturing and fragmentation of mitochondria, similar to RFA. Additionally, the damage is enhanced with acoustic cavitation (microbubble formation by the ultrasound waves), which can also reflect the ultrasound wave and further focus on the heating area [23].

With the ultrasound waves, dependent on the acoustic wavelength and direction, it is possible to create mid myocardial lesions with less damage to the epi/endocardium (demonstrated by Engel et al., though only in canine models) [24].

HIFU has been limited due to its rapid lesion formation and thus a high risk of collateral injury during cardiac ablation, demonstrated in multiple human studies later on [25, 26]. However, its ability for ablation without direct contact and focus on deeper tissue continues to be used in other treatments such as prostate cancer or fibroids.

19.8 Quality of Life Improvement

One major end-point that is important to patient satisfaction with regard to arrhythmia ablation relates to quality of life. However, the difficulty associated with assessment of quality of life in those with arrhythmias, specifically atrial fibrillation, is significant due to the high variability in symptomatology including examples such as a vague chest discomfort, shortness of breath, light-headedness, lower extremity edema, chest pain, heart failure, anxiety related to symptoms or disease sequelae, or days lost to medical follow-up [27].

The AXAFA study, a prospective randomized outcome assessment study, looked at quality of life with respect to arrhythmia recurrence after atrial fibrillation ablation, which showed that a decrease in recurrence resulted in improved functional status, quality of life, and cognition [28], highlighting the importance of an effective ablation modality. Similarly, the CABANA and CAPTAF trials were randomized control trials, which assessed the quality of life among patients with atrial fibrillation after ablation and pulmonary vein isolation, respectively, vs. medical therapy. The CAPTAF trial included over 155 patients, whereas the CABANA trial included over 2000 patients. Both trials similarly demonstrated robust improvement in quality of life after 12 months in comparison to medical therapy [29, 30].

19.9 Conclusion

Radiofrequency and cryothermal energy remain the most common forms of energy use in cardiac ablation. However, as newer energy sources are introduced, safety and efficacy must be considered to increase the quality of life. Emerging technologies, including pulse-field ablation, promise safety; however, long-term data has not yet consistently been demonstrated. Even as other forms of energy ablation appear less efficacious from the cardiac standpoint, their use can still be seen in other areas of medicine. The bio physiologic basis behind their concepts may be useful in the future as technology continues to advance with a promise to improve patient outcomes and quality of life.

References

1. Joseph JP, Rajappan K. Radiofrequency ablation of cardiac arrhythmias: past, present and future. QJM. 2012;105(4):303–14. https://doi.org/10.1093/qjmed/hcr189.
2. Ghzally Y, et al. Catheter ablation. In: StatPearls. StatPearls Publishing LLC; 2021. www.ncbi.nlm.nih.gov/books/NBK470203/.
3. Rottner L, Bellmann B, Lin T, Reissmann B, Tönnis T, Schleberger R, Nies M, Jungen C, Dinshaw L, Klatt N, Dickow J, Münkler P, Meyer C, Metzner A, Rillig A. Catheter ablation of atrial fibrillation: state of the art and future perspectives. Cardiol Ther. 2020;9(1):45–58. https://doi.org/10.1007/s40119-019-00158-2.
4. Kuck K-H, Brugada J, Fürnkranz A, Metzner A, Ouyang F, Chun KRJ, Elvan A, Arentz T, Bestehorn K, Pocock SJ, Albenque J-P, Tondo C. Cryoballoon or radiofrequency ablation for paroxysmal atrial fibrillation. N Engl J Med. 2016;374(23):2235–45. https://doi.org/10.1056/NEJMoa1602014.
5. January CT, Wann LS, Calkins H, Chen LY, Cigarroa JE, Cleveland JC, Ellinor PT, Ezekowitz MD, Field ME, Furie KL, Heidenreich PA, Murray KT, Shea JB, Tracy CM, Yancy CW. 2019 AHA/ACC/HRS focused update of the 2014 AHA/ACC/HRS guideline for the management of patients with atrial fibrillation. Heart Rhythm. 2019;16(8):e66–93. https://doi.org/10.1016/j.hrthm.2019.01.024.
6. January CT, Wann LS, Alpert JS, Calkins H, Cigarroa JE, Cleveland JC, Conti JB, Ellinor PT, Ezekowitz MD, Field ME, Murray KT, Sacco RL, Stevenson WG, Tchou PJ, Tracy CM, Yancy CW. 2014 AHA/ACC/HRS guideline for the management of patients with atrial fibrillation. J Am Coll Cardiol. 2014;64(21):e1–e76. https://doi.org/10.1016/j.jacc.2014.03.022.
7. Haemmerich D. Biophysics of radiofrequency ablation. Crit Rev Biomed Eng. 2010;38(1):53–63. https://doi.org/10.1615/CritRevBiomedEng.v38.i1.50.
8. Nelson K, Jutric Z, Georgiades C. Physics and physiology of thermal ablations. In: Georgiades C, Kim HS, editors. Image-guided interventions in oncology. Berlin: Springer International Publishing; 2020. p. 1–13. https://doi.org/10.1007/978-3-030-48767-6_1.
9. Zezo. Biophysics and pathophysiology of radiofrequency lesion formation. Thoracic key. 2019. Accessed 24 Nov 2021. https://thoracickey.com/biophysics-and-pathophysiology-of-radiofrequency-lesion-formation/.
10. Wissner E, Metzner A. Biophysics of modern ablation techniques and their limitations. In: Kibos AS, Knight BP, Essebag V, Fishberger SB, Slevin M, Țintoiu IC, editors. Cardiac arrhythmias. London: Springer; 2014. p. 361–7. https://doi.org/10.1007/978-1-4471-5316-0_28.
11. Bouganim N, Freiman A. History of cryotherapy. Dermatol Online J. 2005;11(2):9. https://doi.org/10.5070/D34F62H9VT.
12. Avitall B, Khan M, Krum D, Hare J, Lessila C, Dhala A, Deshpande S, Jazayeri M, Sra J, Akhtar M. Physics and engineering of transcatheter cardiac tissue ablation. J Am Coll Cardiol. 1993;22(3):921–32. https://doi.org/10.1016/0735-1097(93)90212-J.
13. Jin E-S, Wang PJ. Cryoballoon ablation for atrial fibrillation: a comprehensive review and practice guide. Korean Circ J. 2018;48(2):114. https://doi.org/10.4070/kcj.2017.0318.
14. Zezo. Catheter cryoablation: biophysics and clinical applications. Thoracic key. 2019; Accessed 24 Nov 2021. https://thoracickey.com/catheter-cryoablation-biophysics-and-clinical-applications/.
15. Avitall B, Kalinski A. Cryotherapy of cardiac arrhythmia: from basic science to the bedside. Heart Rhythm. 2015;12(10):2195–203. https://doi.org/10.1016/j.hrthm.2015.05.034.
16. Gage AA, Baust JM, Baust JG. Experimental cryosurgery investigations in vivo. Cryobiology. 2009;59(3):229–43. https://doi.org/10.1016/j.cryobiol.2009.10.001.
17. Dukkipati SR, Cuoco F, Kutinsky I, Aryana A, Bahnson TD, Lakkireddy D, Woollett I, Issa ZF, Natale A, Reddy VY. Pulmonary vein isolation using the visually guided laser balloon. J Am Coll Cardiol. 2015;66(12):1350–60. https://doi.org/10.1016/j.jacc.2015.07.036.
18. Bordignon S, Chun K-RJ, Gunawardene M, Schulte-Hahn B, Nowak B, Fuernkranz A, Schmidt B. Endoscopic ablation systems. Expert Rev Med Devices. 2013;10(2):177–83. https://doi.org/10.1586/erd.12.86.
19. Reynolds MR, Zheng Q, Doros G. Laser balloon ablation for AF: a systematic review and meta-analysis. J Cardiovasc Electrophysiol. 2018;29(10):1363–70. https://doi.org/10.1111/jce.13698.

20. Chu E. HRS 2021: top five takeaways. Cardiology. 2021;50(8):30–1.
21. Frandsen SK, Gissel H, Hojman P, Tramm T, Eriksen J, Gehl J. Direct therapeutic applications of calcium electroporation to effectively induce tumor necrosis. Cancer Res. 2012;72(6):1336–41. https://doi.org/10.1158/0008-5472.CAN-11-3782.
22. Haines DE, Bradley CJ. The promise of pulsed field ablation. EP Lab Digest. 2019;19:1–5.
23. Singh S, Nair KKM, Koruth JS, d'Avila A, Danon A. The role of high-intensity focused ultrasound in ablation of atrial fibrillation and other cardiac arrhythmias. Res Rep Focus Ultrasound. 2015;3:11. https://doi.org/10.2147/RRFU.S81794.
24. Engel DJ, Muratore R, Hirata K, Otsuka R, Fujikura K, Sugioka K, Marboe C, Lizzi FL, Homma S. Myocardial lesion formation using high-intensity focused ultrasound. J Am Soc Echocardiogr. 2006;19(7):932–7. https://doi.org/10.1016/j.echo.2006.02.012.
25. Schmidt B, Chun KRJ, Metzner M, et al. Pulmonary vein isolation with high-intensity focused ultrasound: results from the HIFU 12F study. Europace. 2009;11:1281–8.
26. Neven K, Schmidt B, Metzner A, et al. Fatal end of a safety algorithm for pulmonary vein isolation with use of high-intensity focused ultrasound. Circ Arrhythm Electrophysiol. 2010;3:260–5.
27. Sridhar AR, Colbert R. Quality of life after atrial fibrillation ablation: measuring the most important end-point. Heart. 2020;106(24):1876–7. https://doi.org/10.1136/heartjnl-2020-317547.
28. Piccini JP, Todd DM, Massaro T, Lougee A, Haeusler KG, Blank B, de Bono JP, Callans DJ, Elvan A, Fetsch T, Van Gelder I, Gentlesk P, Grimaldi M, Hansen J, Hindricks G, Al-Khalidi H, Mont L, Nielsen JC, Noelker G, Kirchhof P. Changes in quality of life, cognition and functional status following catheter ablation of atrial fibrillation. Heart. 2020;106(24):1919–26. https://doi.org/10.1136/heartjnl-2020-316612.
29. Mark DB, Anstrom KJ, Sheng S, Piccini JP, Baloch KN, Monahan KH, Daniels MR, Bahnson TD, Poole JE, Rosenberg Y, Lee KL, Packer DL, CABANA Investigators. Effect of catheter ablation vs medical therapy on quality of life among patients with atrial fibrillation: the CABANA randomized clinical trial. JAMA. 2019;321(13):1275–85. https://doi.org/10.1001/jama.2019.0692.
30. Blomström-Lundqvist C, Gizurarson S, Schwieler J, Jensen SM, Bergfeldt L, Kennebäck G, Rubulis A, Malmborg H, Raatikainen P, Lönnerholm S, Höglund N, Mörtsell D. Effect of catheter ablation vs antiarrhythmic medication on quality of life in patients with atrial fibrillation: the CAPTAF randomized clinical trial. JAMA. 2019;321(11):1059–68. https://doi.org/10.1001/jama.2019.0335.

Correction to: Aesthetic Treatments with Focused Ultrasound

Mary Nielsen

Correction to:
Chapter 11 in: Robert L. Bard (ed.), *Image-Guided Aesthetic Treatments*, https://doi.org/10.1007/978-3-031-36266-8_11

This book was inadvertently published with the incorrect word "Softwave" instead of the correct term "Sofwave" on page 149. This has now been amended across all versions of the book.

The updated version of this chapter can be found at
https://doi.org/10.1007/978-3-031-36266-8_11

R. L. Bard (ed.), *Image-Guided Aesthetic Treatments*,
https://doi.org/10.1007/978-3-031-36266-8_20

MIX
Papier aus verantwortungsvollen Quellen
Paper from responsible sources
FSC® C105338

If you have any concerns about our products,
you can contact us on
ProductSafety@springernature.com

In case Publisher is established outside the EU,
the EU authorized representative is:
Springer Nature Customer Service Center GmbH
Europaplatz 3, 69115 Heidelberg, Germany

Printed by Libri Plureos GmbH
in Hamburg, Germany